Diseases of the goat

Diseases of the goat

John Matthews BSc BVMS MRCVS

Chalk Street Services Ltd, The Limes
Chelmsford, Essex, UK

4TH EDITION

WILEY Blackwell

Contents

Preface to the fourth edition

It is now 25 years since the first edition of *Diseases of the Goat* was published as *Outline of Clinical Diagnosis of the Goat* and 7 years since the third edition was published. The original concept was to provide a reasonably priced text that would provide useful and practical information for veterinary surgeons, whether they were in farm animal, mixed or small animal practice, and that would also be of use to students and goatkeepers. Despite the plethora of information that is now available on the Internet, I still believe that the book provides a valuable source of information that is readily accessible, whether kept in the car, surgery or on the farm.

The identification of a new disease in ruminants throughout Northern Europe, caused by Schmallenberg virus, which followed the arrival of blue tongue virus earlier in the century, and outbreaks of tuberculosis, long thought by British goatkeepers to be of no importance in goats, which occurred in both commercial and show herds, emphasised the fact that no country is an island, let alone an individual farm, so I have included more information on exotic diseases in this edition. In response to requests from readers of the third edition, I have expanded the chapter on poisonous plants to make it more relevant for readers out-with the United Kingdom and included information on predators, euthanasia, post-mortem techniques and fracture repair. As in the previous editions, I have tried to include new references that are likely to be relevant to the veterinarian in practice and updated the information throughout the book.

I hope that this new edition will continue to provide general practitioners with the support they need when dealing with caprine patients.

Acknowledgements

As with the previous editions, I am extremely grateful to my wife Hilary, who has provided encouragement and support during the compilation of this edition and given valuable advice on goat husbandry.

Tony Andrews, David Harwood, Peter Jackson, Katherine Anzuino and Leigh Sullivan have supplied photographs that are reproduced with their permission and I am pleased to acknowledge their contribution and that of their colleagues involved with the clinical cases to which they relate. Peter Cox supplied photographs for the cover.

I am pleased to acknowledge the contribution of the many members of the Goat Veterinary Society and the American Association of Small Ruminant Practioners, whose tips and advice, which they have willingly shared with other veterinary surgeons and goatkeepers, I have incorporated in this edition.

Author's note

For many medical conditions, there are no drugs available that are specifically licensed for use in goats. Dose rates are quoted in the book for many unlicensed drugs. These drug rates have been obtained from published reports, data held on file by the drug manufacturers and from personal experience. Whenever possible, the clinician should use drugs that carry a full product licence, both for goats and for the condition being treated. In all cases where unlicensed drugs are used, milk should not be used for human consumption for a minimum of 7 days and meat for a minimum of 28 days following the administration of the drug. Not all the drugs mentioned have a current licence for food-producing animals in the United Kingdom. It is the reader's responsibility to ensure that he/she is legally entitled to use any drug mentioned.

CHAPTER 1

Female infertility

The normal female goat

In temperate regions, female goats are seasonally poly-oestrus. Most goats are totally anoestrus in the northern hemisphere between March and August, although fertile matings have been recorded in all months of the year. Anglo-Nubian and pygmy goats in particular have extremely long breeding seasons. Recently imported goats from the southern hemisphere may take time to adjust to a new seasonality. The breeding season is initiated largely in response to decreasing day length, but is also dependent on temperature, the environment (particularly nutrition) and the presence of a male. Decreasing day length also stimulates reproductive activity in the buck. Table 1.1 details the reproductive aspects of the goat.

Investigation of female infertility

> Because of the seasonal pattern of breeding, infertility must be investigated as early as possible in the breeding season.

The investigation of female infertility in the goat presents major difficulties when compared with the cow because of the inability to palpate the ovaries and because of the seasonal pattern of breeding – does are often presented towards the end of the season, limiting the time available for remedial measures. Figure 1.1 lists possible causes of infertility in the doe.

Table 1.1 Reproduction in the goat.

Breeding season	September to March (northern hemisphere)
Puberty	5 months
Age at first service	4 to 6 months (male)
	7 to 18 months (female)
Oestrus cycle	19 to 21 days (dairy goats)
	18 to 24 days (Pygmy goats)
Duration of oestrus	24 to 96 hours (usually 36 to 40 hours)
Ovulation	24 to 48 hours after start of oestrus
Gestation length	150 days (145 to 156 days)
Weight at first mating	60–70% of predicted adult weight
	~30 kg for meat goats
	30–40 kg for dairy goats

Initial assessment

The preliminary history should consider:
- Individual or herd/flock problem.
- Feeding, including mineral supplementation.
- Management practices – hand-mating, artificial insemination (AI), buck running with does.
- Disease status of herd/flock.

If there is a *herd problem*, investigate:
- Male infertility (Chapter 3).
- Intercurrent disease – parasitism, footrot, etc.
- Nutritional status – energy or protein deficit, mineral deficiency (phosphorus, copper, iodine, manganese).
- Stress – overcrowding, recent grouping of goats.
- Poor heat detection.
- Services at incorrect time.

Diseases of the Goat, Fourth Edition. John Matthews.
© 2016 John Wiley & Sons, Ltd. Published 2016 by John Wiley & Sons, Ltd.

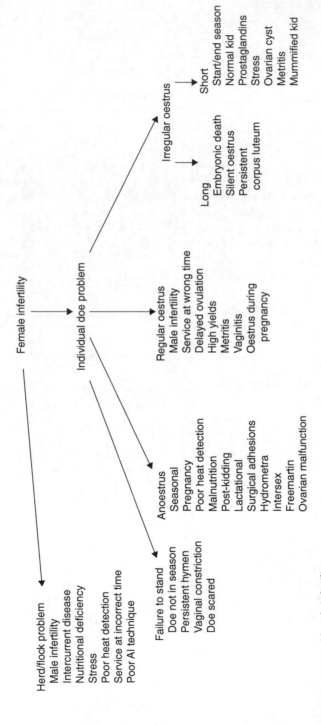

Figure 1.1 Causes of female infertility.

Assessment of individual doe

General assessment

- Conformation.
- Body condition.
- Dentition.
- Clinical examination.

Any obvious clinical signs such as debility, anaemia or lameness should be investigated and corrected where possible before commencing specific therapy aimed at correcting a reproductive disorder.

In the UK overfeeding is probably a greater cause of infertility than poor condition.

Specific examination

- Specific examination of the reproductive and mammary systems. Include, where necessary, examination of the vagina and cervix with a speculum to identify anatomical abnormalities.

Specific history

- Date of last kidding/stage of lactation.
- Daily milk yield.
- Presence or absence of obvious oestrus signs.
- Length of oestrus cycles.
- Date of last service.
- Willingness to stand for male.
- Kidding difficulties last time – malpresentation/manipulation, metritis, retained placenta, abortion, mummified fetus, stillbirths.

Further investigations

- Specific laboratory tests:
- Progesterone assay
- Oestrone sulphate assay
- Bacteriological examination of vaginal or uterine samples
- Feed analysis
- Real-time ultrasound scanning
- Laparoscopy or laparotomy.

Individual infertility problems

Individual infertility problems will generally fall into one of four categories:

1 **Difficulty at service**.
2 **Anoestrus.**
3 **Irregular oestrus cycles**.
4 **Regular oestrus cycles**.

Difficulty at service

- Doe not in season.
- Doe scared – common with maiden animals, particularly if a large buck is used on a small doe.
- Persistent hymen or vaginal constriction.

Anoestrus

> Always consider the possibility of an undetected pregnancy (even if the owner insists that no mating has occurred) before attempting treatment, particularly with prostaglandins.

The causes of anoestrus are listed in Table 1.2 and discussed below.

- *Seasonal*. Most goats are totally anoestrus between March and August.
- *Pregnancy*.
- *Poor heat detection*.

Although some dairy goats show only minor behavioural changes during oestrus, oestrus detection is generally easier than in Angora goats, with most does showing obvious signs of tail wagging, frequent bleating, urination near the buck, swelling of the vulva and a mucous vaginal discharge. The signs are generally accentuated in the presence of a male or even a 'billy rag', that is a cloth that has been rubbed on the head of a buck and stored in a sealed jar.

Oestrus can be determined visually by means of a speculum. At the onset of heat, the cervix changes from

Table 1.2 Causes of anoestrus.

Seasonal
Pregnancy
Poor heat detection
Malnutrition
Post-kidding anoestrus
Lactational anoestrus
Adhesions following surgery
Hydrometra
Intersex
Freemartin
Ovarian malfunction

its normal white colour, becoming hyperaemic, and the cervical secretions are thin and clear. The secretions rapidly thicken, becoming grey/white and collecting on the floor of the vagina. Conception is best when mating occurs at the stage at which the cervical mucus is cloudy and the cervix is relaxed.

Unlike cows, most does will not stand to be ridden by other females even when in oestrus. Riding behaviour is sometimes seen as an expression of dominance in the herd or as part of the nymphomaniac behaviour of goats with cystic ovaries. Many young bucks will mount and serve females that are not in true standing oestrus if the female is restrained, although older bucks are more discriminating. The doe will stand to be mated only when she is in oestrus.

In the milking doe, a rise in milk production may occur 8 to 12 hours before the start of oestrus and milk production may fall below normal during oestrus.

When the buck is running with the flock or herd, sire harnesses with raddles or marker paste will aid oestrus detection. A marked vasectomised ('teaser') buck can be used to detect (and help initiate) the start of oestrus in a group of does.

- *Malnutrition.* An energy or protein deficit due either to poor nutrition or intercurrent disease may cause anoestrus. Deficiencies of minerals such as cobalt, selenium, manganese, zinc, phosphorus, iodine and copper and deficiencies of vitamins B12 and D are all reported to cause infertility.
- *Post-kidding anoestrus.* Many does will not show signs of oestrus for 3 months or more after kidding, even if kidding takes place during the normal breeding season.
- *Lactational anoestrus.* Some high yielding does do not exhibit marked signs of oestrus. These animals may respond to prostaglandin injections with careful observation for oestrus 24 to 48 hours later. Animals that do not respond may need a further injection 11 days later.
- *Adhesions following surgery.* The goat's reproductive tract is sensitive to handling and adhesions will occur unless very high standards of surgery are maintained during embryo transplant or other surgical procedures. Talc from surgical gloves will produce a marked tissue reaction.

False pregnancy (hydrometra, cloudburst)

False pregnancy occurs when aseptic fluid accumulates in the uterus in the absence of pregnancy, but in the presence of a persistent corpus luteum, which continues to secrete progesterone. The incidence of false pregnancies is fairly high, particularly in some strains of dairy goats and incidences of between 3 and 30% have been reported in commercial herds.

Aetiology

- A persistent corpus luteum following an oestrus cycle in which pregnancy did not occur. This may occur in any sexually mature female but is particularly common in goats in their second year of a lactation ('running through') without being mated. Certain families seem prone to develop the condition.
- A persistent corpus luteum following embryonic death with resorption of the embryo.
- Occurrence is increased following use of progestagen sponges and treatment with equine chorionic gonadotrophin (eCG).

Clinical signs

- The doe acts as if pregnant, with enlargement of the abdomen and a degree of udder development if not milking (Plate 1.1). Milking does may show a sharp drop in yield and this may result in a significant economic loss if the condition is not corrected.
- Fetal fluids collect in the abdomen (*hydrometra*) and the doe may become enormously distended, although the amount of fluid varies from 1 to 7 litres or more.
- When the hydrometra occurs following embryonic death, the false pregnancy generally persists for the full gestational length, or longer, before luteolysis occurs, progesterone secretion ceases and the fetal fluids are released (*cloudburst*). Some does milk adequately following a natural cloudburst.
- When the false pregnancy occurs in a doe which has not been mated, the release of fluid often occurs in less than the normal gestation period, the doe may cycle again and a further false pregnancy may occur if she is not mated. Subsequent pregnancies are not generally affected, but the doe is likely to develop the condition again the following year. The expelled fluid is generally clear and mucoid. The vulva and perineum become moist and the tail sticky (Plate

1.2). Some goats that spontaneously cloudburst early, before a large amount of fluid has accumulated, have a bloody discharge. The abdomen decreases to a normal non-pregnant size and bedding appears wet. Some does continue to squirt small amounts of fluid for a couple of days and in fat does this could be confused with cystitis.

- If the false pregnancy follows fetal death, fetal membranes and possibly a decomposed fetus are present; otherwise no fetal membranes are formed.

Diagnosis

- Realtime ultrasound scanning of the right ventrolateral abdominal wall in early false pregnancy, or of either flank later, shows large fluid-filled hyperechoic compartments with the absence of fetuses or caruncles (Plate 1.3). The uterus is separated into compartments with thin tissue walls, which undulate when balloted. White flecks may be seen in the fluid. Scanning should take place at least 40 days after mating to avoid confusion with early pregnancy and is easier before 70 days. *Pyometras* (rare) also present as fluid filled uteri but are more hyperechoic.
- Elevated milk or plasma progesterone levels are consistent with pregnancy, but with low milk or plasma oestrone sulphate levels at >45 days.
- X-ray at 70–80 + days fails to show fetal skeletons in an anoestrus doe with a distended abdomen.
- Pregnancy specific protein is negative in pseudopregnancy.

Treatment

- As pseudopregnancy is maintained by the presence of a corpus luteum, treatment is by prostaglandin injection:

   Dinaprost, 5–10 mg i.m.or s.c. or Clorprostenol, 62.5–125 μg i.m. or s.c.

   Dinaprost has a direct effect on uterine muscle and may be preferable to clorprostenol.A second injection of prostaglandin 12 days after the first may cause evacuation of further uterine fluid and, it is suggested, may make the condition less likely to recur.
- An oxytocin injection a few days after treatment with prostaglandin stimulates uterine contractions and aids involution:

   Oxytocin, 2–10 units, 0.2–1.0 ml i.m. or s.c..

   Pituitary extract (posterior lobe), 20–50 units, 2-5 ml i.m. or s.c. or 2–10 units, 0.2–1.0 ml i.m. (preferred) or s.c.
- The prognosis for future fertility is good, with 85% of goats becoming pregnant if mated during the same breeding season.

Other conditions causing anoestrus

- *Hydrops uteri.* A false pregnancy may need to be distinguished from hydrops uteri. Hydrops uteri is an unusual condition of pregnant goats caused by an abnormal accumulation of fluid in either the amniotic (hydamnios) or allantoic (hydrallantois) sacs. Distension of the uterus is caused by accumulation of fluid, which may be greater than 10 litres, leading to bilateral, rapidly progressive abdominal distension. Other clinical signs, similar to those of pregnancy toxaemia, are a result of compression of other organs by the fluid – lethargy, inappetence, decreased defaecation, recumbency, tachycardia and dyspnoea.

   Ultrasonography can be used to distinguish between false pregnancy (hydrometra), where the uterus is distended with fluid but no fetuses, membranes or cotyledons are present, and hydrops uteri, where fluid, fetuses, membranes and cotyledons are present. Most fetuses of animals with hydrops uteri have congenital defects and are underdeveloped, but may appear normal although not viable.

   Treatment is by caesarian section or by induction of parturition with prostaglandins, but cardiovascular support with intravenous fluids should be provided because of the danger of hypotension from the sudden loss of large volumes of fluid.
- *Intersex (pseudohermaphrodite).* An intersex is an animal that shows both male and female characteristics. In goats the dominant gene for absence of horns (polled condition) is associated with a recessive gene for intersex. Thus an intersex is normally polled with two polled parents. Intersex is a recessive sex-linked incompletely penetrant trait resulting from the breeding of two polled goats – intersex goats are homozygous for the polled (hornless) gene and homozygous for the intersex gene.

   A mating between a homozygous (PP) polled male and a heterozygous (Pp) polled female will produce 50% intersexes; a mating between a heterozygous (Pp) polled male and a heterozygous (Pp) polled female will produce

25% intersexes. In theory, mating two homozygous (PP) polled animals should produce 100% intersexes, but the gene has incomplete penetrance.

Affected animals are genetically female with a normal female chromosome complement (60 XX), but phenotypically show great variation from phenotypic male (Plate 1.4) to phenotypic female (Plate 1.5). Some animals are obviously abnormal at birth with a normal vulva but enlarged clitoris or a penile clitoris. The gonads are generally testes or ovotestes, which may be abdominal or scrotal and phenotypic males may have a shortened penis (hypospadias), hypoplastic testes or sperm granuloma in the head of the epididymis. Other animals may reach maturity before being detected and may present as being anoestrus. A phenotypically female animal may have male characteristics due to internal testes.

Intersexes with female appearance are sometimes presented as kids or goatlings with a history of anoestrus. Although the vulva is normal, there is no true vagina or cervix, the clitoris may be enlarged and the anogenital distance may be > 3 cm. The presence or absence of a vagina of proper length should always be investigated in anoestrus kids. The absence of a vagina can be demonstrated by gently inserting a lubricated plastic rod, for example a ballpoint pen, into the vulva (Plates 1.6 and 1.7) or endoscopically. Care should be taken not to mistake a persistent hymen for a shortened vagina.

Intersexes with male appearance may have a penis or penis-like structure just below the anus. These animals may have urine scalding down their hind legs or have dysuria. Urine may accumulate in the perineal area causing dermatitis. In some cases, the urethra does not pass through the vestigial penis/clitoris and surgery may be required to establish an effective urethral opening. Localised hypospadia has been described in some cases.

- *Freemartins (XX/XY chimeras).* Most female kids born co-twin to males are normal females, because placental fusion is much less common than in cattle. A freemartin is a female rendered sterile in utero when her placenta and that of her twin male fuses in early gestation, allowing vascular anastomosis between the allantoic membranes, exchange of cells and hormones between the two foetuses and XX/XY chimaerism. The developing genital tract of the female is influenced by the male and results in hypoplasia of the female gonads. A freemartin may be polled or horned. There is some evidence that the condition is slightly more common when the female shares the uterus with two or more male fetuses. Externally freemartins appear female but internally show a variable degree of masculinisation:
  - o Heavy masculinisation, Gonads resemble testes and may contain tubules and interstitial tissue.
  - o Light masculinisation. Oocytes have been found in the gonads.
- *Whole body chimera.* The rarest type of caprine intersex, which arises from the fusion of two embryos, produces a true hermaphrodite with an XX/XY karyotype and gonads of both sexes.
- *Ovarian malfunction.* Ovarian inactivity is poorly understood in the goat, but some anoestrus goats will respond to treatment with gonadotrophin releasing hormone [GnRH]:
  Buserelin, 0.020 mg i.m., s.c. or i.v. or Gonadorellin, 0.5 mg i.m.
  Other goats will respond to treatment with prostaglandins, suggesting a *persistent corpus luteum* or *luteinised cystic ovaries.*
  Ultrasound scanning can be used to examine the ovaries but is not as easy as in cattle, because the reproductive tract cannot be manipulated manually so it is impossible to scan all the surfaces of the ovary. Both transrectal (using a lubricated 5 or 7.5 MHz linear transducer) or transabdominal (using a 5 MHz transducer) scanning can be carried out with the goat in a standing position. The bladder is located as a landmark and the transducer rotated to the left or right until the ovary is visualised. The ovary appears as a tissue-dense, circular to oblong structure cranial to the bladder. Follicles are non-echogenic fluid-filled structures that appear as black circular sacs.
  Increased use of laparoscopic techniques may aid the diagnosis of these conditions.

Irregular oestrus cycles (see Table 1.3)

Long oestrus cycles
- *Embryonic death.* Early embryonic death with loss of the corpus luteum will produce a subsequent return to oestrus following resorption of the embryonic material. Following embryonic death, a percentage of does will not return to oestrus but develop hydrometra.
- *Silent oestrus.* Some does will exhibit oestrus early in the season and then show no further oestrus signs for

Table 1.3 Irregular oestrus cycles.

Long	Short
Embryonic death	Start/end of season
Silent oestrus	Normal kid behaviour
Persistent corpus luteum	Prostaglandins
	Premature regression of the corpus luteum
	Stress
	Ovarian follicular cyst
	Metritis
	Mummified kid
	Ovarian tumour

some months. These goats may be cycling silently and will respond to treatment with prostaglandins.

- *Persistent corpus luteum*. Failure of the corpus luteum to undergo luteolysis at the correct time will delay the return to oestrus. Treat with prostaglandins (see this chapter).

Short oestrus cycles (<18 to 21 days)

- Short anovulatory cycles of about 7 days are common at the *start of the breeding season* and occasionally occur at the end of the breeding season.
- *Kids* commonly show short cycles during their first breeding season.
- Very short oestrus cycles have been recorded following administration of *prostaglandins* to abort does. A normal oestrus pattern returns after 3 to 4 weeks.
- *Premature regression of the corpus luteum* is recognised as a problem in goats undergoing oestrus synchronisation for embryo transplant. In some cases this will be a result of stress (see below). In other cases, the cause is unknown.
- *Stress* will often cause groups of goats to show short cycles of around 7 days, presumably because of premature regression of the corpus luteum. For this reason goats being brought together for a breeding programme, for example for embryo transplant, should be grouped at least 3 months before the start of the programme.
- *Ovarian follicular cysts* produce oestrogens, which result in a shortened oestrus cycle of between 3 and 7 days or continuous heat. Eventually the oestrogenic effects produce relaxed pelvic ligaments and the goat displays male-like mounting behaviour. The diagnosis can be confirmed by laparoscopy or laparotomy.

Treatment is exceptionally difficult in goats because the relatively short breeding season means that by the time treatment is completed the doe has already entered seasonal anoestrus. Medical treatment is only successful if commenced early:

Chorionic gonadotrophin 1000 U, i.m. or i.v. or

Gonadotrophin releasing hormone (GnRH): buserelin, 0.020 mg i.m., s.c. or i.v. or gonadorellin, 0.5 mg i.m.

Surgical treatment to exteriorise and rupture the thick wall of the cyst should be considered in valuable animals.

- *Ovarian tumours* are rare in goats, with granulosa theca cell tumours being the most common type. Clinical signs include short cycles, nymphomania and male behaviour. Examination of the ovary laparoscopically or with rectal or transabdominal ultrasound usually shows an enlarged ovary that may be cystic.
- *Endometritis* may cause short cycling or return to oestrus at the normal time.
- *Vaginitis*: see 'Regular oestrus cycles'.
- The presence of fetal bone remaining from a *mummified kid*, which is not expelled at parturition, will act as a constant source of stimulation and result in short oestrus cycles. There may be a history of bones and fetal material being expelled at kidding or subsequently.

Regular oestrus cycles (see Table 1.4)

- *Male infertility* (Chapter 3).
- *Service at the wrong time*.
- *Delayed ovulation/follicular atresia*. There is little scientific evidence describing these conditions in goats, but in practice a 'holding' injection given at the time of

Table 1.4 Regular oestrus cycles.

Male infertility
Service at the wrong time
Delayed ovulation
High yielders
Metritis
Vaginitis
Oestrus during pregnancy

service or AI will aid fertility in some animals by stimulating ovulation on the day of service:

Chorionic gonadotrophin, 500 U i.m. or i.v.

Gonadotrophin releasing hormone (GnRH): buserelin, 0.010 mg i.m., s.c. or i.v.

Gonadorellin, 0.25 mg i.m.

- *High yielding females.* Some high yielding females may have suboptimum fertility, possibly due to a pituitary dysfunction resulting from the heavy lactation. Maturation of follicles, ovulation and formation of the corpus luteum may be promoted by chorionic gonadotrophin, 500 U i.m. or i.v.
- *Metritis.* A low-grade metritis may result in the failure of the embryo to implant and subsequent return to service at the normal time.
- *Vaginitis.* Vaginitis occasionally occurs, particularly after the removal of vaginal sponges, and may result in short oestrus cycles or repeated return to service at a normal cycle length. In New Zealand, Australia and the United States, *caprine herpesvirus 1 (CpHV-1)* causes vulvovaginitis with short oestrus cycles and resulting infertility. Initial clinical signs are oedema and hyperaemia of the vulva with a slight discharge, which becomes more copious over the next few days. Multiple, shallow erosions with yellow to red-brown scabs develop on the vulvar and vaginal mucosa. Lesions heal spontaneously in about two weeks but may recur. Infection may be subclinical.

The virus is transmitted venereally and in the male produces penile hyperaemia and erosions of the preputial and penile epithelium. There is prolonged shedding of the virus by the preputial route.

CpHV-1 is also responsible for lethal systemic infections in one to two week old kids and for subclinical infections of the respiratory tract in adults.

- *Oestrus during pregnancy.* A few goats exhibit regular oestrus signs during pregnancy although this is less common than in cattle. Ovulation does not occur and the signs of oestrus are usually rather weak. Accurate pregnancy diagnosis is important before attempting treatment, particularly with prostaglandins.

Pregnancy diagnosis

> Non-return to service is not a reliable method of pregnancy diagnosis. Many does do not outwardly cycle throughout the breeding season and the non-return may be due to seasonal anoestrus or false pregnancy. Neither is mammary development in primiparous goats a reliable method of pregnancy diagnosis as maiden milkers are common. Nor is abdominal distension.

Although animals may have behavioural changes during late pregnancy (for example, a 'dog sitting' position is normal for some pregnant goats (Plate 1.8), these are very variable. Accurate pregnancy diagnosis is essential to distinguish between pregnant goats, those with false pregnancies and those that are not cycling.

A vasectomised and harnessed teaser male running with the does will detect return to service, that is non-pregnancy, but should not be relied upon as some males will mount females that are not cycling. *Always* undertake an accurate pregnancy diagnosis before using prostaglandins to induce oestrus. Table 1.5 lists the methods available.

Table 1.5 Techniques available for pregnancy diagnosis in the doe.

	Days	Fetal numbers	Accuracy (%)	Usefulness
Vasectomised male	>20	No	65–90	Moderate
Abdominal palpation	60–115	No	60–90	Moderate
Progesterone assay	18–22	No	90–95	Moderate
Oestrone sulphate assay	>50	No	>95	High
Pregnancy specific protein B	>26	No	>95	High
Realtime ultrasound	28–100	Yes	95–100	High
Doppler ultrasound	60–90	No	85–90	Moderate
Radiography	>70	Yes	>90	Low

Oestrone sulphate assay

Oestrone sulphate concentrations in milk and plasma increase steadily during pregnancy and can be used to diagnose pregnancy 50 days post-service. This test will distinguish between true pregnancy and hydrometra, but occasional false negatives do occur, particularly if the sampling is close to 50 days, and repeat sampling may be indicated before the induction of oestrus with prostaglandins to avoid the possibility of aborting a pregnant doe.

Ultrasonographic scanning

Realtime ultrasonographic scanning has the added advantage of giving some indication of the number of kids being carried, thus enabling a better estimate of the nutritional requirements of the doe during pregnancy. The technique is virtually 100% accurate in determining pregnancy and 96 to 97% accurate in determining twins and triplets. Good operators can distinguish hydrometra, resorbed fetuses and other abnormalities as well as live kids (Table 1.6). Goats can be scanned transabdominally or transrectally. Sector scanners are best for transabdominal scanning but linear scanners can be used and are better for transrectal scanning. Transrectal ultrasound techniques are preferred for very early pregnancies and permit diagnosis 4 to 5 days earlier than transabdominal techniques.

Transabdominal scanning is usually carried out with the goat standing. A 3.5 or 5 MHz transducer is suitable for most of the pregnancy, but may not penetrate as far as the foetus in late gestation, although caruncles will be visible. Before about 90 days a 5 MHz transducer gives the best results; in later pregnancy, a 3.5 MHz probe is preferable. Scanning can be used from 28 days post-service when a fluid-filled uterus can be identified, but is best used between 50 and 100 days of pregnancy. Cotyledons can be distinguished from about 40 days and individual foetuses by 45 to 50 days. By 100 days individual fetuses more than fill the entire screen, making accurate determination of numbers difficult (Table 1.7). The most common error is to underestimate the number of fetuses.

The transducer is placed on the right side of the restrained standing doe in the relatively hairless area

Table 1.7 Transabdominal ultrasound scanning for pregnancy diagnosis.

Day of gestation	Ultrasound findings
28	Fluid-filled uterus
30–35	Fetal heart beats detectable
40	Cotyledons visible (doughnuts or c-shaped structures)
45–50	Individual fetuses first identifiable
45–90	Accurate determination of multiple kids
	Gestational age corresponds to crown rump length, biparietal diameter and chest diameter
>100	Identification of number of fetuses becomes difficult because individual kids fill the screen; fluid and fetuses shift cranially

Table 1.6 Abnormal finding on ultrasonographic examination of the uterus.

Abnormality	Ultrasound findings
Recent abortion	Margins of the enlarged uterus observable, with caruncles often visible but with no fetus or fluid
Hydrometra	Anechoic or hypoechoic fluid-filled uterus, often with membranous strands visualized in the lumen of the uterus or apparent septae within the lumen of the uterine horn
Pyometra	Fluid-filled uterus; fluid more hyperechoic than hydrometra, often has a swirling appearance
Retained mummified foetus	Hyperechoic bone shadows in the absence of fluid contrast
	Lack of fluid contrast, dense bony shadows, or cranium or ribs in an organized foetal mass
	Usually smaller than expected foetal mass
	No sign of viability of fetus
Macerated foetus	Hyperechoic bone shadows in the absence of fluid contrast
	Overriding bony densities, usually linear or curvilinear images, with no sign of normal fetal architecture

just cranial and dorsal to the udder, with the transducer beam aimed towards the opposite brim of the pelvis (towards the pelvic inlet) and the abdomen scanned by slowly sweeping cranially. The uterus is normally dorsal or cranial to the bladder. Early in pregnancy (30 to 45 days), the uterus lies towards the pelvis inlet, but later is usually against the right abdominal wall. Clipping the area helps in fibre or long-coated goats. The area should be as clean as possible and large amounts of ultrasound gel used.

Transrectal scanning can be carried out from 25 days. Faeces are removed from the rectum and the lubricated 5 or 7.5 MHz linear transducer is advanced gently until it is adjacent to the reproductive tract. Initially the animal should be examined in a standing position, which is generally less stressful for the animal, but if the uterus is not identifiable the doe can be placed in dorsal recumbency.

Foetal viability can be evaluated during ultrasono-graphic examination, the presence of fetal movement or heartbeat indicating a live fetus. The fetal heart beat can be detected 35 days into the pregnancy by transabdominal ultrasonography (earlier by transrectal ultrasonography). Lack of echogenicity of amniotic fluid, the proper amount of fluid for the gestational stage and normal foetal posture and movement are signs of a healthy fetus. Fetal size incompatible with the expected gestational age may indicate earlier fetal death, as may increased fluid echogenicity, 'floating' membranes, collapsed fetal posture and failure to detect a heartbeat or fetal movement. Hyperechogenicity of the cotyledons is a common finding in a non-viable pregnancy.

Age determination is most accurately carried out early in gestation. Gestational age can be subjectively assessed based on size of the fetus and cotyledons, or the size of the amniotic vesicle in early gestation. Between 40 and 100 days, the length of the fetuses and the fetal head width or biparietal diameter (BPD) correlate closely with gestational age (see Table 1.8 and Figure 1.2). Later in pregnancy, the variation in size of fetuses is too great to permit accurate age determination.

Determination of fetal gender is by visualisation of the male/female genital tubercle or male scrotum. Best results are obtained between 55 and 75 days. Accuracy is decreased when multiple kids are present, because the spontaneous movement and repositioning of the foetuses during the examination makes visualising individual foetuses difficult.

Table 1.8 Correlation of fetal length with age of fetus.

Gestation (days)	Fetal length (mm)
45	40
60	100
90	250

Pre-breeding examination is important, especially in herds with out-of-season breeding programmes, for routine examination of does before assignment to breeding groups will allow detection of animals that would not respond to synchronisation, treatment of abnormal does and identification of does for potential culling. Abnormal findings by ultrasound can be followed by a vaginal speculum exam or other diagnostic procedures.

Doppler ultrasound techniques

Doppler ultrasound techniques can detect the fetal pulse after about 2 months' gestation, using either an intrapelvic probe or an external probe placed on a clipped site immediately in from the right udder or lateral to the left udder using ultrasound gel or vegetable oil to improve contact. Between 60 and 120 days' gestation the accuracy in detecting non-pregnancy is more than 90%, but the method is unreliable in detecting multiple fetuses.

Pregnancy specific protein B

Pregnancy specific protein B (PSPB) is produced by the placenta and is identifiable in plasma or serum, using an ELISA test, from 26 days after mating and then throughout pregnancy, dropping rapidly after parturition, but still detectable for several weeks. It has an accuracy rate of >95% – false positives are likely to be caused by loss of the embryo, rather than inaccuracy of the test. A positive result therefore means that the animal is pregnant or has recently been pregnant (or aborted or resorbed). If it is suspected that a doe has or may have resorbed or aborted, a second blood sample several weeks later would distinguish between pregnancy (continuing high protein level) or non-pregnancy (precipitous drop in protein level). Goats carrying multiple fetuses have higher PSPB concentrations than those carrying singles but there is sufficient overlap to prevent accurate identification of

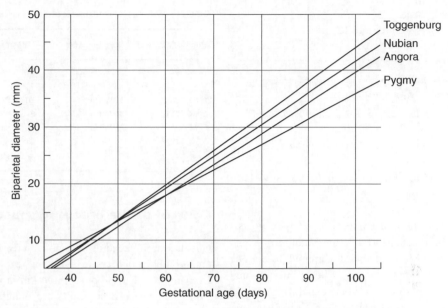

Figure 1.2 Biparietal diameter and gestational age of goats (from Haibel *et al.*, 1989).

single from multiple fetuses. The test is marketed in the United States by BioTracking, Moscow, ID.

Progesterone assay

Progesterone secreted by the corpus luteum of a pregnant goat can be detected by radioimmunoassay or by ELISA methods in milk or in plasma. Progesterone levels remain high throughout pregnancy.

Random sampling will not lead to accurate pregnancy diagnosis because the corpus luteum of the normal oestrus cycle and that of hydrometra also produce progesterone. A sample taken 24 days after mating will give nearly 100% accuracy in determining non-pregnancy but only about 85 to 90% accuracy in determining pregnancy because of factors such as early embryonic death and hydrometra. *A low progesterone level always indicates non-pregnancy*.

Radiography

Fetal skeletons are detectable by radiography between 70 and 80 days, although the technique is more useful after 90 days. An enlarged uterus may be detected at 38 days and over.

Rectoabdominal palpation

In the non-pregnant goat a plastic rod inserted in the rectum can be palpated at the body wall. Between 70 and 100 days post-service, the pregnant uterus prevents palpation of the rod. However, the technique produces unacceptably high levels of fetal mortality and risk of rectal perforation.

Ballotment

Ballotment of the right flank or ventrally is a time-honoured goatkeepers' technique for pregnancy diagnosis, but in the author's experience it is extremely unreliable. Fetal movements can often be observed in the right flank of the doe during the last 30 days of gestation.

Use of prostaglandins

Unlike other ruminants where placenta-derived progesterone becomes significant, the goat depends on corpus-luteum-derived progesterone throughout pregnancy, and is thus susceptible to luteolytic agents, including prostaglandins, throughout the whole of the pregnancy. Prostaglandins can be used for:

- Timing of oestrus.
- Synchronization of oestrus.
- Misalliance.
- Abortion.
- Timing and synchronization of parturition.

■ Treatment of hydrometra.
■ Treatment of persistent corpus luteum.

> Prostaglandins can be used to terminate pregnancy throughout the whole gestation period.

Suggested doses of prostaglandins in dairy goats are:

Dinaprost, 5–10 mg i.m. or s.c. or Clorprostenol, 62.5–125 µg i.m. or s.c.

Smaller doses will produce luteolysis in Angora goats. The effect of prostaglandin administration is seen between 24 and 48 hours (generally around 36 hours) post-injection, provided the animal being injected has an active corpus luteum, that is between days 4 and 17 of the normal oestrus cycle or during pregnancy. For induction of parturition where live kids are required, prostaglandins should not be used alone before day 144 of gestation, because prostaglandins bypass the steps involved in producing fetal lung surfactant. Before day 144, dexamethasone should be used and will produce parturition in about 48 to 96 hours (Figure 1.3).

Where rapid termination is required and the viability of the kids is not critical, for example when the doe is collapsed, prostaglandins can be used at any stage of gestation. There is generally no problem with retained fetal membranes following induction with prostaglandins or dexamethasone.

Table 1.9 Methods for controlling oestrus cycles.

Transitory Period	Breeding season	Out of breeding season
Buck effect	Prostaglandin injection(s)	Lighting regimes
Progestagen sponge or CIDR + PMSG	Progestagen sponge or CIDR + PMSG	Progestagen sponge or CIDR + PMSG Lighting regime + Melatonin

Control of the breeding season

Out-of-season breeding is being increasingly used to enable milk producers to maintain regular supplies of fresh milk and to produce three kid crops in 2 years from fibre goats. Best results are obtained when the techniques are used to extend the breeding season, that is by early or late season breeding, rather than in deep anoestrus. Table 1.9 shows methods available for controlling oestrus cycles.

Introduction of a buck or teaser male (buck effect)

Introduction of a buck or teaser male produces oestrus before the start of the breeding season, with loose synchronisation of oestrus. The introduction of a teaser or entire male into a group of does, which have been deprived of the sound, sight and smell of a male for at least 4 to 6 weeks during the transitional period before

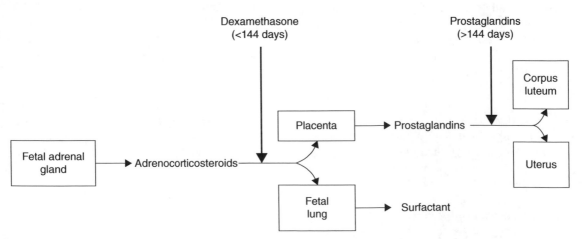

Figure 1.3 Induction of parturition.

the start of the normal breeding season, will produce oestrus cycles within 3 to 10 days, but the first one or two oestruses may be silent, without any sign of behavioural oestrus. A silent oestrus may be followed by a fertile oestrus 21 days later or the first silent oestrus may be followed by a short cycle and a second silent oestrus or fertile oestrus after about 5 days, following premature regression of the corpus luteum.

The fertility of the females after exposure is variable – the closer to the breeding season, the higher the fertility.

Prostaglandin injections

During the normal breeding season, the luteolytic effect of prostaglandins can be used to induce oestrus in animals with a corpus luteum, that is between days 4 and 17 of a normal oestrus cycle. Return to oestrus occurs between 24 to 48 hours post-injection, generally about 36 hours; 60–70% of the herd should respond to a single injection.

> Dinaprost, 5–10 mg i.m. or s.c. or Clorprostenol, 62.5–125 µg i.m. or s.c.

For synchronisation of oestrus, two injections should be given 9 to 11 days apart.

Lighting regimes

Lighting extends the breeding season into the spring, with synchronisation of oestrus. Does respond to a shortening daylength by ovulation and oestrus. Keeping goats under an artificially long daylight regime during the winter months, followed by a sudden change to normal daylength in the spring, enables out-of-season breeding to be achieved from April to June during the normal anoestrus period.

From 1 January, 20 hours of artificial light are given daily for 60 days. After 60 days, the goats are returned to normal lighting. Oestrus occurs 7 to 10 weeks later. The oestrus period may be shorter than normal (often only 8 to 10 hours compared to the normal 24 to 96 hours) and the signs of oestrus are not very obvious, so best results are obtained if the males are run with the females. Sudden introduction of the male to the females after their return to normal daylength increases the percentage of successful matings.

The lights must be of sufficient number and intensity to simulate daylight and suppress melatonin – 200 lux is provided by one 36 watt fluorescent light per $18\,m^2$ of floor space with lights at a height of about 2.75 m. The males should undergo light treatment at the same time as the females. With this regime, kidding rates of 50 to 60% can be expected, although up to 90% has been obtained.

Theoretically, it is not necessary to provide continuous lighting for the extended long day period. In sheep, a long day effect can be obtained by providing one extra hour of light during the night, provided it is given 7 to 8 hours before dawn. However, equivocal results have been obtained with goats, so the practical application of short light pulses remains to be established. One regime is to provide additional light between 6 a.m. and 9 a.m. (fixed dawn) and between 10 p.m. and midnight.

Progestagen-impregnated intravaginal sponges

Progestagen-impregnated intravaginal sponges enable:
- Oestrus synchronisation within the breeding season.
- Extension of the breeding season.
- Out-of-season breeding.

Two types of impregnated sponge are currently available in the UK:

> Medroxyprogesterone, 60 mg (Veramix Sheep Sponge, Zoetis) and Flugestone acetate, 20 mg (Chronogest, MSD)

Applicators are available for insertion of the sponges, but because the goat's vagina is more delicate than that of sheep, it is generally better to insert the sponges manually with a gloved hand using a small amount of antiseptic cream. If the animals are handled gently, the incidence of vaginitis or vaginal adhesions is low, but oxytetracycline powder may be used at insertion.

The principal of progestagen synchronisation is that:
- Gonadotrophin releasing hormone (GnRH) and gonadotrophin release is inhibited because of the negative feedback of the progestagen on the hypothalamus/pituitary.
- When the progestagen is suddenly withdrawn, there is a rebound effect with the sudden release of GnRH, and thus gonadotrophin, provided that there is no residual luteal function, which is itself secreting progesterone.
- Thus the progestagen must be administered for at least 12 days, but preferably longer (up to 20 days),

or used in conjunction with prostaglandins given 48 hours before sponge removal.

Improved pregnancy rates are generally obtained with shorter periods of progestagen treatment, particularly in large goats, as the hormonal levels in the sponges are designed for sheep. Progestagens are used for 9–12 days with prostaglandin treatment 48 hours before removal of the sponges (see Table 1.10). Removal of the sponges promotes oestrus in 95 to 100% of animals in the transitionary and normal breeding periods, but in only about 70% of animals outside these periods.

Two days before sponge removal, or at sponge removal if during the breeding season, a dose of follicle stimulating hormone, that is serum gonadotrophin (PMSG), is administered s.c. or i.m. to ensure optimum ovulation. The dose depends on the size of the goat, its yield and the season when the sponges are being used (Table 1.11). If

high doses of serum gonadotrophin are used, superovulation may occur, with resultant multiple births.

There are usually very strong signs of oestrus following sponging. The presence of a male improves the response. Oestrus occurs 24 to 72 hours after sponge removal (generally 30–36 hours). This is dependent upon several factors, which include:

- Social cues.
- Day length and ambient temperature.
- Whether the goat has been routinely cycling and producing regular pulsatile amounts of LH.
- Age of animal.
- Amount and type of chorionic gonadotropin or follicle stimulating hormone given before or at sponge or CIDR removal.

Table 1.10 Regimes for sponging goats.

Breeding season

Day 0	**Day 9**	**Day 11**	**Day 12–13**
Sponge inserted	Prostaglandin injection	Sponge removed + serum gonadotrophin injection	Onset of oestrus

Out of breeding season

Day 0	**Day 9**	**Day 11**	**Day 12–13**
Sponge inserted	Serum gonadotrophin injection	Sponge removed	Onset of oestrus

Transitory period

Day 0	**Day 9**	**Day 11**	**Day 12–13**
Sponge inserted	Prostaglandin injection + serum gonadotrophin injection	Sponge removed	Onset of oestrus

Table 1.11 Serum gonadotrophin treatments for sponged goats.

	Time of injection of serum gonadotrophin	**Dose of serum gonadotrophin (i.u.) (PMSG)**	
		Production of milk/day <3.5 kg	**> 3.5 kg**
Out of season (March–June)	48 hours before sponge removal	600	700
Transitory period	48 hours before sponge removal	500	600
Breeding season (September–February)	At sponge removal	400	500

Table 1.12 Optimum time for artificial insemination following sponge removal.

Fixed time (once)	Between 43 and 46 hours after sponge removal
Fixed time (twice)	30 and 50 hours after sponge removal
Fixed time (laparoscopically)	48 to 52 hours after sponge removal
After oestrus detection	12 to 24 hours after the onset of oestrus

- Whether the doe can smell a buck or is being physically teased with a vasectomized or epidydimectomised buck.

Although there is some breed variation, the doe typically ovulates between 19 and 23 hours after going out of heat. The optimum times for artificial insemination using frozen semen are shown in Table 1.12. Fixed time AI results in pregnancies but the rate is reduced when compared to insemination based on oestrus detection. Sufficient males should be available if natural mating is used in a synchronised herd, for example 1 male to 10 females during the breeding season and more for out-of-season breeding.

> Conception rates during the transitory period or out-of-season will be lower than for mating within the breeding season. Fertility will improve closer to the start or end of the breeding season. Many factors can influence fertility including breed, age and weight of the doe, month of treatment, buck selection and management.

Because the sponges are not licensed for goats, there is no defined milk withhold period but synthetic progesterones like medroxyprogesterone are known to be excreted into the milk in large quantities whilst the sponge is in place and for at least 3 days afterwards.

Controlled internal drug release

Suitable progesterone-impregnated intravaginal controlled internal drug-releasing devices (CIDRs) are available in many countries, although at present not the UK, for oestrus synchronisation in goats. CIDRs, silicon rubber elasomers moulded over a nylon spine, are inserted into the vagina like a sponge and similarly release a controlled amount of progesterone into the bloodstream, placing the treated does in the luteal phase of the oestrous cycle. The level of progesterone in milk from healthy goats after CIDR insertion for 19 days is similar to or less than those endogenously produced during dioestrus or pregnancy.

CIDRs available in the United States, Australia and New Zealand (Eazi-Breed CIDR, Zoetis) contain 0.3 g of a natural progesterone and similar timing and hormone regimes to sponges are used.

During the breeding season they are inserted and left in place for 14 to 18 days. The majority of does will be in oestrus approximately 48 hours after device removal. For AI using frozen semen, it is recommended that pregnant mare serum gonadotrophin (PMSG) 200 to 400 IU is given 48 hours before device removal. The use of vasectomised bucks is recommended prior to insemination. Insemination using a laparoscopic or cervical technique should be performed within 48 hours after device removal.

During the transitional periods, at the start and end of the breeding season, PMSG injections should be given at CIDR removal to help promote ovulation.

Out of season, if the does are not cycling, only a short period of progesterone is required to initiate follicle production. CIDRs are inserted for 7–9 days, followed by PMSG when the CIDR is removed. Breeding behaviour will likely occur without the PMSG, but the does do not ovulate and therefore the conception rate is very poor.

Outside the normal breeding season, buck fertility is usually much reduced. When using sponges and CIDRs, it is important to recognise this limitation and to use an increased male to female ratio, possibly with hand mating, or use AI. Reduced numbers of pregnancies and decreased numbers of feti/doe are common at this time. Does generally only cycle once, so failure to exhibit oestrus should not be used as an indicator of pregnancy.

Good record keeping will help improve conception rates using natural service and AI:

- Season of year/doe already cycling or not.
- Amount and type of chorionic gonadotropin given.
- Time of sponge or CIDR removal.
- Time to first signs of oestrus (hours).
- Time to end of oestrus; doe will no longer stand for buck (hours).
- Natural service or AI; fresh or frozen semen.
- Time AI carried out after sponge or CIDR removal (hours).

- Number of does confirmed pregnant.
- Number of progeny produced.

Melatonin

Animals measure day length using melatonin secreted during the hours of darkness by the pineal gland. In sheep, treatment with melatonin provides a short day/long night signal that will advance the breeding season. Goats appear to need exposure to long days, provided by artificial light, before they will respond to melatonin. Twenty hours of artificial light from 1 January for 60 days followed by a return to natural light, combined with melatonin treatment by subcutaneous implant, will advance the breeding season by 2 to 3 months. Males should be light-treated under the same regime as the females and their fertility may be further increased by melatonin treatment. The males should be removed from the herd at the start of the melatonin treatment and kept apart (out of sight, sound and smell) until they are reintroduced 35 to 40 days later. Fertile oestrus will occur from 2 to 6 weeks after the introduction of the males (i.e. from late April to June), with peak mating activity occurring 3 to 4 weeks after introduction (during May) and peak kidding during November.

If light treatment is not used, it is recommended that does should not be implanted before mid-May.

Melatonin can also be used in cashmere goats to delay the shedding of fleece, so obviating the need for winter shearing when weather conditions require goats to be housed and there is increased risk of post-shearing deaths.

Melatonin, 18 mg implant, s.c. behind ear

Further reading

General

Bretzlaff, K.N. and Romano, J.E. (2001) Advanced reproductive techniques in goats. *Vet. Clin. North Amer., Food Anim. Pract.,* **17**, 421–434.

Evans, G. and Maxwell, W.M.C. (1987) *Salomon's Artificial Insemination of Sheep and Goats.* Butterworths, London.

Howe, P.A. (1984) Breeding problems in goats. *Proc. Univ. Sydney Post Grad. Comm. Vet. Sci.,* **73**, 511–514.

Jackson, P. (2004) Aspects of reproduction in the doe goat. *Goat Vet. Soc. J.,* **20**, 9–12.

Johnson, B.M., Nuti, L.C. and Wiltz, D. (1994) Ultrasonic examination of the caprine ovary *Vet. Med., Food Anim. Pract.,* May, 477–480.

Mews, A. (1981) Breeding and fertility in goats. *Goat Vet. Soc. J.,* **2** (2), 2–11.

Noakes, D. (2003) Some aspects of normal and abnormal reproduction in goats. *Goat Vet. Soc. J.,* **19**, 14–22.

Peaker, M. (1978) Gestation period and litter size in the goat. *Br. Vet. J.,* **134**, 379–383.

Skelton, M. (1978) Reproduction and breeding of goats. *J. Dairy Sci.,* **61**, 994–1010.

Ward, W.R. (1980) Some aspects of infertility in the goat. *Goat Vet. Soc. J.,* **1** (2), 2-–5.

Caprine herpes virus

Camero, M. *et al.* (2015) Caprine herpesvirus type 1 infection in goat: not just a problem for females. *Small Ruminant Res.,* **128**, 59–62.

Control of the breeding season

Abecia, J.A., Forcada, F. and González-Bulnes, A. (2011) Pharmaceutical control of reproduction in sheep and goats *Vet. Clin. North Am. Food Anim. Pract.,* **27** (1), 67–79.

Abecia, J.A., Forcada, F. and González-Bulnes, A. (2012) Hormonal control of reproduction in small ruminants. *Anim. Reprod. Sci.,* **130**, 173–179.

Corteel, J.M. *et al.* (1982) Research and development in the control of reproduction. In: *Proc. III Int. Conf. Goat Prod. and Dis.,* Arizona, **1982**, pp. 584–591.

Evans, G., Holt, N., Pedrana, R.G. and Pemberton, D.H. (1987) Artificial breeding in sheep and goats. *Proc. Univ. Sydney Post Grad. Comm. Vet. Sci.,* **96**.

Geary, M.R. (1982) Use of Chronogest sponges and PMSG. *Goat Vet. Soc. J.,* **3** (2), 5–6.

Haibel, G.K. (1990) Out-of-season breeding in goats. *Vet. Clin. North Amer.: Food Anim. Pract.,* **6** (3), 577–583.

Henderson, D.C. (1985) Control of the breeding season in sheep and goats. *In Practice,* **7**, 118–123.

Henderson, D.C. (1987) Manipulation of the breeding season in goats – a review. *Goat Vet. Soc. J.,* **8** (1), 7–16.

Leboeuf, B. *et al.* (2003) Efficacy of two types of vaginal sponges to control onset of oestrus, time of preovulatory LH peak and kidding rate in goats inseminated with variable numbers of spermatozoa. *Theriogenology,* **60** (7), 1371–1378.

Rowe, J.D. *et al.* (2010) Progesterone milk residues in goats treated with CIDR-G(®) inserts. *J. Vet. Pharmacol. Ther.,* **33** (6), 605–609.

Fetal age determination and sexing

Amer, H.A. (2010) Ultrasonographic assessment of early pregnancy diagnosis, fetometry and sex determination in goats. *Anim. Reprod. Sci.,* **117** (3–4), 226–231.

Haibel, G.K., Perkins, N.R. and Lidi, G.M. (1989) Breed differences in biparietal diameters of second trimester Toggenburg, Nubian and Angora goat fetuses. *Theriogenology*, **32** (5), 827–834.

Santos, M.H.B *et al.* (2007) Early fetal sexing of Saanen goats by use of transrectal ultrasonography to identify the genital tubercle and external genitalia. *AJVR*, **68**, 561–564.

Hydrometra

Hesselink, J.W. (1993) Incidence of hydrometra in dairy goats. *Vet. Rec.*, **132**, 110–112.

Hesselink, J.W. (1993) Hydrometra in dairy goats: reproductive performance after treatment with prostaglandins. *Vet. Rec.*, **133**, 186–187.

Pieterse, M.C. and Taverne, M.A.M. (1986) Hydrometra in goats: diagnosis with realtime ultrasound and treatment with prostaglandins or oxytocin. *Theriogenology*, **26**, 813–821.

Souza, J.M.G. *et al.* (2013) Hormonal treatment of dairy goats affected by hydrometra associated or not with ovarian follicular cyst. *Small Ruminant Res.*, **111** (1–3), 104–109.

Hydrops uteri

Jones, S.L. and Fecteau, G. (1995) Hydrops uteri in a caprine doe pregnant with Goat–sheep hybrid fetuses. *JAVMA*, **206** (12), 1920–1922.

Morin, D.E., Hornbuckle, T., Rowan, L.L. and Whiteley, H.E. (1994) Hydrallantois in a caprine doe. *JAVMA*, **204** (1), 108–111.

Intersexes

Hamerton, J.L., Dickson, J.M., Pollard, C.E., Grieves, S.A. and Short, R.V. (1969) Genetic intersexuality in goats. *J. Reprod. Fert. Suppl.*, **7**, 25–51.

Laparoscopy

Van Reven, G. (1988) Laparoscopy in goats. *Goat Vet. Soc. J.*, **9** (1/2), 24–32.

Ultrasonography

DesCôteaux, L. (ed.) (2010) *Practical Atlas of Ruminant and Camelid Reproductive Ultrasonography*, pp. 181–199. Wiley-Blackwell, Iowa.

Erdogan, G. (2012) Ultrasonic assessment during pregnancy in goats – a review. *Reprod. Domestic Animals*, **47**, 157–163.

Rowe, J.D. (2014) Use of reproductive ultrasound for goat herd management. *AABP Proceedings*, **47**, 104–107.

CHAPTER 2

Abortion

> The most common cause of abortion is 'unknown'.

The cause of most cases of abortion is never determined, but it is estimated that only 50% of abortions are infective in origin. Determining the cause of a small ruminant abortion can be a somewhat subjective decision. The identification of an infectious agent, using a highly sensitive test such as the polymerase chain reaction (PCR), does not always indicate disease causation for organisms that may be normal resident microflora. Examination of the products of abortion, acid-fast stains, bacterial and viral culture and other diagnostic tests may give a better picture of the likely cause of the abortion. A list of the possible causes of abortion is provided in Table 2.1.

'Abortion outbreaks' are generally diagnosed more easily than abortion in an individual animal because diagnostic material is more readily available and because individual abortions are more often due to non-infective causes. Even when infection is responsible for the abortion, fetal infection and/or death may have occurred weeks, or even months, before the actual abortion occurs and routine diagnostic procedures may be unable to identify the cause.

Initial advice to owners

- Instruct the owner to save all the products of abortion for further examination – fetus/fetuses, fetal membranes. The diagnosis will probably depend on laboratory investigation of aborted material.
- Advise isolation of the aborted doe until a diagnosis is reached and/or uterine discharges have ceased.

- Warn of possible zoonoses, particularly during pregnancy. Care should be taken when handling aborted products – wear gloves. Any aborted material not required for laboratory examination should be burned or buried. Dogs and cats should be kept away from the aborted material.

Initial assessment

The preliminary history should consider:
- Individual or flock/herd problem.
- Possible exposure to infected animals – mixing with bought-in stock, etc.
- Homebred or bought-in does.
- Feeding, for example silage.
- Vaccination.
- Known disease status.
- Whether abortions have occurred in previous years.

Specific enquiries should cover:
- The length of gestation/timing of abortion (see Table 2.2).
- The general breeding history – return to service, etc.
- The incidence of abortion, still births, weak kids.
- The age of does that are aborting.
- Signs of illness in the aborted does.
- Drugs used on herd, for example prostaglandins.
- Access to possible poisons.
- The possibility of stress on the doe – handling, transport, etc.

Clinical examination

The doe should be fully examined for signs of disease. Aborting does may be ill and the clinical signs may aid diagnosis, but because abortion may occur some

---

Diseases of the Goat, Fourth Edition. John Matthews.
© 2016 John Wiley & Sons, Ltd. Published 2016 by John Wiley & Sons, Ltd.

Table 2.1 Causes of abortion.

Luteolysis	Infection
■ Trauma	■ Enzootic abortion
■ Stress	■ Toxoplasmosis
	■ Listeriosis
Iatrogenic	■ Campylobacter
■ Prostaglandins	■ Q-fever
■ Corticosteroids	■ Leptospirosis
	■ Salmonellosis
Poisoning	■ Tickborne lever
■ Plant	■ Border disease
■ Wormers	■ Brucellosis
	■ Neosporosis/sarcocystosis
Nutrition	■ Caprine herpesvirus 1
■ Starvation	■ Any bacteria responsible for
■ Vitamin A deficiency	bacteraemia
■ Manganese deficiency	■ Foot and mouth disease
	Fetal developmental abnormalities

Table 2.2 Timing of abortion.

Abortion throughout gestation	Abortion in late gestation
■ Toxoplasmosis	■ Listeriosis
■ Chlamydia	■ Campylobacter
■ Leptospirosis	■ Q-fever
■ Prostaglandins	■ Salmonellosis
■ Stress	■ Border disease
■ Tickborne fever	■ Corticosteroids
■ Foot and mouth disease	■ Multiple fetuses
■ Bluetongue	■ Energy deficit
	■ Mineral deficiency

time after infection, many aborting does will show few additional clinical signs. Abortion may follow acute septicaemia and pyrexia caused by conditions not normally associated with abortion, for example enterotoxaemia. A blood sample should be taken for laboratory investigation.

The aborted fetuses and placentae should be examined grossly before submitting to the laboratory. If a number of does have aborted, samples from several animals should be submitted because of the possibility of more than one infectious agent being involved.

Laboratory investigation

Ideally, material from every abortion should be submitted for laboratory analysis but this may not be economically feasible. Clusters of abortions should always be investigated as should sporadic abortions affecting >2% of the herd.

The diagnostic laboratory should have as complete a case history as possible, including:

- Number of infected animals.
- Age of infected animals, stage of gestation at which abortion occurred.
- A description of placental and fetal lesions.
- Clinical signs in the aborting does.
- Knowledge of any intercurrent diseases on the farm.

Submission of correct specimens is essential for accurate diagnosis:

- *Placenta* including several cotyledons – fresh or fixed in formol saline.
- *Fresh fetuses* (refrigerated but not frozen).

The preferred samples are fetus *and* placenta collected into an intact polythene bag (one per doe). Mummified fetuses are of little diagnostic value. If unable to submit whole fetuses:

- Fetal lung and liver – fresh and fixed
- Fetal abomasal contents – fresh; collect aseptically using a vacutainer tube and needle
- Fetal heart blood or thoracic fluid – fresh; collect into a plain vacutainer tube using syringe/pipette
- Fetal brain – fixed.

The gross appearance of placentae and fetuses may be suggestive of a particular aetiology, but are rarely pathognomonic, and adequate samples permit the demonstration of pathogens by microscopy, direct culture or virus isolation.

- *Serum from aborted animals.* At least 10 animals or 10% of the herd in 'abortion storms'. Maternal serology is suitable for enzootic abortion and *Toxoplasma*, both of which are better diagnosed by submission of fetal and placental material as above. Paired serum samples, with the second sample 14 days after the first, are often of more use than single samples.
- *Fetal serum.* The presence of antibodies in fetal serum allows a definitive diagnosis as the uterus should remain sterile during gestation.
- *Vaginal swabs* may be of value if placentae or fetuses are not available.

Samples should be double-bagged for transport with fetuses and placenta from individual does kept separate. If being sent by post, samples should be packed according to postal regulations, preferably in rigid containers with screw-top lids and sealed in leakproof inner packaging such as a plastic bag with sufficient absorbent material to soak up the entire contents if leakage occurs.

Infectious causes of abortion

There are important differences between sheep and goats in the behaviour of some infectious organisms that cause abortion. Because the epidemiology of these conditions is different in the two species, the control measures taken to limit the spread of disease in sheep will not necessarily be applicable to goats. More than one infective agent may be involved in an 'abortion storm'

Enzootic abortion (chlamydial abortion)

Abortion occurs at any stage of pregnancy (unlike sheep where abortion is restricted to the last 2 to 4 weeks) because of the luteolytic effect from endometrial inflammation. The incubation period is as short as 2 weeks, so infection and abortion may occur within one pregnancy, even if infection occurs late in pregnancy (see Table 2.3).

Aetiology
- *Clamydophila abortus* (formerly *Chlamydia psittaci*), an intracellular organism containing both RNA and DNA.

Transmission
- Ingestion of the organism shed in faeces but more generally from aborted material as *Chlamydophila* are not very resistant in the environment. Shedding in vaginal secretions may begin as early as 9 days before abortion and last as long as 21 days after abortion.

Table 2.3 Chlamydial abortion in goats compared to sheep.

Abortion may occur *at any stage of pregnancy*, rather than in the 3rd trimester as in sheep
Colonization of the placenta can occur *at any stage of pregnancy*
The *time from infection to abortion can be as little as two weeks*; in sheep it may be
many months later, mostly during the next pregnancy
The *doe may become ill* with septicaemia and pneumonia following abortion

- Carrier does or males in endemic herds and bought-in does continue the spread of infection. Kids born live will also carry the infection, although they remain negative serologically, and may shed organisms when they kid themselves.

Clinical signs
- Often abortion is the only clinical sign and the doe rapidly recovers, but severe illness with metritis, keratoconjunctivitis and pneumonia has been reported.

Post-mortem findings
- Placenta – intercotyledonary placentitis often with a covering of yellow purulent material, giving a leathery appearance. Advanced autolysis occurs.
- Fetus – no specific gross lesions occur; the fetus may be autolysed or fresh.

Diagnosis
- Examination of smears from the placenta, the mouth or nostrils of the foetus or the vagina of the doe using modified Ziehl–Neelsen stain demonstrates red-staining elementary bodies.
- The standard serological test is the complement fixation test. Does have significant antibody titres to chlamydial antigens after abortion. Titres of at least 4/32 are considered positive and indicative of infection in the current season. Paired serum samples taken 2 to 3 weeks apart can aid diagnosis. Antibodies can also be detected in fetal serum. Vaccination titres are usually low.
- The Western blot (WB) test can be used to confirm the diagnosis but is not suitable for screening large numbers of samples.
- Isolation of the organism from placenta or fetal tissue in tissue culture or in embryonic eggs – an extremely labour-intensive technique.
- Other tests used in some laboratories include ELISA, PCR and immunofluorescence with monoclonal antibodies.

Treatment and control
- Segregate aborting animals for 2 weeks until the excretion of chlamydia has ceased.
- Dispose of aborted material and disinfect the area.
- Cull any live kids born to infected does.

- Treat all pregnant goats in the herd with tetracyclines for 10 days and move them to uncontaminated pasture halfway through treatment:

  > Dairy goats: 20 mg long-acting oxytetracycline/kg i.m. every 3 days
  > Fibre goats: as dairy goats, or 400–450 mg oxytetracycline/head/day orally

- Consider a vaccination programme, but only where infection is already present in the herd. Attenuated live and inactivated vaccines are licensed in the United Kingdom for use in sheep but not goats. Live vaccines must only be used in non-pregnant animals; the inactivated vaccine can be used during pregnancy. Vaccination of healthy females at least 4 weeks before should prevent infection but may not prevent abortion in goats already infected. However, there is some evidence in sheep that use of the inactivated vaccine during an outbreak may reduce the number of abortions. In sheep, vaccination will provide protection for up to three lambings post-vaccination, depending on the vaccine. Vaccination should continue indefinitely as vaccination does not eliminate infection. Inactivated vaccines do not pose a zoonotic risk and can be safely handled by women of child-bearing age.
- Fertility is usually normal in pregnancies subsequent to the abortion, but immunity may wane after about 3 years.

Public health considerations

- The organism is excreted in body fluids including milk. Pregnant women are particularly at risk from contact with aborted material and from drinking unpasteurised milk.

Toxoplasmosis

Aetiology

- *Toxoplasma gondii*, an obligate protozoan parasite of endothelial cells.

Transmission

- Infective oocysts are passed in the faeces of cats, which act as the definitive host, multiplying and disseminating infection and contaminating stored foodstuffs or pastures. An asexual phase occurs in intermediate hosts, which include mammals and birds and a reservoir of infection for susceptible cats exists in birds and wild rodents, which may pass the infection vertically between generations. Cats then amplify and spread the infection.
- Goats act as intermediate hosts, becoming infected by ingesting foodstuffs contaminated with cat faeces containing oocysts and the resulting asexual developmental stage, the tachyzoite, actively enters host cells and multiplies. An immune response is detectable after about 12 days post-infection and the infection is either cleared or bradyzoites (tissue cysts) are formed. When a pregnant goat is infected, the tachyzoites travel to the placenta, causing a placentitis.
- Direct contact with the products of abortion – does eat placentae containing bradyzoites and tachyzoites.
- Transplacental infection of kids. Very low levels of infection may result in abortion.

Clinical signs

- Pyrexia and lethargy may occur in the doe about 2 weeks after infection, but the doe will be clinically normal at the time of abortion. Occasional fatalities occur in adult goats – post-mortem findings include nephritis, cystitis, encephalitis, hepatitis, enteritis and abomasitis.
- Goats exposed to infection prior to mating will not abort.
- Resorption, fetal death and mummification occur if infection is during the first third of pregnancy.
- Abortions, stillbirths and weak kids are produced if infection occurs later in pregnancy.
- Normal but infected kids may be produced to does affected in late pregnancy. Up to 80% of females may be infected and abort.

Post-mortem findings

- Placenta – yellow or white focal lesions, 1 to 3 mm in diameter on the cotyledons, with the intercotyledonary areas not affected.
- Fetus – there are usually no specific gross lesions on the fetus.

Diagnosis

- Diagnosis is aided by the clinical picture, the presence of the characteristic small white necrotic foci in placental cotyledons, the possible presence of a mummified fetus and on fetal serology and histopathology.

- Indirect fluorescent antibody (IFA) test on fluid collected from the fetus thorax or abdomen.
- ELISA and latex agglutination tests are used to detect antibodies in fetal and maternal serum. Polymerase chain reaction (PCR) tests specific for *T. gondii* are available in some laboratories.
- Serological examination of dam (complement fixation test) may be confusing due to high serological levels in the normal population. Antibody titres can persist for years and vaccination produces similar titres. Rising titres between paired samples is indicative of infection and a low titre means that the abortion was not due to *Toxoplasma*.

  Where dams are seropositive from exposure but have not aborted because of recent *Toxoplasma* infection, tissues will be PCR negative.
- Serological examination of live kids before suckling will demonstrate high specific antibodies.
- Histological examination of fetal tissues – brain, lung, liver, heart, kidney and spleen – shows necrotic foci surrounded by inflammatory cells and a non-suppurative mengioencephalitis typical of protozoan infection.
- Immunohistochemistry (IHC) can be used on formalin-fixed tissues to demonstrate antigen in bradyzoites and tachyzoites.

Treatment and control
- Animals remain infected for life.
- Sheep that have experienced abortion do not generally abort the following year, but it has been suggested that infected goats *may* sometimes abort in subsequent pregnancies, so it *may* be advisable to cull infected does.
- Chemoprophylaxis is likely to be of limited value in goats because of the risk of abortion during subsequent pregnancies, but decoquinate, 2 mg/kg bodyweight daily, can be added as a premix to commercial rations from mid-gestation to reduce perinatal losses. Monensin sodium, 15 mg/kg bodyweight daily, is also effective but banned from use in many countries, including the United Kingdom.
- Infection can be prevented by stopping the access of cats to grain stores, feeding troughs and hay barns.
- Products of abortion should be destroyed as soon as possible.

- Oocysts may persist on pasture or in soil for over a year and are very resistant to most disinfectants.
- Cats acquire immunity to reinfection and do not subsequently present a threat to livestock unless they become immunosuppressed. Preventing cats breeding on the premises will prevent the spread of the disease via the intermediate host – younger cats generally pose the greatest threat.
- Rodent and bird control will reduce the reservoir of infection that exists for susceptible cats.
- Vaccination. A vaccine containing living tachyzoites of *Toxoplasma gondii* is licensed in the UK for use in sheep but not goats; a single injection 3 to 4 weeks prior to mating gives a minimum of two seasons' protection. Vaccination will not introduce infection into the herd.

  The vaccine against toxoplasmosis can be given at the same time as the live vaccine against *Chlamydophila abortus* produced by the same manufacturer or at the same time as the inactivated vaccine against *C. abortus*. The vaccines should be given on opposite sides of the neck using different equipment.

Public health considerations
- Toxoplasma tachyzoites are passed in the milk of infected docs, so there is a risk to children and pregnant women from drinking infected milk as well as from handling aborted material. Aborted material should never be handled with bare hands.

Listeriosis

See Chapter 11.

Although two species *Listeria monocytogenes* and *Listeria ivanovii* are associated with abortion in sheep, only *L. monocytogenes* causes abortion in goats.
- Abortion results from infection early in gestation; abortion occurs from the 12th week but generally in late pregnancy.
- Infection later in gestation results in still births; some kids are born alive but die soon afterwards.
- Retained placentae and metritis are common after abortion.

Post-mortem findings
- Placenta – placentitis with cotyledons and intercotyledonary areas affected.

- Fetus – necrotic grey-yellow foci 1 to 2 mm in diameter in the liver and sometimes the lung.

Diagnosis

- The organism is easily grown and identified in the laboratory as a Gram-positive beta-haemolytic bacillus and can be isolated from the fetal stomach, uterine discharges, milk and the placenta.
- Fluorescent antibody examination of aborted material.

Treatment and control

- Clinically ill animals can be treated with ampicillin or potentiated sulphonamide.
- Aborted does are considered immune and should be retained in the herd.

Campylobacter (vibriosis)

Aetiology

- Comma-shaped Gram-negative bacteria. *Campylobacter* fetus (formerly *Vibrio* fetus). *Campylobacter jejuni* is a significant cause of abortion in the United States.

Transmission

- Ingestion of organisms from aborted material.
- Some does remain permanent carriers and are thought to be the main source of novel infection for herds.
- Wildlife can act as vectors.

Clinical signs

- Abortion in the last 4 to 6 weeks of gestation; some infected goats do not abort but produce weak kids at full term. These kids usually die within a few days.
- Does may be pyrexic and lethargic with diarrhoea for a few days either side of the abortion, but often the goat appears clinically normal.
- A post-abortion mucopurulent vaginal discharge is usual.
- Males are infected but do not show clinical signs.

Post-mortem findings

- Placenta – changes minimal.
- Fetus – may have doughnut-shaped foci of 10 to 20 mm diameter in the liver; the fetus is usually autolysed.

Diagnosis

- Direct Gram smears of fetal abomasal contents and placenta. The organism appears as curved, Gram-negative rods.
- Culture of fetal abomasal contents under microaerophilic conditions on selective media.
- Immunohistochemistry (IHC) can be used on formalin-fixed tissues to demonstrate *C. fetus* antigens.

Treatment and control

- Segregate aborting animals immediately and then cull them because of the possibility of a carrier state.
- Cull any live kids born.
- Dispose of abortion material and contaminated material by burning or burying.
- Treat the remainder of the herd with penicillin/dihydrostreptomycin or long-acting tetracycline 20 mg/kg every 48 hours during the outbreak or tetracycline 200–300 mg /head/day in feed before and during the kidding season. Tetracycline resistance appears quite common in *Campylobacter jejuni* isolated from sheep in parts of the United States.
- Vaccination. Killed, adjuvanted vaccines are available in North America and New Zealand, but are not available in the United Kingdom.

Public health considerations

- *Campylobacter* causes acute gastroenteritis in humans, usually by faecal contamination from diarrhoeic or apparently healthy goats. Faecal contamination of raw goats milk produced human disease in an outbreak in the United Kingdom.

Q-fever

Q-fever occurs in domesticated and wild animals throughout the world and is an important zoonosis. Clinical signs of disease are very uncommon, but abortions can occur in cattle, sheep and goats. The disease is considered endemic in livestock in Australia and, although it is almost never diagnosed as a clinical problem in animals, people working closely with animals are routinely vaccinated. An outbreak in the Netherlands in 2007–2009 was linked to abortions in dairy goat herds and thousands of goats were culled as a public health measure.

Aetiology

- Very small intracellular parasite *Coxiella burnetii*, a member of the Rickettsia family.

Transmission

- *C. burnetii* is highly infectious. Only one organism is required to produce infection under experimental conditions.
- By ingestion after direct contamination with abortion material or the urine, faeces and milk of an infected animal. Cattle, sheep, goats and wildlife may be infected and infection can be spread between species.
- By inhalation or through injured skin after contact with the organism.
- By infected ticks (unconfirmed in the United Kingdom).
- Healthy carrier goats spread the infection. Goats and cows shed the organism in milk and vaginal secretions for months or years, whereas sheep are more likely to shed in faeces. The organism is persistent in the environment and can infect any type of animal – cats, dogs, rabbits, insects – so a farm will stay contaminated.
- The organism can survive for weeks in the environment, surviving best in dry and dusty conditions, where it can attach to dust particles. It is extremely stable and highly contagious in the dried state, remaining dormant for 50+ years under the right conditions. One organism is said to be able to infect a human by the aerosol route.

Clinical signs

- Most infected goats are healthy carriers, but some aborting animals will be clinically ill with a retained placenta.
- Abortion occurs in the last month of pregnancy and stillborn or weak infected kids may be born at term.
- Further abortions have been shown to occur at a further two subsequent pregnancies.

Post-mortem findings

- Placenta – placentitis with clay-coloured cotyledons and intercotyledonary thickening; indistinguishable from that seen with *Chlamydophila abortus* abortion.
- Fetus – autolysed with no specific lesions.

Diagnosis

- Smears from the placenta or fetal stomach contents stained with a modified Ziehl–Neelsen stain show acid-fast pleomorphic coccobacilli.
- Immunohistochemistry on formalin-fixed sections of the placenta can be used to demonstrate *C. burnetii* antigens. Conventional histopathology and IHC are considered to have good specificity but poor sensitivity.
- A complement fixation test on the dam's serum shows the antibody level rising about a week after infections and persisting for a month. Titres of >1/10 are considered positive.
- ELISA and indirect fluorescent antibody (IgG phase 1 and 2 antigens) tests are available in some laboratories; both the specificity and sensitivity of serology are considered inferior to IFA.
- Realtime polymerase chain reaction (PCR) tests specific for *C. burnetii* are useful if tissues are available. PCR can utilise a variety of tissues – placenta, fetal lung, meconium, liver and abomasal content and maternal uterus, vaginal mucosa (tissue or swab) and whole blood.
- Culture is not routinely used for diagnosis due to the zoonotic risk.

Treatment and control

- Tetracyclines will probably control an outbreak and reduce abortions, but do not prevent shedding or reduce the zoonotic risk.

  Oxytetracycline, 20 mg/kg, 2 injections, the first at around 105 days' pregnancy and the second 2 weeks later

- A inactivated vaccine is available in Europe (Coxevac, CEVA) and could be used in the United Kingdom in the event of a disease outbreak. The effectiveness of the vaccine in goats has been determined in two field studies with pregnant goats exposed to *Coxiella burnettii*. The studies conducted in cattle and goats showed that Coxevac reduces bacteria shedding (which is a major factor in spreading the disease) in vaginal discharge and milk, whilst in goats Coxevac reduced bacteria shedding in faeces and the placenta as well. The studies in goats also showed a lower proportion of abortions in the goats that were vaccinated compared with unvaccinated goats. The duration of protection was established to be 280 days in cattle and one year in goats. In goats it is very common to see a palpable reaction of 3 to 4 cm diameter at the injection site, which may last for 6 days. The reaction reduces and disappears without need for treatment. In goats, it is also very common to observe a slight increase of rectal temperature for 4 days post-vaccination without other general signs. The withdrawal period for Coxevac for meat and milk is zero days.

Public health considerations

- The disease is most important as a human infection. Infection usually results from inhaling the resistant spore form on dust particles contaminated with fetal, placental and uterine fluids, faeces or urine, but also by drinking infected milk or eating unpasteurised dairy products (the organism migrates into the cream, survives freezing and likes acidity). The organism is killed by pasteurisation. Animal hides, wool and fur are potential sources of infection for abattoir workers. Infection can also occur via tick bites or skin abrasions.
- Outbreaks can occur in urban areas when there is windborne spread from nearby livestock premises.
- Disease often occurs in people without signs of disease in infected animals. Herd immunity tends to be excellent after an outbreak so abortions stop but shedding still continues.
- When working with an infected herd, good personal hygiene is essential, particularly during kidding. Hands should be washed frequently and disposable overalls should be worn or clothing changed and washed before leaving the premises. Personal protective equipment, including facemasks and goggles should be worn for high risk activities such as handling abortion materials, pressure washing or working in very dusty livestock areas.
- Products of kidding. Placentas, aborted fetuses, contaminated bedding, etc., should be removed immediately and disposed of by incineration, burial or autoclaving. Contaminated bedding should be wetted down to prevent the generation of aerosols.

- Manure should be composted well and not spread as it is more contagious in the dry state.
- It is very difficult to eliminate organisms from the environment, even with the removal of organic material and disinfection with quaternary ammonium products.
- Infected animals are safe to eat if thoroughly cooked but the slaughter of positive animals may pose a risk of infection to abattoir workers.
- Vaccination in routinely carried out in some countries for groups of workers potentially at risk from infection. A Q-fever vaccine is available in Australia and is 83 to 100% effective in preventing the disease. However, the vaccine can only be given to individuals 15 years of age and over. Prior to immunisation, a blood and a skin test is recommended to see if the individual has previously been exposed to Q-fever – either naturally or by previous vaccination. Vaccinating those already exposed to Q-fever can result in severe reactions. Vaccination will not prevent disease in someone who has already been infected but is in the incubation period of the disease.

Leptospirosis

See Chapter 17.

Leptospirosis is a rare cause of abortion in goats. Abortions are reported to occur only following septicaemia in acute infections.

Diagnosis

- Serology: microscopic agglutination test (MAT); ELISA.
- Isolation and identification of *Leptospira* spp. in the doe's urine, placenta, or fetal fluids and kidney tissues.

Salmonellosis

Aetiology

- Numerous *Salmonella* serotypes have been reported to cause abortion in sheep and goats, including *S. abortus ovis*, *S. typhimurium*, *S. dublin* and *S. montevideo*. Sources of infection include birds, cattle and human sewage, but the interval between infection and abortion means that identifying the source of infection may be difficult.

Clinical signs

- Some serotypes, including *S. typhimurium* and *S. dublin*, cause systemic illness with diarrhoea in addition to abortion, stillbirths or very weak live kids, which die shortly afterwards. The fetuses are autolytic and oedematous with lesions characteristic of septicaemia.
- *S. abortus ovis* causes sporadic abortions in middle to late gestation. Abortion is also the main presenting sign of *S. montevideo* infection.
- Abortion material is heavily contaminated with salmonellae and acts as a source of infection for other animals.
- Metritis and retained fetal membranes are common following abortion and does may die from septicaemia.

Diagnosis

- Diagnosis is established by bacterial isolation from the abomasum and other fetal organs or from vaginal swabs. Serotyping is carried out at a *Salmonella* reference laboratory.

Treatment and control

- Antibiotic treatment of sick and in-contact pregnant does should be based on the antibiotic sensitivity of bacterial isolates.
- An inactivated *S. dublin* and *S. typhimurium* vaccine is licensed for cattle in the United Kingdom and could be used off-licence for goats in the face of an outbreak of salmonellosis.

Tickborne fever

Anaplasma phagocytophilum (formerly *Ehrlichia phagocytophilia*) causes tickborne fever in sheep, cattle and goats in the United Kingdom and can cause severe economic losses in some locations due to reduced weight gain and milk yields, abortions and secondary infections. *Anaplasma phagocytophilum* is also responsible for human granulocytic anaplasmosis, a severe febrile illness increasing in incidence in the United States and Europe.

Aetiology

- *Anaplasma phagocytophilum* is an intracellular parasite of the Rickettsia family, transmitted by the tick vector *Ixodes ricinus*.
- *A. phagocytophilum* in feral goats in the United Kingdom has been reported from Scotland and Northern Ireland, where it may be a significant wildlife reservoir.
- Very little work has been done regarding the prevalence of *Anaplasma* infections or their clinical significance in sheep and goats in North America. *A. phagocytophilum* is present in the northeast of the United States, together with an appropriate vector, *Ixodes scapularis*. In the west, *Ixodes pacificus*, the western black-legged tick, is a suitable vector. It is not known whether or not clinical illness, similar to tickborne fever in the United Kingdom, is caused by North American strains of *Anaplasma*.

Epidemiology

- In endemic areas most nymphs and adult ticks are infected and thus virtually all ruminants and deer exposed to ticks also become infected, generally very early in life, and so do not encounter infection for the first time when pregnant. Exposure of pregnant does to infection results in abortion. Feral goats may potentially be a significant wildlife reservoir of the disease.

Clinical signs

- Pyrexia, lethargy, weight loss (often not recognised).
- Abortion and metritis.
- Temporary infertility in male goats.

In addition, infection may increase the pathogenicity of other diseases such as tick pyaemia, louping ill, listeriosis and pasteurellosis.

Anglo-Nubian goats react more severely than other breeds of British goats.

Diagnosis

- Detection of the organism in polymorphonuclear leucocytes in Giemsa-stained blood smears.
- Examination of the brains of aborted fetuses reveals eosinophilic multifocal leucomalacia and glial nuclear loss.
- Demonstration of rising antibody titres in paired serum samples using ELISA.

- PCR to detect the parasite in heparinised blood samples from infected does.

Control
- Susceptible pregnant animals should not be exposed to tick-infected pastures.
- *A. phagocytophilum* is sensitive to tetracyclines.

Border disease (hypomyelinogenesis congenita, hairy shaker disease)

Border disease virus (BDV) causes abortion, stillbirth and infertility in small ruminants and probably has a worldwide distribution.

Aetiology
- Pestivirus, serologically related to bovine viral diarrhoea virus (BVDV-1 and BVDV-2).
- BDV has been segregated into several phylogenetic groups, BDV-1 to BDV-7, and further genotypes may be characterised in the future.
- Pestiviruses have been isolated from only a few naturally infected goats and field cases are rarely reported.

Epidemiology
- Persistently infected cattle and sheep are believed to be the main reservoirs of pestiviruses (Border disease and BVD) that infect goats. Bovine virus diarrhoea virus (BVDV) is easily spread between cattle and goats during cohabitation and the virus can spread transplacentally to the caprine fetus.
- Direct animal contact by ingestion or aerosol is the main source of infection; sheep, goats, deer and possibly pigs are potential sources of infection.
- Surviving infected kids will remain carriers.
- Although the oronasal route is probably the most common means of natural dissemination, spread is possible via the use of common needles or ear-tagging or castrating equipment previously used on a persistently infected animal, even of another species.

Clinical signs
- Most clinical cases involve abortion and poor viability of newborn kids.
- Infection during early pregnancy can result in fetal death and resorption with return to service after an extended period.

- Abortion, stillbirths, barren does, fetal death, maceration and mummification result from infection after about the 70th day of gestation.
- Small weak kids occur with varying degrees of tremor and skeletal abnormalities, although hairy coat abnormalities as seen in lambs rarely, if ever, occur. Kids with cerebellar hypoplasia may be unable to stand or present with seizures or opisthotonus.
- When goats are experimentally or naturally infected, persistently infected offspring occur less frequently than in sheep. Immunological competence in goat fetuses seems to occur 20 days later than it does in sheep, corresponding to about 80 to 100 days of gestation. Because infection of goats before the time of immune competence usually kills the fetus, the prevalence of persistent infection in goats is very low.
- Infection in non-pregnant goats is often subclinical.
- One Austrian goat that was naturally infected with BVDV-1 showed poor body condition, stiff gait and difficulty in rising, and subsequently died of fibrinopurulent pneumonia.
- BDV in goat herds with diarrhoea has been reported from eastern China.

Post-mortem findings
- Kids – affected kids show hydrocephalus and cerebellar hypoplasia.
- Placenta – severe necrotising caruncular placentitis.

Diagnosis
- Live animal. Virus isolation and serology from kid or doe blood by ELISA and PCR. Experimental infections of mature goats produce neutralizing antibodies that are detectable for at least 4 years.
- Post-mortem. Antigen can be detected in fresh samples of thyroid, kidney, brain, spleen, intestine, lymph nodes or placenta; virus can be isolated from post-mortem material sent in virus transport medium; heart blood can be used for serology; histopathology of brain and spinal cord shows hypomyelinogenesis and immunohistochemical labelling can be used.

Control
- Infections with pestiviruses in goats do not appear to be a problem and do not usually require any control, but the small potential to be a reservoir of infection for cattle and sheep needs to be considered when planning eradication programmes.

Brucellosis

Brucella abortus

Goats can be infected with *Brucella abortus* and hence are included in dairy cow testing programmes, but the incidence of infection is minute in all parts of the world. In infected goats abortion is rare and mastitis common. Serological testing of goats for brucellosis is reported to have severe limitations.

Brucella melitensis

Goats and sheep are most susceptible to *Brucella melitensis*, which occurs mainly in southern Europe and Middle Eastern countries. It is absent from the United Kingdom, but sporadic outbreaks have been reported in the United States. The disease is important as a major zoonosis producing Malta fever in humans who drink infected milk. It is contagious to cattle and less commonly affects pigs and horses.

Brucella melitensis is a notifiable disease in the United Kingdom. Suspect *Brucella melitensis* when there are late abortions (2 months), stillbirths, weak neonates, mastitis, orchitis, lameness and hygroma.

The disease is most likely to be introduced by the importation of infected animals, semen or embryos. The European Union requires sheep and goats imported on to an officially free holding to originate from a free holding and be subject to testing in isolation before the movement. Contaminated milk and milk products are a zoonotic risk. Pasteurization kills the bacteria.

Epidemiology

- Goats excrete the organism in milk, urine and faeces and in vaginal discharges for 2 to 3 months.
- Kids carried to term become carriers and can shed the organism.
- Infection enters the adult animal through the nasopharynx, conjunctivae or upper alimentary tract by direct or aerosol contamination following abortion, when very large numbers of organisms are excreted. Venereal infection occasionally occurs.
- Brucellosis is usually introduced into the herd by the purchase of an infected animal or by sharing common grazing.

Clinical signs

- Abortion is the main clinical sign and usually occurs during the last months of gestation. The organism is excreted in uterine and vaginal secretions, urine, faeces and milk after parturition or abortion.
- Abortion occurs particularly in the first pregnancy and subsequent pregnancies may proceed to term with the birth of live but weak kids.
- Systemic disease with pyrexia, lethargy, weight loss, diarrhoea, mastitis, metritis, fall in milk yield and lameness may occur.
- Males may develop orchitis.

Post-mortem findings

- The placenta is normal on gross examination.

Diagnosis

- Isolation of the organism from a culture of the placenta or fetal stomach.
- Serological tests include ELISA, SAT, CFT and Rose Bengal tests, but cross-reactions with other bacteria are common, leading to false positives.

Vaccination

- A live vaccine (Rev 1) is considered to be highly effective in small ruminants and is used globally where the disease is endemic. It is generally used in kids 3–6 months of age, although it can be used in adults. Vaccination of pregnant animals results in abortion. The recommended strategy is the mass vaccination of all animals in the first year, followed by the annual vaccination of all newborn animals.
- Vaccination programmes are being used to control brucellosis in areas where the disease is endemic and have been shown to be cost-effective, but complete eradication of the disease is difficult and, without adequate disease surveillance, the disease can rapidly spread from small residual foci.
- It is not possible to distinguish between bacterial titres due to natural infection and vaccination. Rev 1 titres persist for a long time following vaccination.

Public health implications

- Milk and milk products, such as unpasteurised cheese, are potential sources of human infection.

Neosporosis

Neospora is a major cause of fetal loss in cattle that parallels that of *T. gondii* infection in sheep and goats.

While neosporosis is likely to be an uncommon cause of abortion in goats, experimental infection is readily induced in them. Furthermore, clinical signs and pathological lesions in sheep and goats are similar to those induced in them by *T. gondii*, although there are subtle histopathological differences. The incidence of the organism in goats in the United Kingdom is unknown.

Aetiology

- *Neospora caninum*, a protozoan parasite with a life cycle similar to *Toxoplasma gondii*. Dogs and wild canids act as definitive hosts, where sexual reproduction occurs.
- Cattle are the major intermediate hosts, where asexual reproduction occurs; sheep, goats, horses, deer, dogs and foxes are also occasionally affected.

Transmission

- Sporocysts are passed in dog faeces and are later ingested by the goat.
- Infection need not occur during pregnancy to cause abortion; vertical (transplacental) transmission from the dam to the fetus occurs and can occur repeatedly in the same animal.

Clinical signs

- Abortion, stillbirth and weak kids. Dams generally show no other clinical signs.

Diagnosis

- Serological examination by immunofluorescent antibody test (IFAT) and ELISA.
- Histological examination of brain and heart – characteristic non-suppurative Encephalitis.
- Immunohistochemistry on formalin-fixed tissues to demonstrate antigen.
- Parasites found in tissues by specific staining (immunoperoxidase (IPX) test).

Treatment

- No drugs have been shown to prevent transplacental transmission.

Control

- There are currently no effective control measures against the parasite. However, as it is now known that dogs can shed *Neospora* oocysts, it is important that dogs be kept away from feed and water and should be prevented from eating aborted foetuses, placental tissue or dead young, which may harbour infection.

Sarcocystosis

Aetiology

- *Sarcocystis capracanis*, a protozoan parasite using the goat as an intermediate host, with the dog as the definitive host.
- Other species-specific prey–predator life cycles have been demonstrated for goat–dog (*S. hircicanis*) and goat–cat (*S. moulei*). Goats are the intermediate host for *S. orientalis*, but are unaffected (dogs are probably the final host).
- *Sarcocystis* relies on the predator–prey relationship of animals. Oocysts are passed through the faeces of an infected animal and undergo sporogony. Lysis of the oocysts releases sporocysts into the environment, where they are ingested by an intermediate host such as a goat. Sporozoites are then released in the new host and migrate to muscle tissue where they undergo asexual reproduction. Once the intermediate host is eaten by the definitive host, such as a dog, the parasite undergoes sexual reproduction to create macrogamonts and microgamonts. They create a zygote, which develops into an oocyst that is passed through the faeces, completing the life cycle.
- The incidence of the organism in the United Kingdom is unknown. It is likely that sarcocystiosis is underdiagnosed as a problem and that better diagnostic methods are needed to show the true extent of the losses caused.

Clinical signs

- *Sarcocystis* spp. infections are quite prevalent in farm animals, following ingestion of food or water contaminated with sporocysts; however, clinical sarcocystiosis is much less commonly diagnosed than toxoplasmosis and neither is it normally associated with fetal infection or abortion in either sheep or goats. Most animals are asymptomatic, and the parasite is only discovered at slaughter.
- Clinical signs depend on the number of sporocysts ingested. They are non-specific and include pyrexia, anorexia, lethargy, haemolytic anaemia, jaundice,

nervous signs and abortion due to maternal failure – the placenta and fetus are not infected; weak kids may be born alive.

Diagnosis

■ Diagnosis is difficult as infection is so common and clinical signs are absent, mild or non-specific. Serology may be useful in some situations and histopathology/immunohistochemistry is valuable for confirming the cause of death.

Post-mortem findings

■ Non-specific findings; petechial haemorrhages in many organs.
■ Haemorrhages in heart and skeletal muscle.
■ Immunofluorescent and immunoperoxidase techniques are used to identify meronts in endothelial cells including the maternal caruncle.

Control

■ Livestock become infected by sporocysts from the faeces of carnivores. Because most adult cattle, sheep and many pigs harbour cysts in their muscles, dogs and other carnivores should not be allowed to eat raw meat, offal or dead animals. Supplies of grain and feed should be kept covered; dogs and cats should not be allowed in buildings used to store feed or house animals.

Public health considerations

■ Human infection is rare but can happen when undercooked meat is ingested.

Other organisms

Any bacterial infection that results in bacteraemia can occasionally cause abortion, for example *Mannheimia haemolytica* (formerly *Pasteurella haemolytica*) and *Trueperella pyogenes* (formerly *Corynebacterium* pyogenes).

Other organisms that have been implicated in abortion are as follows.

Bacillus spp.

Bacillus species occur ubiquitously and are normal components of cut grass. They proliferate in poor quality silage on exposure to oxygen. Abortion outbreaks in cattle fed on big bale silage have been attributed to *B. licheniformis* and *B. licheniformis* is occasionally implicated in caprine abortions.

Yersinia pseudotuberculosis

Yersinia pseudotuberculosis infection in goats has been associated with:

■ Enteritis and/or typhlocolitis.
■ Systemic abscessation.
■ Conjunctivitis.
■ Hepatitis.
■ Mastitis.
■ Placentitis, abortion, perinatal mortality, endometritis, infertility.

Late- and full-term abortions and early neonatal deaths have been reported following enteric infection and subsequent bacteraemia. Reported lesions were necrosuppurative placentitis with intralesional bacterial colonies, and bacterial embolisation with necrosuppurative fetal pneumonia, hepatitis and, less frequently, splenitis and nephritis.

Mycoplasma spp.

M. mycoides and *M. agalactiae* are reported to cause vulvovagintis and abortion, with abortion occurring during the first third of pregnancy. Aborting females shed the organism in milk and amniotic fluid and the organism can be found in the placenta and the liver and spleen of the fetus.

Caprine herpes virus

Caprine herpesvirus 1 (CpHV-1) is responsible for lethal systemic infections in one to two week old kids and for subclinical infections of the respiratory and genital tract in adults. CpHV-1 may also cause infertility, abortions, returns to service and genital lesions (see Chapter 1).

The virus has been linked to sporadic abortion storms following introduction of the virus to herds by latent carriers. Virus isolation, fluorescein-conjugated antibody staining and histological examination of fetuses can be used to identify herpes virus abortion, but serology is of limited use because positive results indicate exposure, which may not be recent. Serology may help identify goats that could become latent carriers of the virus.

Kids born alive may remain unaffected by the virus and are thus at low risk of being infected with the virus, although kids may have maternal antibodies for several months after birth.

Bluetongue virus

Goats are generally less severely affected by the bluetongue virus than sheep (Chapter 10) and the virus is an unlikely cause of abortion in goats. Infection of sheep during pregnancy can cause fetal death and resorption, abortion or live 'dummy' lambs with developmental defects including hydranencephaly (absence of cerebral hemispheres).

Orthobunyaviruses

See Chapter 8.

Orthobunyaviruses, including Akabane virus (Australia, Japan, Israel, South Africa, the Middle East), Cache Valley virus (United States, Canada, Mexico) and Schmallenberg virus (Northern Europe, including the United Kingdom), can cause an increased incidence of abortions and congenital malformations classified as arthrogryposis hydranencephaly syndrome (AHS) in fetuses and neonatal kids. These include stillbirth, premature birth, mummified fetuses, arthrogryposis, joint malformations, scoliosis, torticollis, kyphosis, lordosis, hydrocephalus, hydranencephaly, microcephaly and cerebellar dysplasia, behavioural abnormalities and blindness. Adult goats are otherwise generally asymptomatic so pregnant animals may remain healthy but abort or deliver mummified fetuses and stillborn or deformed kids. An apparently normal kid can be born twin to a mummified kid or one with severe deformities. Pre-colostral titres in the kid's serum or fetal fluids confirm the diagnosis.

Foot and mouth disease

Abortion is less likely than in sheep but can occur as a result of pyrexia (Chapter 6).

Rift Valley fever (RVF)

RVF is a vector-borne disease of sheep and goats characterised by high rates of abortion and neonatal mortality. Cattle and wild mammals are also susceptible and it is a major zoonosis. Susceptibility of different breeds to RVF varies considerably. Morbidity and mortality can approach 100% in naïve adults and young animals.

Suspect RVF when pregnant goats abort and kids under 1 week die suddenly. Other animals may be jaundiced with haemorrhagic diarrhoea.

The disease could be imported with infected mosquitos, via wild life introduced as exotic pets, illegal imports or bush meat, although the disease is unlikely to become established in the United Kingdom under present climatic conditions. Imports of live sheep and goats into the European Union from affected countries are banned.

Present distribution

Endemic in sub-Saharan Africa with occasional incursions into northern Africa and the Middle East, including Saudi Arabia, and recently South Africa.

Aetiology

- Single-stranded RNA virus of the family Bunyaviridae within the genus *Phlebovirus*, spread by various mosquitos. Transovarian transmission is an important epidemiological feature and infected eggs can survive in soil for years before being released during rainy seasons. In endemic areas RVF virus regularly circulates between wild ruminants and haematophagous mosquitoes; disease is usually inapparent.

Clinical signs

Very short incubation period, as short as 12 hours in kids and 2 days in adults. In an endemic area, infections in non-pregnant animals may be subclinical.

Neonatal kids:
- Weakness, lethargy, anorexia
- Abdominal pain
- Rapid, abdominal respiration
- Death in 24–36 hours
  Older kids and adults:
- Sudden death
- Pyrexia, inappetance, lethargy
- Jaundice in some animals
- Abortion storms with rates approaching 100%
- Agalactia
- Vomiting
- Mucopurulent nasal discharge
- Dysentery
- Haematuria
- Death

Post-mortem findings
- Jaundice
- Focal hepatic necrosis
- Multiple haemorrhages
- Intrathoracic and intraabdominal oedema

Diagnosis
- Virus isolation or demonstration of the viral genome, PCR.
- Serology – virus neutralisation, ELISA, haemagglutination inhibition.
- Histopathology – characteristic cytopathology of the liver of affected animals and immunostaining allows the specific identification of the RVF viral antigen in infected cells.

Wesselsbron disease
Wesselsbron disease and Rift Valley fever share many clinical and pathological features. However, Wesselsbron disease is usually milder, producing much lower mortality, fewer abortions and less destructive liver lesions. It is seen mainly in sheep, but goats, cattle, pigs and horses can also be infected. Newborn lambs and goat kids are most susceptible. In lambs and kids, the clinical signs include pyrexia, anorexia, weakness and an increased respiratory rate and mortality may occur in 30% of affected lambs. Infections in adult goats are usually inapparent and limited to pyrexia, but pregnant goats may abort.

Wesselsbron disease is caused by the Wesselsbron virus, an arthropod-borne virus in the genus *Flavivirus* of the family Flaviviridae. It has been isolated from vertebrates and arthropods from many sub-Saharan African countries, and serologic surveys provide evidence of its occurrence in other countries.The infection rate appears to be high in ruminants in endemic regions of Africa. In cattle, sheep and goats, the seroprevalence may be as high as 50%. Animals of all ages seem to be susceptible to infection.

Non-infectious causes

Medication
Prostaglandin administration will produce abortion at any stage of the gestation. *Phenothiazine* used as a worm drench is reported to cause abortion in late pregnancy as will *corticosteroids* given in late pregnancy. *Levamisole*,

administered in the last two months of pregnancy, has been implicated in late-term abortions.

Trauma and stress

> As the doe is dependent on corpus-luteum-derived progesterone throughout pregnancy, anything that causes luteolysis will produce abortion.

This means that goats may be more susceptible than other species to abortion from trauma or stress. Any condition that causes release of prostaglandins, and thus luteolysis, will cause abortion.

Heat stress can cause fetal hypoxia, hypotension and endogenous corticosteroid release with subsequent abortion.

Developmental abnormalities
Very few deformed fetuses are produced, but a fetus with developmental abnormalities may be aborted. An hereditary defect of Angora does in South Africa led to chronic hyperadrenocorticism, death of the fetus and then its expulsion.

Multiple fetuses
Abortions or early parturition appear more common in Anglo-Nubian goats, which commonly carry three, four or more fetuses. In these cases, placental insufficiency probably leads to fetal expulsion.

Poisons
Plant poisonings are occasionally implicated in abortion, for example *Astragalus* spp. and *Lathyrus* spp., but are unlikely to be of significance in the United Kingdom. Toxic plants can also produce fetal abnormalities (see Chapter 21).

Poisonings from non-plant sources also occasionally occur, generally causing abortion by producing a systemic illness.

Malnutrition
Energy deficit. Frank starvation will cause abortion, particularly if the energy input is insufficient during the last third of pregnancy.
Mineral deficiencies. Mineral deficiencies, for example, selenium, copper and iodine, generally cause the

birth of dead or weak kids at full term, rather than abortion, but manganese deficiency has been shown to cause abortion at 80 to 105 days of gestation.

Vitamin deficiencies. Prolonged vitamin A deficiency has been shown to cause abortion, stillbirth, illthrift, retained placenta and night blindness due to the absence of visual purple in the retina. However, vitamin deficiency is extremely unlikely, even in severe drought.

Mycotoxins

Mycotoxins have been implicated in abortions in other species of ruminants due to oestrogenic activity (see Chapter 21) and may affect goats.

Further reading

General

East, N. (1983) Pregnancy toxaemia, abortions and periparturient diseases. *Vet. Clin. North. Amer.: Large Anim. Pract.,* **5** (3), November, *Sheep and Goat Medicine,* 601–618.

Harwood, D.G. (1987) Abortion in the goat, an investigative approach. *Goat Vet. Soc. J.,* **8** (1), 25–28.

Hazlett, M.J. *et al.* (2013) A prospective study of sheep and goat abortion using real-time polymerase chain reaction and cut point estimation shows *Coxiella burnetii* and *Chlamydophila abortus* infection concurrently with other major pathogens. *J. Vet. Diag. Invest.,* **25** (3), 359–368.

Holler L.D. (2012) Ruminant abortion diagnostics. *Vet. Clin. North Amer.: Food Anim. Pract.,* **28** (3), 407–418.

Mears, R. (2007) Abortion in sheep. 1. Investigation and principal causes. *In Practice,* **29,** 40–46.

Mears, R. (2007) Abortion in sheep. 2. Other common and exotic causes. *In Practice,* **29,** 83–90.

Merrall, M. (1985) The aborting goat. In: *Proceedings of a Course in Goat Husbandry and Medicine,* November 1985, Vol. **106,** pp. 181–198, Massey University.

Menzies, P.I. (2011) Control of important causes of infectious abortion in sheep and goats. *Vet. Clin. North Amer.: Food Anim. Pract.,* **27** (1), 81–93.

Moeller, R.B. Jr, (2001) Causes of caprine abortion: diagnostic assessment of 211 cases (1991–1998). *J. Vet. Diagn. Invest.,* **13,** 265–270.

van Engelen, E., Luttikholt, S., Peperkamp, K., Vellema, P. and van den Brom, R. (2014) Small ruminant abortions in The Netherlands during lambing season 2012–2013. *Vet. Rec.,* **174** (20), 506.

Border disease

Krametter-Froetescher, R. *et al.* (2008) Descriptive study of pestivirus infection in an Austrian goat. *Vet. Rec.,* **163,** 193.

Li, W. *et al.* (2013) Detection of border disease virus in goat herds suffering diarrhea in eastern China. *Virology J.,* **10,** 1–7.

Lken, T. (2000) Border disease in goats. In: *Recent Advances in Goat Diseases* (ed. Tempesta, M.). International Veterinary Information Service, Ithaca, NY (www.ivis.org).

Rosamilia, A. *et al.* (2014) Detection of border disease virus (BDV) genotype 3 in Italian goat herds. *The Veterinary Journal,* **199** (3), 446.

Brucellosis

Brucellosis in Sheep and Goats (*Brucella melitensis*) (2001) Report of the Scientific Committee on Animal Health and Animal Welfare. Available at: ec.europa.eu/food/fs/sc/ scah/out59_en.pdf.

Blasco, J.M. and Molina-Flores, B. (2011) Control and eradication of *Brucella melitensis* infection in sheep and goats. *Vet. Clin. North Amer.: Food Anim. Pract.,* **27** (1), 95–104.

MacMillan, A.P. (1999) Brucellosis in goats. *Goat Vet. Soc. J.,* **18,** 38–40.

Poester, F.P., Samartino, L.E. and Santos, R.L. (2013) Pathogenesis and pathobiology of brucellosis in livestock. *Rev. Sci. Tech. Off. Int. Epiz.,* **32** (1), 105–115.

Campylobacter

Anderson, K.L., Hammond, M.M., Urbane, J.W., Khoades, U.K. and Bryner, J. H (1983) Isolation of *Campylobacter jejuni* from an aborted caprine fetus. *JAVMA,* **183,** 90–92.

Caprine herpes virus

Chénier, S. Montpetit, C. and Hélie, P. (2004) Caprine herpesvirus-1 abortion storm in a goat herd in Quebec. *Can. Vet. J.,* **45** (3), 241–243.

McCoy, M.H. *et al.* (2007) Serologic and reproductive findings after herpesvirus-1 storm in goats. *JAVMA,* **231,** 1236–1239.

Chlamydial abortion

Appleyard, W.T. (1986) Chlamydial abortion in goats. *Goat Vet. Soc. J.,* **7** (2), 45–47.

Nietfield, J.C. (2001) Chlamydial infections in small ruminants. *Vet. Clin. North Amer.: Food Anim. Pract.,* **17** (2), 301–314.

Rodolakis A. (2001) Caprine Chlamydiosis. In: Tempesta M. (Ed.), *Recent Advances in Goat Diseases* (ed. Tempesta, M.). International Veterinary Information Service, Ithaca NY (www.ivis.org).

Stuen, S. and Longbottom, D. (2011) Treatment and control of chlamydial and rickettsial infections in sheep and goats. *Vet. Clin. North Amer.: Food Anim. Pract.,* **27** (1), 193–202.

Neosporosis

Eleni, C. *et al.* (2004) Detection of *Neospora caninum* in an aborted goat foetus. *Vet. Parasitol.*, **123** (3–4), 271–274.

Plant poisoning

Panter, K.E., Welch, K.D., Gardner, D.R. and Green, B.T. (2013) Poisonous plants: effects on embryo and fetal development. *Birth Defects Research Part C: Embryo Today: Reviews*, **99**, 223–234.

Q-fever

Arricau Bouvery, N., Souriau, A., Lechopier, P. and Rodolakis, A. (2003) Experimental *Coxiella burnetti* infection in pregnant goats: excretion routes. *Vet. Res.*, **34**, 423–433.

Emery, M.P. *et al.* (2014) *Coxiella burnetti* serology assays in goat abortion storm. *J. Vet. Diag. Invest.*, **26** (1), 141–145.

Guatteo, R., Seegers, H., Taurel, A.E., Joly, A. and Beaudeau, E. (2011) Prevalence of *Coxiella burnetti* infection in domestic ruminants: a critical review. *Vet. Microbiol.*, **149**, 1–16.

Hatchette, T.F. (2001) Goat-associated Q fever: a new disease in Newfoundland. *Emerging Infectious Diseases*, **7**, 413–419.

Hogerwerf, L. *et al.* (2011) Reduction of *Coxiella burnetii* prevalence by vaccination of goats and sheep, The Netherlands. *Emerg. Infect. Dis.*, **17** (3), 379–388.

McCaughey, C. (2014) Q fever: a tough zoonosis. *Vet. Rec.*, **175** (1) 15–16.

Mearns, R. (2011) Q fever – a threat? *Goat Vet. Soc. J.*, **27**, 39–46.

Roest, H.I.J. *et al.* (2013) Q fever in pregnant goats: humoral and cellular immune responses. *Vet. Res.*, **44**, 67.

Stuen, S. and Longbottom, D. (2011) Treatment and control of chlamydial and rickettsial infections in sheep and goats. *Vet. Clin. North Amer.: Food Anim. Pract.*, **27** (1), 193–202.

Waldhalm, D.G., Stoenner, H.G., Simmons, E.E. and Thomas, A.L. (1978) Abortion associated with *Coxiella burnetii* infection in dairy goats. *JAVMA*, **173**, 1580–1581.

Tickborne fever

Silaghi, C., Scheuerle, M.C., Friche Passos, L.M., Thiel, C. and Pfiste, K. (2011) PCR detection of *Anaplasma phagocytophilum* in goat flocks in an area endemic for tick-borne fever in Switzerland. *Parasite*, **18** (1), 57–62.

Toxoplasmosis

Buxton, D. (1989) Toxoplasmosis in sheep and other farm animals. *In Practice*, **11**, 9–12.

Buxton, D. (1998) Protozoan infections (*Toxoplasma gondii, Neospora caninum* and *Sarcocystis* spp.) in sheep and goats. *Vet. Res.*, **29** (3–4), 289–310.

Dubey, J.P., Miller, S. and Desmonts, G. (1986) *Toxoplasma gondii* induced abortion in dairy goats. *JAVMA*, **188**, 159–162.

Herbert, I.V. (1986) Sarcocystosis and toxoplasmosis in goats. *Goat Vet. Soc. J.*, **7** (2), 25–31.

Yersinia pseudotuberculosis

Giannitti, F., Barr, B.C., Brito, B.P., Uzal, F.A., Villanueva, M. and Anderson, M. (2014) *Yersinia pseudotuberculosis* infections in goats and other animals diagnosed at the California Animal Health and Food Safety Laboratory System: 1990–2012. *J. Vet. Diagn. Invest.*, **26** (1), 88–95.

CHAPTER 3

Male infertility

Investigation of male infertility

The examination of bucks for breeding should be included as a routine part of herd health plans. The examination primarily involves a thorough clinical examination, together with the palpation and visual inspection of the external genitalia. In addition, assessment of semen may be necessary during infertility investigations, or to check vasectomized bucks after surgery. See Figure 3.1 for the causes of male infertility.

Initial assessment

The preliminary history should consider:
- Individual or flock/herd problem.
- Management practices – handmating/buck running with does.
- Feeding, including mineral supplementation.
- Workload of the bucks.
- Age of bucks.

If more than one buck is involved consider:
- Overuse of bucks, particularly if used out of season or on synchronised groups of does. One buck can mate with over 100 does over a season, but a ratio of one mature buck to about 70 does or two bucklings (two toothbucks) to 70 does is more satisfactory. A well-grown kid could serve up to 30 does in a season.
- Low sexual drive – if bucks are used out of season on light-treated or sponged does.
- Disease status – parasitism, footrot, etc.
- Nutritional status.
- Poor heat detection.

If there is a problem with an individual goat, the specific history should determine whether the problem is:
- Return to service of females.

- Failure to serve at all.
- Failure to serve properly.

Assessment of individual buck

General assessment
- Body condition – condition score
- Leg and feet
  - Arthritis
  - Weak pasterns
  - Poorly trimmed feet
  - Stance and gait
- Lymph nodes

Specific examination
Observe sexual activity using a doe in season as a teaser (prostaglandin treatment of doe during the breeding season can be used to induce oestrus at a time suitable for examination).
- Libido.
- Failure to mate.
- Examine and palpate the external genitalia:
  - Check the scrotum and contents.
  - Measure the scrotal circumference; unlike sheep, there are no clearly defined guidelines for scrotal circumference and testicular size in goats, but a mature dairy buck should have a scrotal circumference of > 36 cm. Scrotal circumference is directly correlated to body weight and testosterone concentration. It can vary with the seasons, usually at its largest during the autumn breeding season (September to November) and can decrease by 2 to 3 cm during the summer. The circumference should be measured at the greatest circumference of the scrotum.
  - The testes should move freely in the scrotum.
  - Note the size, shape, consistency and symmetry of the testes.

Diseases of the Goat, Fourth Edition. John Matthews.
© 2016 John Wiley & Sons, Ltd. Published 2016 by John Wiley & Sons, Ltd.

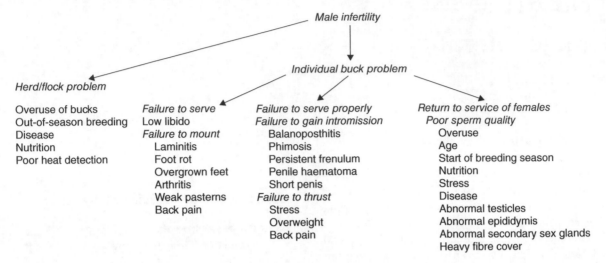

Figure 3.1 Causes of male infertility.

o Presence, size and normality of head and tail of the epididymis; measure the epididymal diameter.

o Spermatic cord.

o Prepuce and preputial orifice for evidence of trauma or infection.

o Check for the presence of the urethral process; absence does not affect fertility but its removal indicates a history of urolithiasis (Chapter 14). Extending the penis from the prepuce in an unsedated goat can be difficult; check when the goat is urinating or spraying or when collecting a semen sample.

■ *Ultrasonographic examination* of the testicles can demonstrate focal areas of increased echogenicity indicating mineralisation, evidence of testicular degeneration and information on palpable scrotal abnormalities. The normal testicle has a homogenous appearance with a central hyperechoic line (the mediastinum testis); hyperechoic areas can indicate fibrotic changes, while hypoechoic areas are fluid-filled cystic structures. Degenerate testicles have a heterogenous pattern and more hyperechoic areas. The epididymis and spermatic cord can be examined for fibrosis and cystic structures. The tail of the epididymis is normally more heterogenous and less echogenic than the testicle.

Breeding soundness examination

Bucks being assessed for breeding soundness should be examined as above to check their general health, as well as a specific examination of the external genitalia, together with semen collection and evaluation (see below). They should also be checked for other known genetic defects – hernias, supernumerary tests and jaw malformation.

Scrotum

Scrotal dermatitis, abscesses, fly strike and trauma can all lead to temporary or permanent testicular degeneration and reduced fertility.

Testes

The testes should be bilaterally symmetrical, large, oval and firm during the breeding season. The highest quality sperm is usually produced by the bucks with the largest testicles. Normal testicular tissue feels firm and resilient on palpation. Asymmetry suggests injury, disease or anatomical abnormality.

Cryptorchidism

Cryptorchidism may be unilateral or bilateral. Unilateral cryptorchids are generally fertile, but semen quality may be affected; bilateral cryptorchids are sterile. A genetically female intersex (Chapter 1) may be a cryptorchid. In Angora goats, cryptorchidism has been shown to be inherited as a recessive trait.

Enlarged testes

- An inguinal hernia causing distension of the scrotum may be confused with enlarged testicles.
- *Orchitis*, or inflammation of the testes, may be unilateral or bilateral, acute or chronic. In the acute condition, the testes will be swollen and painful and the buck will be pyrexic, lethargic and unwilling to move (Plate 3.1). In chronic orchitis, fibrous adhesions may limit movement within the scrotum and the testicles become atrophied and fibrous. Ultrasonographic examination of the scrotum using a 5 MHz linear scanner will aid differentiation between orchitis and epididymitis.
- *Neoplasia* is an uncommon cause of infertility in bucks, but seminomas, adenomas and carcinomas have been reported and should be detectable by ultrasonography.
- *Haematoma*, or intratesticular haemorrhage, may cause enlargement of a testis.

Small testes

- *Testicular hypoplasia*
  - Underdeveloped testes occur particularly in polled males as part of the intersex condition (qv). The condition is generally bilateral, occasionally unilateral.
  - Severe malnutrition will also produce small testes.
- *Testicular atrophy* occurs as a sequel to scrotal trauma, orchitis, sperm granuloma or systemic disease, if the goat is debilitated and as part of the ageing process in some bucks. With fibrosis the testicle feels very firm on palpation.
- *Testicular degeneration*, where the testes feel soft and doughy due to tubular degeneration.

Conditions of the spermatic cord

- *Varicocoele* presents as a hard swelling in the dorsal part of the pampiniform plexus; caused by dilation and thrombosis in the internal spermatic vein. The exact aetiology is unknown but may be hereditary. Diagnosis is by palpation and ultrasound. The condition can result in lameness and can be associated with poor quality sperm. There is no treatment and affected bucks should be culled.

Abnormal epididymis

- *Sperm granulomas* are palpable as hard knots at the head of the epididymis although the testes are normal in consistency. The condition occurs particularly in polled males as part of the intersex condition (Chapter 1), but can also arise from an infection causing epididymitis. If the condition is bilateral, the buck is sterile. Sperm granulomas result from the complete or partial blockage of one or more efferent ductules draining into the epididymis, so that the ductule becomes distended with inspissated sperm, eventually rupturing and releasing sperm into the stroma of the epididymis. The resulting inflammatory response results in granuloma formation and back pressure leads to testicular degeneration. The granulomas in the head of the epididymis and the reduced size of the testicle are both palpable.
- *Epididymitis* uncommonly occurs in goats as a result of infection with a variety of pathogens, or, following trauma, resulting in swelling of the epididymis with inflammation, hyperplasia and obstruction of the epididymal ducts (Plate 3.2).

Penis/prepuce

Balanoposthitis

- Inflammation of the penis and prepuce often leads to scar tissue and adhesions. The acute inflammation and the resulting fibrosis both cause infertility.
- *Caprine herpesvirus 1 (CpHV-1)* causes balanoposthitis in goats in New Zealand and Australia, with hyperaemia of the penis and ulceration of the prepuce.
- *Orf* (Chapter 9) occasionally infects the prepuce.
- Mycoplasmas and ureaplasms *may* be involved.

Persistent frenulum

The adhesions between the penis and prepuce, which are present in the prepubertal male kid, normally disappear by about 4 months of age, but occasionally persist.

Phimosis

Phimosis is seen as an inability to extrude the penis at service. It may result from trauma and balonoposthitis, but is occasionally congenital.

Paraphimosis

Paraphimosis is the inability to withdraw the penis into the prepuce, resulting in the penis becoming swollen and oedematous. It is associated with trauma, infection and balanoposthitis. If of recent occurrence, the penis can be replaced under sedation and maintained in place with a purse-string suture. Suitable antibiotic/corticosteroid ointment will sooth and lubricate the passage. The tension on the suture should allow free passage of urine. More chronic cases have a poorer prognosis if the penis is excessively traumatised.

Short penis

A short penis results in inability to protrude the penis beyond the prepuce. The condition is not treatable. Short penile length, *hypospadia* (opening of the urethral orifice on the ventral aspect of the penis) sperm granulomas and hypoplastic testicles can be associated with interex in goats.

Haematoma of the penis

Haematoma of the penis follows trauma, such as caused by headbutting.

Examination of semen

- Collection of semen:
  - Using an artificial vagina gives better quality semen than electroejaculation; if possible use a doe in oestrus as a teaser.
  - Electroejaculation should only be used on an anaesthetized animal.
  - The best semen samples are obtained during the breeding season.
  - Some idea of sperm motility can be gained from a vaginal semen sample examined on a warmed slide.
- Examination of semen: volume, motility, numbers, morphology, absence of inflammatory cells/debris, live:dead ratio (Table 3.1).

Table 3.1 Normal semen characteristics.

Semen	
o Volume (ml)	0.5–1.5
o Concentration (×106/ml)	1500–5000
o Total sperm (×106)	750–7500
o Good motility (%)	70–90 (distinct swirling wave motion)
o Normal morphology (%)	80–95
o Dead or abnormal sperm	<20%

o Volume. Read from the graduated collecting tube; a greater volume is normally obtained by electroejaculation than with the artificial vagina.

o Density. Visual appraisal of the ejaculate density gives an approximate estimate of concentration; accurate counts can be made with a haemocytometer (Table 3.2).

o Wave motion is a function of the concentration of sperm and their activity. It is affected by temperature, so it is important to avoid cold shock, particularly under field conditions (examine a drop of semen at 100× magnification) (Table 3.3).

o Motility is defined as the percentage of sperm moving forward (examine a drop of semen under a cover slip at 400× magnification).

o Add 1 drop of semen to 3–5 drops of fresh nigrosin/eosin stain, make a smear and examine under an oil immersion lens. Allows assessment of sperm density, the live:dead ratio (live sperm are colourless as they repel stain) and the normal:abnormal ratio. A high percentage of morphological abnormalities is associated with either sexual immaturity or degenerative changes.

o Make a stained smear with Leishmann's or 'Diff-Quick'. Check for the presence of neutrophils. Their presence indicates infection.

Table 3.2 Visual appraisal of semen density.

Appearance	Sperm density	Comment
Very thick creamy	>4 000 000 sperm/mm^3	Probably fertile
Thick creamy	4 000 000 sperm/mm^3	Probably fertile
Creamy	3 000 000 sperm/mm^3	Probably fertile
Thin creamy	2 500 000 sperm/mm^3	Probably fertile
Thick milky	2 000 000 sperm/mm^3	Probably fertile
Milky	1 000 000 sperm/mm^3	Low fertility
Cloudy	<100 000 sperm/mm^3	Probably infertile
Watery	<50 000 sperm/mm^3	Probably infertile

Table 3.3 Semen motility.

Motility	Comment
None	Sperm dead, infertile
Slow wave motion	<50% active, low fertility
Distinct waves with motion	70–80% active, probably fertile
Dark waves with motion	>89% active, fertile

Individual buck problems

Failure to serve at all
Low libido

- Season. The normal breeding season in the northern hemisphere is September to March, but many bucks are now expected to work out of season following light or sponge treatment of does. If possible, bucks should be stimulated, for example, by light, at the same time as the does. Most bucks will mate at any time of the year, but some reduction in libido must be expected out of season.
- Poor condition. Intercurrent disease such as parasitism, energy or protein deficit.
- Hereditary. Sexual drive is hereditable.
- Presence of other males. Competition may increase libido or a dominant male may suppress libido in subordinates.

Note: many (particularly older) bucks will only serve a female that is definitely in season. Some bucks will only serve each female once within a short period of time, rather than twice as expected by dairy goatkeepers.

Failure to mount

- Skeletal or muscular lesions:
  - foot problems: laminitis, footrot, overgrown feet
  - arthritis
  - weak pasterns
  - back pain.

Failure to serve properly
Failure to gain intromission

- Conditions of prepuce: phimosis due to trauma or infection, persistent frenulum (rare), adhesions/scarring.

Note: a very young male kid (<4 months) may have difficulty protruding the penis because of the normal adhesions between penis and prepuce.

- Conditions of penis: adhesions/scarring, haematoma, short penis.

Failure to thrust

- Stress:
  - too many people 'assisting'
  - tiredness
  - strange surroundings.
- Overweight.
- Back pain.

Return to service

Return to service is generally caused by poor sperm quality.

- Overuse, particularly out of season and if large numbers of does are synchronised; reduced sperm density may take 6 weeks or more to recover.
- Age. Old or young animals may have reduced sperm density and/or poor quality semen.
- Start of the breeding season. Maximum sperm production occurs several weeks after the onset of the breeding season.
- Nutrition. Young males are particularly sensitive to poor nutrition including protein and energy deficits and vitamin deficiency (particularly vitamin A). The role of trace elements is not well documented, but copper, manganese, cobalt, zinc and phosphorus deficiencies may affect sperm production.
- Stress.
- Intercurrent disease. Pyrexia will reduce sperm density through damage to the epididymis and testes, causing permanent damage in some cases and a minimum of 6 weeks to recover. The spermatogenic cycle is about 22 days in the goat and normal fertility is not restored until a full spermatogenic cycle is completed.
- Abnormal testicles.
- Abnormal epididymis.
- Abnormal accessory sex glands, for example seminal vesiculitis results in ejaculates containing large numbers of white cells with no palpable orchitis or epididymitis.
- Heavy fibre cover. An unshorn Angora with heavy fleece may have reduced fertility due to an increase in scrotal temperature and the effect on spermatogenesis. Even after shearing, 6 to 8 weeks will be required before return to full fertility.
- *Gynaecomastia* (see Chapter 13). Although the fertility of males with gynaecomastia is not normally affected, a large 'udder' adjacent to the testicles can increase scrotal temperature and reduce fertility. A mastectomy can be considered in these animals.

Further reading

General

Greig, A. (1987) Infertility in the male goat. *Goat Vet. Soc. J.*, **8** (1), 1–3.

Merman, M.A. (1983) Male Infertility. *Vet. Clin. North Amer.: Large Anim. Pract.*, **5** (3), 619–635.

Gynaecomastia

Janett, F., Stckli, A. Thun, R. and Nett, P. (1996) Gynecomastia in a goat buck. *Schweiz. Arch. Tierheilkd*, **138** (5), 241–244.

Jaszczak, K. *et al.* (2010) Cytogenetic, histological, hormonal and semen studies in male goats with developed udders. *Animal Science Papers and Reports, Institute of Genetics and Animal Breeding, Jastrzębiec, Poland*, **28** (1), 71–80.

Wooldridge, A.A. *et al.* (1999) Gynecomastia and mammary gland adenocarcinoma in a Nubian buck. *Can. Vet. J.*, **40** (9), 663–665.

Semen quality and examination

Ahmad, N. and Noakes, D.E. (1996) Seasonal variation in the semen quality of young British goats. *Br. Vet. J.*, **152**, 225–236.

Evans, G. and Maxwell, W.M.C. (1987) *Salamon's Artificial Insemination of Sheep and Goats*. Butterworths, London.

Ultrasonography

Ahmad, N., Noakes, D.E. and Subandrio (1991) B-mode real time ultrasonographic imaging of the testis and epididymis of sheep and goats. *Vet. Rec.*, **128**, 491–496.

Ahmad, N., Noakes, D.E. and Middleton D.J. (1993) Use of ultrasound to diagnose testicular degeneration in a goat. *Vet. Rec.*, **132**, 436–439.

DesCôteaux, L. (ed.) (2010) *Practical Atlas of Ruminant and Camelid Reproductive Ultrasonography*, pp. 181–199. Wiley-Blackwell, Iowa.

CHAPTER 4

The periparturient goat

Management of the doe during pregnancy, and between kidding and peak lactation, is essential for the health of the animal and the economic success of the goat farmer. This is the critical period in the goat cycle and the period when most problems occur. Goats should remain fit but not fat – a body condition score of 3 is ideal. Body condition at kidding plays a pivotal role in determining subsequent health, production and reproductive performance. Both overfeeding and underfeeding in late pregnancy increase the risk of metabolic disorders. In the United Kingdom over-fat does and multiple foetuses rather than underfeeding cause most periparturient problems (Table 4.1). In extensively kept animals, kidding in the Spring, cold weather can result in poor pasture growth, poor body condition in late pregnancy and an energy/protein deficit leading to starvation and pregnancy toxaemia. Similarly, in animals with an extended breeding cycle, with breeding twice a year, kidding may coincide with periods of poor feed availability.

The gestation period for the goat is approximately 150 days, but 80% of fetal growth occurs during the last 6 weeks of pregnancy, so additional nutrients are not required until this time. During the third trimester of pregnancy, the nutritional requirements of the doe for crude protein and energy increase above those required by a non-productive adult by about one and half times for does carrying a single kid and two times for those carrying twins. Breeds like the Anglo-Nubian, which often produce three or more kids, face a greater challenge than breeds where singles or twins are the norm. In addition, many animals will still be growing and/or lactating. The requirement for calcium and phosphorus is similarly increased. At this time of increasing nutritional demand, dry matter consumption is depressed because the growing kids restrict abdominal space and rumen fill. Abdominal volume is further reduced in

Table 4.1 Problems with over and under feeding.

Obese goats	Thin goats
Depressed appetite	Pregnancy toxaemia
Pregnancy toxaemia	Abortion
Vaginal prolapse?	
Rectal prolapse	
Ruptured uterine artery	
Maternal dystocia from reduced pelvic size	Kids with reduced birthweight
Fetal dystocia from oversized kids	
Inappetance/anorexia	Lower milk yield
Post-parturient toxaemia	Ketosis/acetonaemia
(fatty liver syndrome/ketosis)	Kids with reduced weight gains

goats carrying large amounts of abdominal fat. A similar, or even greater, increase in nutritional requirement occurs during the transition from late gestation into lactation. A goat at peak lactation can produce its own weight of milk in 10 days.

The dry period

As with cows, a 6 to 8 week dry period is generally recommended before parturition, although some research work indicates that this is not necessary. However, short dry periods may have a negative impact on the quantity and quality of colostrum produced as well as affecting the subsequent lactation. Milking should be stopped abruptly – stopping production of prolactin and reducing milk secretion. In high yielders the udder may become quite large until the pressure stops milk production, but within a few days the udder

Diseases of the Goat, Fourth Edition. John Matthews.
© 2016 John Wiley & Sons, Ltd. Published 2016 by John Wiley & Sons, Ltd.

will shrink and become softer. Pressure of milk causes an inflammatory response so leucocytes collect in the udder helping to prevent infection. Milking once daily for a week before drying off may help reduce milk production in very high yielders. Udders should *never* be partially milked out as this increases the susceptibility to infection. Teat dipping for a week after stopping milking will help prevent infection during drying off. Routine use of dry goat therapy is not recommended unless there is a history of mastitis during the previous lactation. There are no intramammary preparations licensed for goats in the United Kingdom, so dry cow products must be used in accordance with the cascade. Drug withholding times for intramammary preparations may be much longer than in the cow and drug residues may persist for some time into the next lactation.

Management during late pregnancy

Voluntary food intake can be reduced at this time by stress (changes in groupings, transportation, yarding, shearing, absence of the owner, weather), so it is important to provide the goats with a stable, calm environment, maintaining fixed groups to avoid stress on the less dominant animals. Concomitant disease (lameness, poor dentition, gastrointestinal parasites) and nutritional deficiency (vitamin B12/cobalt) will also reduce appetite. Table 4.2 shows the routine husbandry tasks that need undertaking in the dry period.

Anthelmintic treatment during the dry period reduces the parasite burden on the dam and reduces the potential exposure for the kids. Animals should be checked for external parasites and treated accordingly; lice are a common problem in winter and can cause anaemia in kids; chorioptic mange is common in housed goats.

Where appropriate, specific trace element deficiencies, such as selenium, should be addressed at this time (see Chapter 8).

A booster vaccination against Clostridial disease (tetanus and enterotoxaemia) should be given to the does 4 to 6 weeks before kidding to ensure maximum transfer of immunity to the kids and the does should be moved to the kidding area at least 2 weeks before the kidding date.

Kidding areas should be cleaned and rested between kiddings, which will help reduce the incidence of mastitis, metritis and kid septicaemia. Maternity areas should be clean, well ventilated, well bedded, quiet and provide secure footing. Animals should be encouraged to exercise. Routine foot trimming at this time is less stressful than after parturition and promotes increased mobility.

Feeding during late gestation

Both underfeeding and overfeeding in late pregnancy increase the risk of metabolic and other problems (Table 4.3). The doe needs to be on a relatively low plane

Table 4.2 Routine husbandry tasks before kidding.

Maintain fixed groupings	Avoids undue stress on less dominant goats
Move to the kidding area at least 2 weeks before the kidding date	Maternity areas should be clean, well ventilated, well bedded, quiet and provide secure footing
Kidding area should be cleaned and rested between kiddings	Reduces the incidence of mastitis, metritis and kid septicaemia
Clostridial vaccination: tetanus + enterotoxaemia	4 to 6 weeks before kidding to ensure maximum transfer of immunity to kids
Hoof trim	Promotes increased mobility
	Less stressful than after kidding
Anthelmintic treatment	Avoids need to throw milk away
	Reduces burden on dam
	Reduces exposure for kids
Check for external parasites: lice + chorioptic mange	Lice are a common problem in winter and can cause anaemia in kids
	Chorioptic mange is common in housed goats in winter

Table 4.3 Feeding in late pregnancy.

Aim	To avoid over fat or over thin does
	To maintain body condition score 3
Forage	Feed high quality forage *ad libitum*
	Hay intake will be approximately 1.5 to 2.5 kg/100 kg body weight
	Offer fresh forage several times daily
	Allow for 20+ % wastage to encourage maximum intake
	Dry matter intake can be increased by offering green forage
	Woody browse will help maintain rumen function
Concentrate	Increase concentrate part of ration gradually over the 8 weeks before kidding
	Introduce the lactation ration before kidding to avoid feed refusal and to allow rumen bacteria to adapt
	High energy diets enable requirements to be met with a lower dry matter intake
Mineral and vitamins	Ensure the concentrate ration is correctly supplemented with minerals and vitamins
	Home mixed rations may need a suitable supplement
	Check calcium/phosphorus balance if large amounts of brassicas or sugar beet pulp are being fed.
	70 kg doe requires 6.0 g calcium and 4.2 g phosphorus/day
	Excess calcium intake increases the risk of milk fever
	Offer suitable mineral lick

the rumen papillae to increase their surface area in response to the increased absorption of volatile fatty acids, a process that takes around 14 days. This helps to minimise the move towards negative energy and protein balances, reduces the potential for rumen acidosis and avoids food refusal associated with a sudden diet change. If fetal numbers have been determined by ultrasound scanning, the goats can be grouped and fed according to the litter size. Angora goats have higher protein and energy requirements than dairy goats at the same stage of pregnancy and lactation, so the dry and transition periods can be critical. For extensively kept goats, kidding should be planned for a time when pasture is rapidly growing and is high in protein and energy.

High forage intake during late pregnancy appears to stimulate high forage intake during lactation, whereas overfeeding concentrates in late pregnancy confers little benefit and may even be detrimental to future milk yield. Offering goats a choice of forage at this time, coupled with clearing and refreshing racks and troughs regularly, will promote an increase in roughage intake. Where animals are fed a total mixed ration in a passageway, intake will be increased by regularly pushing the feed up to the goats, as they will be encouraged to investigate and eat.

Feeding in early lactation

On a body weight for weight basis, goats are much heavier producers than cows. All heavily lactating goats, particularly young first kidders, will lose weight despite the availability of an adequate diet. Goats lose about 1 kg adipose tissue/week for the first month post-partum and 0.5 kg/week for a further month. Peak milk yield (about 4 to 8 weeks post-parturition in most breeds) occurs before peak appetite (about 10 weeks post-kidding). A positive energy balance is not reached until 6 to 8 weeks after kidding. From about the fourth month of lactation dairy goats begin to regain live weight. These changes are not mirrored by changes in condition score as goats carry little subcutaneous fat. High yielding does require roughage and concentrates of good quality as the demand for energy and protein is high. Despite the increased demand for nutrients, the dry matter intake is likely to be limited and similar to late pregnancy, particularly during the first two to three

of nutrition 6–8 weeks before kidding to encourage udder involution at drying-off, then an increasing plane of nutrition from about 5 weeks pre-partum. The amount of non-digestible fibre (NDF) in the diet is the major limiting factor determining nutrient intake in the doe at this time; the NDF intake capacity for late pregnant ruminants is around 0.8% of body weight. It is essential to supply good quality roughage *ad libitum* during this time to maximise dry matter intake and the rumen residence time, whilst at the same time increasing the amount of concentrates fed to about 0.5 to 1.0 kg/day by parturition. The lactation ration should be introduced before kidding to eliminate checks through diet change around kidding (Table 4.3). A gradual increase in the amount of concentrates fed allows time for the rumen microorganisms to acclimatise, so optimum fermentation is achieved, and for

Table 4.4 Feeding in early lactation.

Aim	To obtain a high nutrient intake to minimise loss of body weight and promote a high milk yield
	To formulate the ration to supply adequate nutrients to enable the genetic potential of the goat to be expressed
	To avoid metabolic problems like laminitis and ruminal acidosis
Forage	Feed high quality forage *ad libitum*
	Offer fresh forage several times daily
	Allow for 20+% wastage to encourage maximum intake
	Maintain 50% forage in total diet dry matter
Concentrate	Increase level gradually by about 0.1 kg/day during the first weeks of lactation
	0.5 kg concentrate (16–18% CP) for each litre of milk produced
	High energy, high protein (18–22% CP) in heavy milkers
	Split concentrate feed into 3 or 4 feeds a day if possible
	Avoid giving > 0.5 kg at a single feed to prevent rumen acidosis and maintain a stable population of rumen microorganisms
Minerals and vitamins	As for late pregnancy

weeks. Ideally, long roughage should still comprise 50% of the total dry matter intake (Table 4.4). Voluntary feed intake increases steadily after parturition and usually reaches a peak during the third month of lactation, but this varies considerably. Milk yield is highly correlated with ME intake, with the correlation increasing as the lactation progresses. Intake is maximised by ensuring good quality feed is available at all times; where animals are fed a total mixed ration, selective feeding will result in better quality components being eaten first, leaving poorer components such as maize stalks until last. 'Pushing out' from the feed-passage face and removing the last 4–7% of the ration fed will ensure a more balanced intake.

Most experimental nutrition trials have been carried out on relatively low yielding animals of relatively small stature and information is sparse on larger, high yielding goats.

Periparturient toxaemia

> In the United Kingdom, overfat does and multiple fetuses rather than underfeeding cause most periparturient toxaemias.

Periparturient toxaemia (*pregnancy toxaemia, post-parturient toxaemia*) (Table 4.5) occurs in response to insufficient intake of energy to meet the increasing demands of pregnancy or lactation. Suboptimum food intake, for whatever reason, is the main predisposing factor.

Pregnancy toxaemia occurs in the last 4 to 6 weeks of pregnancy when energy intake is insufficient to meet the increasing demand. Compression of the rumen by the fetuses decreases voluntary food intake and the change in physiological state prior to kidding further depresses appetite. In extensively kept goats, undernutrition through inadequate food supply, poorly balanced rations or heavy worm burdens is a major contributing factor but, in the United Kingdom, many dairy goats that develop pregnancy toxaemia have been overweight. Intra-abdominal fat deposits reduce the rumen capacity and thus food intake. During periods of negative energy balance (pre- and post-kidding) excessive quantities of fat are mobilised from body depots. Non-esterified fatty acids (NFAs) are released to provide a source of energy and are oxidized for fuel and converted to ketone compounds. When NFAs are present in large amounts, some are converted back into triglycerides and stored as fat droplets in hepatocytes. Fatty infiltration of the liver results in hepatic dysfunction, reducing gluconeogenesis, resulting in a further breakdown of adipose tissue.

In early lactation, most does suffer a mild ketonaemia as the energy demands of lactation are not met adequately by the diet. In most animals, an equilibrium is established and the ketosis remains subclinical, but a more severe energy deficit through inadequate food supply, poorly balanced rations or heavy worm burden may lead to an acute clinical *ketosis* or *acetonaemia*.

About 2 to 4 weeks after kidding, goats that have large fat deposits at kidding may develop a *post-parturient toxaemia* similar to pregnancy toxaemia or *fatty liver disease* of cows.

Although goats can use products from rumen fermentation, such as volatile fatty acids, for most of their

Table 4.5 Periparturient toxicosis.

	Pregnancy toxaemia	Pregnancy toxaemia	Post-parturient toxaemia Fatty liver syndrome
When	Last 4–6 weeks of pregnancy	Last 4–6 weeks of pregnancy	2 to 4 weeks post-partum
Which animals	Fat goat	Thin goat	Fat goat
Predisposing factors	Pet goats in small pens	Angora, cashmere	High milk production
	Overconditioned show goats	Extensively grazed	Overconditioned show goats
	Goats on maize silage	Multiple foetuses	Goats on maize silage
	Multiple fetuses	Stress – fear, weather, housing, shearing	
	Lack of exercise		
Aetiology	Decrease in voluntary food intake	Starvation	Decrease in voluntary food intake
	Rapid mobilisation of fat reserves and subsequent hepatic lipidosis		Rapid mobilisation of fat reserves and subsequent hepatic lipidosis
Biochemical findings	Metabolic acidosis	Metabolic acidosis	Metabolic acidosis
	Hypoglycaemia	Hypoglycaemia	Hypoglycaemia
	Ketonaemia	Ketonaemia	Ketonaemia
	Hyperglycaemia terminally with dead fetuses		

energy requirements, the nervous system, kidneys, mammary gland and fetus have a direct requirement for glucose. Glucose requirement peaks during late pregnancy and early lactation. If a glucose deficiency occurs, excessive fat breakdown begins in an attempt to maintain blood glucose levels, resulting in abnormally high levels of ketones and fatty degeneration of the liver, with depression of all liver functions.

Laboratory tests

- Ketostix, Multistix, Acetest tablets or Rothera's reagent can be used to detect ketones in urine or milk.
- The urine ketone tests are semiquantitative tests based on the degree of colour change that occurs when sodium nitroprusside reacts with acetoacetate and, to a lesser degree, acetone. The sensitivity and specificity with the urine strip Ketostix (Bayer) have been shown to be 90 and 86%, respectively, at the trace level (approximately 490 µmol/litre of acetoacetate), making this the best test for urine. β-Hydroxybutyrate (BHB) does not react at all with nitroprusside. The Precision Xtra (Abbott) monitoring system uses an enzyme that detects only BHB, the most common ketone body in blood.
- Most milk ketone tests also utilise the sodium nitroprusside reaction with acetoacetate. In general, these tests have poor sensitivity (40% and many false negatives) and good specificity (100% with few false positives). The Keto-Test (Elanco) is a milk-dip test strip that changes colour in the presence of abnormally high concentrations of circulating BHB. It has been shown to have greater sensitivity and specificity compared to other milk tests.

- A blood sample can be submitted for an energy profile – glucose, BHB, non-esterified fatty acids, ketones.
- Plasma glucose concentrations are too variable on their own to confirm the diagnosis. Hypoglycemia is not a consistent finding as marked hyperglycaemia occurs terminally in goats with pregnancy toxaemia. It is postulated that fetal death removes the suppressing effect of the fetus on hepatic gluconeogenesis. CSF glucose levels may be more accurate than blood; they remain low even when serum glucose rebounds in advanced cases after fetal death.
- Non-esterified fatty acid concentrations are also variable, but can be elevated above 0.4 mmol/litre, indicating likely hepatic lipidosis resulting in impaired hepatic function. Changes in liver enzyme levels are not generally useful for diagnosis.
- Determination of levels of BHB in blood is considered the 'gold standard' for monitoring and identifying subclinical ketosis pre-kidding. BHB is a more reliable indicator of disease severity than blood glucose levels. Products targeted at diabetics, such as the Abbott

Precision Xtra or the Nova Max, can be used to take a blood sample and measure the ketone levels directly. The Precision Xtra has been validated for use in goats.

BHB levels: normal <0.8 mmol/litre, subclinical ketosis >0.8 mmol/litre, clinical disease >3.0 mmol/litre (commonly > 5.0 mmol/litre)

■ A sample of late-gestation does can be tested for BHB levels to determine the extent of the risk in the rest of the herd/flock. Generally, 10–20 does should be sampled (3–20% of the pregnant herd). The mean value of the results obtained gives an indication of the risk: low risk 0–0.7; moderate underfeeding 0.8–1.6; and severe underfeeding (high risk) 1.7–3.0 mmol/litre.

Pregnancy toxaemia
Clinical signs
■ Initially inappetence (eats browsings/hay, refuses concentrates); later complete anorexia.
■ Lethargic, unwilling to move; walks with difficulty.
■ Lower limbs may swell, the feet look larger than normal and the hair appears to stand on end perpendicular to the coronary band.
■ Weight loss.
■ Occasionally nervous signs – tremor around the head and ears, reduced vision or blindness, head pressing, stargazing, eventually recumbency, coma with or without abortion, death.

Treatment

> Termination of pregnancy is generally the only successful treatment for pregnancy toxaemia.

Drug doses are given in Table 4.6. Drugs licensed for use in farm animals in the United Kingdom should be used in accordance with the Cascade.

In the absence of abortion or parturition, treatment for pregnancy toxaemia is generally unsatisfactory, particularly when fat animals are involved. Pregnancy can be terminated by inducing parturition, by removing the kids by caesarian section, or by rapid removal of the kids by non-sterile caesarian section under local anaesthesia, followed by euthanasia of the doe. Using dexamethasone, rather than prostaglandins, to induce parturition

may be beneficial in improving the survival rate of the kids, as well as having a gluconeogenic effect in the dam, but is slower. A compromise is to give the corticosteroid injection, followed by a prostaglandin injection 24 hours later.

The owner and veterinary surgeon are often faced with a dilemma – terminate pregnancy early to save the dam or wait until the kids are nearer to full-term to try to get live kids. Delay, of course, carries the risk of losing both dam and kids. If there is doubt concerning the viability of fetuses, fetal movement can be demonstrated during the last month of gestation by ultrasonography, although near-to-term fetal heartbeats can be more difficult to detect. There is evidence that hypoglycaemia might indicate that the fetuses are alive and hyperglycaemia that the fetuses are dead.

■ *Encourage the goat to continue eating* (anything!). Usually the best response is to browsings and green food (e.g. ivy in winter). Goats that continue to eat may survive; totally anorexic animals will die.
■ *Stimulate appetite* with products such as B vitamins, rumen stimulants and proprietary twin-lamb disease remedies.
■ Provide *glucogenic agents*:
  ○ 20% Glucose solution, 200 ml, part i.v. or i.p., the rest s.c.
  ○ Glycerine (glycerol), 60 ml in warm water orally, twice daily for 4 to 5 days.
  ○ Ketocol (Leeders) is a commercial preparation of glycerol, which is more palatable than propylene glycol, 50 ml in 500 ml of warm water or by drench twice daily, given as a bolus rather than sprayed on feed.
  ○ Propylene glycol, 200 ml orally twice daily for 4 to 5 days.
■ *Stimulate gluconeogenesis*:
  ○ Dexamethasone, 25 mg, 12.5 ml i.m. (will produce abortion in late pregnancy).
  ○ Dexamethasone, 25 mg + protamine zinc insulin, up to 40 U, s.c., twice daily. Insulin has an antipolytic effect as well as affecting peripheral glucose utilisation, but is not licensed for farm animals in the United Kingdom.
  ○ Anabolic steroids (where allowed by regulatory bodies).
■ *Flunixin meglumine.* Adding flunixin (2.5 mg/kg, i.m. SID) to the standard protocol for the treatment of pregnancy toxaemia may improve feed intake and

Table 4.6 Drugs used in the periparturient goat.

Drug	Dose	Comments
Calcium borogluconate 20%	80–100 ml i.v. (give s.c. in stressed animal)	Calcium should not be added to fluids with
Calcium borogluconate 20%	25 ml/litre of intravenous fluids	sodium bicarbonate in them
Glucogenic agents		
20% Glucose solution	200 ml, part i.v. or i.p., the rest s.c.	More palatable than Ketol
Glycerine (glycerol)	60 ml in warm water orally, twice daily for 4 to 5 days	Give as bolus rather than added to ration
Ketocol	50 ml in 500 ml warm water or by drench twice daily	
Propylene glycol (Ketol)	200 ml orally twice daily for 4 to 5 days	
Gluconeogenesis		
Dexamethasone, 25 mg	12.5 ml i.m.	Will cause abortion in about 48 hours
Dexamethasone, 25 mg + protamine	12.5 ml i.m.	Insulin is not licensed for use in farm
zinc insulin	Up to 40 U, s.c., twice daily	animals in the UK
Prostaglandins		
Dinaprost	5–10 mg i.m. or s.c.	Will induce parturition in about 36 hours
Clorprostenol	62.5–125 µg i.m. or s.c.	
Oxytocin	5–10 U i.m. or s.c.	
NSAIDs		
Meloxicam	2 mg/kg loading dose then	Every 36 hours
	0.5 mg/kg s.c. or i.v.	
Flunixin	2.2 mg/kg i.v. daily	For 5 days maximum
Carprofen	1.4 mg/kg s.c. or i.v.	Repeat once after 48–72 hours
Ketoprofen	3 mg/kg i.m. or i.v.	Daily for 3–5 days
Tolfenamic acid	2–4 mg/kg s.c. or i.v.	Repeat once after 48 hours
Analgesics		
Pethidine	10 mg/kg i.m. or s.c.	
Butorphanol	0.3–0.5 mg/kg i.v., i.m. or s.c.	
Buprenorphine	0.01 mg/kg i.m. or s.c.	
All drugs should be used in accordance with the Cascade or local regulations		

the success rate for the delivery of live kids and the survival of the dam. The mechanism of action is unknown.

- *Fluid therapy*. In more severe cases, aggressive fluid therapy, including dextrose and bicarbonate for ketoacidosis, is necessary. Potential metabolic complications include persistent hyperglycemia, hypokalemia, dehydration or overhydration/hypervolemia. Solutions with dextrose should be administered judiciously to avoid inducing glucose diuresis.

Any fluid deficits from *dehydration* should be corrected first, using a balanced isotonic electrolyte solution. The fluid deficit can be calculated using the formula:

Body weight (kg) × % dehydration = fluid deficit
in litres

The percentage of dehydration can be calculated from Table 4.7.

- *Energy requirements*. The negative energy balance can be corrected by adding dextrose and amino acids to the isotonic electrolyte solution:

5 litres of balanced isotonic fluid + 500 ml 50% dextrose + 1 litre 8.5% amino acids

Administer at maintenance fluid rate – weight of fluid = 5% of body weight (1 kg = 1 litre), that is about 50 ml/kg/day or 2.5 litres/day for a 50 kg animal. Monitor:

o Blood and/or urine glucose

o The level of hydration, PCV and total protein to avoid fluid overload.

Table 4.7 Fluid loss and associated clinical signs.

Percentage fluid loss based on body weight	Clinical signs
0–5	Mild, barely detectable, increased thirst Capillary refill ˜ 2 seconds
5–10	Moderate, mouth dry, skin remains erect when pinched, tacky mucous membranes Capillary refill 3–4 seconds
10	Severe, body cold, eyes shrunken, comatose Capillary refill > 4 seconds

Then 20 mmol of potassium can be added per litre of fluid to help prevent hypokalemia, given at a maximum infusion rate of 0.5 mmol/kg/hour.

- *Ketoacidosis*. Goats with pregnancy toxemia, especially those showing neurologic signs, should be suspected of having ketoacidosis. The acidosis should be corrected using sodium bicarbonate according to the formula:

  Body weight (kg) × base deficit × 0.3 = mmol bicarbonate needed

  where 0.3 is the extracellular fluid volume (ECFV) for an adult goat. Then 1 ml of 1.26% sodium bicarbonate solution = 0.15 mmol of bicarbonate and can be administered at a rapid rate without problems. If the serum bicarbonate level is not known, the correction must be empirical. In severe acidosis, a base deficit of 10 nmol/l can be safely assumed.

- *Hypocalcemia* (see later in this chapter) may coexist in goats with pregnancy toxemia. Calcium can be supplemented at 25 ml of calcium borogluconate per litre of fluids or alternatively 80–100 ml of calcium borogluconate 20%, with magnesium hypophosphate 5% and dextrose 20%, can be given i.v. Calcium should not be added to fluids with sodium bicarbonate in them. Fruit-flavoured antacid tablets provide a ready, palatable source of oral calcium carbonate, which can be used to increase the calcium intake of less severely affected does. The suggested dose is 1 g/50 kg body weight every 12 hours, that is 2 tablets of a standard tablet containing 500 g.

- **Mild acidosis** can be treated by dosing with sodium bicarbonate (500 ml of a 5% solution). Small doses of sodium bicarbonate (100 to 150 ml) will stimulate the oesophageal groove to close, aiding the oral administration of other fluids.

Post-mortem findings

- Emaciated carcase or large amounts of abdominal fat.
- Yellow-orange enlarged liver, which is greasy and friable.
- Adrenal glands may be enlarged.
- Aqueous humour: 3-OH butyrate concentration > 2.5 mmol/l
  CSF: 3-OH butyrate concentration >0.6 mmol/l

Prevention

- Sensible nutrition throughout pregnancy – good quality roughage with concentrate feeding increasing during the last trimester. If fetal numbers have been determined by ultrasound scanning, the goats can be grouped and fed according to the litter size.
- Avoid overfat and overthin does.
- Maintain fixed groupings during the last trimester to avoid undue stress on less dominant goats.
- Encourage exercise on a daily basis.
- Rumen protected choline added to rations during the transition period appears beneficial in preventing and treating fatty liver in dairy cows and proprietary mixtures of B-group vitamins and methyl group donors (rumen protected choline, niacin, vitamin B12, biotin, folic acid and thiamine) are fed to cattle to support liver function, reducing the accumulation of triacylglycerides and clearing mobilised fat. These may also have a role to play in the dairy goat and there is some experimental support for the ability of rumen protected chlorine to reduce plasma β-hydroxybutyrate levels and hepatocellular lipid accumulation in the periparturient period and in increasing milk production, fat percentage and fat and protein yield, but further work is required. Feeding niacin (vitamin B3, nicotinic acid), 6 g daily for the last 60 days of gestation, has been recommended to reduce the risk of pregnancy toxaemia and lactational ketosis by reducing fatty acid mobilisation.
- Monensin sodium is licensed for dairy cows in the United States and is fed to increase the amount of propionate available for gluconeogenesis by influencing the ratio of volatile fatty acids, but could not be fed in the United Kingdom as it is classed as a growth promotor.

Post-parturient toxaemia (fatty liver syndrome)

Clinical signs

- Initially inappetence (eats browsings/hay, refuses concentrates); later complete anorexia.
- Milk yield initially depressed and then drops markedly.
- Lethargic.
- Chronic weight loss over several weeks.
- Eventually recumbency, coma and death. Most goatkeepers will request euthanasia before this stage is reached.

Treatment

- As for pregnancy toxaemia.
- Other supportive therapy:
  - Multivitamins, particularly A/D.
  - Vitamin E/selenium preparations may help hepatic metabolism in post-parturient toxaemia.
  - Restoration of normal rumen microflora. Use natural yoghurt or probiotics or drench rumen contents from a healthy animal.
- Diazepam, 0.05 mg/kg, 0.01 ml/kg i.v., will stimulate feeding for about 30 minutes.

Post-mortem findings

- As for pregnancy toxaemia.

Lactational ketosis (acetonaemia)

On a body weight for weight basis, goats are much heavier producers than cows. All heavily lactating goats, particularly young first kidders, will lose weight despite the availability of an adequate diet, around 150 g/day for the first month and 70 g/day for the second month. These changes are not mirrored by changes in the condition score as goats carry little subcutaneous fat. From the fourth month onwards multiparous goats put on about 40 g/day and primaparous goats 80 g/day.

In early lactation, when the demands of the lactation for energy are not met adequately by the food intake, does suffer a mild ketonaemia and do not achieve a positive energy balance until 6 to 8 weeks after kidding. In most animals an equilibrium is established and the ketosis remains subclinical, but intermittent periods of indigestion may occur, particularly if high levels of concentrate feeding lead to increased rumen acidity and decreased rumen motility, and milk production and activity may be irregular. Towards the time of peak lactation, goats may develop an acute clinical ketosis or acetonaemia. In the absence of frank starvation, this is commonest in primaparous does from high-yielding families.

Clinical signs

- Inappetance (eats browsings/hay, refuses concentrates).
- Rapid loss of condition.
- Milk yield drops.
- Mild ataxia.
- Constipation – hard, small droppings with pointed ends; mild abdominal pain.
- Acetone smell to breath.

Note: left-sided displacement of the abomasum (see Chapter 14) produces a secondary ketosis and clinical signs similar to primary acetonaemia.

Laboratory diagnosis

- Ketostix, Multistix, Acetest tablets or Rothera's reagent can be used to detect ketones in urine or milk.
- A blood sample can be submitted for an energy profile - glucose, β-hydroxybutyrate, non-esterified fatty acids, ketones. Serum 3-OH butyrate concentrations > 3.0 mmol/litre support the diagnosis and are commonly > 5.0 mmol/litre.

Prevention

- Clinical ketosis can be avoided by reducing the energy deficit in early lactation by encouraging food intake and feeding a balanced diet containing adequate levels of good quality fibre and increasing levels of concentrates. Concentrate levels should be increased gradually by about 0.1 kg/day during the first weeks of lactation to avoid other metabolic problems like laminitis and ruminal acidosis.

Treatment

- Corticosteroids.
- Other treatments as for pregnancy toxaemia.

Prognosis

- Good; animals with this form of ketosis respond well to treatment.

Hypocalcaemia (milk fever)

Most clinical cases of hypocalcaemia occur after kidding when the increased demands of lactation for calcium cannot be met quickly enough (see later in this chapter), but hypocalcaemia may occur in conjunction with pregnancy toxaemia and subclinical disease may be present at any stage of the periparturient period. Many goats will benefit from calcium therapy when presented with other periparturient diseases and *all recumbent or comatose goats should be treated as potentially hypocalcaemic and given calcium.*

Abortion

See Chapter 2.

Bloody mucoid discharges from the vulva can occasionally be produced by other conditions rather than abortion or parturition with dead kids. Plate 4.1 shows the discharge from a non-pregnant pygmy goat with apparent abdominal distension (obese!) and discharge emanating from a blood-filled bladder.

Dead kids without immediate abortion

Retention of a dead or mummified kid is not uncommon in goats. Kids may be retained for several months before the doe produces a macerated kid or bones. Small pieces of bone may be retained in the uterus and cause infertility. Occasionally, mummified kids are found incidentally at post-mortem (see also Chapter 1).

Vaginal prolapse

> Adequate analgesia and control of straining should be primary considerations when dealing with periparturient problems.

Vaginal prolapse is relatively common and likely to recur during subsequent pregnancies with probable increasing severity, but some goats prolapse only once. Most goats generally kid normally without subsequent prolapse of the uterus.

Aetiology
- An increase in intrapelvic pressure in late pregnancy initiates straining by the doe, forcing the vagina through the vulva. Factors implicated in increasing the likelihood of prolapse include:
  - Multiple fetuses.
  - Conformation of the dam – musculature, pelvic anatomy, possible hereditary component.
  - In goats, overfatness is generally not significant.
  - Starvation. Hypoproteinaemia results in the loss of body collagen.

Clinical signs
- The degree of prolapse is variable, from a minor protrusion of the vagina through the vulval lips when lying down to a complete prolapse of the vagina and cervix in which the bladder may also be prolapsed (Plate 4.1).
- The contents of the vaginal prolapse can be visualised using ultrasonography with a 5 MHz transducer and either a linear array or sector scanner.

Treatment
- Minor prolapses. If the area is clean, untraumatised and returns to its normal position when the doe stands up, no treatment is necessary.
- Larger prolapses will need replacing after thorough cleaning. Analgesia with a suitable NSAID, for example flunixin meglumine, 2.2 mg/kg and the use of caudal epidural anaesthesia (Chapter 24) to provide analgesia and control straining are essential before replacement of the prolapse is attempted (Plate 4.2).
- Various retention techniques have been used. Plastic or alloy intravaginal retainers are commonly used in sheep, but often cause vaginitis and further straining and are difficult to attach to short-coated dairy breeds. The Buhner suture (Figure 4.1) uses 5 mm umbilical tape, which is laid down subcutaneously on both sides of the vulva, using a large half-curved needle, starting below the ventral vulval commissure, passing through the lateral fibrous tissue to emerge dorsal to the dorsal commissure, then passing down through the fibrous tissue of the opposite side to emerge below the ventral commissure again, where it is tied with a double bow. Splashing lidocaine or bupivacaine into the vaginal vault as the vulva is closed helps prevent straining. The retaining suture must be released to allow kidding

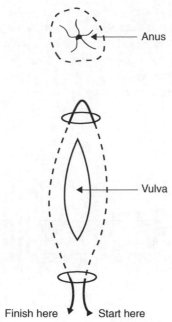

Anus

Vulva

Finish here ◥ Start here

Figure 4.1 Buhner suture.

to take place, so the doe needs regular checks once the pelvic ligaments relax.

■ Post-surgically, broad-spectrum antibiotic cover should be given for 5 days.

■ Consider early induced parturition with prostaglandins if the goat is distressed. Induction of parturition also allows the retaining suture to be removed at the optimum time.

■ Prolapse of the intestines through a vaginal rupture may occur if a portion of the intestines is forced into the pelvis.

Evisceration through a vaginal tear

Evisceration of the intestines through a vaginal tear rarely occurs in heavily pregnant does during the last month of gestation. There is no treatment and euthanasia should be carried out immediately on humane grounds.

Rectal prolapse

Rectal prolapse is rare, but may occur on its own or follow vaginal prolapse if straining continues. Effective caudal analgesia often allows the rectal tissue to return to its normal position. Larger prolapses may need manual reduction, with a purse string suture of 5 mm umbilical tape placed subcutaneously, leaving an anus of about 1.5 cm diameter. Very large rectal prolapses may need amputating under caudal epidural anaesthesia (Chapter 24).

Uterine torsion

Uterine torsion, which is very uncommon in the doe, may need distinguishing from incomplete dilation of the cervix. It may involve the vagina or only the cervix or the body of the uterus. Attempted correction by rolling is usually unsuccessful and correction is usually made after removal of the kids by caesarian section.

Rupture of the prepubic tendon

Rupture of the prepubic tendon is rare, but can occur in older multiparous goats during the last few weeks of pregnancy or occasionally following trauma. The rupture occurs on the left side and presents as a swelling immediately cranial to the pubis. Affected does are unlikely to kid naturally and will need manual assistance at kidding or a caesarian section. The doe should be euthanised if it survives kidding.

Normal parturition

The average gestation period of the doe is 150 days, with a range of 145 to 156 days, but the vast majority of does kid between 149 and 151 days. Does carrying multiple kids tend to kid earlier than does with a single kid. The sacrotuberous ligaments, extending from the base of the tail to the ischial tuberosity, relax before kidding, generally indicating that parturition will occur within the next 12 to 24 hours; in some does, however, relaxation occurs earlier than this. Normal parturition is divided into 3 stages:

1 *First stage labour*, which lasts between 3 and 12 hours, occurs when uterine contractions push the fetuses, fetal fluids and placentae against the cervix, causing it to dilate. In multiparus does, first stage labour is usually shorter than in primaparous does. During this

time, the doe shows behavioural changes, usually seeking a place away from other goats, getting up and lying down, turning and talking to her abdomen. A thick string of mucus appears at the vulva as the cervical plug dissolves. The cervix dilates completely in response to internal pressure as the fetus(es) change position in preparation for birth. The soft tissue components of the pelvic canal soften and become more distensible.

2 *Second stage labour* typically lasts about an hour and finishes when the last kid is born. Contraction of abdominal muscles and diaphragm (straining) cause the allantochorion ('water-bag') to protrude through the vulva lips and with further straining to rupture, releasing clear fluid. The amnion and fetus are then engaged in pelvic cavity and further straining causes expulsion of the first kid. The amniotic sac does not always rupture during the birth and, if not removed from the kid's nostrils by the licking of its mother or human intervention, may result in asphyxiation of the kid. The interval between births of further kids is usually between 10 and 60 minutes; intervention should be considered after 1 hour.

3 *Third stage labour* involves expulsion of the fetal membranes (usually within 4 hours after the expulsion of the last kid) and uterine involution.

A light, odourless, reddish vaginal discharge (*lochia*) is normal after kidding for about 14 days or more and should not be confused with metritis. The discharge sticks to the tail and many owners clip and wash the tail to make the doe more comfortable.

Uterine involution and re-epithelialisation are normally completed between 18 and 25 days, with the most rapid involution occurring during the first and second weeks after parturition as a response to myometrial contractility, which plays a major role in clearing out the lochial debris. The completion of uterine involution and resumption of ovarian activity depends on a number of factors, including breed, season of parturition, nutrition and lactation.

Prolonged gestation

If parturition has not occurred by 155 days, parturition should be induced with prostaglandins (Chapter 1) and will result in kidding in about 36 hours. Hypocalcaemia (Chapter 11) should always be considered and treated where necessary. Common causes of prolonged gestation are:

- Non-pregnancy!
- False pregnancy (Chapter 1)
- A single large kid
- Dead kids
- Hypocalcaemia.

Dystocia

> The uterus tears easily. If the correction of a malpresentation is prolonged or delivery difficult, a caesarian section is indicated.

Initial assessment

The preliminary history should consider:

- Is the expected kidding date of the doe known and if so is she at full term?
  - If the doe is kidding early, care is required in case this is a possible abortion and presents a zoonotic risk (abortion is discussed in Chapter 2).
- How long has the doe been trying to kid? Have any kids been born yet?
  - Prolonged second stage labour may be due to:
    - fatigue.
    - malpresentation of the fetus – transverse, posterior or breech presentations or the simultaneous presentation of more than one fetus.
- Is straining present or not? One of the commonest causes of non-progression of parturition is a breech or transverse presentation, where the kid does not engage in the pelvis and fails to stimulate contractions.
- Have fetal membranes been seen and when did they appear?
- Has the owner examined the doe intrapelvically and with what result?

General assessment of the doe

- General condition:
  - An alert bright doe represents a good risk.

o An exhausted, depressed or sick doe is a poor risk both for kidding or caesarian section and removal of kids by non-sterile caesarian section, with appropriate analgesia, followed by immediate euthanasia of the doe may be the best option on both welfare and financial grounds.

■ Breed and size of the goat:

o Most pygmy goats are too small to permit manual correction of malpresentations or to deliver oversized kids and will need a caesarian section.

■ Condition score:

o An overfat doe may have a single, large fetus with fat in the pelvis and relative fetal oversize.

o A thin doe may have multiple fetuses or pregnancy toxaemia.

■ Udder development:

o Poor udder development may indicate premature kidding or abortion.

o If there is an apparent lack of colostrum, the feeding of any live kids born needs to be considered.

Specific examination

■ Appearance of the vulva:

o Tight suggests that the doe is possibly not ready to kid yet.

o Relaxed suggests the doe is ready to kid, but fetuses are possibly not engaged in the pelvis.

o Swollen, bruised or traumatised suggests interference by the stockperson (Plate 4.3).

■ Is any part of the fetus visible?

o The condition of the fetus may give an indication of its viability and that of its siblings.

o An oedematous fetus indicates a dystocia of several hours duration.

■ Are fetal membranes visible?

o Membranes should appear healthy; autolysis suggest dead fetuses or abortion.

■ Vaginal/uterine discharge?

o Colour, blood, meconium staining?

■ Smell?

o An unpleasant odour indicates that at least one kid has been dead for several hours.

o A putrid smell suggests that the kids have been dead for more than a day.

Vaginal examination

All obstetrical examinations should be done as gently as possible with copious amounts of lubricant gel.

■ How easy is it to insert a hand into the vagina?

o If the vulva and vagina are tight, the doe is probably not ready to kid.

o An assessment can be made about the possible ease of kidding. If inserting a lubricated hand is difficult, it will be equally difficult to deliver a kid.

■ Condition of the vagina:

o A dry, tacky vagina that is beginning to contract around the fetus suggests the doe has been attempting to kid unsuccessfully for some time and increases the risk of uterine rupture during delivery, even with the use of adequate lubricant; these kids are usually dead.

o A bruised, swollen or torn vagina suggests previous interference by the stockperson.

o If the examination causes the doe undue pain, an epidural anaesthetic should be administered (Chapter 24).

■ Is the cervix dilated fully, partially or not at all?

o If partially dilated, can it be dilated manually with care? Gentle manual dilation of the vulva, vagina and cervix may be necessary where the fetus has not engaged correctly in the pelvis, for example with a transverse presentation. Overenthusiastic stretching of the cervix may result in tearing and haemorrhage. If haemorrhage occurs, it may be possible to gently pull the cervix caudally towards the vulva and exteriorise it sufficiently to identify and ligate the bleeding vessel.

o If the cervix cannot be dilated (*incomplete cervical dilation* (*ringwomb*)):

◆ Is the goat ready to kid? Inexperienced goatkeepers may ask for assistance early during first stage labour when the first abdominal movements are seen. Some (most?) cases of incomplete cervical dilation represent too early an intervention and the best treatment is patience and tincture of time!

◆ Is the goat pregnant? A mucoid vaginal discharge does not always indicate parturition. Plate 15.4

shows the discharge from a non-pregnant pygmy goat with a bladder filled with blood.

◆ Is parturition premature? This could indicate the start of an abortion outbreak. Diseases such as toxoplasmosis affect hormone production by the placenta.

◆ Hypocalcaemia (see later in this chapter) may result in apparent failure of cervical dilation and should always be considered, but is not common in goats at the time of parturition.

◆ Are the kids dead? If the kids are dead, there may be inadequate hormonal preparation for parturition. Sometimes the cervix is actually closing after failure of parturition to occur at the correct time, because of pregnancy toxaemia, uterine inertia or fetal malpresentation.

True ringwomb, where the cervix fails to dilate sufficiently to allow parturition, is rare. It has been suggested that one cause of ringwomb may be the absence of the final preparturient surge of prostaglandin, which may be responsible for the induction of relaxin, a glycoprotein hormone that softens the cervix in some species, although relaxin has not yet been studied in the doe.

Treatment of ringwomb is always problematical:

◆ Prostaglandins may produce kidding in about 4 hours: dinaprost, 5–10 mg i.m. or s.c. or clorprostenol, 62.5–125 μg i.m. or s.c.

◆ Dilation may be promoted by treatment with vetrabutine hydrochloride, 2 mg/kg (at present not licensed for ruminants in the United Kingdom).

Failure of cervical dilation with live kids is an indication for caesarian section: when a goat with a non-dilated cervix is in advanced second stage labour, a decision must be made to either carry out a caesarian section or euthanise the doe.

■ If the cervix is dilated, the kid(s) can be palpated and an assessment made of the possible cause of the dystocia, that is malpresentation of a single kid, more than one kid presented at the pelvic inlet, relative foetal oversize, etc. With experience it is usually possible to tell if it will be possible to deliver the kid(s) vaginally.

The 30–30–30 rule

If the doe has been in obvious labour for 30 minutes, check her internally. If everything – posture, position and presentation – appears correct, wait for another 30 minutes before intervening further. If it has been more than 30 minutes since the birth of one kid and there is another one present, it is time to deliver the next one.

Correcting the dystocia

Epidural anaesthesia is indicated for any protracted kidding to reduce stress on the doe.

Generally, dystocia is due to postural, positional or presentational defects and only occasionally due to an oversize fetus. Overfat does, particularly goatlings, and pygmy goats have reduced pelvic capacity, limiting the ability to manipulate the kid. Maternal causes of dystocia are shown in Table 4.8 and fetal causes in Table 4.9. *Any* deviation from the normal anterior presentation, dorsal position and extended posture may cause problems and postural defects are more common with multiple kids (too little room as the kids present simultaneously) and premature or aborted kids. Transverse presentations are quite common with multiple births and prevent the fetus engaging in the pelvic canal. The uterus of the goat is more readily damaged than that of the ewe. Adequate lubrication and dilatation of the canal is essential or rupture of the cervix, with dorsal tearing of the uterus and possibly uterine haemorrhage, will occur.

The L + 4R rule for kiddings

Lubrication **R**ecognition **R**epulsion **R**emoval **R**e-examination

Most dystocias of fetal origin can be corrected by retropulsion, manipulation and traction on the head and limbs. Before attempting to deliver a kid, it is essential to check that the limbs and head present in the pelvic canal belong to a single kid. It is always easier to deliver a kid in posterior presentation. Kids can often be delivered with only one forelimb extended forward and the other leg still flexed at the shoulder. In most cases, kids can be delivered without using ropes on the legs, but if the head needs to be manipulated a kidding rope around the head is essential and can be used to ease the

Table 4.8 Maternal causes of dystocia.

Birth canal	Abdomen	Uterus
Pelvic size	**Failure of abdominal contractions**	**Inertia**
Immaturity	Old age	*Myometrial defect*
Inadequate nutrition and growth	Debility	Systemic illness
Primaparous does	Absence of fetus in pelvic inlet	■ pregnancy toxaemia
Small doe	Pain	■ hypocalcaemia
■ breed, e.g. pygmy	Obesity	■ septicaemia
■ conformation	Rupture of abdominal muscles	
Obesity	■ hernia	Overstretching
Fracture		Exhaustion
	Ruptured uterus	■ large litters
	Uterine torsion	■ fetal dystocia
	Stress	■ fetal monsters
		Stress
Constriction of soft tissue		
Scar tissue		
Congenital defects		
Obesity		
Prolapse		
Tumour		
Failure to dilate		
Cervix		
■ prematurity		
■ intervention too early		
■ ringwomb		
Vulva		
■ primaparous does		
■ fibrosis/scarring		

Table 4.9 Fetal causes of dystocia.

Oversize	Malpresentation	Fetal death
Singletons	*Any* deviation from the normal	Infection
Male kids	anterior presentation,	Pregnancy toxaemia
Prolonged gestation	dorsal position and extended	Malnutrition
Congenital birth defects	posture	Congenital lesion
	Presentation	
	Posterior	
	Transverse	
	Simultaneous – 2 or more kids	
	Position	
	Ventral	
	Lateral	
	Posture	
	Front legs deviated	
	Hind legs deviated (breech)	
	Head deviated	

head into the pelvis and through the vulva. Applying traction to the forelegs without securing the head will result in the head deviating sideways and make the situation worse. With a large kid (or small pelvis), the head should be pulled into the pelvis first and the legs pulled under it (use ropes if necessary).

> Always check for additional kids after each kid is delivered.

Routine kid care

Clip (cut umbilical cord short if too long)
Dip (umbilical cord in iodine)
Strip (squirt colostrum from each teat to check colostrum present and teats functional)
Sip (make sure each kid gets colostrum)

Drug treatment

See Table 4.6.

- Clenbuterol, 0.8 μg/kg, can be used to produce myometrial relaxation during kidding or caesarian section. In countries where clenbutarol is illegal, adrenaline (epinephrine) has been used to relax the uterus; 1 ml (1 mg) of 1:1000 adrenaline i.m.
- Oxytocin can be used to stimulate uterine muscle contractions during parturition, provided there is no obstructive dystocia and can also be given to stimulate uterine contraction removal of the kids and milk let-down; oxytocin, 2–10 U i.m. or s.c.
- Parenteral antibiotics should be given whenever there has been manipulation within the uterus.
- Non-steroidal anti-inflammatory drugs should be given if the doe is toxaemic or sore. Carprofen, 1.4 mg/kg repeat once after 24 hours s.c. or i.v.; Flunixin meglumine, 2.2 mg/kg SID for 3–5 days\break i.v.; Ketoprofen, 3 mg/kg SID for 3–5 days i.m. or i.v.; Meloxicam, 2 mg/kg initially then 0.5 mg/kg every 36 hours s.c. or i.v.; Tolfenamic acid, 2–4 mg/kg repeat once after 48 hours s.c. or i.v.
- Calcium borogluconate should be given to any doe suspected of being hypocalcaemic. Calcium borogluconate 20% (or better calcium borogluconate, magnesium and phosphorus), 80–100 ml slowly i.v., s.c. or half by each route. The response to calcium by the s.c.

route is very rapid in the goat and may be preferable if the goat is stressed by handling.

Is a caesarian section necessary?

Goats tolerate caesarian section far better than prolonged manipulation of the fetuses. Opting for early surgery may save the life of the dam and the kids, so it is essential to make a quick decision as to whether vaginal delivery is likely to be successful. Caeserian section is indicated when vaginal delivery would cause excessive trauma to the dam or kids when the kids are alive or recently dead. Techniques for caesarian section are discussed in Chapter 26.

Dead kids that are infected or decomposed are best removed by *embryotomy* rather than by caesarian section, because of the risk of uterine fluid leaking into the abdomen with subsequent peritonitis. The prognosis for the doe in these circumstances is good provided she is not toxic or systemically ill, if serious damage is not done to the cervix or vagina and if the uterus is not ruptured. Broad spectrum antibiotics and NSAIDs should be administered with fluid therapy where necessary.

Hypocalcaemia (milk fever)

Frank clinical signs of hypocalcaemia are not common in the United Kingdom, although it is probable that subclinical disease is more widespread and many goats will benefit from calcium therapy when presented with other periparturient diseases, such as mastitis, metritis, etc. The disease is most common in young, high-yielding first kidders in the first few weeks after parturition but may occur in late pregnancy, during parturition and at any stage of lactation, particularly in heavy milkers, and in any age of an adult goat. Older goats are more likely to suffer from hypocalcaemia around and during parturition.

Aetiology

- There is a fall in the serum calcium and phosphorus levels in all goats at kidding due to the onset of lactation; a greater fall occurs in goats that develop hypocalcaemia around parturition, due to a failure in the calcium homeostatic mechanisms to meet the increased demand for calcium.
- In heavy milking goats, an absolute deficiency of calcium at any stage of lactation will precipitate the disease.

Clinical signs

- Often only slight tremors and twitching, with some hyperexcitability and slight ataxia, or even lethargy, inappetence and poor milk yield with no obvious nervous signs.
- More severe cases show marked ataxia and incoordination or fits followed by paresis, paraplegia, recumbency and coma, which may last several hours.
- An eclamptic form occasionally occurs during lactation, for example after a change to better pasture, with pyrexia (41.1 °C), marked muscular tremors, excitement, rapid panting respirations, collapse and death.
- All recumbent or comatose goats should be treated as potentially hypocalcaemic and given calcium.

Diagnosis

- Clinical signs.
- Rapid response to calcium therapy.
- Serum calcium measurements (normal 2.2 to 2.6 mmol/l).

Treatment

- Calcium borogluconate 20% (or better calcium borogluconate, magnesium and phosphorus), 80–100 ml slowly i.v., s.c. or half by each route. The response to calcium by the subcutaneous route is very rapid in the goat and may be preferable if the goat is stressed by handling.
- Relapses may occur, in which case extra phosphorus as well as calcium may be beneficial.

Note: many toxic conditions, for example enterotoxaemia and mastitis, may show a temporary response to calcium therapy.

Hypomagnesaemia

Hypomagnesaemia is uncommon in goats, but occasionally occurs early in lactation in goats grazing on rich pasture. Pregnant goats on poor pasture may also develop the disease.

The clinical signs and treatment of hypomagnesaemia are discussed in Chapter 12.

Transit tetany

A combination of hypocalcaemia and hypomagnesaemia can occur in stressed animals in late pregnancy. The clinical signs and treatment of transit tetany are discussed in Chapter 12.

Trauma to the vulva

Difficult and assisted kiddings will lead to varying degrees of vulval trauma – swelling, bruising, lacerations (Plates 4.3 and 4.4) – which may require local treatment with antiseptic ointments and antibiotic sprays and parenteral treatment with antibiotics and NSAIDs.

Metritis

> A light, odourless, reddish vaginal discharge (*lochia*) is normal after kidding for 14 days or more and should not be confused with metritis.

Metritis, which is most likely to follow manual kiddings following dystocia, retained fetal membranes, retained kids and abortions, is indicated by a dark, sticky, usually smelly discharge that may contain pus (Plate 4.5). The doe may be pyrexic and anorexic with a reduced milk yield and signs of abdominal pain. Does that progress to chronic metritis may be infertile (see Chapter 1).

Treatment

- Any underlying disease should be treated.
- Broad-spectrum antibiotics, for example oxytetracycline 20 mg/kg, initially i.v., then s.c., or antibiotics with a good efficacy against anaerobic bacteria, for example procaine penicillin 10 mg/kg; NSAID; oxytocin.
- Dexamethasone given i.v. is reported to produce a more rapid response when given in conjunction with intravenous antibiotics.

Endometritis

Endometritis ('whites') is much less common than in cattle. A mucopurulent vaginal discharge is evident on vaginal examination about 3 weeks after kidding. Affected animals are not clinically ill, but have a relatively odourless white vaginal discharge (Plate 4.6).

Failure to treat the condition will result in subsequent fertility problems. Broad spectrum antibiotics, such as cephalosporins and oxytetracycline, active against *Actinobaccillus pyogenes* and gram-negative anaerobes, should be administerd parenterally and used to wash out the vagina. Most goats will kid outwith the breeding season and so are unlikely to have an active corpus luteum, meaning that, unlike in cattle, prostaglandins will be of no use in immediate treatment.

Pyometra

Pyometra is an uncommon sequel to metritis and is also reported to occur in females of breeds that cycle after parturition during the normal anoestrus season (Anglo-Nubians, pygmy goats and Nigerian dwarfs), resulting in a persistent corpus luteum.

Clinical signs include anoestrus and occasionally a purulent vaginal discharge. Ultrasound scanning shows a fluid-filled uterus, which is more hyperechoic than seen with a hydrometra.

Retained placenta

> If the doe is still straining, check for another kid.

A retained placenta is much less common than in the cow. Induction of parturition with prostaglandins does not lead to retention. Does regularly eat their own (and other goats) placentae; many reportedly 'retained placentae' have, in fact, been eaten by the goat! (Plate 4.7). Fetal membranes should normally be passed within 4 hours of kidding and veterinary attention should be sought if they are not passed within 12 hours, if the goat is unwell or there is a suspicion of a retained kid. After this time, contraction of the uterus and closure of the cervix will prevent manual removal. However, if the doe is bright, eating and non-pyrexic, there is no need for immediate action and the doe can be safely monitored by the owner for behavioural changes, including mismothering, and a rise in rectal temperature.

In many cases, membranes, which are hanging from the vulva a few hours after kidding, can be easily removed by slow, gentle traction, but forced manual removal should not be attempted. A firmly attached placenta should be cut off close to the vulva. The placenta will detach by day 5 or 6 and the remnants passed along with the lochia. Retained placentae can be caused by selenium and vitamin A deficiencies or hypocalcaemia, or follow infectious abortions (toxoplasmosis, chlamydiosis), dystocia or caesarian section. Often the cause for the retention is not obvious. Induction of parturition with prostaglandins does not lead to an increased incidence of retained fetal membranes.

Injections of oxytocin, 5–10 U, 2–6 times daily or prostaglandin, dinaprost, 5–10 mg i.m. or s.c. or clorprostenol, 62.5–125 µg i.m. or s.c. may aid removal of the membranes. Stroking the dorsal vaginal wall (feathering), using a gloved finger, will cause an oxytocin release. Cleaning the teats with a warm, wet cloth, clearing the teat orifices and removing a few streams of colostrum from each teat also releases oxytocin and assists a neonate to nurse more easily, thus accomplishing two tasks at once without introducing any outside bacteria into the vagina.

Antibiotic cover should be given routinely (oxytetracycline is suitable) and tetanus antitoxin given to unvaccinated goats.

Retained kid

> Vaginal examination of a sick doe post-kidding should be carried out routinely.

Retained kids after parturition are more common and potentially more serious than a retained placenta. The kid may be delivered normally after a few days, but retention of a non-mummified kid will often result in an acute toxaemia with pyrexia, so most affected does will become lethargic and anorexic, with a dramatic drop in milk yield, abdominal pain and death in about 3 days if the condition is not recognised. Some does will strain, but many will not and a manual examination of any sick doe post-kidding should be considered routine. If the cervix is closed and an internal examination of the uterus is not possible, transabdominal scanning of the standing doe with a 5 MHz sector scanner, or radiography, will confirm the diagnosis.

It may be possible to ballot the retained kid in the abdomen. The pregnant uterus lies towards the ventral surface of the abdomen and the kid can be balloted upwards with a fast vertical movement – stand behind the doe facing in the same direction as the animal; bend over from the waist and place the palms of the hands flat on the abdominal wall directly cranial to the udder; then pull quickly vertically upwards towards the goat's back. Smaller animals can be straddled as if riding a horse backwards to help prevent the doe moving sideways.

Rupture of the uterus

Rupture of the uterus usually occurs dorsally in the body of the uterus just cranial to the cervix. Repair of a dorsal tear is extremely difficult either by a left flank abdominal incision or vaginally. However, in many cases, contraction of the uterus will seal the defect and the doe may not only survive, but breed and kid satisfactorily in subsequent years. The main dangers are shock and peritonitis – the fetal membranes should be removed as completely as possible, high levels of intravenous antibiotics given and pain relief given, for example flunixin meglumine, 2.2 mg/kg i.v. Intravenous fluid therapy will increase the goat's chance of survival.

Ruptured uterine artery

A ruptured uterine artery is rare but may accompany a ventral tear of the uterus or occur during a difficult kidding, with or without human intervention. It may also occur spontaneously during late pregnancy, particularly in overweight does, due to stretching of the artery because of the weight of the uterus. Fatal intraperitoneal haemorrhage can occur without obvious vaginal haemorrhage.

Uterine prolapse

Uterine prolapse is also rare, but may occur a few hours after kidding, often subsequent to a retained placenta or as a result of continued straining because of pain and inflammation in the reproductive tract. If the placenta is still attached, it should be gently removed before thorough cleaning and replacement of the uterus under epidural anaesthesia (see Chapter 24). Using xylocaine in the epidural will block sensation and help prevent straining for 8 hours or more as opposed to 1–2 hours for lignocaine alone. Covering the prolapsed uterus in a thick coat of sugar reduces the oedema, shrinking the uterus to make it easier to replace. A small amount of warm water dribbled over the sugar starts the osmotic gradient.

The horns of the uterus must be fully extended when replaced. Filling the uterus with warm water or saline, using a thin-necked bottle or intravenous drip set, helps ensure that the uterine horns are fully extended and the uterus returns to its correct position in the abdomen. Retention sutures are not generally necessary if the replacement is complete, but a purse string suture is sometimes used (see 'Vaginal prolapse' in this chapter). Antibiotics, procaine penicillin or oxytetracycline should be given i.m. or s.c. for 3–5 days, together with an NSAID to reduce inflammation. A doe that prolapses her uterus is unlikely to do so the following year.

Urine scald

Trauma to the vagina and vulva at kidding can lead to dribbling of urine around the vulva and caudal hind legs (Plate 4.8). Severe urine scald will lead to a secondary contact bacterial dermatitis (see Chapter 11).

Mastitis

See Chapter 13.

Laminitis

See Chapter 7.

Further reading

General

East, N.E. (1983) Pregnancy toxaemia, abortions and penparturient diseases. *Vet. Clin. North Amer.: Large Anim. Pract.*, **5** (3), 601–618.

Edmondson, M.A., Roberts, J,F,, Baird A.N., Bychawski, S. and Pugh, D.G. (2012) Theriogenology of sheep and goats. In: *Sheep and Goat Medicine*, 2nd edition (eds Pugh, D.G. and Baird, A.N.), pp. 150–231. Elsevier-Saunders, Maryland Heights, MO.

Groenevelt, M. (2012) Periparturient problems in the goat. *Goat Vet. Soc. J.*, **28**, 80–85.

Caesarian section

Mueller, K. (2011) Caesarian section in the doe. *Goat Vet. Soc. J.*, **27**, 34–38.

Dystocia

Winter A. (1999) Dealing with dystocia in the ewe. *In Practice* **21**, 2–9.

Fluid therapy

Jones, M. and Navarre, C. (2014) Fluid therapy in small ruminants and camelids. *Vet. Clin. North Amer.: Food Anim. Pract.*, **30** (2), 441–453.

Nutrition

AFRC Technical Committee on Responses to Nutrients, Report No. 10 (1998) The Nutrition of Goats, CAB International, Wallingford.

Chamberlain, A.T. (2010) Dry goat nutrition. *Goat Vet. Soc. J.*, **26**, 31–35.

Morand-Fehr, P. (2005) Recent developments in goat nutrition and application: a review. *Small Ruminant Research*, **60**, 25–43.

National Research Council (2007) *Nutrient Requirements of Small Ruminants: Sheep, Goats, Cervids, and New World Camelids*, The National Academies Press, Washington, DC.

Pinotti, L. *et al.* (2008) Rumen-protected choline and vitamin E supplementation in periparturient dairy goats: effects on milk production and folate, vitamin B12 and vitamin E status. *Animal*, **2** (07), 1019–1027.

Pinotti, L. (2010) Polyunsaturated fatty acids and choline in dairy goats nutrition: production and health benefits. *Small Ruminant Research*, **88** (2–3), 135–144.

Pinotti, L. (2012). *Vitamin-Like Supplementation in Dairy Ruminants: The Case of Choline, Milk Production – An Up-to-Date Overview of Animal Nutrition, Management and Health* (ed. Professor Narongsak Chaiyabutr), ISBN: 978-953-51-0765-1, InTech, DOI: 10.5772/50770. Available from: http://www.intechopen.com/books/milk-production-an-up-to-date-overview-of-animal-nutrition-management-and-health/vitamin-like-supplementation-in-dairy-ruminants-the-case-of-choline.

Prenatal stress

Baxter, E. (2016) Effects of prenatal stress on mothers and kids. *Goat Vet. Soc. J.*, **32** (in print).

Pregnancy toxaemia

Albay, M.K. *et al.* (2014) Selected serum biochemical parameters and acute phase protein levels in a herd of Saanen goats showing signs of pregnancy toxaemia. *Veterinarni Medicina*, **59** (7), 336–342.

Brozos, C., Mavrogianni, V. and Fthenakis, G. (2011) Treatment and control of peri-parturient metabolic diseases: pregnancy toxemia, hypocalcemia, hypomagnesemia. *Vet. Clin. North Amer.: Food Anim. Pract.*, **27** (1), 105–113.

Doré, V., Dubuc, J., Bélanger, A.M. and Buczinski, S. (2013) Evaluation of the accuracy of an electronic on-farm test to quantify blood beta-hydroxybutyrate concentration in dairy goats. *J. Dairy Sci.*, **96** (7), 4505–4507.

Doré, V. *et al.* (2015) Definition of prepartum hyperketonemia in dairy goats. *J. Dairy Sci.*, **98** (7), 4535–4543.

Lima, M.S., Pascoal, R.A., and Stilwell, G.T. (2012) Glycaemia as a sign of the viability of the fetuses in the last days of gestation in dairy goats with pregnancy toxaemia. *Irish Vet. J.*, **65** (1), 1–6.

Ospina, P.A. *et al.* (2013) Using nonesterified fatty acids and β-hydroxybutyrate concentrations during the transition period for herd-level monitoring of increased risk of disease and decreased reproductive and milking performance. *Vet. Clin. North Amer.: Large Anim. Pract.*, **29** (2), 387–412.

Pichler, M., Damberger, A., Arnholdt, T. *et al.* (2014) Evaluation of 2 electronic handheld devices for diagnosis of ketonemia and glycemia in dairy goats. *J. Dairy Sci.*, **97** (12), 7538–7546.

Zamir, S., Rozov, A. and Gootwine, E. (2009) Treatment of pregnancy toxaemia in sheep with flunixin meglumine. *Vet. Rec.*, **165** (9), 265–266.

Rectal prolapse

Anderson, D. E. and Miesner, M. D. (2008) Rectal prolapse. *Vet. Clin. North Amer.: Food Anim. Pract.*, **24** (2), 403–408.

Vaginal prolapse

Scott, P. and Gessert, M. (1998) Management of ovine vaginal prolapse. *In Pract.*, **20** (1), 28–34.

CHAPTER 5

Weak kids

Weak kids arise from multiple causes (Table 5.1), which may be interrelated. Sensible management before, during and after kidding will improve the kids' chances of survival (Table 5.2).

Initial assessment

The preliminary history should consider:
- Individual or flock/herd problem.
- Kidding routine.
- Post kidding management.
- Beginning or end of kidding period.
- Feeding.
  If a flock/herd problem consider:
- Associated abortions/stillbirths.
- Possible nutritional deficiencies.
  If an individual problem, specific enquiries should cover:
- Weak since birth or developed since?
- Seen to suckle or not.
- Difficult or prolonged birth.
- Kidded inside or outside – possibility of exposure.

Clinical examination

Observe kid and dam together in their normal surroundings
- Mismothering – particularly first kidders.
- Behaviour of siblings.
- Sucking reflex.

Examine dam
- Udder conformation/teat abnormalities.
- Milk let-down.
- Mastitis.
- Vaginal discharge.

Table 5.1 Causes of weak kids.

Prematurity	Exposure
Birth injury	■ Primary hypothermia
■ Trauma	■ Secondary hypothermia
■ Compression	
■ Asphixiation	**Intrauterine malnutrition**
	■ Underfeeding of doe
Congenital defects	■ Trace element deficiencies
	○ Copper
Genetic diseases	○ Iodine
■ Mucopolysaccharidosis	○ Selenium
■ Beta mannosidosis	■ Congenital infection
Post-natal malnutrition	○ Toxoplasma
■ Failure to suck	○ Chlamydophilosis
■ Doe unwilling/unable to feed	○ Campylobacter
Post-natal infections	**Floppy kid syndrome**
■ Septicaemia	
■ Navel infections	
■ Pyaemia	
■ Enteritis	
■ Joint ill	

Table 5.2 Improving the survival of the newborn kid.

- Correct nutrition of the pregnant doe, particularly during the last 6 weeks of gestation
- Monitor parturition and correct dystocias as soon as possible
- Supervise all kids to ensure that they suck within 1 hour of birth
- Stomach tube all kids that are weak or not able to suckle their dam
- Give 50 ml/kg of colostrum or colostrum substitute within 4 hours of birth
- Monitor dam to ensure she is mothering the kid without excessive pawing and is allowing the kid to suckle
- Separate doe from other goats if she is not settling with her kid(s)
- Dip all kids' navels in strong iodine solution at birth and again 4 hours later
- Maintain clean kidding environment
  ○ Vaccinate does against clostridial disease to ensure good passive immunity for kids

Examine kid

- Alert?
- Check for congenital lesions.
- Nervous signs.

Prematurity/low birth weight

Birth weights of kids are very variable, ranging from over 7 kg for a single male down to 2 or 3 kg in multiple births. Birth weight is important as the larger the kid at birth the faster the growth rate.

Kids up to 14 days premature have a good chance of survival and kids up to 21 days premature can often be reared with intensive care. Premature kids may have respiratory problems due to inadequate lung surfactant being produced. This is particularly the case if parturition is induced with prostaglandins before about day 144 of gestation.

Birth injury

At birth the kid undergoes some quite profound changes to enable it to adapt to its new environment. With the exception of the development of the rumen the major physiological changes are over in a few days after birth and any associated signs of maladjustment appear by this time. It is quite possible that the kid will have to compensate for the deleterious effects of parturition itself:

- *Trauma* from the physical forces of parturition or from traction in an assisted birth.
- *Compression* of the kid's thorax as it passes through the pelvis, causing compression of the lungs.
- *Asphyxia* from pressure on the umbilical cord during passage through the pelvic cavity or from reduced efficiency of the placenta during uterine contractions.

Birth injury can result directly in the death of a kid if the damage is severe enough, for example from abdominal haemorrhage due to liver rupture, or difficulty in breathing, or may lead to death from starvation/hypothermia by impairing feeding and movement.

Intrauterine malnutrition

Inadequate placental development, as a result of maternal malnutrition, intrauterine infection or other cause, will result in poor fetal development and low birth weights because of poor transfer of oxygen, electrolytes and nutrients. The newborn kid is also more prone to hypothermia as chronic fetal hypoxia inhibits the capacity for thermoregulation.

Underfeeding of the doe

Correct feeding of the doe throughout pregnancy is essential. Placental development is directly related to the nutrition of the doe, so that low birth weights follow directly from maternal underfeeding. Underfeeding, particularly during the final 6 weeks of pregnancy, will result in small kids with low levels of fetal liver glycogen and fat and the birth of hypoglycaemic kids with poor energy reserves. Gross underfeeding may result in abortion or stillbirths. Does should be in good body condition (score 2.0–3.0) and well fed during the last 6 weeks of pregnancy.

Trace element deficiencies

Copper deficiency (enzootic ataxia, swayback)
Aetiology

- Copper deficiency is a disease of grazing animals or animals fed grass-based diets and home-produced cereals. Zero-grazed animals receiving a concentrate ration are unlikely to be affected.
- It is either the result of copper-deficient soils (*primary copper deficiency*) or generally in the United Kingdom as a result of a conditioned deficiency with reduced copper utilisation by the grazing animals, because of interaction with other minerals (*secondary copper deficiency*), for example pasture top-dressing with molybdenum and sulphur, which reduce the availability of copper, or heavy lime applications, which increase pasture molybdenum intake and thus reduce the copper intake. Molybdenum and sulphur interact with copper in the rumen to form insoluble copper thiomolybdates.
- Excess iron and sulphur in the diet can result in copper deficiency, even though copper intake appears to be adequate.
- Although the clinical signs and pathological lesions are similar to those in lambs, in goat herds clinical cases tend to be sporadic rather than a flock problem as in sheep and there is less correlation between copper levels and clinical disease.

- Fibre goats appear to be more susceptible to deficiency than dairy goats (and are also more prone to copper toxicity).
- Although it has been suggested that meat goats have a higher requirement for copper than dairy goats, this remains to be established from supplementation trials on multiple goat meat farms.
- Young rapidly growing animals have higher copper requirements than adults and milk is a poor source of copper. Copper deficiency occurs in kids when their mothers are showing no signs of copper deficiency.
- Heavy worm burdens can affect copper uptake by altering the pH of the alimentary tract, making copper less soluble. Solubility of copper in the abomasum may be reduced by up to 70% and the subsequent uptake of dissolved copper by the liver by up to 50%.

Clinical signs

1 **Congenital form**
   o The kid is affected at birth (Plate 5.1). Some kids may be of low viability and succumb to hypothermia without showing marked neurological signs.
2 **Delayed form**
   o Clinical signs do not appear until the kid is several weeks or even months old.
   o Bright, alert, willing to suck and eat.
   o Muscle tremors, head shaking.
   o Progressive hind limb ataxia, progressing to paralysis.
   o Adult goats in the same herd may have anaemia, decreased milk production, discoloured hair, diarrhoea, poor fleece quality and fail to thrive.
   o Other kids may show growth retardation, increased susceptibility to infections, poor fleece quality and susceptibility to fractures (distinguish from parasitism, cobalt deficiency or inadequate nutrition).

Diagnosis

- Clinical signs.
- *Plasma* copper levels >9 µmol/litre adequate. Interpretation in individual animals is difficult as blood levels in the normal range are commonly found in goats with low liver values. Plasma levels should be interpreted on a herd basis. Do all the tested animals have copper levels >9 µmol/litre?

Whole blood contains superoxide dismutase (SOD)/erythrocyte copper, ceroplasmin (CP)/plasma copper and 'free' or albumin bound copper. There will be a difference in the whole-blood copper concentration depending on the laboratory method used.
Note: (1) Serum levels are lower than plasma levels (>7.5 µmol/litre adequate).
       (2) For copper (and other trace elements), laboratories use diagnostic ranges rather than reference ranges, that is testing is designed to determine whether animals require more copper.
- Cerebrospinal fluid (CSF) within normal limits.
- Histological examination of the CNS.
- Liver copper levels:
   o Liver copper levels > 40 mg/kg DM indicate that copper supplementation is not needed.
   o Liver copper levels < 40 mg/kg DM suggest that copper supplementation may be necessary.
   Low liver copper levels may occur in some kids without enzootic ataxia and some apparently affected kids appear to have normal levels (due to subsequent supplementation?).

Post-mortem findings

- Generally no gross pathology of the nervous system.
- Demyelination of cerebellar and spinal cord tracts.
- Cerebellar corticol hypoplasia; necrosis and loss of Purkinje cells of cerebellum.
- Chromatolytic necrosis in brain stem nuclei and spinal cord.
- May be skeletal abnormalities – brittle bones, healing rib fractures.

Treatment

> Although copper toxicity is less likely in goats than sheep, the diagnosis should always be confirmed before any copper supplementation takes place. Animals should be monitored closely for signs of toxicity.

Treatment is often unsuccessful except early in the disease, but may prevent further deterioration in the delayed form.
Overdosage with copper causes toxicity (Chapter 15) so supplementation should be used with care. Although they provide an unknown and unregulated copper dose

over a period of time, copper oxide needles given orally are generally safer than injections.

■ Injection:

Adult goats: 25 mg, i.m.

If kids are injected, small doses (<5 mg), repeated if necessary, are safer than a single large dose.

■ Oral:

Copper oxide needles 1 g/10 kg in gelatin capsules, that is one 2.5 or 2 g gelatin capsule for kids of 20 to 40 kg body weight and two 2.5 or 2 g capsules or one 4 g capsule for a 50 kg adult.

■ Copper sulphate solutions, 35 mg copper sulphate/kid, given by mouth every 2 weeks; should be mixed with milk to minimise the astringent effects on the gastric mucosa.

Prevention

■ Soil and plant analysis for copper and its antagonists molybdenum, sulphur and iron and correction by fertiliser applications under professional advice.

■ Copper supplementation to does during pregnancy:

o Injection: 25 mg, i.m., 10 weeks prior to kidding.

o Oral: copper oxide needles, 1 g/10 kg in gelatin capsules, that is one 2.5 or 2 g gelatin capsule for kids of 20 to 40 kg body weight and two 2.5 or 2 g capsules or one 4 g capsule for a 50 kg adult. The copper oxide particles become trapped in the abomasum, slowly releasing absorbable copper for about 6 months. Liver reserves are increased much more effectively than by copper injections.

o Water additives: copper tablets.

o Food supplements: copper sulphate, for addition to feed at 254 g/kg; dose: up to 2 g/head.

Supplementation of the doe will prevent swayback, reduce kid mortality and improve early growth rates, but to ensure adequate later growth and prevent delayed swayback, kids should be dosed at about 2 to 3 weeks of age.

Iodine deficiency (goitre)

> Enlarged thymic glands are common in dairy kids and must be distinguished from goitre.

Goitre is commonly misdiagnosed by goatkeepers when kids have any enlargement in the throat region (see Chapter 9). In particular, thymic swellings, which are common, regularly lead to a misdiagnosis. True iodine deficiency is probably rare in the UK and limited to known geographical regions. Angoras appear to be more susceptible than dairy goats or sheep.

Aetiology

■ Natural deficiencies of iodine; primary deficiency is associated with low soil or water iodine concentrations and is limited to specific geographical areas.

■ Goitrogenic feeds, for example kale and cabbage, produce a secondary iodine deficiency by accumulation of isothiocyanates, which prevent the accumulation of iodine in the thyroid gland.

Clinical signs

■ Abortion.

■ Stillbirths or very weak kids born at term or slightly early with thin sparse hair coat; susceptible to cold stress, respiratory problems.

■ Enlarged thyroid glands (goitre) in the affected kids produce palpable swellings posterior and ventral to the larynx (more discrete than thymic glands involving the distal rather than proximal cervical region). The thyroid may weigh between 10 and 50 g compared to the normal weight of 2 g.

■ A subclinical deficiency may result in small weak kids without obvious goitre.

■ Older goats in the herd may show decreased production, poor growth rate and reduced appetite.

■ Iodine deficiency may also result in subfertility.

Diagnosis

■ Fetal thyroid histology:

o Thyroid hyperplasia with little or no colloid formation.

■ Fetal thyroid iodine content:

o Low thyroid concentrations (<1200 mg/kg DM) suggest decreased iodine availability.

■ Thyroxine (T4) assay on blood of adult animals:

o Only low in moderate and severe iodine deficiency.

o Affected by age, physiological status and disease and is thus not a reliable test for iodine deficiency.

o Ruminants store iodine very effectively in the thyroid and maintain thyroid hormone secretion through moderately long periods when iodine intakes are deficient.

- Plasma inorganic iodine (PII):
  - A measure of current iodine supply in the diet, but gives no indication of historical dietary intake. In cattle, <105 ng/ml is considered marginal and <51 ng/ml is considered low.
  - PII may still be normal with moderate dietary levels of iodine but high goitrogen intake. Goitrogens affect iodine uptake and metabolism within the thyroid so PII remains apparently adequate but inadequate thyroid hormone production results in low circulating T4. T4 and PII should be used together to investigate the cause of iodine deficiency.

Prevention and treatment

- Iodised saltlicks or loose iodised salt in the diets of older goats will prevent development of iodine deficiency. Alternatively, dose with potassium iodide 2 months and 2 weeks before kidding – dissolve 20 g of potassium iodide in 1 litre of water and dose at a rate of 10 ml per 20 kg body weight.
- 30 ml of 7% strong iodine (7% tincture of iodine) can be applied to the back of the doe during late pregnancy, instead of dosing with potassium iodide.
- Affected kids can be treated with 3 to 5 drops of Lugol's iodine in milk daily for 1 week. Alternatively, 1 ml/3 kg of 7% strong iodine can be applied to the back of the kid.
- Avoid goitrogenic feeds such as kale.

Treatment of goats incorrectly diagnosed by the owner as being iodine deficient can lead to *iodine toxicity*, which produces anorexia, lacrimation, coughing, dandruff in the coat and weight loss.

Selenium deficiency

Kids may occasionally show signs of white muscle disease (Chapter 8) at birth.

Congenital infections

Weak kids may be born as part of clinical syndromes involving abortions and stillbirths, such as toxoplasmosis, chlamydophiliosis and campylobacter (Chapter 2). Infection of the pregnant doe causes a placentitis that impairs transfer of nutrients to the foetus. Where the infectious agent crosses the placental barrier, as with toxoplasmosis, further signs of disease, such as abnormal sucking behaviour, may also impair the ability

of the kid to survive. Infection with some species of *Salmonella* and border disease virus may result in kids being born weak or with signs of neurological disease due to previous bacteraemia or viraemia.

Inherited diseases

Mucopolysaccharidosis IIID

Mucopolysaccharidosis IIID is an inherited lysosomal storage disease of Nubian goats and their crosses in the United States; Anglo Nubian goats in the United Kingdom are not carriers for the disease. The trait is recessive, so that carrier goats with only a single copy of the abnormal gene are clinically normal. Individuals that are homozygous for the defective gene are clinically affected.

Aetiology

- The affected goats have a deficiency in *N*-acetylglucosamine 6-sulfatase (G-6-S) activity that results from a single nonsense mutation in the 5′ region of the gene coding for the expression of this enzyme, which is required for the catabolism of glycosaminoglycans (GAG). Uncatabolised GAG accumulate in lysosomes, producing marked cytoplasmic vacuolation in the central nervous system and other tissues. *N*-acetylglucasamine and heparin sulphate accumulate in the tissues and urine.

Clinical signs

- Affected goats show delayed motor development, growth retardation and early death, although the severity of the disease is variable because of phenotypic variation.
- Marked neurological deficits may be present at birth or progressive neurological signs may appear in older goats. Neurological signs include the inability to stand, abnormal gait, persistent head tremor and intermittent hyperextension of the forelimbs. Animals may become deaf or blind.
- Less severely affected kids may be smaller than normal at birth and grow slowly. Kids may appear to grow normally for a few months and then stop growing. There is decreased muscle mass and a 'slab-sided' appearance, sometimes with blocky heads.
- Immune function appears to be compromised, so that animals may be more prone to infection.

Diagnosis

- A real-time PCR single nucleotide polymorphism assay is available that can distinguish affected goats. This enables carrier animals to be detected and eliminated from breeding programmes.

Beta mannosidosis

Beta mannosidosis is an inherited lysosomal disease of Nubian goats, Anglo Nubian and their crosses attributable to an autosomal recessive gene, which has been reported in Australia, New Zealand, the United States, Fiji and Canada, but not the United Kingdom. Because of the absence of the enzyme beta-mannosidase, kids are unable to stand from birth due to carpal contractures and hyperextended fetlocks (see Chapter 8).

Myelofibrosis

Myelofibrosis is an inherited disease of pygmy goats in California, attributable to an autosomal recessive gene. Kids are normal at birth, but become weak and inactive as early as 2 weeks of age (Chapter 18).

Congenital defects

Congenital defects are relatively uncommon in goats. Some, such as atresia ani and cleft palate, will be incompatible with satisfactory growth and development, unless they can be corrected surgically. Others will limit the ability of the kid to suckle and may lead to starvation, unless the condition is recognised and remedial measures taken.

Contracted tendons as a result of positional constraints in utero are relatively common. Except in severe cases, physiotherapy is usually sufficient to correct the problem. Excessive laxity and overextension of the leg joints is also a common temporary problem, which is usually self-correcting in a few days.

Congenital cardiac disease

Kids are infrequently clinically diagnosed with structural cardiac abnormalities. A *ventricular septal defect* (*VSD*) is the commonest reported congenital heart defect in kids. An *Ebstein's anomaly* (tricuspid valve dysplasia) and *atrial septal defect* were identified using echocardiography in a pygmy goat.

Clinical signs associated with congenital heart defects include exercise intolerance, lethargy, weakness, reduced growth rate and varying degrees of dyspnoea at rest or with exercise. The commonest murmur is a pansystolic murmur heard over the tricuspid valve on the right side of the thorax or bilaterally.

The normal heart rate for a kid is 120–140 beats/minute (adult rates of 70–100 beats/minute are attained by 3 months of age).

Small ventricular septal defects are occasionally identified in adult animals as incidental findings not apparently associated with clinical disease.

Portosystemic shunt

Stunted kids with intermittent neurological signs may have a portosystemic shunt, which, although uncommon, has been identified in kids of various breeds.

Post-natal malnutrition

Unless the kid is removed at birth and hand-reared, it is completely dependent on the doe for food. The kid has very limited energy reserves and a high energy requirement and so is totally dependent on the early intake of colostrum to maintain life. If the kid is unable to suckle easily, or the doe is unable or unwilling to feed the kid, the kid should be removed, dried, stomach tubed and then bottle-fed as necessary.

Post-natal infections

In the first few hours after birth, the kid is susceptible to infection from a number of infective agents, which gain access via the navel or mouth, resulting in infection of the navel, septicaemia, pyaemia, enteritis and joint ill. Possible organisms involved include *Escherichia coli*, *Clostridium perfringens* type B, *Staphylococcus aureus*, *Streptococcus* spp., *Corynebacterium* spp., *Salmonella* and rotavirus.

Many other organisms are potential pathogens. Infection is more likely in intensive kidding systems, particularly towards the end of the kidding period.

Floppy kid syndrome (metabolic acidosis without dehydration in kids)

Floppy kid disease (FKS) is a metabolic acidosis without dehydration, first reported in 1987. Affected kids are normal at birth, but develop sudden onset of profound muscular weakness (flaccid paresis or paralysis or ataxia) at 3 to 10 days of age. Kids show decreased muscle tone, anorexia and apathy.

Aetiology

- The cause is unknown; many kids may be affected at one time, but it is not known if the condition is infectious or contagious. Most cases occur late in the kidding season. The condition is reversible, suggesting a transient initiating cause.
- Morbidity tends to increase towards the end of the kidding season and ranges from 10 to > 50% in affected herds.
- Intensive milk feeding may predispose to this condition, but the condition also occurs in kids reared on their dam and in kids fed pasteurised and unpasteurised milk.
- It can occur in any breed, although Anglo-Nubians seem to be over-represented in the United Kingdom.
- *Clostridium botulinum*, *Escherichia coli* and *Caprine herpesvirus* have been proposed as candidate aetiological agents. These agents have not been definitively proven or excluded as potential causative agents.

Clinical signs

- The kid is normal at birth but develops sudden onset of profound muscular weakness (flaccid paresis or paralysis) or ataxia at 3 to 10 days of age (Plate 5.2).
- Affected kids show no signs of diarrhoea, respiratory disease or other signs referable to a specific organ system.
- The kids cannot use their tongues to suckle but can swallow.
- Spontaneous recovery, even of severely affected kids, may occur, but mortality can reach 30 to 50% in untreated cases.
- Most kids respond well to treatment, but there may be delayed recovery (4 to 6 weeks) of neuromuscular function. Occasional relapses may occur.
- In a group of kids, close attention should be paid to kids of a similar age. If one animal has noticeable signs, there may be others with mild ataxia or

muscular weakness. Early treatment improves the likelihood of recovery.

Note: any other profoundly weak or acidotic kid will appear floppy or limp so that the condition needs differentiating from white muscle disease, botulism, colibacillosis, septicaemia and enterotoxaemia.

Laboratory investigation

- Affected kids have a profound metabolic acidosis with a pH as low as 7 (normal 7.4 to 7.44), low bicarbonate and a base deficit of 20 mmol or more; sodium and chloride levels are normal but potassium is decreased in some kids.
- There are no detected repeatable biochemical abnormalities referable to specific organ systems (except mild renal changes in some cases).
- Serum concentrations of D-lactate are significantly higher in FKS kids (>7 mM) than in normal kids (approximately 0.3 mM) and the neurological signs have been ascribed to increased plasma D-lactate concentrations. In one study, the plasma concentration of L-lactate was significantly lower in the affected kids (0.67 versus 1.60 mM). However, there was no linear relationship between the anion gap and the D-lactate concentration, so other, unidentified, factors must be partially responsible for the increased anion gap.
- FKS kids had a significantly greater number of colony-forming unit (CFU) counts for enterococci, streptococci, staphylococci and lactobacilli than healthy kids. These groups of bacteria include several D-lactate-producing species, which makes dysbacteriosis a likely cause of the increased plasma D-lactate concentration in FKS. The cause of the dysbacteriosis is unclear.

Treatment

- Correction of the acidosis by administration of sodium bicarbonate (half a teaspoonful of baking soda) or liquid antacid such as Peptobismol or Gaviscon (30 ml).
- Mildly affected kids respond to oral bicarbonate or antacids if given at the onset of the disease. Some kids respond to one treatment, but others may require repeated administration of bicarbonate with supportive care and nursing. Milk can be fed by stomach tube.
- More severely affected kids require intravenous isotonic (1.26%) sodium bicarbonate to correct the

Table 5.3 Estimation of sodium bicarbonate required to correct electrolyte imbalance.

(Body weight in kg) $\times$ 0.5 $\times$ base deficit = mmol bicarbonate required

0.5 is the extracellular fluid volume (ECFV)
Base deficit = normal serum bicarbonate − patient's serum bicarbonate

Normal serum level = 25 nmol/litre
1 ml of 1.26% sodium bicarbonate = 0.15 mmol bicarbonate
One teaspoon of sodium bicarbonate provides 64 mmol of HCO_3

electrolyte imbalance, following electrolyte estima-tion where possible (Table 5.3) – approximately 125 to 200 ml over 1 to 3 hours.

If the serum bicarbonate level is not known, the correction must be empirical. In mild acidosis, the base deficit is about 5 mmol/litre; in severe acidosis, the base deficit is 10 nmol/litre or more. The volume of 1.26% bicarbonate required may range from 125 to 200 ml and this should be given over 1 to 3 hours. Overtreatment with intravenous bicarbonate causes clinical depression so it is better to be conservative when estimating the base deficit and finish correcting the acidosis with oral sodium bicarbonate.

- Antibiotic therapy can be used empirically because of the possiblity of an underlying bacterial cause – trimet-hoprim and sulfonamide, 24 mg/kg i.m. or s.c. daily for 3 days; long-acting amoxicillin, 15 mg/kg i.m.

Exposure

Primary hypothermia

Primary hypothermia is caused by direct exposure of kids to cold, wet, windy weather so that heat loss exceeds heat production. Small kids have a relatively large surface area relative to body weight and rela-tively small energy reserves and so are more prone to hypothermia than large kids.

Secondary hypothermia

Most kids who die from hypothermia succumb to sec-ondary hypothermia, where the neonates are unable to suckle and replenish their body reserves in weather that is insufficiently cold to kill through primary hypother-mia. Thus, mismothering, agalactia, birth injury, failure of milk letdown by the mother, etc., can all lead to death from secondary hypothermia.

Treatment depends on age and body temperature, so the degree of hypothermia should always be measured by means of a rectal thermometer. Hypothermic kids over 5 hours old will be hypoglycaemic and must have the hypoglycaemia reversed by intraperitoneal admin-istration of glucose (discussed later) before warming. If the hypoglycaemia is not reversed, the increased cerebral metabolism, produced by warming, will lead to convulsions and death.

A kid of any age, 37–39 °C:
- Dry the kid.
- Give colostrum by bottle or stomach tube.
- Return to the mother if she is interested in mothering the kid.

Hypothermic kids under 5 hours old, temperature <37 °C:
- Dry thoroughly.
- Warm to >37 °C over 30 to 60 minutes.
- Give colostrum by bottle or stomach tube.

Hypothermic kid over 5 hours old, temperature <37 °C, able to hold its head up:
- Dry thoroughly.
- Warm to >37 °C over 30 to 60 minutes.
- Give glucose or 20% glucose solution by stomach tube.

Hypothermic kid over 5 hours old, temperature <37 °C, unable to hold its head up:
- Dry thoroughly.
- Hypothermic kids over 5 hours old will be hypogly-caemic.

Do not warm until the hypoglycaemia is reversed using *10 ml/kg of 20% glucose* by intraperitoneal injection, that is large kid (single) 50 ml, medium kid (twin) 35 ml, small kid (triplet) 25 ml. Glucose normally comes as a 40% solution, which needs diluting 1:1 with sterile water (recently boiled water from the kettle is adequate in an emergency, once it has cooled to blood heat).

Holding the kid by its front legs, inject 1 cm to the side and 2 cm behind the umbilicus (i.e. towards the anus), with the needle directed at a 45° angle towards the rump, using a 50 ml syringe and 19 g 25 mm needle.

Hyperthermic kids are best warmed in controlled temperature hot air boxes with air at 37–40 °C, using a domestic fan heater. A household thermometer near the kid should be used to monitor the temperature. Heat lamps do not allow the rate of warming to be controlled and may cause skin burns or overheating. Heat lamps are, however, suitable for maintaining the environmental temperature, once the kid is revived and fed.

Colostrum

> After birth, feeding colostrum is the single most important event in any kid's life.

Each kid should receive colostrum within the first 6 hours of birth, preferably during the first hour, either directly from the dam or by bottle or stomach tube (discussed later). Within hours of parturition, the kid's ability to utilise the colostrum is reduced and the quality of the colostrum from the doe becomes poorer, as she begins to produce normal milk. Colostrum should be fed at a rate of *50 to 75 ml/kg* three times during the first day. Anything that increases the kid's requirement for heat production, such as chilling, increases the demand for colostrum. Housed kids require about 210 ml/kg during the first day, while kids outside in inclement weather require around 280 ml/kg/day (Table 5.4). Failure to absorb adequate amounts of colostrum leads to high mortality rates in young kids.

Colostrum has many functions:

- Laxative: aids excretion of the meconium and stimulates the digestive system.

Table 5.4 Colostrum requirements for newborn kids.

Weight of housed kid	First feed	Daily requirement
3 kg	150 to 200 ml	600 ml
4 kg	200 to 300 ml	850 ml
5 kg	250 to 475 ml	1100 ml

- Nutritional: provides carbohydrates and proteins, whilst the high fat content is an excellent energy source, rich in fat soluble vitamins (β-carotene, retinol and α-tocopherol).
- Protective: colostrum is a rich source of immunoglobulins, Ig. There are three major classes of immunoglobulins, IgG, IgM and IgA. Immunoglobulin G is further subdivided on physiochemical properties into IgG1 and IgG2. The Ig antibodies provide the kid with passive immunity until its own immune system begins functioning at about 3 weeks of age. High levels of antibodies, particularly IgG1, are produced by the dam in the weeks before parturition and preferentially transported into the colostrum. This process may start as many as 8 weeks before parturition, so that a short dry period may markedly depress the immunoglobulin concentration in colostrum. Similarly, colostrum from aborted goats is likely to be of poor quality.
- The newborn kid is capable of transporting intact Ig molecules from the colostrum across the intestinal wall into its bloodstream, where it becomes circulating antibody protecting against general infection. This ability to absorb intact antibodies declines rapidly in the hours after birth, although it may be longer in the kid than the calf or lamb. The concentration of antibody in colostrum declines rapidly after the first 6 to 12 hours after birth. Pre-partum milking to relieve udder congestion, oedema or discomfort mimics these changes and the immunoglobulin concentration will be much lower by the time of parturition. Even leakage of colostrum from the udder before kidding will result in lower immunoglobulin levels.
- There are both individual and breed variations in the level of antibodies in colostrum. Older does have a wider immunological experience than young does and provide a wider spectrum of protective antibodies to their kids. Because the dairy breeds produce larger amounts of colostrum than non-dairy breeds, the IgG concentration in their kids' serum is often considerably higher.
- Colostrum also contains small amounts of IgA and IgM, providing some local protection, particularly in the intestine.
- The half-life of passively acquired antibodies is approximately 12 days, with most kids still having detectable antibodies for 5 to 6 weeks. High levels

Table 5.5 Factors preventing adequate colostral transfer to the newborn kid.

Maternal factors	Management factors	Kid factors
Short dry period	Milking before parturition	Weakness
Abortion/prematurity	Leakage of colostrum	Anoxia
Breed	Overcrowding	Prematurity
Parity	Lack of supervision	Competition for teats
Yield	Failure to stomach tube	
Litter size		
Udder shape		
Mothering ability		

of antibody can prevent an adequate response to vaccination.

- Contains hormones, growth factors, cytokines, enzymes, polyamines and nucleotides, which are able to exert biological effects and may influence gastrointestinal tract development and function.
- Helps prevent hypothermia.

Even when the dam has plenty of colostrum of good quality, various factors can prevent adequate uptake of colostrum by the kid (Table 5.5). Prolonged parturition or caesarian section may result in a weak or anoxic kid that is disinclined to search for the teat, and a mother that is unable to mother the kid. First kidders may inadequately stimulate the kids to the suck or indeed even refuse to stand to be suckled. Kidding unsupervised in overcrowded conditions may lead to mismothering. Kids have difficulty suckling goats with pendulous udders or conical teats.

Wherever possible the kid should receive its mother's colostrum, but if this is not available, frozen stored colostrum, cow's colostrum or commercial lamb colostrum substitute can be used. Colostrum or milk from other herds should never be used if there is a danger of introducing diseases such as caprine arthritis encephalitis virus. After the first day, the kid can receive goat's milk or milk replacer. Cow, lamb and calf milk replacers can all be successfully used to rear kids.

Frozen colostrum from the first milking of mature CAE negative does can be stored for 12 months or more and fed to kids whose own dams are unable to supply sufficient colostrum. Yoghurt pots or pint milk containers are convenient for storage. Containers should be labelled with the date and the name of the donor. Colostrum from mature does has a higher level of antibodies and provides greater passive immunity than that from first kidders. Only colostrum taken during the first 12 hours of kidding should be stored. There appears to be a strong correlation between the Ig concentration of colostrum and its specific gravity; s.g. > 1.029 is preferable. The colostrum should be allowed to thaw gradually, without applying direct heat, to avoid destroying the antibodies. Once thawed, the colostrum should be used immediately. Microwave thawing should not be used as it reduces the immunoglobulin concentration, as does repeated freezing and thawing.

Fermented colostrum can also be stored. Surplus colostrum is stored in a cool place in a clean container like a plastic dustbin with an open top, which allows the colostrum to breathe, but covered with gauze or muslin to prevent contamination from flies. Fresh colostrum can be added as it becomes available. Stir the colostrum daily. It will ferment but can be used for about 3 months. Mix one part hot water to three parts colostrum and feed as for fresh colostrum.

In herds where CAE, Johne's disease or mycoplasmosis control measures are in place, either the colostrum should be heat-treated for 30 minutes at 63 °C in a conventional 'batch' pasteuriser (see Chapter 23) or an alternative source of colostrum supplied:

- For cow colostrum, consider heat treatment as cow colostrum could transmit diseases such as salmonellosis and cryptosporidosis. It may also produce anaemia by destruction of the kid's red blood cells. Cow colostrum will not confer passive immunity to diseases such as enterotoxaemia, tetanus, caseous lymphadenitis and orf.
- Commercial colostrum substitutes may be of limited value if inadequate passive immunity is produced in the kids.

Feeding by stomach tube

Attempting to bottle feed a weak or comatose kid may lead to regurgitation and inhalation pneumonia. Any kids that are not sucking well should be fed by stomach tube using a lamb stomach tube and 60 ml syringe. An 18-French feeding tube or a urethral catheter long enough to reach the last rib can be utilised in an emergency.

Moisten and warm the tube and pass it straight into the kid's mouth. The end of the tube can be felt passing down the neck, external to the trachea. Inset the tube to the level of the last rib and inject the colostrum slowly. Kids should be fed at the rate of 50 ml/kg or until the stomach feels full.

Further reading

General

Anon (1982) Detection and treatment of hypothermia in newborn lambs. *In Pract.*, **4** (1), 20–22.

Bales, A. (1987) Feeding lambs by stomach tube. *In Pract.*, **9** (1), 18–20.

Bales, A. and Small, J. (1986) *Practical Lambing*. Longman, London.

Matthews, J.G. (1985) Care of the newborn kid. *Goat Vet. Soc. J.*, **6** (2), 64–67.

Matthews, H. (2009) Kid rearing in small herd. *Goat Vet. Soc. J.*, **25**, 99–103.

Papworth, S.M. (1981) The young kid. *Goat Vet. Soc. J.*, **2** (2), 12–15.

Colostrum

Bentley, J. Colostrum management for the dairy goat kid. Available at: https://www.extension.iastate.edu/dairyteam/sites/www.extension.iastate.edu/files/dairyteam/DairyGoatColostrumManagementFactsheet.pdf.

White, D.G. (1993) Colostral supplementation in ruminants. *Comp. Cont. Ed. Pract. Vet.*, **15** (2), 335–342.

Congenital heart disease

Laus, F., Copponi, I., Cerquetella, M. and Fruganti, A. (2011) Congenital cardiac defect in a pygmy goat (*Capra hircus*). *Turk. J. Vet. Anim. Sci.*, **35** (6), 471–475.

Copper disorders

Laven, R. (2014) Do my goats need more copper? *Goat Vet. Soc. J.*, **30**, 69–73.

Livesey, C.T. (2011) Copper disorders in ruminants. *Goat Vet. Soc. J.*, **27**, 56–70.

Suttle, N.F. (ed.) (2010) *Mineral Nutrition of Livestock*, 4th edition, Chapter 11: Copper, pp. 255–305. CAB International, Wallingford, Oxford.

Floppy kid syndrome

Bleul, U. *et al.* (2006) Floppy kid syndrome caused by D-lactic acidosis in goat kids. *J. Vet. Internal Med.*, **20** (4), 1003–1008

Bleul, U. *et al.* (2013) Quantitative analysis of fecal flora in goat kids with and without floppy kid syndrome. *J. Vet. Internal Med.*, **27** (5), 1283–1286.

Lorenz, I. and Arrcangelo, G. (2014) D-lactic acidosis in neonatal ruminants. *Vet. Clin. North. Amer.: Food Anim. Pract.*, **30** (2), 317–331.

Neurogenetic disorders

Clavijo, A. *et al.* (2010) Diagnosis of caprine mucopolysaccharidosis type iiiD by real-time polymerase chain reaction-based genotyping. *J. Vet. Diagn. Invest.*, **22**, 622–627.

Jones, M.Z. *et al.* (1998) Caprine mucopolysaccharidosis-IIID: clinical, biochemical, morphological and immunohistochemical characteristics. *J. Neuropathol. Exp. Neurol.*, **157** (2), 148–157.

Windsor, P.A., Kessell, A.E. and Finnie, J.W. (2011) Review of neurological diseases of ruminant livestock in Australia. VI: postnatal bovine, and ovine and caprine, neurogenetic disorders. *Australian Vet. J.*, **89**, 432–438.

Portosystemic shunt

Kinde, H. *et al.* (2014) Congenital portosystemic shunts and hepatic encephalopathy in goat kids in California. *J. Vet. Diagn. Invest.*, **26** (1), 173–177.

CHAPTER 6

Inadequate growth rate

Initial assessment

The preliminary history should produce an overall picture of the management system and information on the specific problem. Consider:

- Individual or flock/herd problem.
- Birth weight and weaning weights if available.
- Kidding and weaning percentages.
- Kids reared on dam or artificially.
- Age of kids when ill-thrift first noticed.
- Age of kids at weaning.
- Feeding of weaned kids.
- Management and feeding of lactating does.
- Body condition of does.
- Age distribution of does (particularly maidens and aged animals).
- Disease history of kids, particularly diarrhoea and pneumonia.
- Trace element supplementation of does and kids.
- Pasture fertilisation and lime applications.
- Anthelmintic treatments – dose rates and types of drench.

Clinical examination

- Examine the herd for evidence of parasitism or undernutrition:
  - Body condition – weights of kids should be checked.
- Individual kids (and their dams) should be examined in detail for evidence of clinical disease:
  - Diarrhoea
  - Respiratory problems
  - Lameness
  - Anaemia
  - Submandibular or ventral oedema.

- Individual does may have evidence of mastitis, metritis, teat lesions or other chronic disease resulting in a low milk yield.

Laboratory investigations

Specific laboratory tests undertaken will depend on the suspected causes(s) of poor growth.
  Blood tests:
- Haematology – haemoglobin, PCV.
- Serum biochemistry – plasma proteins, liver enzymes.
- Trace elements – copper, selenium, vitamin B12.
  Faecal tests:
- Worm egg counts (Chapter 14). If anthelmintic resistance is suspected a faecal egg count reduction test should be carried out.
- Coccidial oocyst counts.

Post-mortem examination

Post-mortem examination of poorly thriving kids can provide information on:

- Abomasal damage + presence of *Haemonchus* and *Teladorsagia* nematodes. Total worm counts may be required to assess their significance and recent treatment with an anthelmintic could have reduced their numbers.
  It also permits:
- Trace element estimations (copper, selenium, vitamin B12) on the liver.
- Histological examination of the gastrointestinal tract, liver, etc.

Diseases of the Goat, Fourth Edition. John Matthews.
© 2016 John Wiley & Sons, Ltd. Published 2016 by John Wiley & Sons, Ltd.

Pre-natal growth

The effects of the *in utero* environment and fetal programming on post-natal performance have been investigated in sheep and it appears that maternal nutrition during pregnancy, maternal size, parity of the ewe and the number of lambs, amongst other factors, contribute to birth weight and thus weaning size (see below).

Birth to weaning

Aim: rapid growth to economically produce a healthy well-grown kid with good rumen development.

Target weight gain: *180–200 g/day* (range 140–250 g/day on different rearing systems), that is *1.5 kg/week* in a well-managed system.

Birth weights

Birth weights are very variable, ranging from over 7 kg for a single male down to 2 or 3 kg in multiple births. An average birth weight of >3.5 kg is desirable for any kid being reared as a replacement (optimum birth weights: singles 4.5 kg, twins 4 kg, triplets 3.5 kg, quadruplets or more 3 kg). Birth weight is important as the larger the kid at birth the faster the growth rate.

Low birth weights may arise as a result of:
- Undernutrition of the dam during the last trimester of pregnancy:
  o Check body condition scores of the does.
- Multiple births:
  o Limited placental placentation is available for each developing fetus.
- Prematurity as a result of infectious agents such as *Toxoplasma*, *Chlamydophila*, etc., causing subcritical placentitis:
  o Associated abortions and/or barren does.
- Prematurity for any other reason.

Pre-weaning performance should be evaluated by regular weighing and evaluating the daily live weight gain. Regular weighing of the growing kids allows early corrective measures to be taken, such as batching of small kids, delaying weaning, increasing concentrate feeding and giving anticoccidial treatment.

Weight corrections are possible within certain limits by increasing the energy and protein intake but, below certain levels, culling may be indicated.

Weigh kids at birth, weaning, 4 months, mating.

Poor growth in individual kids <4 weeks being reared on their mother

There are many causes of poor growth in individual unweaned kids including:
- Inadequate milk supply:
  o Poor nutrition of the dam – inadequate supplementary feeding before and after parturition, overstocked pasture.
  o Low milk yield.
  o Inadequate milk for multiple kids.
  o Mastitis.
  o Any infectious disease resulting in a drop in milk yield.
  o Post-parturient conditions such as metritis and laminitis.
- Inability of the kid(s) to suckle:
  o Mismothering or rejection – occurs most commonly in housed goats under conditions of high stocking density when they are unable to isolate themselves from the rest of the herd during first stage labour; in goats kept under extensive conditions, disturbance of kidding may disrupt maternal bonding; rejection may occur after handling goats for worming, etc.
  o Teat lesions – pain may cause dam to stop kid suckling.
  o Competition for teats – kid may be stopped from sucking by stronger siblings.
- Failure of the kid to suckle:
  o Congenital lesions – cleft palate.
  o Mouth lesions – orf (see Chapter 9).
  o Disease – septicaemia, joint ill.

Poor growth in groups of kids <4 weeks being reared on their mother

- Inadequate milk supply:
  o Poor nutrition of goats during late pregnancy and early lactation. Investigate nutrition before and after kidding. Underfeeding during the last third of pregnancy resulting in restricted udder development and reduced lactation yield may be more important

than mild undernutrition during early lactation. Underfeeding does in late pregnancy will also reduce the amount of colostrum available for the kids.

- Disease:
  - ○ Coccidiosis. Although diarrhoea is likely to be a major presenting sign, some kids may be tucked-up with rough coats and lethargy (see Chapter 14).
  - ○ Copper deficiency. In growing kids, copper deficiency may result in poor live weight gain. Other clinical signs include rough hair coat, anaemia, conjunctivitis, diarrhoea, conjunctivitis and increased susceptibility to bacterial infections and fractures. Newborn kids in the herd may have swayback and older kids enzootic ataxia (see Chapter 5).
  - ○ Orf lesions on the does' teats and kids' lips may restrict suckling (see Chapter 10).

Poor growth in groups of kids <4 weeks being artificially reared

- Problems with the milk replacer (see below).
- Disease:
  - ○ Coccidiosis.
  - ○ Copper deficiency.
  - ○ Orf.

Artificial rearing of kids

As the raison d'être for most dairy goats is the production of milk for the household or sale, kids will generally be removed from their mothers at a few days of age and raised on whole milk or milk replacer (Plate 6.1).

Kids can successfully be removed at birth, if the kid is sickly, one of a multiple litter, the dam is ill or, in the case of some first kidders, aggressive to her young, but it is usual to leave the kid on its dam (Plate 6.2) for at least four days of age to encourage maximum colostrum intake (Chapter 5). Removal of the kid at day 5 enables disbudding to take place on the 4th day and the kid to be returned to its dam for a further 24 hours before final separation, thus minimising the stress factor for the kid. Should any problems occur post-disbudding, the kid will respond better to maternal rather than human stimulation.

What milk?

There appears to be very little difference in the growth rate of kids reared by their dams and kids reared artificially, unless they are weaned at an early age (<35 days) when dam-fed kids are heavier. Kids will grow equally well on goat milk or good quality milk replacer. The key factor determining growth rate is the quality of the milk (fat content and dry matter content).

- Feeding whole milk is more popular for small-scale goatkeepers (with no caprine arthritis encephalitis problems in their herds) than feeding milk replacer. Kids fed on whole milk generally have fewer digestive problems and less bloating than those fed on milk replacer.
- Feeding milk replacer allows the goats' milk to be marketed and, provided management is good, is a practical alternative to whole milk at a much cheaper cost. Table 6.1 gives a suitable analysis for milk replacer for kids.
- Kids perform best on replacers where the protein is 100% milk protein, so that, in general, better results are obtained with milk replacers that contain a high skimmed milk powder content (>45% analysis) than with cheaper alternatives.

  Whey/soya-based products, which contain high levels of lactose, are cheaper but less digestible, more likely to cause bloat and diarrhoea, are often a false economy and should be avoided.
- The fat (oil) content of the replacer is basically used by the goat as an energy source. The type of fat does not appear to be as important as the type of protein – kids have been reared successfully on animal and vegetable fat.
- Milk substitutes for calves and lambs normally contain 22–26% protein and 12–24% fat. Goat's milk has a similar composition and energy value to cow's milk, whereas sheep's milk has a higher fat and protein content but a much lower lactose content; 22% protein is a perfectly adequate level for kid rearing.

  Fat levels depend on quality rather than the total %, but are optimal at 16–22%. It is advisable not to exceed 22% fat in the milk replacer for the first few weeks of feeding and never to exceed 30%.

Table 6.1 Milk replacer for rearing female dairy kids.

High skimmed milk powder (>45%)
22% protein, 16–22% fat (oil)
125g/litre (12.5% DM)

- Growth performance is similar on goat, lamb or calf milk replacer, provided it is of good quality. However, sheep and goat milk replacers are generally more expensive than cow replacers.
- Milk replacers that give good results for calves are likely to be equally suitable for kids, but should be fed at a 50% increase on the recommended rate for calves.
- All milk replacers should be fed at a concentration of 125 g/litre or 12.5% dry matter.
- Male kids being reared for meat will grow faster if fed at 150 g/litre but this increases the total cost (although not the cost per kg).
- Some replacers are formulated to be fed warm, others cold. Some contain growth promotants, which may improve feed conversion efficiency and thus increase weight gain.

Problems with milk replacers

Most problems with milk replacers are caused by management failures leading to poor milk clot formation in the abomasum, resulting in poorly digested milk reaching the small intestine.

- Failure to follow the manufacturer's instructions:
  o Failure to mix the powder adequately – use a whisk or electric mixer.
  o Incorrect mixing temperature:
    ◆ Milk clotting time in the abomasum is increased; a reduction of 6 °C will double the time taken for the clot to form.
    ◆ Fat is poorly dispersed, which results in a valuable energy component being lost and fat floating on the surface of the milk sticks to the nose and muzzle of the kid, causing hair loss.
    ◆ Proteins and minerals are wasted by sinking to the bottom of the mixing container.
    ◆ Poor oesophageal groove closure, so milk passes into the rumen.
  o Diluting the milk powder; the correct strength milk powder should *always* be fed.
- Poor quality milk substitutes with low or zero levels of skimmed milk powder.
- Powder overheated during manufacture.

Very strict hygiene should be observed, with all feeding and mixing equipment thoroughly cleaned on a regular basis, using dairy detergent or dilute hypochlorite solutions.

> **When feeding kids milk replacer**
>
> Feed the correct *amount* of properly *mixed* milk, at the correct *strength* and the correct *temperature*.

Warm or cold milk?

- Milk can be fed cold (refrigerated), at room temperature or warm (34–40 °C). Warm milk is usually used with bottle feeding or for simple group-feeding units where the quantity fed is restricted to set amounts at set times of the day. With automatic feeding units, feeding cold or cool milk prevents kids from drinking large quantities of milk at a time, reducing digestive problems and bloat. Milk dispensing machines feeding warm milk utilise a lot of milk replacer and so are more expensive.
- Cold milk feeding can be introduced from about a week of age. Initially, the change to cold milk will reduce the kid's intake but this will increase to normal after a short period. Cold feeding is less labour intensive than feeding warm milk and hygiene is easier to maintain as bacterial growth is reduced, so the equipment requires less frequent cleaning.

How much milk?

- There are as many feeding regimes for kids as there are goatkeepers. Depending on the production system, kids are fed milk from birth to as little as 6 weeks or less in some early weaning systems or six months or longer when the kid is reared by its mother. Tables 6.2 to 6.4 indicate feeding schedules for 12, 10 and 6 week weanings, respectively.
- Although, at first, the size of the abomasum is a limiting factor, as the abomasum expands the upper desirable daily intake of around 2 litres/kid/day is reached between the 7th and 10th days. If allowed to, older kids on *ad lib* systems will take 3 litres or more/day

Table 6.2 Feed schedule for 12 week weaning.

Age (weeks)	Daily milk feeds
1	4 ×
2–6	3 ×
6–10	2
10–12	1 ×
13	No milk

Table 6.3 Feed schedule for 10 week weaning (Mowlem, 1984).

Age (weeks)	Daily milk feeds
1–6	3 × 750 ml
7–8	2 × 850 ml
9	2 × 570 ml
10	1 – 570 ml
11	No milk

Table 6.4 Feed schedule for 6 week weaning (Mowlem, 1984).

Age (weeks)	Daily milk feeds
1–4	*Ad libitum*
5	Half amount consumed on last day of week 4
6	Half amount consumed on last day of week 5
7	No milk

but this is unnecessary, expensive and may retard dry feed intake and rumen development.

■ Kids initially fed more frequently will grow faster than kids fed twice daily.

Poor growth from 4 weeks to weaning

Apart from inadequate nutrition, the major causes of growth setbacks in this age of kid are *parasitic disease – coccidiosis* (check faeces samples for oocysts) and *gastrointestinal nematodes* (check faeces for eggs) (see Chapter 14) – and other *chronic diseases*, particularly pneumonia.

Copper deficiency in growing kids may result in poor live weight gain; other clinical signs include rough hair coat, anaemia, conjunctivitis, diarrhoea, conjunctivitis and increased susceptibility to bacterial infections and fractures. Newborn kids may have swayback and older kids enzootic ataxia (see Chapter 5).

Genetic disease such as *mucopolysaccharidosis* may not be apparent at birth and present as poor growth with decreased muscle mass (see Chapter 5).

Weight at weaning is more important than age at weaning.

■ Kids can be weaned when they have reached about 10 kg, but special care and excellent nutrition is required. The earlier the weaning age, the greater the weaning shock, and a *weaning weight of >15 kg* is preferable.

■ Although kids can be weaned as young as 5 or 6 weeks, a weaning age of 8 weeks is probably preferable in most commercial dairy situations and show kids where early growth is important will often be weaned later at 12 weeks and a weaning weight of >19 kg. In extensively managed herds, kidding over about a six week period, kids can be weaned at 13 weeks after the start of kidding.

■ Prolonging milk feeding beyond 12 weeks may restrict rumen development and the future productivity of the goat.

■ In a commercial system, any kid weighing less than 12 kg at 8 weeks should be culled. For kids between 12 and 15 kg, weaning should be delayed and milk feeding continued until the kid is 15 kg.

■ There appears to be no reason to wean kids abruptly. Less weaning stress is produced by gradual withdrawal of milk by restricting the amount fed and the number of feeds per day.

Pre-weaning solid feeding

At birth, the digestive system of the kid is very similar to that of the dog or human. The abomasum and small intestine have major roles in digestion, as the rumen is small, rudimentary and non-functional and the kid is totally dependent on milk to provide its nutritional needs, as kids cannot digest solid feed until the rumen develops.

Kids will pick at straw and hay from about 10–14 days of age. At first this is rejected, but gradually increasing amounts are swallowed. Some of these solid feeds remain in the rumen, leading to the development of the microbial population and beginning the change from the pre-ruminant phase, dependent on the abomasum for digestion, to the ruminant as the rumen–reticulum and large intestine increase rapidly in size. Fibrous foods, in particular, encourage rumen growth and the development of the muscles of the rumen wall. Rumination is obvious by about the third week of life. However, somewhat counterintuitively, there is a substantial body of scientific evidence that fermentation of forage does not influence the epithelial development of the rumen. Rather it is the fermentation of sugar and starch sources that generates propionate and butyrate volatile fatty acids. Butyrate is metabolised by the rumen epithelial cells, stimulating their development and growth. It is essential that the kid is consuming adequate amounts of concentrate before weaning. As the developing rumen has only a limited capacity, only good quality forage should be fed during the pre-weaning period and an adequate daily concentrate intake must be encouraged before allowing access to forage. Overfeeding of forage before weaning delays rumen papillae development, delaying the transition to a ruminating animal.

At 8 weeks, a weaned kid has a reticulorumen capacity five times as large as suckling kids of the same age. In the adult goat, the rumen has about ten times the volume of the abomasum.

At weaning, kids must be consuming adequate amounts of high quality food:

- Bed on clean *straw*.
- Offer good quality fibrous *hay ad lib*. The intake should be at least *200–300g/day/kid* at weaning. Kids are very selective and wasteful with poor quality hay. The hay should be offered in some type of wall-mounted rack, never in a net, as kids easily become entangled and may strangle themselves or break a leg. The mesh in racks should be of such a size as to prevent heads becoming trapped.
- By weaning, kids can be started on *silage* if available.
- After the second week of life introduce *concentrates*. The ration should contain a minimum of *11 MJ of metabolic energy* and *180g crude protein /kg dry matter (18%)*, with adequate vitamins and minerals. This can be a proprietary feed or a mixture of ¾ cereals + ¼ soya + mineral/vitamin mix.
- Any feed formulated for calf or lamb rearing is suitable for kids. Although it is often easier to start kids on a coarse mixture, they pick at the mix and leave the protein/mineral pellets. Introducing grower or milk cubes as early as possible or starting with lamb starter pellets, followed by cubes, will reduce wastage.
- Between 2 and 4 weeks, maximum feed intake starts to be efficiently regulated by energy density. Initially concentrates should be offered *ad lib* and changed regularly to maintain the kids' interest and prevent soiling.
- 0.5 kg weight gain can be expected for each 1.8–3.2 kg of feed consumed.
- At weaning, kids should generally be eating *70–80g* of concentrate feed/day and some older kids will eat considerably more. For early weaned kids, 30–50 g is sufficient.
- Wherever possible, food containers should be raised from the floor to limit faecal soiling.
- Clean *water*, changed once or twice daily, must be available at all times as soon as the kids start eating solid food.

Housing

Although kids can be successfully reared in groups of up to 25 kids per pen, rearing kids in smaller groups of *6–10 per pen* means that individual kids are more easily observed, making management easier. Rearing large numbers of kids together before weaning requires a high standard of management and kids in large groups are more prone to digestive and respiratory problems and growth setbacks.

Overcrowding must be avoided, as goats at the top of the dominance hierarchy will consume more than their allotted ration, with a risk of acidosis developing, whilst subordinate goats will be deprived:

- *0.6 m²/kid* is required if the kids are to remain in the same pen until weaning.
- *12–15 cm/kid* of trough space is required up to 8 weeks and *30 cm/weaned kid*.

Grazing

Goats require tall (up to 7 cm), high quality pasture to achieve high intakes and perform well. Recommendations are to graze no closer than 4 cm in winter. At this height, doe performance is limited slightly but subsequent kid birth weight and survival are not reduced and sufficient pasture is available for feeding during lactation. Does will not readily graze below 2 cm. Kidding should be timed to coincide with reasonable pasture growth, that is later in the year than for sheep.

The kids should be introduced to grass gradually and turnout should preferably be on to 'clean' pasture, that is pasture which no goats grazed the previous year. High rates of kid growth are achieved on leafy, green pasture with a residual grazing height of about 5 cm.

Kids are more susceptible than adult goats to gastrointestinal worms and especial care should be taken to prevent them acquiring a significant worm burden (see Chapter 14).

- Turnout on to rich spring pasture can cause digestive upsets, disturb the balance of the rumen microflora and produce checks in weight gain.

■ Over-reliance on grass can result in low live weight gains, particularly in the late summer when the quality and quantity of the grass decline, so supplementary feeding of roughage and concentrates will be necessary.

■ Overstocking:
  ○ Poaching and spoilage, particularly in wet weather, can reduce both the availability and palatability of grazing.
  ○ Overgrazing will also increase the risk of coccidiosis and ingestion of nematode larvae.

■ Late kids may not grow well and remain permanently stunted. This is often due to a combination of the poor quality of the summer pasture available to the dams and to the kids after weaning and pasture contamination with gastrointestinal nematodes.

Weaning shock

■ Weaning is potentially stressful for all kids and can be accompanied by reduced growth, failure to grow or even loss of weight, depending on the age and weight of the kids and the intake of solid food before weaning. The magnitude of weaning shock seems to be more related to the weight than the age of the kid. Kids with a high intake of solid feed experience less growth check than those with lower intakes.

■ Male kids are reportedly more susceptible to weaning shock than females.

■ Healthy kids experience less weaning shock than those being challenged by diseases like coccidiosis.

Poor growth after weaning

> Poor growth after weaning is essentially a management problem.
> Weights should continue to be monitored after weaning.

Goats kidding at under 2 years will continue to grow during their first, and probably up to their third, lactation.

The productivity of goats is maximised when they are fed diets of high digestibility, which encourage a high level of digestible energy intake and contain sufficient nitrogen and trace minerals to enable rapid growth. Table 6.5 gives target weights for dairy goats and Table 6.6 target weights for fibre and meat goats.

Feeding good quality roughage with a high roughage to concentrate ratio will:

■ Encourage rumen development.
■ Produce a strong well grown frame.
■ Maintain steady growth.

Table 6.5 Target weights for dairy goats.

Birth (kg)	6 months (kg)	1 year (kg)	18 months (kg)	Mature (kg)
3.0–4.5	Does 25–40	Does 45–60	Does 50–75	Does 55–105
	Bucks 30–45	Bucks 50–70	Bucks 60–80	Bucks 75–120

Table 6.6 Target weights for fibre and meat goats. From Thompson (1990).

	Birth (kg)	6 months (kg)	1 year (kg)	18 months (kg)	Mature (kg)
Angora Australasian	2.5–3.0	Does 15–20	Does 22–27	Does 27–35	Does 40–50
		Bucks 18–25	Bucks 28–35	Bucks 40–50	Bucks 55–65
Angora South African/Texan	2.8–3.3	Does 18–25	Does 28–33	Does 35–45	Does 50–60
		Bucks 23–30	Bucks 35–45	Bucks 45–55	Bucks 70–90
Cashmere/ Cashgora	2.5–.0	Does 13–18	Does 20–25	Does 25–30	Does 35–65
		Bucks 16–23	Bucks 25–33	Bucks 35–45	Bucks 50–60
Meat breeds	3.5–4.5	Does 25–30	Does 35–45	Does 45–55	Does 55–65
		Bucks 30–35	Bucks 50–60	Bucks 60–70	Bucks 80–100

After weaning, housed kids should be grouped into batches of up to 15 animals, according to size and weight. The level of feeding, particularly the amount of concentrate, can then be adjusted to the condition of the kids to produce a desirable growth rate for each group. Overfeeding concentrates will result in an overfat goat with poor rumen development.

Rearing similar sized animals together, and allowing adequate trough space per kid, prevents bullying and results in even growth throughout the group.

Before mating, the goats should be in settled, homogeneous groups, so that stress is at a minimum for the critical first month of gestation. Mating should be delayed in any kids that have not reached the requisite weight.

Extensively reared weaners should be grazed on high quality pastures, utilising fresh pastures at the beginning of any rotational system (before being grazed by older animals) and hay aftermath if available.

Poor performance at this stage of growth may be multifactorial in origin. The main causes of poor growth are:

- Nutritional:
  o Inadequate or inappropriate forage and/or concentrates. Only high quality forage and grains/concentrates should be fed to weaners; review the feeding regime and quality of forage being fed.
  o Poor grazing or overstocked pasture after weaning. Check the amount of pasture available and grazing history since weaning. The kids' rumens have insufficient capacity to deal with poor quality forage. If the nitrogen content of the feed is very low, the kid will have to use muscle protein to maintain rumen microbial digestion and will lose weight.
- Disease:
  o Chronic gastrointestinal parasitism. Check faecal egg counts (but recently wormed animals may have negative counts) and consider anthelmintic resistance. Take blood samples for pepsinogen and albumin content (may indicate chronic gastric damage) and haematology (anaemia from Haemonchosis). Monitoring daily live weight gain has a key role in sustainable parasite control. Reduced live weight gains, as well as clinical signs of diarrhoea or anaemia, are indicative of possible heavy worm burdens.
  o Other chronic diseases, for example pneumonia, will limit growth.

o Trace element deficiencies. Deficiencies of cobalt (Chapter 8) and copper (Chapter 5) are both possible causes of poor growth in this age group in grazing animals. If conserved forage is from the same pastures that are being grazed, any micronutrient deficiency will be aggravated.

- ◆ Cobalt deficiency. Clinical signs most commonly observed in growing kids after weaning are lethargy, poor appetite, small size, and poor body condition despite adequate nutrition. *White liver syndrome*, attributed to cobalt deficiency, has been described in New Zealand in grazing Angora and Angora-cross goats between 4 and 18 months of age (generally 4 to 6 months), although it has not been described in the United Kingdom or the United States. It is a form of fatty liver disease, resulting in widespread fatty changes in the liver. As well as the signs of cobalt deficiency described above, a secondary hepatic encephalopathy may develop. Photosensitisation, as described in sheep, has not been reported in goats.
- ◆ Copper deficiency. In growing kids, copper deficiency may result in poor live weight gain.
- ◆ Iodine, selenium and phosphorus deficiencies will also cause ill-thrift.

o Severe ectoparasite infestations.

> Gastrointestinal helminthiasis or coccidiosis can mask an underlying trace element deficiency, particularly cobalt deficiency.

1. Weaning to mating at 7 months

Aim: steady growth to mating weight optimise rumen development to produce a kid of >25 kg (preferably 35–40 kg for dairy kids, that is 50 to 54% of the mature weight) at mating.

Target weight gain: 2 to 4 months *150 g/day* 4 to 7 months *100—110 g/day*

Goats kidding at <25 kg have a very poor kidding performance.

By 4 months of age each kid will be eating *800 g/day hay* and *400 g/day 16% crude protein (CP) concentrate*.

At mating, each kid will be eating *1.2 kg/day hay + straw + 400–700g 16% CP concentrate*. The amount of concentrate required will depend on the quality of the hay.

Although the young kidded goat will need extra feeding to enable her to continue her body growth during her first lactation (10–15 kg in goats kidded at 1 year), in dairy goats, the extra feed is more than compensated for by the value of milk produced. Correctly managed, the kid will mature into a well-grown animal whose lifetime milk yield should exceed that of a goat kidding at 2 years.

2. Weaning (3 months) to mating at 10 months (traditional 'early kidding')

Aim: steady growth optimise rumen development to produce a kid 60% adult weight at service, that is >42 kg.

Target weight gain: *110–120 g/day*

3. Weaning (3 months) to mating at 19 months

Aim: steady growth optimise rumen development prevent goatling becoming excessively fat before mating.

Target weight gain: *110–120 g/day* to 12 months

After 12 months, the amount of concentrate should be carefully regulated to maintain growth, whilst preventing the goatling from becoming obese.

Further reading

General

AFRC Technical Committee on Responses to Nutrition Report No. 10 (1998) *The Nutrition of Goats*. CAB International, Wallingford, UK.

Baxter, E. (2016) Effects of prenatal stress on mothers and kids. *Goat Vet. Soc. J.*, **32** (in print).

Committee on the Nutrition Requirements of Small Ruminants, National Research Council (2007) *Nutrition Requirements of Small Ruminants, Sheep, Goats, Cervids and New World Camelids*. The National Academies Press, Washington, USA.

Kenyon, P.R. and Blair, H.T. (2014) Fetal programming in sheep – effects on production. *Small Ruminant Research*, **118**, 16–30.

Lambert, M. G. (1990) Goat grazing behaviour and management research in New Zealand. *Proc. Univ. Sydney Post. Grad. Comm. Vet. Sci.*, **134**, 59–64.

McGregor, B.A. (1990) Nutritional management. *Proc. Univ. Sydney Post. Grad. Comm. Vet. Sci.*, **135**, 105–130.

Mowlem, A. (1984) Artificial rearing of kids. *Goat Vet. Soc. J.*, **5**, 25–30.

Thompson, K.G. (1990) Planned animal health and management in fibre goats. *Proc. Univ. Sydney Post. Grad. Comm. Vet. Sci.*, **135**, 19–25.

White, D.G. (1993) Colostral supplementation in ruminants. *Comp. Cont. Ed. Pract. Vet.*, **15** (2), 335–342.

CHAPTER 7

Lameness in adult goats

> The most common cause of lameness and the most important welfare issue is poor foot care.

As in most other farm animals, the majority of cases of lameness in goats involve the foot. Conformation problems such as weak pasterns or cow-hocks will predispose to uneven hoof growth, and environmental factors such as excessively wet conditions that soften the horn may lead to excessive horn growth and increase susceptibility to infection. However, *the cornerstone of lameness prevention within a herd remains regular routine foot trimming*.

In goats, pain is recognised as one of the main signs associated with most lesions of the feet, so lameness in goats is a welfare issue and can be a particular problem where routine foot care is neglected.

The chronic pain state associated with lameness can be associated with significant production losses – reduced milk yield and growth impairment – because of the inability/unwillingness to feed.

> In adult goats, most causes of lameness are associated with the feet.

Initial assessment

The preliminary history should consider:
- Individual or flock/herd problem.
- Sudden or gradual onset of lameness.
- Duration of lameness.
- Static or progressive lameness.
- Any predisposing factors, such as excessively wet conditions.

Clinical examination

The animal should be examined at rest and while moving from a distance of a few feet for:
- Weight bearing.
- Stance.
- Stiff, painful or abnormal gait.
- Swelling around joints.
- Obvious wounds, swellings, etc.
- Conformation.
- Overgrown or abnormally appearing feet.

A detailed examination should then localise the seat of the lameness by:
- Cleaning and trimming the feet where necessary.
- Palpation.
- Manipulation.

Additional information can be obtained from radiography or laboratory examination as indicated.

Further assessment

- *Radiography* may prove useful in the investigation of lameness:
  o Fractures, particularly those distal to the elbow and stifle joints.
  o Arthritis.

  Goats are generally amenable to handling, but sedation or general anaesthesia may be required to allow correct positioning of limbs.
- *Ultrasonography*, using a 7.5 MHz linear array scanner, can provide additional information:
  o Thickness of joint capsules and the extent and nature of any joint effusions (compare with contralateral joint where this is normal).

Diseases of the Goat, Fourth Edition. John Matthews.
© 2016 John Wiley & Sons, Ltd. Published 2016 by John Wiley & Sons, Ltd.

Treatment

■ Precise diagnosis of the cause of lameness is required for effective treatment and control. Specific treatment should be instigated as soon as a diagnosis has been made; effective treatment should produce both resolution of the lesion and a return to normal gait.
■ Ensure feet are correctly trimmed.
■ Lameness in goats is often very painful; instigate pain relief/anti-inflammatory treatment as indicated. Non-steroidal anti-inflammatory drugs are effective for the provision of daily pain relief. For short-term use, injectable NSAIDs licensed for cattle are suitable (see Table 7.1). For long-term use, oral preparations – tablets, liquid or granules (Table 7.2) – have proved useful, although not specifically licensed for small ruminants. The dose should be reduced

Table 7.1 Injectable NSAIDs.

Drug	Dose	Route
Carprofen	1.4 mg/kg repeat once after 24 hours	s.c. or i.v.
Flunixin meglumine	2.2 mg/kg s.i.d. for 3–5 days	i.v.
Ketoprofen	3 mg/kg s.i.d. for 3–5 days	i.m. or i.v.
Meloxicam	2 mg/kg loading dose then 0.5 mg/kg s.c. or i.v. every 36 hours	s.c. or i.v.
Tolfenamic acid	2–4 mg/kg repeat once after 48 hours	s.c. or i.v.
Phenylbutazone[a]	4 mg/kg	i.v.

[a]Phenylbutazone is banned from use in food-producing animals in the EU.

Table 7.2 Oral NSAIDs.

Drug	Dose	Route
Carprofen	1–2 mg/kg once daily	Oral
Meloxicam	2 mg/kg initial dose 1 mg/kg daily until pain controlled 0.5–1 mg/kg every other day long term	Oral
Aspirin[a]	50–100 mg/kg every 12 hours	Oral
Phenylbutazone[b]	10 mg/kg for 2 days, then once daily for 3 days, then every other day or as needed	Oral

[a]Aspirin is poorly absorbed from the rumen so relatively high doses are needed. Aspirin is not licensed for use in food-producing animals in the UK.
[b]Phenylbutazone is banned from use in food-producing animals in the EU.

to the lowest effective dose. At lower doses, it may be possible to repeat the dose every 24 hours, but animals should be closely monitored.

Meloxicam is regularly used orally for long-term pain relief in old arthritic goats using a loading dose of 2 mg/kg, followed by 1 mg/kg daily until the pain is controlled, then 0.5 mg/kg daily or 1 mg/kg every other day as necessary. Goats metabolise meloxicam much faster than cattle and sheep, so the drug needs to be given more often because of the shorter half-life. There does not appear to be significant risk of ulceration, even with long-term use, provided the dose is tapered to the lowest that will control pain.
■ Corticosteroids: dexamethasone, 0.1 mg/kg, i.v.
■ Tetanus is a possible sequel to any penetrating infection, particularly of the foot, and adequate antitetanus cover should always be given.

Non-infectious diseases of the foot

Overgrown feet

> The cornerstone of lameness prevention is routine care (Table 7.3) and regular foot trimming (Table 7.4).

Overgrown feet are a particular problem in intensively managed goats, because the normal wear on the hoof associated with exercise on hard ground is limited and because regular hoof care in large herds is very labour intensive. In smaller herds feet are usually trimmed monthly or every 6 weeks; most commercial dairy herds struggle to trim feet every 6 months, so that lack of foot care can become a welfare problem in some herds. Overgrown feet cause an abnormal gait, place increased stress on joints, tendons and ligaments, are painful for the animal and can result in loss of production because of unwillingness to move and feed.

Table 7.3 Care of the goat's foot.

Keep the feet dry	If indoors, use dry straw on top of good concrete
Keep the feet moving	On hard but not abrasive surfaces
Keep the feet properly trimmed	As regularly as necessary

Table 7.4 Foot trimming procedures.

1 Clean all dirt and grit from the foot
2 Remove all loose horn including ingrowing walls and interdigital flanges
 o Overgrown outer wall turns inwards under the sole trapping dirt and grit
 o Overgrown inner wall produces flanges that can trap dirt in the interdigital cleft, predisposing to foot rot and other infections
3 Level the heels and lower if necessary
 o In overgrown feet, the outer heel is often significantly higher than the inner heel
 o Both heels should be the same height and low enough to allow proper shaping of the foot
4 Pare the sole from the new heel level forward to the toe, trimming the walls to match if necessary
 o The outer claw generally grows more (deeper and longer) than the inner claw and so will require additional trimming
 o Care should be taken to avoid cutting too far and drawing blood or cutting so far that the feet become tender
5 Remove any overgrown or upturned toe that still remains
 o It is better to shape the sole from heel to toe, rather than chopping off the end of the toe. This gives a more normal alignment of the pedal bone and flexor tendons
6 Remove all underrun horn
 o Expose and remove if possible all degenerate and infected tissue
 o Widen all cracks into 'U' shaped valleys
 o Widen all holes in the horn into craters
7 The final result should be a flat smooth surface from heel to toe
 o The sole should preferably be slightly concave towards the interdigital space so that dirt is not trapped between the claws
 o When viewed from the side, goat hooves should be parallelograms with the coronary band parallel to the sole and the front of the claw parallel to the rear
8 If soft tissue is exposed
 o Spray with tetracycline aerosol or dip each foot in a pot containing formalin at about 4% concentration
 o Bandage the foot if necessary and keep dry for 7–10 days
 o Change bandage if foot gets wet

Feeding and metabolic foot disease

In cattle, *rumen acidosis* (Chapter 15) is considered a major factor in poor hoof quality and non-infectious diseases of the hoof and, by extrapolation, increased foot problems in the goat are likely to arise from dietary practices that chronically reduce rumen pH as a result of composition of the ration or incorrect feeding:

■ *Diet composition* – diets with inadequate fibre, diets high in rapidly fermented feeds, forages with low particle size, selective feeding.
■ *Inappropriate feeding* – rapid change to high concentrate diets after parturition, feeding large amounts of concentrate in a short time, feeding forages and concentrates separately, improperly total mixed rations.

Goats should be fed to maintain a stable rumen pH of approximately 5.8 to 6.5.

Recent work on lameness in commercial herds in the UK has found acidic pH levels in goats with treponeme infections, together with hoof lesions such as sole ulceration and haemorrhage, leading to the suggestion that the treponeme infection may be secondary to hoof changes caused by subacute ruminal acidosis (SARA), but further work is required to clarify the situation.

Hoof health can also be affected by dietary supplementation:

■ *Biotin* is essential for keratin–protein synthesis in hoof tissue; diets that acidify the rumen decrease the microbial synthesis of biotin. Levels of 3–4 mg/day have been recommended for animals with a history of hoof disease.
■ *Copper* and *zinc* are both involved in keratin synthesis.
  Zinc methionine, 0.5 mg daily, and zinc sulphate, 250 mg/day, have been used to treat hoof problems.
  Adequate levels of copper should be maintained in the diet and the dietary copper to molybdenum ratio maintained between 4:1 and 6:1.
■ Claw horn is a product of specialised epidermal cells that deposit a range of cytoskeletal and other proteins that contain different proportions of sulphur-containing and other amino acids, in particular cysteine. The dietary supply of cysteine, its precursors and other nutrients will influence

horn growth and hardness. Supplementation of the diet of cashmere and mohair goats with *methionine*, 5 g/30 kg body weight daily, has resulted in increased concentrations of cysteine in their claw horn and increases in the hardness of the horn in the sole and abaxial wall.

White line disease ('Shelley Hoof')

The white line is the junction of the horn of the wall and that of the sole. White line disease involves separation of a portion of the horny outer wall from the underlying sensitive laminae at the white line. It is always the abaxial hoof wall that is affected and the front feet are most commonly affected.

Aetiology

- The aetiological causes of white line disease are not clear; the white line is the cemented junction of the wall and the sole and so is an area of weakness. Minor trauma to the area by stones, rough concrete or gravel may lead to damage and a slight separation, which is then increased by dirt being forced into the space. Wet conditions underfoot will soften the hooves and make damage more likely. If the separation between the wall and sole is not significant, normal hoof growth may carry debris back to the surface, where it is shed, and the lesion can resolve. If further impaction of dirt occurs, the lesion will progress until the horn of the hoof wall in the adjacent area separates completely from the sole.

Clinical signs

- The condition is often noticed at routine foot trimming, particularly during the wetter months of the year. Early lesions include thickening, softening and slight separation of the wall from the laminae and this later progresses to complete horn separation, with the formation of a pocket that becomes filled with dirt and debris, eventually putting pressure on the laminae. Where foot care is deficient, the condition may progress until the animal is lame. If infection occurs in the area, pus will collect and track to the coronary band, forming a foot abscess.

Treatment

- Early foot trimming to pare away loose horn, leaving a characteristic half-moon shape of keratinised

laminae, will resolve the problem before lameness occurs. Extensive deficits can be packed with hoof putty after cleaning.

Horn separation

In most cases, horn separation is probably a sequel to white line disease (see above), but the exact relationship between the two conditions requires clarification. Horn separation can also follow trauma to the wall of the hoof. Footrot and contagious caprine digital dermatitis will also lead to horn separation.

Sole horn lesions

Primary sole horn lesions, including sole ulcers, are rarely reported as a cause of lameness in goats. In the United Kingdom, most commercial dairy herds are kept indoors in straw yards, reducing exposure to predisposing factors such as extensive time on concrete or stone tracks. However non-infected sole lesions do occur. The roles of subacute ruminal acidosis (SARA) in goats fed high levels of concentrates and hormonal changes around kidding in these animals need further investigation.

Treponeme species have been identified from the feet of lame goats where the majority of the lesions seemed to start from the sole and it is postulated that a primary claw horn lesion becomes secondarily infected with treponemes.

Foreign body penetration of the sole

Puncture of the sole by a foreign body such as a stone or nail results in immediate lameness in the affected leg and occasionally a goat is presented with a foreign body, for example a nail, still embedded in the foot or interdigital area. If the foreign body is removed, the penetration site opened up and drainage established, recovery will occur rapidly, but neglect may lead to abscess formation.

Abscess of the sole

Abscess of the sole is an uncommon, painful lesion of uncertain aetiology, probably as a result of trauma to the sole and possibly a precursor to sole ulceration and the formation of a granulomatous lesion. Pain is evident over an area of the sole and pus is released when the foot is trimmed. Treatment consists of careful foot trimming, cleaning of the area and topical or parenteral use of antibiotics.

Granulomatous lesions of the sole

Granulomatous lesions of the sole have been described in a herd of milking goats. Although the aetiology is unclear, it is probable that granulomatous lesions are a sequel to direct trauma to the sole and subsequent ulceration, which is slow to heal. Treatment consists of resection of the granulation tissue at the level of the solar horn, removing all underrun horn and careful foot trimming.

Fracture of the distal phalanx

A fracture of the distal phalanx or pedal bone produces an acute lameness in one foot. Radiography is required to confirm the diagnosis. Resolution may occur if movement is restricted for at least 6 weeks by a waterproof cast.

Laminitis (aseptic pododermatitis)

Aetiology

Laminitis is a metabolic disorder of the corium and germinal layer of the foot, produced by a degeneration of the vascular supply to the corium.

- *Acute laminitis* occurs in response to endotoxin release during ruminal acidosis or toxic conditions.
- *Subacute* and *subclinical laminitis* are produced by overfeeding over a longer period.
- *Chronic laminitis* develops where an acute or subacute laminitis is not recognised or satisfactorily treated because horn formation is disturbed.
- Trauma to the hoof may also predispose to laminitis.
- A genetic predisposition may exist in some families.

Occurrence

Acute laminitis may occur:

- After any toxic condition, such as mastitis, metritis, retained fetal membranes or pneumonia.
- A few days after kidding with or without one of the above conditions.
- As a sequel to acidosis:
  o in females fed high-energy diets
  o in silage-fed goats with continued ingestion of acid silage.
- Laminitis is also seen with systemic viral diseases such as foot-and-mouth disease and bluetongue.
  Subacute and *subclinical laminitis* occur:
- In goatlings and kids as young as 8 weeks where high protein/energy concentrate rations (together with inadequate fibre?) are fed.

- In does overfed for the level of production.
- In male goats fed on milking rations, particularly during the summer months when they are not working. Mammary development and milk production in bucks, particularly British Saanens, or Saanens from high-yielding families, are also accentuated at this time by overfeeding and there is a danger of mastitis developing (see Chapter 13).

Chronic laminitis occurs as a sequel to acute, subacute or subclinical laminitis and is common in goats kept as pets, such as pygmies, which have been inappropriately and/or overfed over a prolonged period.

Clinical signs

Acute laminitis results in the sudden onset of a tender foot or feet (generally both front feet, but occasionally all four feet), with a disinclination to walk, prolonged recumbency or walking on knees, and a shifting of weight distribution when standing to spare the affected feet, teeth grinding and other signs of pain, pyrexia, and a fall in milk yield. The coronet of the affected foot feels hot, but the toe cold.

> Subclinical laminitis is a common and often unrecognised disease of dairy goats.

Subacute and *subclinical laminitis* are only differentiated by degree. In subacute laminitis minor gait abnormalities occur whereas in the subclinical condition no gait changes are present and the feet do not feel hot.

Subclinical laminitis is a common and underdiagnosed disease of dairy goats, particularly kids and goatlings, which leads to the development of horn abnormalities in older animals.

Haemorrhage of the wall, heel and particularly the sole is evident on routine foot trimming as a fine reddish discoloration which, unlike bruising, is generally not painful.

As in cattle, subclinical laminitis leads to the development of other lamenesses because poor quality horn is produced with changes in horn growth, particularly of the sole, so that the shape of the claw is changed and there may be marked differences in height and width between the lateral and medial claws.

Note: even in normal feet, the front medial claws will be larger than the lateral claws but this is accentuated when laminitic.

> Chronic laminitis produces very hard feet with thick 'platform soles'.

Chronic laminitis produces a chronically lame goat with feet that, at first glance, appear relatively normal in shape. As it is usually only the front feet that are laminitic, comparing the depth of the front hooves to the depth of hind hooves provides a clear indication of the excessive growth and the amount of hoof that needs to be removed to return the foot to a normal depth.

The horn is very solid, with failure to differentiate clearly into wall and sole, and may be impossible to trim with ordinary foot shears. The feet are extremely deep, often 5 cm or more (hence the term 'platform soles') (Plates 7.1 and 7.2). A rock-hard, very deep foot is pathognomonic of the disease. Front feet are more commonly affected than back feet and both front feet are usually affected. Anglo-Nubian, Anglo-Nubian crosses and pygmy goats seem more prone to the disease than the Swiss breeds of dairy goats. Severely affected animals have a characteristic goose-stepping walk and spend a lot of time on their knees (Plate 7.3). Unlike cattle, overgrown 'sledge runner' feet ('slippering') is not a feature of the disease in goats. 'Slippering' in goats is produced by foot overgrowth due to lack of routine foot care (Plate 7.4). In severe cases of laminitis, the wall and sole may loosen from the corium, with concomitant downward rotation of the pedal bone, but this is much rarer than in the horse.

Treatment and control

- Most cases of laminitis can be prevented by better management, particularly by correct feeding practice.
- Acute cases should be placed on a reduced protein/energy diet, that is hay with a very reduced or no concentrate ration, and a deep bed provided.
- Antibiotic cover should be given to combat any infectious or toxic cause of the condition.
- Pain relief with an NSAID is essential (see 'Treatment' in this chapter).

- The value of antihistamines is uncertain and the use of corticosteroids controversial and probably contraindicated, as in the horse.
- Heat treatment of the feet will help restore the circulation if used during the first few hours when vasoconstriction is occurring. Cold water treatment is of benefit later, and for about 7 days, to reduce the subsequent vasodilation.
- Chronic cases need careful foot trimming to relieve pain by reducing pressure on the sensitive areas. Regular repeat foot care is needed when the foot is grossly overgrown or misshapen. It is often impossible to return the foot to its normal depth even with regular trimming, but frequent attention reduces the degree of discomfort and, with the help of NSAIDs, many goats can be kept comfortable for prolonged periods. The front part of the toes should be left slightly longer than normal and the heel pared down until it can be easily flexed digitally.

Zinc deficiency

Although more usually recognised as a proliferative dermatitis (parakeratosis; see Chapter 11), zinc-deficient goats may have skeletal and hoof abnormalities, resulting in abnormal posture with the back arched and feet close together. The feet may be painful on palpation with deep transverse ridges around the hoof wall.

Tumour

Tumours, including a humeral chondrosarcoma and malignant melanomas involving the interdigital cleft, coronet (Plate 7.5) or the hoof are occasionally reported and cause varying degrees of lameness.

Infectious diseases of the foot

> Goats' feet are more severely affected by wet conditions than those of sheep.

Predisposing conditions for infection

- Prolonged grazing of wet, muddy pastures or housing in wet, dirty yards.
- Overcrowding.
- Introduction of new stock. Infection may be introduced by clinical or subclinical carriers (goats, sheep,

cattle or deer). The carrier state may persist for 2–3 years.

- Poor foot care.
- Poor foot conformation.

Aetiology

- Continuous wetting of the foot and interdigital skin damages the tissues and allows the invasion of the casual organism of interdigital dermatitis, *Fusobacterium necrophorum*, which is widespread in the environment and cannot penetrate healthy, intact skin. Its penetration is aided by other bacteria, such as *Trueperella pyogenes*.
- Interdigital dermatitis may exist as a distinct condition, but in the presence of *Dichelobacter (Bacteriodes) nodosus*, which is introduced by carrier animals, there is a rapid spread of the infection to the hoof and the sole and benign footrot or virulent footrot becomes established. *Dichelobacter nodosus*, which acts synergistically with *F. necrophorum*, has a varying keratinolytic activity that destroys the hoof, permitting further invasion of the foot. When strains with low keratinolytic activity are present damage will be limited and only the mild lesions of benign footrot seen. When the strains have high keratinolytic activity, damage is much more severe and virulent footrot occurs. *D. nodosus* is an obligate anaerobic organism found only in the feet of ruminants affected by footrot and can only survive in the environment for 7–14 days.
- Ten serogroups of *D. nodosus* are currently recognised on the basis of pili carried on their surface and serogroups may be divided into different strains. There is no cross-protection between serogroups.

Diagnosis

- Diagnosis is usually made on the basis of a combination of clinical signs, herd history and the response to treatment; laboratory diagnosis is rarely undertaken, as the fastidious anaerobic nature of *D. nodosus* means that complex media and several weeks are required for characterisation of isolates.

Interdigital dermatitis (scald)

Goats, with longer digits and a deeper interdigital area, show more severe clinical signs of interdigital dermatitis than sheep.

Clinical signs

- A mild to severe lameness is seen in one or more goats with a rapid spread throughout the flock or herd if the predisposing conditions are suitable; animals will be lame in one or more feet, or walking on their knees. Affected animals will lose condition, with a drop in milk yield or shedding of fleece.
- The interdigital area between the claws is inflamed, often with considerable swelling, and there is a characteristic smell. There is no damage to the horn of the hoof. In severe cases there will be ulceration with a purulent discharge.

Treatment

- If there is no footrot on the holding, treat individual animals with antibiotic spray from a distance of 6–8 inches until the lesion is adequately covered and ensure the sprayed area is dry before releasing the goat.
- A severely affected foot can be bandaged and zinc sulphate/vaseline mixtures can be applied locally interdigitally.
- Move to new pasture where there have been no goats or sheep for two weeks.
- If the incidence in the group is high, foot bath the whole group (see below).
- Uncomplicated cases of interdigital dermatitis will resolve quickly if the animals are moved from wet pasture to dry ground or housed and the lesions treated with an antibiotic spray or footbath.
- If there is footrot on the farm, give a high dose of long-acting antibiotic (see treatment of footrot, below).

Footbaths

- With individual goats, dip the feet in a footbath solution daily for 3 days and then weekly for several weeks (Table 7.5).
- With a herd problem, the goats should be run through a footbath on a weekly basis. Goats need to be closely supervised as they are much more adept at avoiding the bath than sheep. The bath should be at least 4 cm deep and the goats should stand in the bath for at least 2 minutes routinely and for 30 minutes when the infection is severe.

Table 7.5 Footbath guidelines.

Supervise the goats carefully to make sure all animals enter the bath for an adequate period –20 minutes for zinc sulphate
The design of the bath is important to prevent the goats from climbing along the race to avoid the liquid; foam mats can be useful
Walk through water first if the feet are muddy
Straw in the bath reduces foaming of zinc sulphate (but inactivates formalin)
If the bath is not under cover, avoid wet conditions to avoid mud, dilution and washing off of the solution
Stand on dry concrete for one hour until feet are dry
Move on to clean pasture after foot bathing
Handle solutions carefully and avoid environmental contamination (particularly important with formalin)

Two solutions are commonly used:

Formalin 2–5%: 2–5 l commercial formalin (formalin 40%) to 100 l of water
Zinc sulphate 10%: 10 kg zinc sulphate to 100 l of water

Formalin is very effective but stings raw tissue and makes the goats less amenable to adequate bathing and also hardens the skin and hoof, possibly preventing the penetration of further solutions. The advantage of formalin over zinc sulphate is that goats can be run through a footbath, without having to stand in it for a long period. *Zinc sulphate solution is the preferred treatment*, although a longer bathing period is required than with formalin and the solution is more expensive. Proprietary preparations contain penetrating/wetting agents, such as ionic detergents and laurel sulphate, to increase the deposition of zinc in the hoof. Ideally, goats should be stood in the solution for a minimum of 20 minutes and then penned on dry ground, such as concrete, for one hour until their feet are dry.

The use of copper sulphate is not recommended as it is toxic to goats and wildlife that drink from the footbath and may stain fleeces.

Footrot

> Footrot is a whole herd problem.

Clinical signs

- These are as for interdigital dermatitis, with initial inflammation of the interdigital skin, but there are lesions in the hoof and sole, with separation of the horn, caused by under-running, which starts at the skin/horn junction towards the posterior part of the interdigital cleft. Separation may spread across the sole and abaxial wall so that in severe cases the hoof will only be attached at the coronet. Pus is present beneath the underrun horn and the horn can be pared away, revealing greyish soft horn with a characteristic foul odour of decomposing tissue. Secondary complications may arise from fly strike or tetanus.
- Unlike sheep, it is impossible to differentiate between benign and virulent footrot on the basis of clinical findings. The strains of footrot that cause benign disease in sheep can cause severe underrunning and interdigital lesions in goats.
- Not all infected goats are lame.

Treatment and control of footrot

> At the beginning of an outbreak, every foot of every goat in the herd should be examined and treated as necessary.

- Regular examination and foot trimming of the whole herd. Lameness prevalence across a herd/flock can be measured on a monthly basis using a simple 6-point locomotion score:

  0 sound, **1** very mild lameness, **2** obvious lameness in an animal that stands and walks on all four legs, **3** obvious lameness in an animal that walks on all four legs but stands on three legs, **4** obvious lameness in an animal that stands and walks on only three legs, **5** obvious reluctance to bear weight on multiple limbs.

- No single management factor will control foot rot, but plans introduced for control of the disease in sheep can be adapted for use in goats (Table 7.6).

Table 7.6 Reducing the impact of infectious foot disease.

Action	Reason	Implementation
Cull badly or repeatedly infected animals	Herd/flock resilience to disease is increased by removing the more severely affected animals	Cull does with misshapen chronic feet Cull goats that get footrot more than twice
Source replacements from herds/flocks that are free from footrot Quarantine incoming animals	Avoid introducing infection to the farm Sheep and cattle should be considered as possible sources of infection and should be similarly quarantined or kept separate from the goats	Develop a quarantine plan and always follow it: Quarantine for at least 4 weeks Footbath on arrival Check feet for disease on arrival and before release from quarantine
Identify and rapidly treat any lame animal	Improves the welfare of individual animals and reduces disease transmission to other animals Reduces disease challenge	Use a lameness scoring system to identify and record lame animals for treatment The first lame goat in a group should be treated within 1–3 days of becoming lame
Avoid propagation of infection on the farm	Avoid spread of infection during gathering, handling, in collection areas and housing Reduces disease challenge	Avoid yarding for long periods Minimise handling events Improve underfoot conditions Handling areas should have a hard surface Consider portable handling areas Apply lime around troughs and gateways Do not breed from badly infected goats
Vaccination	Increase immunity within the herd/flock	Biannual vaccination with footrot vaccine has been useful in controlling disease in sheep but has variable success in goats

- All the feet of all the animals should be examined. Although a minimal paring may be needed to identify some infected animals and grossly overgrown feet will require trimming to establish a more normal shape, *extensive foot trimming appears to delay the healing of footrot in both sheep and goats.*

- Current good practice is to use systemic injections of a long-acting antibiotic, such as Oxytetracycline, 20 mg/kg i.m., or gamithromycin, 6 mg/kg s.c., ensuring that the goat is dosed for the correct weight, together with topical oxytetracycline aerosol sprays or washes. Animals should be rechecked after about 21 days and the treatment repeated where necessary. Antibiotics appear to work just as well with or without footbathing in zinc sulphate and with or without foot paring.

- Foot paring on its own will not prevent or cure foot rot. In addition, overzealous paring, to the extent that bleeding occurs, predisposes the goat to infection with anaerobic bacteria and overexcessive cutting back of the wall results in excessive weight-bearing on the sole, leading to bruising and providing a focus for further infection. Foot shears can act as a medium for transferring disease between animals and should be disinfected regularly. Foot parings, which are infectious, should be disposed of carefully.

- Use pain relief with NSAIDs for the first 24 hours

- Vaccination. *Vaccination alone will not control the disease,* but can be used to assist an eradication programme. Sheep footrot vaccines have been used with very mixed results in goats. Vaccine containing multiple serogroups of *D. nodosus* is necessary, because there is no cross-protection between serogroups and a strong adjuvant is required, because the organism is a poor antigen. Severe local reactions to these oil adjuvanted vaccines have been reported.

Footvax (MSD), 1 ml s.c., two doses at intervals of 4 to 8 weeks; booster doses every 4 to 6 months as required. Pregnant does should not be vaccinated 4 weeks before or after kidding; kids can be vaccinated at 4 weeks of age.

A drug interaction between the vaccine and injected Moxidectin has been implicated in causing massive abortion storms in sheep and the birth of weak, non-viable lambs. Once vaccinated with Footvax, animals should *never again* be treated with Moxidectin injectable.

- Select for resistance. There is some evidence that there are family and breed differences in the incidence of footrot, possibly related to foot conformation.
- Muddy gateways and areas around water troughs should be regularly limed to lower the pH and reduce the ability of the bacteria to survive.

Treponema-associated caprine digital dermatitis

Spirochaetes of the *Treponema* genus have been implicated in the aetiology of bovine digital dermatitis (BDD) and contagious ovine digital dermatitis (CODD) of sheep. *Treponema* species have now been identified in goats with lesions resembling CODD and also in goats with lesions unlike either BDD or CODD.

Aetiology

- *Treponema* species are Gram-negative, spirochaete bacteria. *Treponema medium/Treponema vincentii*-like, *Treponema phagedenis*-like and *Treponema denticola/Treponema putidum*-like spirochaete species have been identified in goats with CODD-like lesions.
- Treponeme species are known to be omnipresent in the environments of cattle and sheep and are probably so for goats, although this remains to be established.
- It is not clear if the treponemes are the primary infection causing the lesions or whether they are secondary infections of an established lesion (of unknown aetiology), which change the nature of the infection and the clinical outcome. It is possible that there is an interaction with other organisms, such as *Fusobacterium necrophorum,* although *Dichelobacter nodosus* is not generally isolated from affected animals.
- Wet conditions, such as standing in collecting yards, may predispose the goats to infection by softening the hoof and promoting white line disease.
- Subacute ruminal acidosis (SARA), leading to subclinical laminitis with changes in the hoof, has been identified as a possible predisposing condition, which enables treponemes in the goats' environment to infect the hoof.

CODD-like disease
Clinical signs

- Initially an ulcerative lesion at the coronary band with extensive under-running of the claw capsule, leading to separation of the claw wall from its underlying tissue and subsequent loss of the horn capsule from the coronary band downwards. The underlying tissue is haemorrhagic and granulomatous (Plates 7.6, 7.7 and 7.8). The under-running may extend to the sole horn, resulting in extensive horn loss on the sole, differing from footrot in that the underlying exposed tissue appears haemorrhagic and granulomatous. The separation of hoof horn at the level of the coronary band accompanied by extensive under-running of the hoof horn capsule is markedly similar to published descriptions of contagious ovine digital dermatitis (CODD) in sheep.
- The separation of the claw at the coronary band contrasts with the separation seen in cases of footrot, where separation of horn occurs at the skin/horn junction towards the posterior part of the interdigital cleft.
- There is severe lameness affecting one digit of one foot in most animals, but both digits of one foot in some goats. The damage to the corium may be so severe that re-growth of the horn is permanently affected.
- The feet of affected animals become severely deformed, with destruction of bone and soft tissues, so that the damage is permanent and, in advanced cases, euthanasia on humane grounds is the only treatment option.

Diagnosis

- Clinical signs.
- Bacterial isolation, but *Treponema* species are fastidious and difficult to culture.
- *Treponema* genus PCR assay and PCR assay for specific *Treponema* phylogroups on punch biopsies from foot lesions.

Treatment, prevention and control

- *Treponema* species are very hard to eliminate once they are introduced on to a holding, so adequate biosecurity and appropriate preventative measures are essential. Although isolation of *Treponema* species is more likely from lame animals and most infected animals are lame, some carrier animals may not show obvious signs of lameness.
- The feet of all goats, including the claw horn and interdigital skin, should be carefully examined before being brought on to the farm. Sheep and cattle may act as a source of infection from treponemes and other infectious agents causing foot diseases and should also be examined carefully. Treponemes can

survive for a short time in slurry and transmission between animals (and species) may occur at pasture.

- Animals should be quarantined on concrete before introduction into the new herd.
- All farms should preferably have their own foot-trimming equipment as, although disinfection will reduce the bacterial load, total elimination of the bacteria is difficult.
- Co-grazing of different species of ruminant should be avoided when any of the animals have clinical signs of infectious disease.
- CODD lesions in sheep have been treated using 1% chlortetracycline footbaths daily for 3 days, after careful trimming of feet to identify any sheep with CODD lesions, together with systemic injection of long-acting amoxicillin trihydrate. The footbath should be deep enough to cover the accessory digits. Other antibiotics used in footbaths for sheep are lincomycin and spectinomycin soluble powder 100 g/200 litres and tylosin soluble powder 100 g/200 litres.
- Parenteral antibiotic treatments, such as long-acting penicillin, may help in mild cases, but will not help advanced cases. Tilmicosin injections have been used in sheep, but should not be used in goats.
- A copper/zinc sulphate paste (Derm Paste, Hoofcare Supplies) has been used topically on early lesions, together with topical oxytetracycline sprays.
- In sheep, a grading system has been proposed for CODD lesions to help identify and describe lesions more precisely and to aid treatment by relating lesion scores to lameness scores. A similar grading system could be used in goat herds.
- Severely affected animals should be euthanized on humane grounds.

Non-CODD like disease

Contagious ovine digital dermatitis (CODD) lesions and the lesions of digital dermatitis in goats with CODD-like disease are reported to start from the coronary band with separation of the claw wall from its underlying tissue and subsequent loss of the horn capsule. Treponeme species have also been identified from the feet of lame goats where *the majority of the lesions seemed to start from the sole*. The majority of affected animals in these herds show non-footrot-like lesions on the sole of the foot, extending from the axial wall to the heel. The lesions present directly on the corium as if the corium had lysed with limited under-running of the horn visible. In more severely affected animals, the whole sole appears to be affected with no healthy corium visible and the horn of the wall detaches from the foot up to 1 cm from the sole, leaving foul smelling and granulomatous soft tissue in the middle of the foot. The interdigital space is rarely infected.

Non-infected sole horn lesions have been identified in animals on the affected farms and may indicate a primary lesion that is subsequently infected by treponemes from the environment.

Septic pedal arthritis/foot abscess

- As a sequel to conditions such as a puncture wound, sole ulceration or white line disease, or following overzealous trimming, deep infection by *Trueperella pyogenes*, *F. necrophorum* or other bacteria may produce an abscess in the heel or more commonly the toe of one claw.
- Septic pedal arthritis results when the infection enters the distal interphalangeal (pedal) joint as a sequel to deep interdigital infection, usually in animals with footrot, and is only rarely associated with puncture wounds. Infection enters the joint through the interdigital joint capsule, which is close to the interdigital space and tracts across the joint to the coronary band.

Clinical signs

- Usually affects individual goats, involving one foot, but herd outbreaks can occur.
- Severe non-weight-bearing lameness. The animal often spends long periods lying down.
- Once septic pedal arthritis has occurred, there is considerable painful swelling of the affected claw, particularly in the interdigital space, the interdigital space widens and the coronary band becomes swollen and painful, with a sinus discharging bloody pus at the level of the coronary band.
- Pyrexia, anorexia.
- Loss of body condition from reduced feeding.

Treatment

- Early treatment by paring to release the pus, bathing with antiseptic solution and poultice, together with systemic antibiotic therapy and pain relief with NSAIDs for about 10 days, will be successful provided the deeper tissues and joints are not involved.
- Where the condition is more severe and there is septic pedal arthritis, considerable deformity of the foot

may occur and antibiotic treatment will be unsuccessful. Joint lavage or amputation of the digit should be considered.

o Joint lavage (see below) promotes ankylosis of the distal interphalangeal joint and provides an alternative to digital amputation for resolution of the lameness. Amputation of the digit can be carried out if the response to joint lavage is not satisfactory as determined by re-examination after 5 days, or if there is still a purulent discharge, there is increased pain or inflammation or the joint is unstable because of extensive ligament damage.

o Amputation can be carried out rapidly in the field, using local anaesthesia (Chapter 26) and is cost effective even in non-pedigree animals.

Pedal joint lavage technique

■ Parenteral antibiotic and analgesic are administered to the goat.

■ A tourniquet is applied above the carpus or tarsus, the area over a superficial vein such as the cephalic or medial radial vein in the fore leg and the lateral saphenous vein or recurrent tarsal vein in the hind leg is shaved and scrubbed and intravenous regional anaesthesia (IVRA) is administered (5–8 ml of 5% procaine or 5 ml of 2% lidocaine using a 20 g needle. Sedation prior to injection is advisable as it limits movement of the limb, aiding injection of the anaesthetic.

■ The foot and lower leg are cleaned and a small area around the coronary band shaved and surgically prepared.

■ Two layers of conforming bandage are pre-placed above the coronary band.

■ A 12 gauge 80 mm cannula is inserted adjacent to the discharging sinus on the lateral wall, just proximal to the coronary band and at right angles to the leg.

■ If required a sample of fluid can be collected for culture/cytology.

■ Sterile isotonic fluid or sterile water is flushed through the cannula and its location is adjusted until the fluid emerges through the sinus at the interdigital space. Flushing should be continued until the fluid is clear.

■ A male luer stopper is placed on the cannula, which is secured in place by a conforming bandage.

■ The joint is then flushed with antibiotic solution, using a 16 gauge 12 mm needle through the luer stopper. Soluble benzylpenicillin is active against likely secondary pyogenic bacteria such as *Trueperella*

pyogenes, but is not licensed for food-producing animals in the United Kingdom. Ceftiofur sodium powder is licensed in cattle in the United Kingdom and North America.

■ The foot is left unbandaged, so that drainage can occur freely at the interdigital space.

■ The joint is flushed daily through the catheter with 10 ml saline followed by the antibiotic solution for 5 days and the catheter is then removed.

■ Topical oxytetracycline spray can be used on the site of cannula insertion and the interdigital area for a few more days.

■ A wooden or plastic block can be applied to the sole of the sound digit to maintain mobility by allowing the goat to stand on one digit during convalescence. This raises the affected claw out of the dirt and shifts the weight on to the good claw allowing the affected claw to rest. The good claw should be trimmed as necessary to give a good bearing surface, then cleaned with spirit so that it is free of particles and grease and allowed to dry. A wooden pre-shaped block can then be applied to the sole, using a quick-setting resin (Demotec).

Orf (contagious pustular dermatitis)

Lesions of orf (Chapter 10) occasionally occur around the coronet or on the legs from licking and may result in lameness.

Mycotic dermatitis (dermatophilosis, strawberry footrot)

Dermatophilus congolense causes 'lumpy wool' and strawberry footrot in sheep and goats. The incidence of both conditions appears to be very low in goats in the United Kingdom, although the condition is easily produced experimentally.

Initially there are raised (paint brush) tufts of hair followed by crusting with pus under the crusts. Removal of the crusts leaves circular, raised, red, granulating lesions on the coronet interdigital space and lower leg as well as on the body, scrotum and head. Lesions on the nose and ears must be distinguished from orf and those on the feet and lower leg from chorioptic mange (Chapter 11). *Dermatophilus congolense* may act synergistically with contagious pustular dermatitis virus.

Predisposing conditions are wet, unhygienic conditions and ectoparasites, which transfer zoospores between animals. Zoospores are generally carried in scabs between animals.

Diagnosis

- Smears, skin biopsy or culture on blood agar.

Treatment

- Dry conditions, broad-spectrum antibiotics; topical applications of 10% zinc sulphate solution or 1% potash alum.

Foot and mouth disease

Foot and mouth disease (FMD) is a highly contagious disease endemic in many parts of the world, although North America has been clear for many years and cases in Western Europe are rare, though often extremely severe when they have occurred. The disease causes a dramatic loss of production, particularly in affected cattle, so that control is necessary on both welfare and economic grounds. It is a notifiable disease in the United Kingdom.

Cloven hoofed animals, including cattle, sheep, goats and pigs, are susceptible and other animals, such as hedgehogs, coypu, rats, deer and zoo animals including elephants, can be infected and transmit the disease.

Aetiology

- Picornavirus with seven distinct virus types (A, O, C, Asia 1, SAT 1, SAT 2 and SAT 3) and approximately 80 specific subtypes. The virus seems to be capable of infinite mutations, so that new different subtypes are constantly appearing.

Epidemiology

The virus can spread through direct or indirect contact:

- Up to 50 miles on the wind if conditions are correct.
- In the saliva, exhaled air, milk and faeces of infected animals.
- Through contact with foodstuffs or other things that have been contaminated by infected animals.
- Virtually any distance by people on skin and clothing.
- On lorries, farm vehicles, etc.
- Horses, wild birds, dogs, cats, poultry, wild game, vermin and other wildlife can carry infected material.

Clinical signs

- FMD causes inflammation of the mouth and of the coronary band.
- *In goats, the disease is usually relatively mild or subclinical. Many infected goats have such mild symptoms that they are easily missed on clinical examination. However, they*

are still infectious to other livestock. Goats are capable of spreading infection for up to nine months after being infected, even though the disease may have passed without any clinical signs being seen.

- Pyrexia (39.5 °C). The rise in temperature is often transient, but if connected with possible signs of FMD in either the same or other goats on the premises, it is a useful non-specific indicator of disease.
- *Lesions in the mouth and around the foot tend to heal very quickly and can easily be missed in goats, which are otherwise well.*
- *Vesicles on the coronary band and interdigital cleft* are much less obvious in goats than in cattle when they are seen. *In a large proportion of infected goats, no foot lesions are seen.*
- *Mouth vesicles* consistently form, but are much smaller than in cattle, and much less painful, so the characteristic drooling of saliva associated with FMD in cattle is absent, although a slight to moderately noticeable bubbling of saliva round the mouth may occur.
- Healing mouth lesions tend to be seen mainly as *white dots on the tongue*, about 1 to 2 mm across, only visible if the animals are 'mouthed', that is examined by opening the mouth and looking.
- In the 2001 outbreak in the United Kingdom, great confusion was caused in sheep and goats by an unknown viral disease, which caused erosions in the front of the dental pad. FMD *never* causes erosions on the front of the dental pad, unless there are erosions elsewhere in the mouth.
- *Vesicles on the udder and teats* are not uncommon in goats, and can be the only ones seen in some animals. Other recorded symptoms of FMD in goats include:
- *Abortion*.
- *Death of young kids*. Peracute death from *myocarditis* may occur in kids less than 2 weeks of age, even though older animals may show no clinical signs.
- Abrupt *reduction in milk yield*.
  All these can be signs of other diseases (Table 7.7).

Diagnosis

- Clinical signs + confirmation by virus isolation.

Control

- Initial control measures in most countries include slaughter of infected and in-contact animals, followed by the disposal of carcases by burial, burning or rendering, in conjunction with strictly enforced movement restrictions.

Table 7.7 Differential diagnosis of FMD lesions.

Mouth lesions	Foot lesions	Neonatal mortality	Teat lesions
Orf	Scald (interdigital dermatitis)	Enterotoxaemia	Orf
Pemphigus foliaceus	Footrot	bluetongue	
Pygmy goat syndrome (seborrhoeic dermatitis)	bluetongue		
Trauma/caustic agents			

- *Vaccination.* FMD vaccines are preparations of inactivated FMD virus of one or several strains combined with an appropriate adjuvant. Little is known about the effectiveness of FMD vaccines in goats. The response to FMD vaccine in the goat appears never to have been fully evaluated, although other vaccines are known to be less efficient in the goat than in other animals and goats are known to respond to FMD vaccination with lower mean antibody titres than cattle.
- *Mass vaccination to prevent infection.* There are many strains of FMD, with little cross-immunity between the main types of the virus and immunity to one type does not confer protective immunity against any of the other types. An effective vaccination programme would require vaccination against a number of strains up to three times a year and this would have to continue indefinitely. The more strains of disease in any vaccine, the less likely it is to achieve the desired level of immunity. The cost would be high if it could be achieved, and it would need a high uptake in any population of animals to be effective.

  In areas where FMD is endemic and vaccination is used routinely, it tends to be the case that one or two strains are endemic, which makes vaccination much more feasible. However, it does not completely eradicate the disease, but merely controls it to a more acceptable level. There is potential for the virus to circulate subclinically and vaccinated animals that have contact with live virus are as likely to become carriers as animals that have recovered from the disease.
- *Vaccination during a disease outbreak.* In Europe, vaccination is only used, under government direction, following a risk assessment about possible spread of the disease and taking into account that vaccination greatly slows the resumption of valuable exports. In effect, vaccination is likely to be needed in areas of high stock density and where the virus has a low infective dose and a high production rate. Control of the outbreak by culling is likely to be more effective where the outbreak is in an area of lower stock density, and with a virus with a high infective dose and low production rate in the animal.

  o *Suppressive vaccination.* Vaccination is used on farms in the zone immediately surrounding infected farms, using the concentrated forms of vaccine that are capable of affording vaccination from aerosol spread within 4 days.

  o *Ring vaccination.* Vaccination of uninfected animals outside the immediate infected area is used to help prevent the spread of disease as a form of firebreak, in conjunction with other control measures.

Lameness above the foot

Weak pasterns

'Weak pasterns' have been a longstanding problem in some families of dairy goats, particularly among Saanens, British Saanens and their crosses. More recently, Angora goats imported from Tasmania and New Zealand have shown similar weaknesses. The condition appears to be inherited as a recessive gene and accentuated by inbreeding. Weak pasterns produce excessive wear on the heels and a long foot with an overgrown toe.

Aetiology

- Weakness of the flexor tendons attached to the pastern joint, the degree of deformity depending on the degree of involvement of the superficial digital flexor tendon, deep digital flexor tendon and the suspensory ligament (see Figure 7.1). Traumatic damage and rupture of the flexor tendons and suspensory ligament (see below) will produce similar conformational changes.

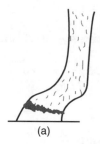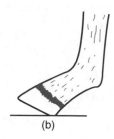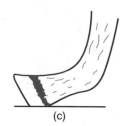

(a)   (b)   (c)

Figure 7.1 Weak pasterns. (a) Superficial digital flexor tendon weakness; (b) superficial and deep digital flexor tendons, weak or ruptured; (c) flexor tendons and suspensory ligament ruptured.

- The condition is accentuated by badly trimmed feet where the heels are cut short and the toes left long. Conversely, well-trimmed feet will ameliorate the condition to some extent. Poor trimming of the feet over a long period will produce the condition even in goats that are genetically sound.
- Older multiparous milking goats often show weakness of the superficial digital tendon.

Clinical signs

- Affected animals may show weakness by the time they are 6 months old, with the condition worsening as the goat gets heavier through growth and pregnancy. Suspect animals will roll on their heels slightly, lifting the toe from the ground when encouraged to shift their weight backwards by pressing on the brisket. The hind legs are more commonly involved, but some animals show marked weakness in the front legs.
- As the condition progresses, the joint adopts a characteristic right-angled bend because of weakness of the superficial flexor tendon, with excessive wear on the heels. With the involvement of the deep flexor tendon the weight is shifted back on to the heels so the toes are raised from the ground, resulting in bruising to the heels. With complete collapse of the joint the weight is carried on the back of the foot without the sole touching the ground.

Accident or trauma

Fractures

Goats being active, inquisitive animals with a propensity to climb, commonly sustain limb fractures, particularly of the lower limbs. Fractures of the limbs are more common in kids than adult goats (see Chapter 8). Goats usually make excellent orthopaedic patients, because of their size, friendly nature and manouverability on three legs.

Fracture management is discussed in Chapter 36.

Tendon and ligament damage

A number of specific causes of lameness have been described.

1. Rupture of the superficial and deep digital flexor tendons

Aetiology

- Trauma to the metacarpal or metatarsal region. A common cause of this injury is a tether becoming entangled around the leg and biting into the flesh. Gross infection of the wound may be present as these cases are often neglected and severe restriction of the blood supply to the distal limb may lead to gangrene.
- Complete rupture of both flexor tendons produces a permanent unsoundness unless surgical repair is carried out. Severe lameness occurs and the animal is unwilling to bear weight as there is overflexion of the fetlock, which touches the ground.
- A complete rupture of the superficial flexor tendon alone leads to slight lameness, with a dropped fetlock and reasonable weight bearing.
- Incomplete rupture of the superficial tendon does not alter the ability to bear weight.

Treatment

- The wound should be thoroughly cleaned and the damage to the tendons assessed.
- Tendon repair can be carried out in a valuable animal using wire, carbon fibre or other suture material.

The prognosis is good if only the superficial tendon is involved, but poor if the deep tendon is damaged.

- The leg should be immobilised in a suitable external cast for at least a month.

2. Rupture of the peroneus tertius muscle
Aetiology
- Trauma from a fall, etc., results in rupture of the muscle, generally at its proximal origin on the stifle.

Clinical signs
- At rest, the limb is weight bearing, but there is a characteristic gait when walking, with the foot dragged and the limb pulled backwards as the hock is extended with the stifle flexed and the Achilles tendon slack and loose.
- There is a painful swelling on the lateral side of the stifle.

Treatment and prognosis
- The progress is favourable, complete rest for about 6 weeks often resulting in recovery.

3. Rupture of the cranial cruciate ligament
Aetiology
- Trauma to the stifle region.

Clinical signs
- During walking, the stifle is fixed, with the heel raised from the ground and weight carried on the tip of the toe. A positive draw forward sign is present.

Treatment
- Surgical treatment is essential or secondary damage to the joint may result in permanent lameness. The caprine stifle is similar anatomically to that of the dog (except for the fabellae) and similar surgical procedures to those used in the dog are suitable.

4. Rupture of the calcaneal tendon
Rupture of the calcaneal tendon results in acute lameness with swelling over the caudal area of the Achilles tendon. Successful primary repair of the tendon has been reported in a kid. In an adult goat repair has been carried out by transposition of the tendon of the peroneus longus muscle.

Luxations

1. Luxation of the scapulohumeral joint
Clinical signs
- The affected fore limb is carried in a semiflexed position, abducted and rotated outward. Attempts at flexion are painful.

Treatment
- Surgery to stabilise the joint.

2. Luxating patella
Patella luxation may be:
- Lateral, congenital and obvious in the young goat (see Chapter 8).
- Medial, acquired as a result of trauma. Acquired lateral luxation may occur but is less common than medial luxation.

Nerve damage

1. Radial nerve injury
Aetiology
- Trauma in the area of the upper limb or axilla.
- Lateral recumbency on a hard surface, for example during anaesthesia.

Clinical signs
- Dropped elbow with flexion of the carpus and fetlock.
- The foot is dragged as the carpus and fetlock cannot be extended.

Treatment
- Corticosteroids and diuretics to reduce the swelling around the nerve.
- Tendon transplantation has been used when the nerve injury was permanent.

2. Lameness after injection
Extreme care should be taken with intramuscular injections, as permanent lameness can result. Temporary lameness in goats is common after injections with irritant substances, such as tetracyclines and enrofloxacin, because of the relatively small muscular masses in the hind leg, particularly in the gluteal region. A more permanent lameness may result from damage to the sciatic or peroneal nerves. Because of the dangers involved in injecting into the limbs, the mid neck region has been recommended as a more suitable injection site (see Appendix 2).

Lameness may also be produced by painful swellings following the subcutaneous injection of irritant drugs (e.g. some oil adjuvanted vaccines) behind the elbow. Intramuscular injections should be avoided wherever possible and the subcutaneous route used for all drugs where so licensed.

2.1. Sciatic nerve injury

Aetiology
- Injections in the gluteal muscle mass.

Clinical signs
- Loss of function in almost all of the hind limb, with loss of skin sensation on the lateral surface of the tibial region and the hock and below.
- The foot is dragged. With each step the leg is pulled upward and forward by contraction of the quadriceps muscles, which are innervated by the femoral nerve.

Treatment and prognosis
- Even severe cases may resolve, but the prognosis is guarded.

2.2. Peroneal nerve injury

Aetiology
- Injections in the caudal thigh region.
- Trauma to the lateral surface of the thigh.

Clinical signs
- Paralysis of the muscles flexing the hock and extending the digits, so that when the foot is brought forward there is knuckling at the fetlock and the hoof is dragged along the ground. If the foot is placed in position, normal weight bearing can occur.

Treatment and prognosis
- Prognosis is generally favourable, with some improvement being seen in about a week.
- Anti-inflammatory drugs and diuretics will reduce swelling in the area of the nerve.
- In cases of permanent injury the fetlock joint can be ankylosed.

Carpal hygroma

Aetiology
- Persistent trauma to the carpal area results in the development of a bursa.

- Common from the routine wear and tear of life but may form part of the caprine arthritis encephalitis syndrome.

Clinical signs
- A firm, non-painful swelling, often bilateral, on the dorsal aspect of the carpal joint.
- The animal is generally not lame.

Treatment
- Acute lesions may resolve without treatment, but chronic conditions are unlikely to resolve.
- Aspiration of the bursal fluid may introduce infection if aseptic precautions are not carefully followed and is likely to produce only a temporary reduction in size.
- Injection with Lugol's iodine will destroy the membrane of the bursa.
- Surgical removal of the bursal sac can be undertaken for cosmetic reasons.

Osteopetrosis

Excessive calcium intake causing deposition in the bones and lameness in bucks and older does has been occasionally reported from the United States, where large amounts of alfalfa hay are fed. In the United Kingdom, where grass hay is normally fed, osteopetrosis is unlikely to present a problem. Excessive calcium in the diet promotes hypercalcitoninism with excessive deposition of calcium into bone with proliferative calcification around joints, which are palpably enlarged with a decreased range of movement. Affected animals should be tested for caprine arthritis encephalititis virus, particularly if there is mineralization of the tendons and joint capsules, because of the similar bony changes that occur with this disease (see later in this chapter).

Osteopetrosis is also seen in animals with enzootic calcinosis from the ingestion of calcinogenic plants containing an active metabolite of vitamin D3, which directly interferes with calcium metabolism (see below and Chapter 21).

Osteoporosis

Osteoporosis has been reported in adult lactating goats with clinical signs of lameness, stiff gait, arched back, weight loss and decreased milk production, which were fed a diet deficient in calcium, phosphorus and vitamin

D in conjunction with malnutrition attributable to gastrointestinal parasitism. Radiographs showed decreased skeletal mineralisation.

Enzootic calcinosis

Ingestion of a number of calcinogenic plants, mostly from the *Solanaceae* family (see Chapter 21), results in loss of condition and weight loss, progressing to emaciation, with a stiff and painful gait and dyspnoea even at rest. In advanced cases, joints cannot be extended completely and animals tend to walk with an arched back. Animals recover rapidly if they are removed in the early stages from dangerous pasture, but mortality is high after prolonged exposure.

Degenerative arthritis (osteoarthritis)

Aetiology
- A non-infectious arthritis resulting from degenerative changes in articular cartilage, together with hypertrophy of cartilage and bone.

Clinical signs
- A chronic lameness of gradual onset in older animals. The joints most commonly affected are the carpus, elbow, hock and stifle and these joints may be palpably enlarged, with crepitus evident on manipulation.
- The goat may have difficulty rising or if only one leg is affected may continuously rest the limb.
- With lack of use, muscle wasting of the affected limb may be evident.

Treatment
- Treatment is discussed earlier in this chapter and in Chapter 22, 'The Geriatric Goat'.

Caprine arthritis encephalitis

Caprine arthritis encephalitis (CAE) is a disease of major importance in many parts of the world including France, Australia and the United States. In the United Kingdom, estimates of the level of infection in pedigree stock are now less than 1% and clinical cases are rarely reported. Since 1983, many goatkeepers have been regularly blood testing for the disease and have adopted suitable control measures, thus drastically limiting the spread of the disease. However, failure to maintain control measures could rapidly lead to an increased incidence of infection. In contrast, although many larger commercial herds have tested all or some of their goats, there are many in which the CAE status is unknown, although the level of clinical disease appears to be very low.

Aetiology
- A lentivirus of the family Retroviridae, caprine arthritis encephalitis virus (CAEV), exists as a single-stranded, icosahedral RNA virus in circulating monocytes. CAEV and Maedi-Visna virus/ovine Lentivirus (MVV, OvLV) are together referred to as *small ruminant lentivirus (SRLV)* because each virus can infect both goats and sheep.
- Various studies have noted breed differences among goats in susceptibility to CAEV, suggesting that there is a genetic basis to susceptibility, but few studies have examined specific genetic regions to identify factors underlying these genetic differences. A genetic marker for susceptibilty to OVLV in sheep has been developed and further genomic regions have been identified as being involved with susceptibility.

Transmission
- Through free virus in the colostrum or milk of infected does. The practice of feeding milk pooled from several does will facilitate spread of the disease throughout the kid population.
- By direct contact between goats by virus-infected monocytes or macrophages shed in body fluids such as saliva, urogenital secretions, faeces and/or respiratory tract secretions. The amount of CAE infected cells found in respiratory, oral, lacrimal and urogenital secretions is low so that prolonged contact is necessary for horizontal transmission to occur. Behavioural traits that could increase the risk of transmission include teat biting and sucking by does and leakage of milk before milking.
- By transfer of blood from an infected to a non-infected goat, e.g. by tattooing or multiple use of needles.
- *In utero* transmission appears to be at a very low level but reported cases of sero-conversion in newborn kids separated from their mother at birth may be explained in some instances by vertical transmission *in utero* or during parturition.

- The virus is very labile in the environment and transmission via pasture or buildings, etc., will not occur.
- Direct cross-species transmission between sheep and goats has not been demonstrated experimentally, but lambs fed milk from CAE-positive goats become infected with the virus and sheep inoculated with virus experimentally became infected and developed lesions of the disease. Experience in Switzerland suggests that seropositive sheep can play an important role in infecting goats and that any eradication or control programme should include sheep as well as goats.
- Goats infected with CAE remain virus carriers for life and many symptomless carriers exist in the population. The virus can thus be unwittingly spread throughout the flock or herd, particularly to the young stock, without the owners being aware of a carrier being present.
- SRLV infect tissues from the male genital tract and lentivirus has been found in semen, which means that horizontal transmission from male to female during natural mating or AI is theoretically possible. SRLV is thought to enter the semen from the circulation via infected macrophages. However, despite infection being found in the seminal plasma and non-spermatic cells (primarily monocyte macrophages), the spermatozoa seem to resist infection and AI seems to represent a minor (but not zero) risk.
- Embryo transfer appears to impose minimal risk, provided the embryos retain their zona pellucida and are washed to the standards developed by the International Embryo Transfer Society (IETS).

Clinical signs

- Lentivirus infections lead to the slow induction of clinical signs and persistent infections. CAEV remains latent until the monocytes containing the virus mature into macrophages, the macrophages then disseminate to other tissues such as the mammary gland, choroid plexus of the brain, synovial membranes, lung and associated lymph nodes.
- Many goats remain symptomless carriers of the virus.
- The clinical signs and lesions of CAE are associated with the viral replication in infected macrophages at the predilection sites and active viral infection induces a strong but non-protective humoral and cell mediated immune response. The disease occurs in five clinical forms.

1. Arthritis

- Generally seen only in yearlings or adult goats, although occasionally in kids as young as 6 months.
- CAE virus affects all synovial membranes including those of joints, tendons and bursae and produces a chronic, progressive synovitis and arthritis with excess synovial fluid.
- Afebrile.
- Good appetite.
- Variable lameness, from slight stillness to extreme pain on standing.
- Gradual loss of condition depending on the degree of lameness.
- The carpal (knee) joints are primarily affected and may be grossly enlarged (Plate 7.9).
- Any other joint may be affected, particularly the shoulder, stifle, hock and fetlock, and the atlantal and supraspinous bursae are often enlarged later in the course of the disease.
- The course of the disease is variable, some animals merely showing slight lameness for a number of years, others showing an acute onset rapidly progressing to restriction of movement.

2. Hard udder

See Chapter 13.
- Clinical signs include gradual fibrosis and induration of the udder.

3. Interstitial pneumonitis

See Chapter 17.
- Early signs include a dry cough, which later progresses to chronic dyspnoea, weight loss and abnormal lung sounds.

4. Encephalitis

See Chapter 12.
- Never recorded in the United Kingdom and comparatively rare elsewhere. Affected kids tend to be between 2 and 6 months of age, but older goats are sometimes affected.
- Neurological signs have occasionally been recorded in adult goats, but are uncommon.

5. Progressive weight loss

See Chapter 9.
- Chronic progressive weight loss is often seen, either in conjunction with other clinical signs or on its own.

Laboratory confirmation

1 **Serology.** Serology is routinely used to identify SRLV infections. Additionally, several methods based on the polymerase chain reaction (PCR) have been developed to detect provirus DNA and, by introducing an additional step of reverse transcriptase (RT-PCR), viral RNA in different diagnostic samples such as milk cells.

o Agar gel immunodiffusion (AGID), enzyme-linked immunosorbent assay (ELISA), radioimmunoprecipitation (RIPA) and western blotting (WB) are all methods used for the serological diagnosis of SRLV infections.

o Routinely virus carriers are identified by using AGID or ELISA to detect antibody to CAEV. Antigens prepared from either CAE or maedivisna viruses can be used in these tests. Due to their complexity and costs WB and RIPA are only used as confirmatory tests.

o The antibodies detected are not protective against disease, but merely an indicator of infection, as only very low levels of neutralising antibodies are produced in response to infection.

o The quality of serological methods is defined by their sensitivity and specificity, but due to the absence of a 'gold standard', the calculation of these parameters is difficult for SRLV diagnostics and there is no agreement between laboratories on the 'best' test to use. AGID is considered highly specific but relatively insensitive and has been replaced by ELISA in many laboratories.

o A positive result means the goat has been infected with the CAE virus and is a potential shedder of the virus, especially if lactating. A negative result means that the goat is either not infected or has been recently infected and is producing amounts of antibody too low to be detected. A suspect result may reflect recently infected animals, young animals who have received colostrum containing antibodies or animals reacting abnormally to the test. Suspect animals should be retested.

o Any goat that is seropositive on a CAE test is infected for life. Infection persists even in the presence of neutralising antibodies because of the ability of the virus to exist as latent proviral DNA.

Conversely, however, a goat that is tested seronegative cannot be assumed free from infection, because: (1) routine tests are relatively insensitive and (2) the period between infection with the virus and seroconversion (i.e. production of detectable antibody) may be prolonged. Goats infected by contact or by drinking infected milk when adult may take 3 or more years to become seropositive. Kids infected postnatally generally seroconvert between 6 and 12 months of age. Some seropositive goats will periodically test seronegative. Animals tested seronegative on AGID or ELISA may test positive using PCR, that is provirus DNA is detectable before antibody production.

o Many goats seroconvert after a period of stress or at parturition. Testing in late pregnancy will not necessarily detect all does that seroconvert after kidding and these animals will produce infected kids.

o Kids that have received infected colostrum have detectable levels of colostral antibody for 2 or 3 months but will subsequently test negative until they seroconvert and produce their own antibodies several months or even years later.

o Antibody levels may fall as the disease progresses so even a clinically diseased animal may test seronegative.

Other tests are available in specialised laboratories but not for routine screening. The use of these more sensitive tests in the future may help detect latently infected animals, thus greatly facilitating eradication programmes:

♦ Detection of provirus DNA (PCR) and viral RNA (RT-PC). In many cases PCR is less sensitive than ELISA tests, but has the advantage of detecting infected animals before seroconversion.

♦ Virus isolation.

o Milk ELISA tests are being developed for bulk milk examination and could be a useful tool to monitor CAE levels in larger herds of unknown status. The ability to detect infection at a low prevalence has been demonstrated.

2 **Examination of synovial fluid**

o Reddish brown synovial fluid with large numbers of cells (1000 to 2000/mm), mainly mononuclear cells (cf. normal goats <500 cells/mm), may contain fibrin tags.

o Locally produced antibody may be detectable in the fluid.

3 **Histological examination (joints)**

o Subsynovial mononuclear cell infiltration and hyperplasia.

o Synovial villus hypertrophy.

o Focal areas of necrosis within the synovial membrane or surrounding connective tissue.

Gross post-mortem findings (joints)

- Hyperplasia of synovial membranes with thickening, fibrosis and, in chronic cases, calcification of joint capsule, tendons and ligaments.
- Periosteal reaction with periarticular osteophyte production.
- Degenerative joint disease with ulceration and erosion of the articular cartilages and destruction of subchondral bone.

Diagnosis

Diagnosis should be based on:

- Serum antibody levels to CAE virus.
- Clinical signs.
- Post-mortem lesions.
- Histopathological change.
- Virus isolation from synovial or brain cells.
- Radiology may aid in determining the severity or progression of arthritic lesions in individual animals and demonstrate pneumonia.

Treatment

- There is no treatment at present for CAE.
- Non-steroidal anti-inflammatory drugs such as flunixin meglamine, meloxicam and carprofen can be used to relieve the pain of arthritis (see Table 7.2).

Prevention and control

> Although the level of CAE in the United Kingdom is now very low, the potential remains for a rapid increase unless routine control measures are maintained.

- Routine tests at 6 to 12 monthly intervals for a minimum of 5 years and preferably more, with no evidence of infection in the herd during that time, are required before a herd can be said to be 'CAE virus free'.
- No kid should receive unpasteurised goats' milk or colostrum from any animal, except its dam. Pooled milk should never be fed to kids. If a doe subsequently proves to be a virus carrier only her own kids will have been infected.
- All adult goats (or in the case of a kid, its dam) should be blood tested before entry into the herd.

- No milk from another herd should be fed under any circumstances.
- Any sheep in contact with the goats should be tested at the same time.

The infected herd/flock

- Cull or isolate all reactors.
- Cull or isolate the offspring of all reactors.
- Infected goats should be separated from non-infected goats by a least 1.8 m. Separate feeding/water utensils should be used.
- Milk infected goats last; keep milk separate from any non-infected milk used for feeding kids.
- As the virus is labile in the environment, infected goats can graze the same pastures as non-infected goats provided the groups are kept separate, that is graze non-infected goats in the morning and infected goats in the afternoon.
- Because the incidence of uterine infection by the virus is very low, removing the kids at birth from reactors by 'snatching', that is preventing suckling or licking by the dam, enables a non-infected kid to be produced in the vast majority of cases.
- Batch-mate and induce parturition using prostaglandins (Chapter 1). Isolate kids, house separately from adult goats, and rear on cows' colostrum and milk or calf or kid milk replacer. If goats' milk or colostrum is fed, it must be pasteurised even if it comes from a supposedly seronegative doe (Chapter 23). Haemolysis very occasionally occurs in kids fed cows' milk (see Chapter 19).

The dangers of producing kids with low colostral antibodies must be weighed against the possible dangers of CAE infection in each herd.

- Kids can be rinsed in warm water and thoroughly dried to remove maternal material. Cardboard boxes can be used to house separate litters of kids for the first few weeks of life; disposable boxes aid in preventing transmission of neonatal pathogens.
- Blood sample kids shortly after birth to detect any possible passive transfer of antibody if the snatching was not done efficiently, then at 6 months and at 3-monthly intervals thereafter to detect possible virus carriers.
- Snatching kids and rearing separately will help to control CAE, caseous lymphadenitis, Johne's disease and mycoplasma.

- CAEV-infected cells have been detected in pre-putial scrapings of bucks and in fresh buck semen. There is a slightly higher risk of seroconversion in does that are mated to CAEV positive bucks. Eliminating oral–genital contact at mating, hand-mating (not loose in a pen) and avoiding the use of bucks with inflammatory reproductive conditions that might increase the likelihood of transferring infected mononuclear cells will minimise the risk if it is necessary to use positive bucks, but hand mating uninfected and infected animals is not risk-free.
- In meat goat and fibre herds where kids are raised on their dam, prevention of infection of herd replacements is accomplished by testing and segregating doe/kid pairs based on CAEV status.

Genetic marker-assisted selection

Recent developments in sheep of a genetic marker test for susceptibility to OvLV and the identification of further genomic regions linked to susceptibility to infection mean that breeding for resistance to SRLVs may become a possibility in the near future, although genetic studies in goats are less advanced.

Control schemes

- In many countries, including the United Kingdom, private or government-sponsored schemes have been introduced to control CAE and have been very successful in dramatically reducing the incidence of the disease in the national herds. The Swiss eradication programme for CAE reduced the prevalence of seropositive herds from 70 to 1% in 15 years, with a reduction in cases with clinical signs to zero.
- Individual herd scheme tailored to control the disease within the herd along the lines previously described.
- British Goat Society Monitored Herd Scheme is a scheme for monitoring the disease status of goat herds by testing but with no restrictions on the movement of goats. All goats attending recognised shows in the United Kingdom must be from CAE negative herds.
- Scotland's Rural College (SRUC) Premium Sheep and Goat Health Scheme monitors the disease status of the herd by regular blood tests and, by restricting movement between herds, aims to maintain herds as CAE free (Premium Sheep and Goat Health Schemes, SRUC, PO Box 5557, Inverness IV2 4YT. Tel: 01463 226995. Available at: http://www.sruc.ac.uk/info/120113/premium_sheep_and_goat_health_schemes).

Lyme disease

Lyme disease (Lyme borreliosis) is a tick-borne spirochaetal disease of animals and humans reported from Europe, North America, China, Japan and Australia. *Ixodes* spp. ticks normally transmit the disease and various vertebrates serve as reservoir hosts for the spirochaete, *Borrelia burgdorferi*. A competent reservoir host acquires Lyme disease spirochaetes when an infected tick (larva, nymph or adult) feeds on it and maintains them to become and remain infectious for feeding ticks. Different genospecies of *Borrelia burgdorferi* are associated with particular reservoir hosts. A host that is competent for one genospecies seems less competent or incompetent for another. Lyme disease spirochetes are eliminated from the ticks when feeding on goats and cattle, reducing the prevalence of infected ticks on a pasture. The mechanism for this is under investigation.

Clinical signs

Goats commonly show serological evidence of infection in endemic areas, but clinical cases are not well documented, with diagnosis often being made after other causes of arthritis have been eliminated. Reported signs include lethargy, pyrexia, joint pain, back pain, stiff neck and unsteady gait.

Laboratory investigation

- IFA as a screening test for antibodies against *B. burgdorferi*.
- Western blot (immunoblot) is qualitative test that detects antibodies produced to the many antigenic proteins of *B. burgdorferi*. Detection of antibodies does not confirm disease.

Treatment

In cattle, antibiotic treatment with oxytetracycline or penicillin for 21 days is recommended. Canine vaccines are not approved for use in goats.

Tumour

Tumours of the limbs, including chondrosarcoma of the humerus, have occasionally been reported as chronic progressive lameness and pain.

Exotic causes of lameness

Brucellosis
See Chapter 2.

Brucella melitensis and *Brucella abortus* can both cause abortions during the fourth month of gestation, as well as mastitis and lameness.

Mycoplasmosis
See Chapter 8.

Polyarthritis occurs as a result of septicaemia following mycoplasma infections. Although arthritis is most common in young kids and yearlings of dairy breeds, all ages and breeds of goats can be infected. The arthritis generally occurs concurrently with other clinical signs of mycoplasma infection, such as abortion, agalactia, pneumonia or keratoconjunctivitis, depending on the mycoplasma species involved. Goats with hot, swollen joints should be examined for other signs of systemic infection that could indicate mycoplasmosis.

Further reading

General

Adams, D.S. (1983) Infectious causes of lameness above the foot. *Vet. Clin. North Amer.: Large Anim. Pract.*, **5** (3), 499–510.

Christodoulopoulos, G. (2009) Foot lameness in dairy goats. *Res. Vet. Sci.*, **86**, 281–284.

Cottom, D.S. and Pinsent, P.J.N. (1988) Lameness in the goat. *Goat Vet. Soc. J.*, **9** (1/2), 14–23.

Galbraith, H. (2000) Protein and sulphur amino acid nutrition of hair fibre producing Angora and Cashmere goats. *Livestock Production Science*, **64**, 81–93.

Hill, N.P., Murphy, P.A., Nelson, A. *et al.* (1997) Lameness and foot lesions in adult British dairy goats. *Vet. Rec.*, **141**, 412–416.

Ingvast-Larsson, C., Högberg, M., Mengistu, U. , Olsén, L. *et al.* (2011) Pharmacokinetics of meloxicam in adult goats and its analgesic effect in disbudded kids. *J. Vet. Pharmacol. Therap.*, **34** (1), 64–69.

Merrall, M. (1985) Lameness in goats. In: *Proceedings of a Course in Goat Husbandry and Medicine*. Massey University, November, Publ. No. 106, pp. 66–77.

Nelson, D.R. (1983) Non-infectious causes of lameness above the foot. *Vet. Clin. North Amer.: Large Anim. Pract.*, **5** (3), November, 1983, 491–498.

Smith, M.C. (1983) Foot problems in goats. *Vet. Clin. North Amer.: Large Anim. Pract.*, **5** (3), 489–490.

Winter, A.C. (2011) Treatment and control of hoof disorders in sheep and goats. *Vet. Clin. North Amer.: Food Anim. Pract.*, **27** (1), 187–192.

Caprine arthritis encephalitis

Adams, D.S., *et al.* (1983) Transmission and control of CAE virus. *Am. J. Vet. Res.*, **44** (9), 1670–1675.

Cortez-Romero, C., Pellerin, J.L., Ali-Al-Ahmad, M.Z., Chebloune, Y. *et al.* (2013) The risk of small ruminant lentivirus (SRLV) transmission with reproductive biotechnologies: state-of-the-art review. *Theriogenology*, **79**, 1–9.

Dawson, M. (1987) Caprine arthritis encephalitis. *In Pract.*, **9**, 8–11.

Herrmann-Hoesing, L.M. (2010) Diagnostic assays ssed to control small ruminant lentiviruses. *J. Vet. Diagn. Invest.*, **22** (6), 843–855.

Knight, A.P. and Jokinen, M.P. (1982) Caprine arthritis encephalitis. *Comp. Cont. Ed. Pract. Vet.*, **4** (6), S263–269.

Leroux, C., Cruz, J.C. and Mornex, J.F. (2010) SRLVs: a genetic continuum of lentiviral species in sheep and goats with cumulative evidence of cross species transmission. *Curr. HIV Res.*, **8**, 94–100.

Nagel-Alne, G.E., Valle, P.S., Krontveit, R. and Sølverød, L.S. (2015) Caprine arthritis encephalitis and caseous lymphadenitis in goats: use of bulk tank milk ELISAs for herd-level surveillance. *Vet. Rec.*, **176**, 173.

Ramsés, Reina, R. *et al.* (2009) Prevention strategies against small ruminant lentiviruses: an update. *Vet. J.*, **182** (1), 31–37.

Rowe, J.D. and East, N.E. (1997) Risk factors for transmission and methods for control of caprine arthritis encephalitis virus infection. *Vet. Clin. North Amer.: Large Anim. Pract.*, **13** (1), 35–53.

Synge, B.A. and Ritchie, C.M. (2010) Elimination of small ruminant lentivirus infection from sheep flocks and goat herds aided by health schemes in Great Britain. *Vet. Rec.*, **167** (19), 739–743.

Thorley, J. *et al.* (2004) Routes of transmission and consequences of small ruminant lentiviruses (SRLVs) infection and eradication schemes. *Vet. Res.*, **35**, 257–274.

White, S.N. and Knowles, D.P. (2013) Expanding possibilities for intervention against small ruminant lentiviruses through genetic marker-assisted selective breeding. *Viruses*, **5**, 1466–1499.

Caprine digital dermatitis

Angell, J.W., Blundell, R., Grove-White, D.H. and Duncan, J.S. (2015) Clinical and radiographic features of contagious ovine digital dermatitis and a novel lesion grading system. *Vet. Rec.*, **176**, 544.

Davies, I. (2011) Treatment options for contagious ovine digital dermatitis. *Vet. Rec.*, **169** (23), 604–605.

Duncan, J.S., Grove-White, D., Oultram, J.W.H. *et al.* (2011) Effects of parenteral amoxicillin on recovery rates and new infection rates for contagious ovine digital dermatitis in sheep. *Vet. Rec.*, **169** (23), 606.

Groenevelt, M., Anzuino, K., Smith, S. *et al.* (2013) Laminitis complicated by treponemes as a major lameness cause in two dairy goat herds. *8th International Sheep Veterinary Congress*, New Zealand, p. 89.

Groenevelt, M., Anzuino,K., Langton, D.A. and Grogono-Thomas, R. (2015) Association of treponeme species with atypical foot lesions in goats. *Vet. Rec.*, **176** (24), 626.

Sullivan, I.E., Evans, N.J., Clegg, S.R. *et al.* (2015) Digital dermatitis treponemes associated with a severe foot disease in dairy goats. *Vet. Rec.*, **176** (11), 283.

Footrot

Hay, L.A. (1990) Footrot and related conditions. *Goat Vet. Soc. J.*, **11** (1), 1–6.

Laven, R. (2012) Use of parenteral long-acting and topical oxytetracycline, without hoof trimming, for treatment of footrot in goats. *New Zealand Vet. J.*, **60** (3), 213–214.

Osteoporosis

Braun, U., Ohlerth, S., Liesegang, A., Forster, E. *et al.* (2009) Osteoporosis in goats associated with phosphorus and calcium deficiency. *Vet. Rec.*, **164**, 211–213.

Septic pedal arthritis

Harwood, D. (2009) An outbreak of septic pedal arthritis in a commercial dairy goat herd. *Livestock*, **14** (7), 19–47.

Lovatt, F. (2012) Joint lavage in the treatment of ovine septic pedal arthritis. *In Pract.*, **34**, 348–354.

Surgery

Anderson, D.E. and St Jean, G. (1996) External skeletal fixation in ruminants. *Vet. Clin. North Amer.: Food Anim. Pract.*, **12** (1), 117–152.

Baron, R.J. (1990) Laterally luxating patella in a goat. *J. Am. Vet. Med. Assoc.*, **191**, 1471–1472.

Hunt, R.J., Allen, D. and Thomas, K. (1991) Repair of a ruptured calcaneal tendon by transposition of the tendon of the peroneus longus muscle in a goat. *J. Am. Vet. Med. Assoc.*, **198** (9), 1640–1642.

Joy, B. and Venugopal, S.K. (2014) Complications in fracture healing using external skeletal fixation in goats. *Int. J. Rec. Sci. Res.*, **5** (7), 1298–1299.

Mueller, K. (2015) Goat orthopaedics – bone sequestrum and fractures. *Goat Vet. Soc. J.*, **31**, 54–59.

Mulon, P.-Y. (2013) Management of long bone fractures in cattle. *In Pract.*, **35**, 265–271.

Purohit, N.R., Choudray, R.J., Chouhan, D.S. and Sharma, C.K. (1985) Surgical repair of scapulohumeral luxation in goats. *Mod. Vet. Pract.*, **66**, 758–759.

Sack, W.O. and Cottrell, W. (1984) Puncture of shoulder, elbow and carpal joints in goats and sheep. *J. Am. Vet. Med. Assoc.*, **185**, 63–65.

Scott, P. (1995) Amputation of the ovine digit. *In Pract.*, **17**, 80–82.

Vogel, S.R. and Anderson, D.E. (2014) External skeletal fixation of fractures in cattle. *Vet. Clin. North Amer.: Food Anim. Pract.*, **30**, 127–142.

Tumour

Schmid, T. *et al.* (2010) Chondrosarcoma in the humerus of a goat. *Vet. Comp. Ortho. Traumatol.*, **23** (4), 273–276.

White line disease

Winter, A and Arsenos, G. (2009) Diagnosis of white line lesions in sheep. *In Pract.*, **31**, 17–21.

CHAPTER 8

Lameness in kids

Trauma

> The kid is an 'accident waiting to happen'.

The most common causes of lameness in kids are the result of accident or trauma, resulting in bruising, sprains, strains or fractures, particularly of the front legs.

Fractures

Fractures occur most frequently in the metacarpal region, followed by the radius/ulna, tibia and metatarsus. In many cases, palpation permits identification of the site of the fracture, but radiography may be required for confirmation if there is little bone displacement.

Fracture management is discussed in Chapter 26.

External fixation with plaster or lightweight resin material is extremely well tolerated. If necessary, internal fixation, using a pin or plate, can be undertaken using techniques similar to those used in the dog (see Table 26.9). Where possible, additional external support is indicated because of the robust use of the leg, which will occur as the fracture heals.

Foreign bodies

Foreign bodies, for example thorns, may penetrate the hoof more easily in kids than in adult goats.

Congenital abnormalities

Overextension of the stifle and hock
Aetiology
- Overextension of the hock and stifle is common in newly born kids and is usually bilateral, although one leg is often more severely affected than the other.

Clinical signs
- The kid has difficulty walking as the leg tends to bow and the stifle and hock joints are unstable.

Treatment
- No treatment is generally necessary as the condition normally corrects itself within a few days, but it is necessary to ensure that the kid is mobile enough to suckle adequately from its dam.

Contracted flexor tendons of the forelimbs

Positional constraints *in utero*, when the size and/or number of kids restricts movement, commonly result in the bilateral contraction of the flexor tendons of the forelimbs, resulting in flexion of the fetlocks so that the animal walks on its fetlocks or with partially flexed fetlocks. The condition may cause dystocia as the front legs cannot extend properly into the pelvis and affected kids may find it difficult to move around and suckle.

Treatment
- Mild cases with only partial flexion of the fetlocks will resolve on their own as the tendons stretch with movement and this can be helped by manually extending the joints to stretch the tendons.
- More severe cases may need splinting to stretch the tendons and allow weight-bearing on the foot. Splinting the affected limb(s) from just above the ground to the elbow or hock (without enclosing the toes) may be necessary to provide continuous pressure on the tendons. The leg should be extended enough to place the tendons under some tension. Splints should be well padded and are initially left in place for 1 to 3 days, then changed with further extension of the limb as necessary. The prognosis is generally good for cases that can be conservatively managed.

Diseases of the Goat, Fourth Edition. John Matthews.
© 2016 John Wiley & Sons, Ltd. Published 2016 by John Wiley & Sons, Ltd.

Angular limb deformities and arthrogryposis

Congenital limb deformities involving the bones and joints are occasionally seen in newborn goats. Congenital arthrogryposis is defined as a syndrome of persistent joint contraction (bilateral rigidity) present at birth, involving one or more of the fore or hind limbs, but most commonly resulting in a bilateral articular rigidity, particularly flexion of phalangeal, metacarpo-phalangeal and carpal joints.

Cases of mild articular rigidity associated with contracted tendons may correct themselves with weight-bearing. Mild deformities can be corrected by manipulation and splinting (see contracted flexor tendons, above). Surgical treatment of severe retractions can be attempted in valuable animals.

Aetiology

- In the United Kingdom, usually as the result of contracted tendons caused by positional constraints *in utero*.
- The teratogenic effects of *plant poisoning* (*Lupinus formosus*, *Astragalus*, *Lathyrus*, *Sophora* and Sudan grass; see Chapter 21) may produce limb deformities.
- An inherited tendon shortening has been reported in Australian Angora goats.
- *Beta mannosidosis* is an inherited lysosomal disease of Nubian and Anglo- Nubian goats and their crosses attributable to an autosomal recessive gene, which has been reported in Australia, New Zealand, the United States, Fiji and Canada, but not the United Kingdom. Because of the absence of the enzyme beta-mannosidase, kids are unable to stand from birth due to carpal contractures and hyperextended fetlocks. Withdrawal reflexes are normal, but movement is accompanied by an intention tremor. Kids may show domed skulls, narrow muzzles, enophthalmos and palpebral fissures. Most kids are deaf. Some kids have intention tremors, pendular nystagmus or bilateral ptosis as part of Horner's syndrome.
- *Arthrogryposis hydranencephaly syndrome* (*AHS*) is caused by infection with an orthobunya virus, including *Akabane virus* (Australia, Japan, Israel, South Africa, the Middle East), *Cache Valley virus* (United States, Canada, Mexico) and *Schmallenberg virus* (Northern Europe, including the United Kingdom). A number of other related viruses exist, including Main Drain virus, Potosi virus and Northway virus in North America and may be responsible for causing disease in ruminants.
  - ○ Orthobunya viruses are arthropod-borne single-stranded RNA viruses that cause intrauterine infection in domestic and wild ruminants. Clinical disease occurs in pregnant animals infected in early pregnancy (28 to 60 days for Schmallenberg and Cache Valley viruses in sheep) during periods of high vector activity. Very early infection can cause embryonic death and return to service.
  - ○ Introduction of a virus to a naive ruminant population can result in severe economic damage, although, in general, goats appear to be much less severely affected than sheep and cattle. Viraemic animals, which are not showing clinical signs, may act as symptomless carriers of the virus, but ruminants do not appear to be long-term carriers of the viruses. Populations of animals exposed to the virus develop immunity to further infection from the same virus and in endemic areas most animals are likely to be immune to disease by the time they reach sexual maturity. There is no cross-protection between different viruses.

Vector

- Ruminants cannot directly affect one another.
- All known orthobunya viruses are spread by arthropod vectors, principally midges (*Culicoides* spp.) and mosquitoes (see bluetongue virus, Chapter 10). Spread of these viruses is linked to the natural movement of insects from infected areas.
- Schmallenberg virus is much more widely and rapidly spread than bluetongue virus because the midges carry ten times the viral load.
- Transplacental transmission has been shown to occur.

Clinical signs

- Adult goats are generally asymptomatic, except for increased incidence of abortions and congenital malformations in kids.
- Fetuses and neonatal kids have congenital malformations classified as *arthrogryposis hydranencephaly syndrome* (*AHS*). These include stillbirth, premature birth, mummified foetuses, arthrogryposis, joint malformations, scoliosis, torticollis, kyphosis, lordosis, hydrocephalus, hydranencephaly, microcephaly and cerebellar dysplasia, behavioural abnormalities and blindness. Specific AHS signs reflect the stage of

gestation when the virus infected the dam and the fetus. The limbs become rigid and distorted because damaged nerves fail to flex and contract the limbs as normal.

- Within a litter, individual fetuses show variable degrees and types of abnormality and some foetuses may appear normal.

Diagnosis

- Antibodies can be identified in serum or EDTA-preserved whole blood by serum neutralisation, ELISA, complement fixation and haemagluttination-inhibition tests, but in adult animals this only demonstrates previous exposure, not the infectious status of the animal. Conversely, lack of seral antibodies rules out the virus as a cause of a malformed fetus or neonate.
- Identification of precolostral or fetal serum antibodies to one of the viruses indicates involvement of the virus.
- Virus isolation in full-term malformed fetuses or neonatal kids is always unsuccessful.
- Real-time and conventional RT-PCR assays are useful for the detection of circulating virus before the peak of viraemia, seroconversion and the development of clinical signs.

Vaccination

- Inactivated vaccines against Schmallenberg virus are approved for use in Europe in sheep and cattle. Vaccination confers a higher level of immunity than natural exposure. The vaccine can be given from 4 months of age in sheep. Sheep (and goats) are given a single dose of vaccine.

Luxation of the patella
Aetiology

- Lateral luxation of the patella is an uncommon problem in goats and is usually congenital. Anglo-Nubian goats are more prone to the condition because of the upright conformation of their hind legs. In Swiss breeds, luxation occasionally occurs as the result of acute trauma in the adult goat and is generally medial.

Clinical signs

- The luxation may be bilateral or unilateral, permanent or intermittent. In its severest form, the stifles

will remain permanently flexed, so that the animal adopts a crouching stance and has difficulty in standing. Where the condition is intermittent there will be periods of acute lameness, which is relieved when the patella is returned to the normal position by manipulation.

Treatment

- Mild intermittent luxation requires no treatment, more severe luxations can be corrected surgically using similar techniques to those used in the dog and severe congenital luxations may necessitate euthanasia.

Spastic paresis

Spastic paresis has been diagnosed occasionally in goats, including a 3 year old male Saanen goat in Czechoslovakia and three male pygmy goats in the United States, of which 2 were related (sire and offspring), but the inheritance of the condition is not understood. Severe joint pain can occasionally lead to abnormalities of gait and posture that can mimic spastic paresis.

Clinical signs

Spastic paresis in goats appears to share many similarities with the disease in cattle:

- Intermittent, unilateral or bilateral spastic contracture of the gastrocnemius muscle leading to hyperextension of one or both hind limbs.
- The hyperextension may be so extreme that the animal is unable to place the foot on the ground and the leg is carried straight behind.
- Marked extension of the tibial-tarsal joints.
- Gastrocnemius muscle is constantly contracted and palpably firm or knotted.
- Back is arched.
- On rising, goats may lift their hindquarters into the air and shift weight to the front limbs for short periods.

Diagnosis

- Selective depression of gamma efferent neurons in the spinal cord by epidural administration of dilute procaine alleviates the condition, indicating that the disorder occurs from overstimulation (or lack of inhibition) of the myotatic (stretch) reflex.

Treatment

- Tibial neurectomy will correct the condition.

Infections

Joint ill (infectious polyarthritis)

Joint ill is a bacterial arthritis of young kids under 3 months of age.

Aetiology

- A number of bacteria may be involved. These are usually environmental contaminants, particularly haemolytic *Streptococcus* spp. and *Staphylococcus* spp. but also *Trueperella* spp. and *Escherichia coli*. Infection occurs through the umbilical cord shortly after birth, as a result of bacteraemia from enteroinvasion, or via the upper respiratory tract or tonsil. Other potential sources of infection with Streptococci include teats, milk and vagina of the dam. *S. dysgalactiae* can survive on dry straw for up to 42 days.

Clinical signs

- Pain and swelling in one or more joints of a neonatal kid, especially carpus, shoulder, hock and stifle, with lameness varying from moderate to non-weight-bearing. Occasionally there is pronounced lameness with minimum joint swelling. In more chronic cases, the affected joint will be stiff or even ankylosed.
- The kid may or may not be pyrexic depending on the stage and type of infection.
- The umbilicus is often inflamed.
- Involvement of the atlanto-occipital joint can produce sudden-onset tetraparesis and recumbency.

Laboratory investigation

- Joint fluid or umbilical swabs can be cultured for bacteria if indicated.
- Synovial fluid from infected joints is usually thick and cloudy with an increased total protein (normal <3 g/litre) with a characteristic pleocytosis, comprised almost entirely of neutrophils. In chronically lame kids, there is little joint effusion and arthrocentesis often yields more blood than joint fluid.

Prevention, control and treatment

- A clean environment at kidding. Bacteria can persist for several weeks in straw in deep-bedded pens, so adding new straw to a dirty pen will not prevent infection and all kidding pens should be cleaned out completely between kiddings.
- Treat umbilical cord with 7% tincture of iodine (Lugol's iodine) or antibiotic spray as soon after birth as possible and then check regularly for signs of inflammation or infection.
- Adequate colostrum (300 ml within 6 hours of birth).
- Treatment is only likely to be successful if given early, administering broad-spectrum antibiotics parenterally and intra-articularly. Wherever possible, antibiotic selection should be based on culture and sensitivity testing. Injections of high doses of parenteral antibiotics for 7 days may effect a cure if combined with careful nursing, but the response to treatment is often poor as progressive and degenerative changes occur within the infected joints. Procaine penicillin (44 000 i.u./kg every 24 hours for at least 5 days) is the antibiotic of choice for Streptococcal infection.
- Procaine penicillin administered to all kids at 36–48 hours of age is effective in the face of a disease outbreak of Streptococcal infection.
- Joint lavage with saline and antibiotic solutions (see Chapter 7), combined with systemic and local antimicrobial treatment, may improve the response to treatment in cases of acute septic arthritis. Joint lavage removes inflammatory exudate, reduces damage to the joint surfaces and helps eliminate infection. Lavage is repeated daily as needed.
- NSAIDs, flunixin, ketoprofen or meloxicam administered intravenously for three consecutive days will relieve pain.
- Good nursing will aid recovery: provide a soft bed, frequently turn any kid unable to stand and massage the affected joints.
- Treating severely affected kids may not be economically or humanely justifiable and euthanasia should be considered. Animals that survive may remain unthrifty.

Erysipelas

Erysipelas polyarthritis is common in lambs in the United Kingdom and has been occasionally reported in kids.

Aetiology

- The bacterium *Erysipelothrix rhusiopathiae* enters through breaks in the skin, for example castration wounds, or via the umbilicus.

Clinical signs

- Pyrexia, anorexia and lethargy, with hot, swollen, painful joints in the acute stage.
  The disease often becomes chronic.

Diagnosis

- Isolation of the organism from joints in acute cases.

Treatment

- High doses of penicillin (44 000 i.u./kg every 24 hours for at least 5 days).
- NSAIDs, flunixin, meloxicam or ketoprofen, intravenously for 3 consecutive days to relieve pain.

Control

- Vaccination of does in herds with a high prevalence of erysipelas polyarthritis.

Tick pyaemia (enzootic staphylococcal infection)

Aetiology

- *Staphylococcus aureus*. The tick *Ixodes ricinus* damages the kid's skin, permitting penetration of the bacteria, which are already present on the skin surface, and resulting in large subcutaneous abscesses and bacteraemia.
- Infection with tick-borne fever may exacerbate the pathogenicity of tick pyaemia. However, not all kids with tick-borne fever develop tick pyaemia.

Clinical signs

- Variable, depending on the site of abscesses, which form in various parts of the body, for example the liver and spinal cord, following the introduction of the bacteria and the resulting pyaemia.
- Hot, swollen, painful joints (particularly carpal joints and hocks), lameness, eventually chronic arthritis, with permanent lameness and poor growth rates.
- Various neurological signs, such as blindness, incoordination, posterior paraplegia.

Treatment

- Early cases can be treated with penicillin.
- Superficial abscesses can be lanced and drained.
- Once severe joint or vertebral lesions are present, treatment is not successful and animals should be euthanised.

Mycoplasma

Mycoplasma spp. have been reported to cause polyarthritis in goats in Europe, Australia and the United States, and with increasing numbers of goats being imported into the United Kingdom, mycoplasma should be regarded as a possible importation hazard. All ages and breeds of goats can be affected, but it is commonest in kids under 6 months and yearlings of dairy breeds. Mycoplasmal arthritis occurs as a result of septicaemia and may be part of a clinical syndrome including septicaemia, pneumonia (Chapter 17), mastitis (Chapter 13) and keratoconjunctivitis (Chapter 20). Congenital forms of arthritis in goat kids reported from Israel have been attributed to *M. mycoides* subspecies *mycoides* and from Greece attributed to *M. agalactiae*.

Aetiology

- *Mycoplasma* spp. such as *M. capricolum*, *M. mycoides* subsp. *capri*, *M. putrifaciens* and *Mycoplasma agalactiae*.

Transmission

- Mycoplasma are usually introduced on to the holding by an asymptomatic carrier.
- Milk is the primary mode of transmission of mycoplasmal infections, either directly from feeding or suckling or indirectly from milk-contaminated buckets or via hands or milk-contaminated clothing.
- Biosecretions from aborted does or goats with pneumonia should be considered at high risk.
- The ear mites *Psoroptes cuniculi* and *Raillietia capri* may carry multiple species of *Mycoplasma* and may represent a natural reservoir for pathogenic *Mycoplasma* spp.
- Even with treatment, recovery from clinical disease is often followed by conversion to an asymptomatic carrier state with intermittent shedding of mycoplasma in milk, most often when animals are stressed, for example at kidding.

Clinical signs

- Outbreaks of arthritis generally in kids and young goats, with acutely swollen joints and pyrexia with or without pneumonia (*M. mycoides*).
- Some herds with endemic mycoplasmosis have relatively little problem until extreme environmental conditions, nutritional problems or concurrent disease, like coccidiosis, favour a clinical mycoplasma outbreak in the herd (juvenile polyarthritis and/or adult mastitis or septicaemia). Mycoplasma infections

can exist in a herd for years between clinical flare-ups. Because special media are required to culture mycoplasma organisms, infections may go undetected until a clinical crisis occurs.

Post-mortem findings
- Purulent or fibropurulent arthritis with haemorrhagic erosions of articular surfaces.
- Lungs collapsed and rubbery.

Diagnosis
- Serology (complement fixation test).
- PCR testing is available for the detection and differentiation of *Mycoplasma* species. However, some closely related species may be misdiagnosed.
- Isolation of the organism from joint fluid in mycoplasma medium.
- Long-term surveillance by culturing milk is necessary to detect infected does.

Treatment
- No antibiotics are effective; although tylosin, 10–50 mg/kg every 8 hours, and other antibiotics like tetracyclines, florfenicol and enrofloxacin have been used to improve the clinical condition, recovered animals often become asymptomatic carriers.

Control
- Closed herds or strict quarantine and screening are recommended to prevent introduction of mycoplasma infections into a herd.
- Once disease has been introduced into the herd, the chronicity of mycoplasma infections and the ability to develop a carrier state make managing the disease difficult.
- Culture each doe's first colostrum for mycoplasma.
- Cull adult carriers as soon as they are identified or as soon as economically feasible.
- Snatch kids at birth and rear on pasteurised colostrum and milk or milk replacer (see CAE control, Chapter 7).
- Rear kids separately from the adult population. 'Clean' kids should not enter the contaminated adult herd and should not share housing, feeders or water troughs.
- Ear cultures and control of ear mites with an ectoparasiticide like ivermectin may be warranted as an added control in some eradication and prevention programmes, but needs species identification, as many mycoplasmas have been isolated from the ears of goats.
- Keep identified positive goats as a separate infected unit until culled.
- 2 metre alleyways should separate clean pens from infected pens.
- Milk positive goats last.

Chlamydia
Clamydophila pecorum (formerly *Clamydia psittaci*) has been reported to cause polyarthritis in young goats in parts of Europe and the United States, but not in the United Kingdom, although the organism has been isolated from sheep joints in this country.

Clinical signs
- Polyarthritis and stiffness as part of an acute febrile illness in a number of kids.
- The joint fluid is not purulent in appearance as the elevation in white blood cells is primarily due to mononuclear cells.

Post-mortem findings
- Fibrinous arthritis with no changes to the cartilage.

Diagnosis
- Smears of joint exudate stained with Giemsa (chlamydial organisms stain purple).
- Immunofluorescence.
- Isolation of chlamydia in embryonating yolk sacs.

Other bacterial arthritides
Other bacteria may occasionally cause arthritis as a result of either septicaemia or direct penetration into the joint from a puncture wound.

Footrot/interdigital dermatitis
See Chapter 7.

Infection with *Fusobacterium necrophorum* and *Dichelobacter nodosus* may become significant in older kids.

Nutritional causes

Calcium, phosphorus and vitamin D deficiency or imbalance
Kids are susceptible to imbalances in the calcium:phosphorus ratio. The calcium: phosphorus

Table 8.1 Daily calcium/phosphorus requirements.

	Gain (g/day)	Calcium (g)	Phosphorus (g)
Maintenance			
50 kg		2.5	1.5
80 kg		4.0	2.4
Production requirements/kg milk		4.0	3.0
Gestation requirements last 2 months		1.5	1.8
Kid daily requirements			
At 1 month old	175	2	1.3
At 2 months old	200	2.7	1.7
At 3 to 5 months old	175	2.9	1.9
At 6 months old	150	3.2	2.0

After Tomas and Turner, 1979; quoted in Baxendell, 1984.

ratio in goat diets should not drop below 1.2:1 and ideally should be around 2:1. Vitamin D is essential for the absorption and metabolism of calcium and phosphorus. On typical diets in the United Kingdom, where grass hay is more commonly fed than lucerne, a relative calcium deficiency is more likely than a calcium excess. Table 8.1 gives the daily requirements for calcium and phosphorus.

Angular limb deformities

Angular limb deformities may be present at birth (qv.), but mild limb deformities are also the most common manifestation of calcium:phosphorus imbalance in goats in the United Kingdom.

Aetiology

- Acquired limb deformities occur in a rapidly growing early maturing kid with a calcium:phosphorus imbalance.
- Angulation of the limb results in epiphyseal compression, producing increased pressure on the growth plate on that side and retarding growth.

Clinical signs

- Outward (lateral) deviation of the fetlock joint (fetlock valgus) is the most common deformity seen in young goats, but more severe imbalances may result in carpal valgus (knock knees) or carpal and stifle varus (bow legs).
- Uneven wear of the feet may occur.
- Lameness.

Treatment

- Correct dietary imbalances.
- Use corrective foot trimming on a fortnightly basis.
- The application of splints in the early stages of carpal varus and fetlock valgus may correct the problem.
- Surgical compression of the growth plate with staples or screws and wire will slow the growth on that side and allow the limb to straighten. Early remedial action is necessary before the natural closure of the growth plates.

Rickets

Rickets is a disease of young growing kids characterised by defective calcification of growing bone.

Aetiology

- Relative or absolute dietary deficiencies of calcium, phosphorus and vitamin D. Rapidly growing kids kept indoors on an otherwise good diet are most likely to be affected.

Clinical signs

- Enlarged painful epiphyses and costochondral junctions.
- Poor appetite and unthriftiness.
- Stiff gait, lameness, unwillingness to stand.
- Arched back.
- Possible bending of the long bones.

Prevention

- Exercise in sunlight with increased vitamin D levels.
- Feed sun-dried hay.
- Calcium and phosphorus supplements where necessary.
- Vitamin D 500 U or vitamins A, D and E 125 000 U.

Treatment

- Correct any calcium/phosphorus imbalance with supplements as necessary.
- Vitamin D 500 U injection.

Osteodystrophia fibrosa
Aetiology

- Like rickets, ostoodystrophia fibrosa is caused by an imbalance of calcium and phosphorus and results from a secondary calcium deficiency due to excess phosphorus feeding, giving a calcium:phosphorus ratio of 1:2.5 or greater.

- Cereals and bran are high in phosphorus. Diets low in fresh green food and good hay but high in cereals and bran predispose to the disease.

Clinical signs
- Unthriftiness.
- Poor appetite.
- Lameness.
- Bilateral swelling of bones of the face and jaw (Plates 8.1 and 8.2).
- Molar and premolar teeth rotated and loose.
- Fractures of long bones.
- Bones soft.

Prevention and treatment
- Correct the calcium:phosphorus ratio in the ration.
- Feed a diet high in green foods; add bonemeal or powdered limestone.
- Severely affected animals with distortion of the mandible should be culled.

White muscle disease
Vitamin E and selenium both have antioxidant functions and can partially substitute for one another in the diet. Vitamin E requirements of the goat may be higher than those of sheep and cattle.

Aetiology
- A selenium/vitamin E deficiency produces a degenerative myopathy, particularly in very young kids born to deficient dams. The clinical signs depend on whether the skeletal muscles (skeletal muscle form) or the heart muscle and diaphragm (cardiac form) are affected or whether both forms may appear together in the same animal.

Predisposing conditions
- Selenium-deficient pastures, where animals are fed on locally produced feed without supplementation.
- Vitamin E deficient diets due to poor quality hay or straw with little concentrate.
- High levels of unsaturated fatty acids, for example fish/soya oils, calf milk with added vegetable fat, cause relative vitamin E deficiency.

Clinical signs
- Kids are affected at birth or up to 6 months of age but generally between 2 and 16 weeks. The most active

kids are often affected first and the disease is often seen 2 to 3 days after turnout.

1. Skeletal muscle form
- Stiffness and reluctance to move, lying down frequently, standing up with Difficulty, crying if forced to move.
- Skeletal muscles firm and painful on palpation (cf. nervous disease), particularly in the hind limbs.
- Non-pyrexic.
- Appetite remains good even if the kid is unable to stand.
- Older kids and adults may show signs of the skeletal muscle form after stress or exercise.

2. Cardiac form
- Sudden death, typically in kids 2 to 6 months old after or during exercise.
- Tachycardia.
- Tachypnoea; hyperpnoea.
- Weakness.
- Severely deficient does may produce stillborn or weak kids that die of acute heart failure after a few days.

Post-mortem findings
- Pale or white streaks in the skeletal muscles, particularly of the hind limbs and lumbar area and the subendocardial muscle of the ventricles of the heart.

Laboratory findings
- Creatine phosphokinase (CPK) and aspartate transaminase (AST) levels are markedly elevated.
- Blood selenium levels are below 50 ppb (normal 158–160 ppb; marginal 50–80 ppb).
- Glutathione peroxidase levels low (<60 U/ml RBCs).
- Liver selenium levels below 500 nmol/kg or vitamin E below 2.5 umol/kg are considered deficient.

Prevention
- Dietary concentrations of 0.l mg/kg dry matter for selenium and 30 to 50 mg/kg dry matter for vitamin E are adequate.
- One month before kidding, inject the does with 3 mg/kg vitamin E and 0.07 mg/kg selenium and/or
- Inject the kids at birth and at 3 to 4 weeks of age with 34 mg vitamin E and 0.75 mg selenium, 0.5 ml s.c., and possibly at 12 to 16 weeks of age with 68 mg

vitamin E and 1.5 mg selenium. Always use subcutaneous injections, as intramuscular injections cause local reactions.

- Slow-release intraruminal boluses containing selenium, 4 to 8 weeks before lambing.
- Add selenium at 100 ppm to feed.
- Oral drench with 5 mg sodium selenite during the last week of pregnancy.
- Oral drench growing kids with selenium combined with anthelmintics, but as the standard inclusion of 0.4 mg/ml of elemental selenium is calibrated for use in lambs given 1 ml/kg body weight of the anthelmintic combination product, it is easy to overdose kids being given the higher doses of anthelmintics recommended for goats, resulting in selenium toxicity (see below).
- Top-dress pasture using slow-release selenium prills (0.5 kg per hectare annually).
- In the United States, the Food and Drug Administration (FDA) regulates the use of selenium as a food additive. Supplemental selenium can only be added to a diet to a total level of 0.3 ppm in the total diet.

Treatment

- Affected kids should be treated with 34–68 mg vitamin E and 0.75–1.5 mg selenium, 0.5–1 ml s.c.

Selenium toxicity

Overdosage with selenium supplements may result in selenium poisoning. The minimum toxic dose by injection is about 0.5 mg/kg (i.e. 50 times the therapeutic dose) but miscalculation can occur if using products developed for cattle. Caution is required when administering parenteral Se/Vit E preparations to kids as overdosage can result in severe respiratory distress and sudden death as a result of myocardial contraction band necrosis.

Acute poisoning can also occur by the single consumption of highly seleniferous plants (see Chapter 21). Several plant species are selenium accumulators, including *Astragalus* (loco weeds and milk vetches), *Onopisis* (goldenweed) and *Zylorhiza* (woody asters).

In the United States, selenium supplementation is controlled by the FDA as selenium is considered a food additive with a legal supplementation rate of 0.7 mg/head/day or 0.3 ppm of the total diet.

Acute poisoning produces severe respiratory distress, diarrhoea, pyrexia, tachycardia, apparent blindness, head pressing, collapse and death from cardiac and respiratory failure within 24–48 hours.

Gross post-mortem lesions included severe pulmonary oedema, hydrothorax and hydropericardium. The primary histopathologic finding is severe, acute and monophasic myocardial contraction band necrosis.

Chronic poisoning may occur with long-term supplementation, or in parts of the world with naturally high selenium levels in the soil, such as the western United States, but is unlikely to occur in the United Kingdom. Chronic poisoning produces lethargy, weight loss, pica, lameness and neurological signs.

Copper deficiency

The ataxia produced by copper deficiency (swayback or enzootic ataxia; see Chapter 5) may be confused with lameness in kids from birth to 4 weeks of age.

Further reading

General

See Chapter 7.

Baxendell, S.A. (1984) Caprine limb and joint conditions. *Proc. Univ. Post. Grad. Comm. Vet. Sci.*, **73**, 370.

Arthrogryposis hydranencephaly syndrome

de la Concha-Bermejillo, A. (2003) Cache Valley virus is a cause of fetal malformation and pregnancy loss in sheep. *Small Ruminant Research*, **49** (1), 1–9.

EFSA (2014) Schmallenberg virus: state of the art. *EFSA Journal*, **12** (5), 3681.

Roger, P. (2015) Schmallenberg virus: an update. *In Pract.*, **37**, 33–37.

Van Maanen,C., van der Heijden, H., Wellenberg, G.J. *et al.* (2012) Schmallenberg virus antibodies in bovine and ovine foetuses. *Vet. Rec.*, **171** (12), 29.

Erysipelas

Wessels, M. (2003) Chronic arthritis and systemic amyloidosis in three goat kids associated with seroconversion to *Erysipelothrix rhusiopathiae*. *Vet. Rec.*, **152**, 302–304.

Fracture repair

Mueller, K. (2010) Goat orthopaedics – bone sequestrum and fractures. *Goat Vet. Soc. J.*, **31**, 54–59.

Mycoplasma

Agnello, S., Chetta, M. Vicari, D. *et al.* (2012) Severe outbreak of polyarthritis in kids caused by *Mycoplasma mycoides* subspecies *capri* in Sicily. *Vet. Rec.*, **170** (16), 416.

DaMassa, A.J., Wakenell, P.S. and Brooks, D.L. (1992) Mycoplasmas of goats and sheep. *J. Vet. Diagn. Invest.*, **4**, 101–113.

East, N.E. (1996) *Mycoplasma mycoides* polyarthritis of goats. In: *Large Animal Internal Medicine*, 2nd edition, pp. 1277–1278. Mosby, St Louis.

Filioussis, G., Giadinis, N.D., Petridou, E.J. *et al.* (2011) Congenital polyarthritis in goat kids attributed to *Mycoplasma agalactiae*. *Vet. Rec.*, **169** (14), 364.

Osteodystrophia fibrosa

Andrews, A.H., *et al.* (1983) Osteodystrophia fibrosa in young goats. *Vet. Rec.*, **112**, 494–496.

Patella luxation

Baron, R.J. (1987) Laterally luxating patella in a goat. *J. Am. Vet. Med. Assoc.*, **191** (11), 1471.

Gahlot, T.K. (1983) Correction of patella luxation in goats. *Mod. Vet. Pract.*, **May**, 418.

Selenium deficiency

Herdt, T.H. and Hoff, B. (2011) The use of blood analysis to evaluate trace mineral status in ruminant livestock. *Vet. Clin. North Amer.: Food Anim. Pract.*, **27**, 255–283.

Suttle, N.F. (ed.) (2010) *Mineral Nutrition of Livestock*, 4th edition, Chapter 11, Copper, pp. 255–305. CAB International, Wallingford, Oxford.

Selenium toxicity

Amini, K. *et al.* (2012) Diagnostic exercise: sudden death associated with myocardial contraction band necrosis in Boer goat kids. *Vet. Pathol.*, **48** (6), 1212–1215.

Spastic paresis

Baker, J. *et al.* (1989) Spastic paresis in pygmy goats. *J. Vet. Int. Med.*, **3** (2), 113.

CHAPTER 9

Chronic weight loss

Initial assessment

The preliminary history should consider:
- Individual or herd/flock problem.
- Similar cases in the herd in the past.
- Management practices:
  - Housing, availability of shelter, general hygiene.
  - Feeding systems.
  - Size of groups, age mix of groups, recent mixing of goats?
  - Horned/disbudded goats.
  - Grazing history.
  - Routine medication: worming, external parasite control.
- Stage of lactation/pregnancy.
- Milk yield.

Table 9.1 lists possible reasons for chronic weight loss.

Clinical examination

> Dairy goats have little subcutaneous fat. Most fat is carried internally in the omentum and perirenal tissues.

Body condition should be carefully assessed by handling the goat. Dairy breeds of goats have different body fat distribution patterns than meat breeds or pygmy goats. Condition scoring, using standard techniques to assess lumbar fat and muscle as used routinely in sheep, is difficult to apply to dairy goats as most of the body fat is carried internally. Apparently thin goats may be found to have a large amount of abdominal fat at post-mortem examination and obese goats have little subcutaneous fat. In Angora goats, scoring is easier but never as accurate as with cattle or sheep. Angoras always feel thin when compared to dairy goats, because they are more slightly built. Careful palpation in thick-fleeced animals is essential to get an accurate impression of body condition.

A condition scoring system that combines lumbar and sternal measurements is more accurate in dairy goats. Sternal scoring gives a better indication of the amount of fat carried by the goat, while the lumbar score indicates body protein. The body condition score is taken as an average of the lumbar and sternal scores.

Lumbar scoring (Figure 9.1)

- Score 0. Extreme emaciation: bones of the skeleton are apparent; junctions between vertebrae are readily perceptible to the touch; skin seems in direct contact with bones.
- Score 1. Very lean: body angular; lumbar vertebrae prominent, with transverse processes readily palpable.
- Score 2. Lean: lumbar vertebrae less prominent; transverse processes easily palpated but with some tissue cover.
- Score 3. Good condition: lumbar vertebrae and transverse processes palpable but with reasonable cover; moderately rounded appearance to body.
- Score 4. Fat: lumbar vertebrae only palpable with gentle pressure and the transverse processes with firm pressure; body smooth and rounded.
- Score 5. Obese: vertical processes cannot be detected even with pressure; there is a dimple in the fat layers where the processes should be; transverse processes cannot be detected; loin muscles are very full and covered with very thick fat.

Diseases of the Goat, Fourth Edition. John Matthews.
© 2016 John Wiley & Sons, Ltd. Published 2016 by John Wiley & Sons, Ltd.

Table 9.1 Differential diagnosis for chronic weight loss.

Primary nutritional deficiency	■ Starvation ■ Trace element deficiency – cobalt, copper, selenium
Inability to utilise available foodstuffs	■ Dentition ■ Mouth lesions ■ Facial paralysis ■ Lameness ■ Blindness ■ Bullying
Unwillingness to utilise available foodstuffs	■ Unpalatable food ■ Males in breeding season
Inability to increase feed intake to match production demands	■ Peak lactation ■ Periparturient toxaemia
Interference with absorption of nutrients/loss of nutrients	■ Gastrointestinal parasitism ■ Johne's disease ■ Liver disease
Interference with rumen/intestinal mobility	■ Chronic rumen impaction ■ Ascites ■ Rumenreticular ulceration ■ Adhesions following surgery ■ Tumour ■ Foreign body
Presence of chronic disorders	■ Pneumonia ■ Peritonitis ■ Enteritis ■ Mastitis ■ Metritis ■ Tuberculosis ■ Caseous lymphadenitis ■ Caprine arthritis encephalitis
Pruritic conditions	■ Lice ■ Sarcoptic mange ■ Scrapie

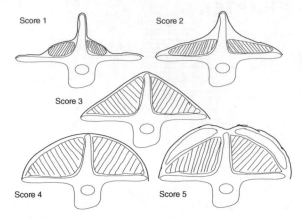

Figure 9.1 Lumbar score.

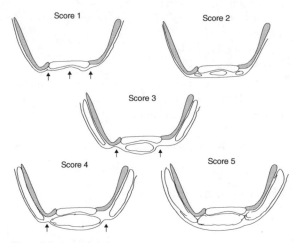

Figure 9.2 Sternal score.

Sternal scoring (Figure 9.2)

■ Score 0. Extreme emaciation: chondro-sternal joints are very prominent; bony surfaces of the sternum are very obvious to the touch; the hardened area of skin lacks mobility.
■ Score 1. Very lean: chondro-sternal joints are rounded but still very easily felt; a hollow in the midline of the sternum is not filled in; the hardened area of skin is loose.
■ Score 2. Lean: chondro-sternal joints are difficult to feel; considerable amount of internal fat, which forms a furrow along the middle of the sternum; subcutaneous fat fills this furrow and extends to lateral borders of the sternum and ends posteriorly at the hollow of the last sternal joint.
■ Score 3. Good condition: bones of the sternum are no longer detectable but the ribs can be felt; thickness of internal fat makes a fatty layer along the lateral edge of the sternum; subcutaneous fat forms a mobile mass that extends in a thin band to the rear in the hollow of the last sternal joint; when the whole sternum is grasped with the hand, two large depressions between these masses and the bone can be detected on each side.
■ Score 4. Fat: neither sternum nor ribs are detectable; a shallow depression can be detected on either side by

palpation; at the rear, the depression on the last sternal joint remains.

- Score 5. Obese: subcutaneous fatty mass is no longer mobile; contours are rounded without depressions on each side; the hollow on the last sternal joint is filled in.

Regular weighing is the most accurate way of monitoring condition in a particular flock or herd.

General examination at rest should include skin (lice, mange), mouth (teeth, lesions), feet (footrot, laminitis), mucous membranes (anaemia), abdomen (ascites, rumen function), auscultation of the thorax (cardiac/respiratory function) and lymph nodes.

Primary nutritional deficiency

Starvation

Starvation is caused by failure to ensure that the ration provides adequate energy and protein to meet the needs of maintenance, growth and production, together with sufficient minerals and vitamins and clean water. It may occur owing to:

- Neglect.
- Inexperience:
  o inappropriate feedstuffs
  o unbalanced ration
  o feed shortage at critical times.

Table 9.2 shows the daily requirements for energy and protein. Obvious dietary deficiencies can generally be easily remedied. Less obvious problems can be investigated by analysing feedstuffs or by *metabolic profiles* of a number of goats in the herd. Suggested profiles are:

- Energy: glucose, ß-hydroxybutyrate, non-esterified fatty acids, ketones.
- Protein: total protein, albumin, urea.
- Trace elements: copper, zinc, iron, selenium, cobalt.

Table 9.2 Daily requirements for energy and protein.

	Energy (MJ)	Protein (g DCP)
Maintenance (80 kg goat)	10	6.5
Plus milk production per litre (3.5% BF)	5.19	48
Pregnancy (average last 2 months)	6	54
Mohair production (6 kg/year)	0.75	18

Trace element deficiency

Specific clinical signs associated with trace element deficiencies are usually only seen in advanced cases. Often the only clinical sign is ill-thrift, so it is important to eliminate the role of nutrition, gastrointestinal parasites and other diseases. Malnourished animals and animals with enteric disease are more susceptible to the effects of trace element deficiencies.

Cobalt deficiency (pine)
Aetiology
- Primary deficiency of cobalt in the diet produces signs of vitamin B12 deficiency with an inability to metabolise propionic acid. Dietary cobalt is converted to vitamin B12 by the microflora of the rumen, released in the abomasum and absorbed in the small intestine. Vitamin B12 is also required for the metabolism of certain S-amino acids, so fibre goats can have a higher requirement than dairy animals.
- A secondary vitamin B12 deficiency may occur with helminth infection.

Incidence
- Certain areas of the United Kingdom, Germany, the Netherlands, New Zealand and Australia are known to be cobalt deficient, as are parts of New England, the upper Midwest and the Southeast in the United States.

Laboratory tests
- Blood cobalt or vitamin B12 levels are a poor guide to cobalt status (it is suggested that 150 to 300 pmol of vitamin B12/litre is considered marginal and over 300 pmol of vitamin B12/litre is adequate) as serum vitamin B12 levels reflect immediate dietary cobalt intake, whereas liver vitamin B12 levels provide a guide to continuous body storage.
- Liver cobalt and vitamin B12 levels provide a useful guide (normal cobalt levels of 0.2 to 0.3 ppm DM).
- Less than 0.1 ppm DM cobalt on a pasture sample suggests cobalt deficiency. Pasture cobalt concentrations are more useful than those of soil. Soil pH above the optimum range of 5.8–6.3 can affect cobalt availability and soil compaction may reduce the pasture uptake of cobalt.

Other elements, including manganese, iron and nickel, can interfere with cobalt uptake by plants.

- The presence in urine of methylmalonic acid (MMA) and forminoglutamic acid (FIGLU) indicates cobalt deficiency.

Clinical signs

- Growing animals have a higher requirement for vitamin B12 than adults and are more severely affected.
- Unthriftiness.
- Inappetence.
- Wasting.
- Emaciation.
- Ocular discharge.
- Anaemia (normocytic, normochromic).
- Reduced milk production.
- Death.

Diagnosis

- Response to cobalt or vitamin.

Treatment and control

- *Vitamin B12 injections*, 250–750 ③g, s.c. or i.m., are a practical and cost-effective method of short-term cobalt supplementation for growing kids and will raise serum and vitamin B12 levels for 1–4 weeks.
- *Oral cobalt sulphate*, 1 mg/kg at monthly intervals; 50 g cobalt sulphate added to 10 litre of water; 5 ml drench to growing kids, 10 ml to does.
- *Trace element ruminal boluses* provide several trace elements and vitamins can provide cobalt supplementation for up to 8 months, but are an expensive treatment for cobalt alone.
- *Cobalt oxide intraruminal bullets* have been used successfully to raise cobalt levels for over 1 year.
- *Anthelmintic preparations* containing cobalt sulphate ('SC drenches') are an effective prophylaxis if used correctly, but inappropriate use of anthelmintics can increase the selection of resistant nematodes.
- Concentrates fed to does should contain appropriate mineral and trace element supplementation.
- Cobalt sulphate, 2 kg/ha, applied as top dressing to pasture every 3 or 4 years (but is generally not cost-effective).
- Spraying cobalt sulphate on pasture at a rate of 175–350 g/ha raises pasture cobalt levels for about 6 weeks and can be used on selected paddocks before kids and does graze.

Copper deficiency

As well as neurological signs (see Chapter 16), copper deficiency may result in growth retardation, emaciation, microcytic anaemia, diarrhoea and increased susceptibility to infection.

Selenium deficiency

Selenium insufficiency can cause ill-thrift and poor growth in kids. More severe deficiency results in weak or premature kids and a degenerative myopathy of skeletal and heart muscles (see 'White muscle disease', Chapter 8).

Inability to utilise available foodstuffs

Dentition

The dental formula of the goat is:

Juvenile 2(Di0/3, Dc0/0, Dp3/3) = 18 deciduous teeth

Adult 2(I0/4, C0/0, P3/3, M3/3) = 32 permanent teeth

In small ruminants, there are no upper incisor or canine teeth and the lower canine tooth functions as a fourth incisor. The dental pad, rostral to the hard palate, replaces the upper incisors to facilitate the tearing of forage and browsing in tandem with the lower incisors. The age at which the permanent teeth erupt is variable. Figure 9.3 shows the dentition of kids and adult goats with approximate time of eruption of teeth. All the deciduous teeth are in place by the fourth week of age. The eruption of the first permanent incisors, at approximately 1 year, is often taken as the time the goat ceases to be a kid and can be important when selling animals for meat or breeding. Both central incisors are fully erupted between 9 and 18 months in dairy breeds and 17 to 19 months in Angoras. The teeth of heavier kids have been observed to erupt sooner than those of lighter kids. Goats over 5 years of age kept extensively show increasing wear of the incisor and molar teeth, so prehension and mastication may become difficult (see Chapter 22, 'The Geriatric Goat'). Uneven wear of molar teeth can result in sharp points, leading to ulceration of the buccal cavity and tongue, often complicated by secondary bacterial infections.

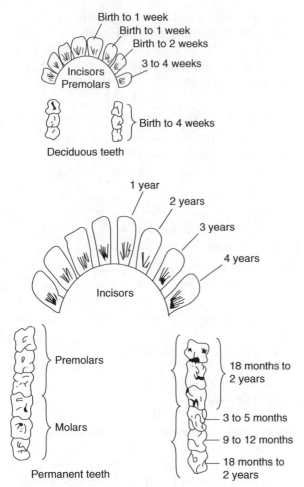

Birth to 1 week
Birth to 1 week
Birth to 2 weeks
3 to 4 weeks
Incisors
Premolars

Birth to 4 weeks

Deciduous teeth

1 year
2 years
3 years
4 years
Incisors

Premolars

Molars

Permanent teeth

18 months to 2 years
3 to 5 months
9 to 12 months
18 months to 2 years

Figure 9.3 Dentition and time of eruption (from Owen, 1977).

Goats may show reluctance to eat, chewing on one side and pouching or dropping of food. Congenital defects such as overshot/undershot jaws (brachygnathism and prognathism) may predispose to dental problems when the lower incisors do not properly appose the dental pad and may directly affect the ability of the goat to feed under range conditions.

Mouth lesions

Painful mouth lesions from infection (e.g. 'Orf', Chapter 10), toxic material resulting in mouth ulceration (e.g. giant hogweed poisoning), necrotic stomatitis from eating abrasive plant material (Chapter 21), drenching gun injuries, or periodontal disease will inhibit eating.

Facial paralysis

Branches of the facial nerve are distributed to the muscles of the ear, eyelids, nose, cheeks and lips. Facial nerve paralysis results in asymmetry of the face with a drooping ear, decrease in size of the palpebral fissure, deviated nose and inability to blink. The goat may drool saliva and cud retention may occur. Listeriosis (Chapter 12) is the commonest cause of facial paralysis in goat, with traumatic injury to the facial nerve, otitis media and other lesions involving the brain stem being less common.

Lameness

See Chapters 7 and 8.

Lameness will reduce grazing or feeding at troughs if the pain is severe. This may be caused by, in particular:
- Chronic degenerative joint disease: CAE, osteoarthritis, etc.
- Foot rot or interdigital dermatitis.
- Laminitis.
- Overgrown feet.

Blindness

See Chapter 20.
- Severe keratoconjunctivitis.
- Vitamin A deficiency.
- Post-cerebrocortical necrosis.
- Lead (blindness is not a prominent sign of lead poisoning in goats.

Bullying

Goats have a well-established rigid social order where the bottom goat(s) may be denied access to food. The problem may be precipitated by:
- Introducing a new goat into an established group.
- Providing insufficient space/goat (3.3 to 9.3 m²/goat).
- Providing insufficient trough space (0.4–0.6 m/goat).
- Having groups of mixed ages.
- Running horned goats with polled or disbudded goats.

Unwillingness to utilise available foodstuffs

Unpalatable feed caused by spoilage, mould, etc., will be refused by goats. Even a change in food, for example a new batch of concentrates, may result in feed refusal for a week or more.

Male goats at the start of the breeding season will often refuse feed, with consequent weight loss.

Inability to increase feed intake to match production demands

The periparturient period

Late pregnancy and lactation place heavy demands on the female. During the last trimester of pregnancy, at a time of increasing nutritional demand, dry matter consumption is depressed because the growing kids restrict abdominal space and rumen fill. Abdominal volume is further reduced in goats carrying large amounts of abdominal fat. *Pregnancy toxaemia* occurs in response to an insufficient intake of energy to meet the increasing demands of pregnancy. A similar, or even greater, increase in nutritional requirement occurs during the transition from late gestation into lactation. A goat at peak lactation can produce its own weight of milk in 10 days. All heavily lactating goats, particularly young first kidders, will lose weight despite the availability of an adequate diet. On a body weight for weight basis, goats are much heavier producers than cows. Goats lose about 1 kg of adipose tissue/week for the first month post-partum and 0.5 kg/week for a further month. Peak milk yield (about 4 to 8 weeks post-parturition in most breeds) occurs before peak appetite (about 10 weeks post-kidding). A positive energy balance is not reached until 6 to 8 weeks after kidding. From about the fourth month of lactation dairy goats begin to regain live weight. These changes are not mirrored by changes in condition score as goats carry little subcutaneous fat.

Most does suffer a mild ketonaemia in early lactation as the demands of the lactation for energy are not met adequately by the diet. In most animals an equilibrium is established and the ketosis remains subclinical. Goats that are not overfat may develop an acute clinical ketosis or *acetonaemia*. Goats that have large fat deposits at kidding may develop a *post-parturient toxaemia* or *fatty liver disease* of cows, presumably in response to impaired liver function. The periparturient period is discussed fully in Chapter 4.

Interference with absorption of nutrients/loss of nutrients

Gastrointestinal parasitism

See Chapters 14 and 18.

> Gastrointestinal parasites are a major cause of weight loss. Assume infection until proved otherwise.

Trichostrongylus spp.: diarrhoea
Teladorsagia (Ostertagi) ostertagi: ill thrift + diarrhoea
Haemonchus contortus: anaemia

Gastrointestinal parasitism should be assumed in all goats with chronic weight loss. (In animals treated with anthelmintics consider underdosing, dosing at incorrect times and resistance, particularly with Benzamidazole products).

A single low faecal egg count is not sufficient to eliminate internal parasitism as a cause of weight loss, as egg counts may not reliably indicate the number of adult worms present.

Moderate infections with immature rumen flukes may cause reduced weight gains or milk production, or ill-thrift. Young and debilitated animals are generally more severely affected than healthy adults. More severe infections cause profuse, projectile, watery diarrhoea with weight loss, dehydration and death in 5 to 10 days.

Johne's disease (paratuberculosis)

> Johne's disease in goats presents as a wasting disease; diarrhoea is not a major sign. In the United Kingdom, it is primarily a disease of commercial herds and probably the biggest cause of death or culling of adult goats.

Johne's disease is of increasing importance in commercial dairy herds in the United Kingdom and is a major reason for culling adult goats (up to 20% per annum), with economic loss from poor milk yields and lost genetic potential. However, it is uncommon in goats kept singly or in small herds.

Aetiology

- Infection with acid-fast bacterium, *Mycobacterium avium* subsp. *paratuberculosis* (*Mycobacterium johnei*) (MAP), producing chronic inflammatory bowel disease.
- Different strains exist, but goats can be infected by both ovine and bovine strains. Cattle strains are recognised as being much more pathogenic to goats than the sheep strains and most clinically ill animals have the cattle strain. Infected goats cohabiting with sheep, and infected with the sheep strain, may remain subclinically infected and potentially act as a reservoir of infection for the sheep. Where fibre goats cohabit with sheep, as in Australia, sheep strains become more significant.
- In individual animals, all the other *M. avium* subspecies (i.e. *M. a. avium* and *M. a. silvaticum*) have been reported to give 'Johne's disease-like' pathology.

Epidemiology

- Excreted in faeces by clinically ill or symptomless carriers.
- Persists in environment for months: in slurry for 1 year, in water for 5–9 months, in soil for up to 4 years; the organism resists freezing, survives boiling for 2 minutes and UV light for 100 hours.
- Many species of wild animals, such as rabbits and birds, can be infected and excrete large numbers of organisms in their faeces.
- Some animals may be intermittent excretors.
- Kids generally infected in the first few weeks of life by faecal contamination of the udder or environment or possibly through infected colostrum (intrauterine transmission and infection via semen have also been demonstrated). About 30% of the offspring of clinical cases are likely to become infected.
- *In utero* infection may occur, particularly in heavily infected does. The rate of intrauterine infection appears to be higher in goats than cattle.
- Ingested organisms remain dormant in the gastrointestinal tract and adjacent lymph nodes, often for many years.
- Clinical disease may be precipitated by stress such as parturition or introduction to a new herd.

- An age-related resistance to infection occurs in cattle and probably also occurs in goats. Although resistance is not 100%, particularly in the face of heavy levels of infection on a farm, animals older than 9 months of age are much less likely to be infected, thus limiting the opportunity for horizontal transmission within a herd. Most infections probably occur within the first 30 days of life. Older animals would only become infected in the face of very heavy contamination of pasture or buildings and, in clean herds, older animals would expect to remain immune to newly introduced infection.

Clinical signs

- Affects adult goats, generally 2 to 3 years old; rarely occurs in younger goats.
- The minimum time from infection to signs of clinical disease in goats is not known but usually between 2 and 4 years.
- Progressive weight loss; may extend from weeks to months, leading to dramatic emaciation (Plate 9.1).
- Appetite maintained initially but later decreases.
- Increasing lethargy and depression.
- Rough hair coat, loss of fibre, flaky skin.
- Diarrhoea only occurs in the terminal stages (Plate 9.2).
- Anaemia develops as the disease progresses.
- Signs of hypoproteinaemia, such as intermandibular oedema.

Diagnosis

> The non-specific signs mean it is impossible to diagnose Johne's disease by clinical examination.
> No single test will detect all infected animals.

- Diagnosis is very difficult in the living animal and it is generally considered to be grossly underdiagnosed.
- Only goats at least 18 months old should be used for diagnostic testing. Although kids are infected at an early age, before this age faecal cultures will be negative as they are unlikely to be shedding the organism, and blood and milk tests will also be negative as they will not be producing antibodies.
- No single bacteriological or serological test is sufficiently accurate to identify all clinical and subclinical

cases or has sufficient specificity to avoid false posi-tives. Testing is unpredictable during latent infection. Titres vary at around the time cases become clinical, so a goat with a positive serological test can go negative and then become positive again.

- *Identification of acid-fast organisms in ileocaecal or mesen-teric lymph nodes* is the best diagnostic test whether at post-mortem or by biopsy.
- *Faecal culture* is the next most reliable ante-mortem test, but requires 8–12 weeks and will not detect less than 100 organisms/g, thereby missing some carriers. If the sample is heavily contaminated a positive result may be detected in a week or two, but it can take two months of incubation or more until the laboratory feels confident that no MAP organisms are present.

Testing pooled faecal samples has been suggested for targeted surveillance and for screening herds of unknown status.

Note: sheep strains are harder to culture than cattle strains and need special culture techniques.

- *Agar gel immunodiffusion* (*AGID*) test correlates reason-ably well with faecal culture; useful for detecting pro-fuse excretors.
- *ELISA* tests are replacing AGID tests in some laborato-ries. Antibody ELISA measures the level of antibody (humeral response) in plasma or serum; gamma inter-feron ELISA measures the level of gamma interferon (cell-mediated immune response), which is the host's earliest response.

AGID is highly specific (>99.5%). An uninfected animal will almost certainly give a negative result, but it has fairly low sensitivity (35% of clinical cases identified), resulting in false negative results in infected animals. It is better for clinical confirmation and detection of advanced cases. Positive test results correlate well with clinical signs.

ELISA tests are also highly specific (93–99%). They are more sensitive than AGID tests, useful for high shedders and better than AGID at detecting animals with no clinical signs but will not detect all subclinical cases.

Milk ELISA tests are useful as a herd test, but not for individuals. Individual goats may be serologically positive in milk during lactation but are generally not positive throughout the lactation. Infected goats' milk will be antibody positive a year before serological tests on blood are positive.

Note: in herds also infected with caseous lymphadeni-tis, CLA goats may be test positive on a serum Johne's ELISA.

> The sensitivity of the serological tests is not high. The ear-lier the stage of infection, the lower the sensitivity and the greater likelihood of false negatives occurring. Serological tests should not be used alone to screen individual animals, unless there is a definitive diagnosis of Johne's disease on the farm when they can be used to identify higher risk ani-mals for management purposes.

- Various DNA techniques are currently being developed. DNA probes can detect repetitive DNA sequences unique to *Mycobacterium avium* subsp.*paratuberculosis* in faeces samples.

A *polymerase chain reaction* (*PCR*) test on faeces is now available routinely in the United Kingdom. It is highly specific (nearly 100%), slightly more sensitive than culture, cheaper and has a much faster turnaround time (five days compared with six to twelve weeks). Care needs to be taken to avoid cross-contamination of samples. Because it is dependent on active shed-ding in the faeces, subclinical infection may be missed and inhibitory factors in goat faeces can cause false negatives.

- *Gamma interferon assays* on whole blood may be bet-ter at detecting subclinical infection than ELISA tests. Specificity of 0.986% was shown in a large sample of Norwegian goats.
- *Complement fixation tests* are inaccurate; false positives and false negatives occur.
- *Intradermal tests* are not recommended; false negatives occur.
- Significantly decreased levels of total protein, albumin and calcium occur in sheep and, although not specific to Johne's disease, may provide a useful preliminary diagnostic screen for emaciated goats in the absence of diarrhoea.

Is MAP present in the herd?

- Test 10% or more of the herd, using ELISA or faecal culture, selecting the thinnest animals for testing. In the United Kingdom, Scotland's Rural College (SRUC) offers a reduced rate for testing pooled faeces samples from 10 goats.

- Culture of 10 faecal samples collected from the ground in areas of high goat traffic, such as collecting yards.
- Use bulk milk ELISA tests.

How many goats in the herd are infected?

- Blood ELISA tests all goats after their second kidding or older.
- Milk ELISA tests all goats after their second kidding or older at drying off.

Does this goat with chronic weight loss have Johne's disease?

- If previous cases have been seen in the herd: ELISA or faecal culture/PCR.
- If infection has never been confirmed in the herd: faecal culture/PCR + post-mortem examination if positive and culture of tissues (ileum and mesenteric lymph nodes).

Post-mortem findings

- Post-mortem findings in goats are generally not as obvious as in cattle as intestinal lesions are less pronounced.
- Emaciation; absence of abdominal fat.
- Mesenteric lymph nodes generally enlarged and oedematous in later stages with foci of caseation. Calcification of mesenteric lymph nodes is commonly seen in goats with Johne's disease and this could also be a feature of TB infection.
- Slight thickening and corrugation of the ileal mucosa and possibly the mucosa of the caecum and proximal colon.
- Even in the absence of gross lesions, sections from the mesenteric lymph nodes, distal ileum and ileocaceal valve should be submitted for histological examination.
- Characteristic granulomatous lesions in the intestinal tract, lymph nodes and possibly liver.
- Massive infiltration of acid-fast bacteria and inflammatory cells into the intestinal mucosa.
- Architecture of intestine destroyed, with significant villus atrophy and villus fusion, leading to a malabsorption syndrome and protein-losing enteropathy.
- Histopathology enables the disease to be classed as either paucillobacillary, with marked inflammatory response and lymphocytes infiltrating the lamina propria of the intestine, but very few acid-fast bacteria

present, or multibacillary, with many acid-fast bacteria present and macrophages the predominant cell type. Intermediate forms between the two extremes are also recognised.

Treatment

- None.

Control

> Once a herd is infected, measures are aimed at damage control, not disease eradication.

- Testing alone will not control transmission of the disease within a herd.
- All tests have limitations.
- Good management is critical.
- Testing and management programs need to be herd specific and in line with the goals and resources available.

1. Establish a diagnosis

- Isolate goats that are losing weight and establish a diagnosis by post-mortem examination.

2. Reduce the level of infection in the herd

- Identify and remove infected animals from the herd as soon as possible:
  o Frequent testing: faecal culture + AGID or ELISA every 6 months; expensive and will not detect infected non-shedders.
- Cull all positive goats and their offspring.
- If the immediate culling of *all* test-positive animals is impractical on financial grounds, any retained infected goats must be clearly tagged and strictly managed until they are eventually culled as they will be shedding MAP in their milk and in their faeces. Heavily infected animals (high ELISA titres) should be culled immediately.
- Cull goats with progressive weight loss *before* they kid.
- Breed replacements from older animals.
- Do not keep kids from known infected does as there is a moderate to high probability that kids born to MAP-infected mothers will acquire the infection, depending on other control measures in place.
- Pooled faecal culture is an economical way to monitor the infection level in the herd.

3. Improve management and hygiene

- Prevent faecal contamination of water and feed troughs.
- Clean pens regularly, using generous amounts of straw.
- Prevent overcrowding.
- Burn the straw litter from infected herds or allow long-term manuring to occur (>1 year) to occur before spreading it on to land, even if the land is not being used to produce food for animal consumption; infected wildlife can act as a reservoir of disease.
- MAP is resistant to most disinfectants. Tools, troughs and feeders should be thoroughly cleaned with soap and water, rinsed and dried before treating with a 'tuberculocidal' disinfectant.

4. At kidding

- Isolate goats at kidding into clean kidding pens in an area separate from the main herd.
- Clean, disinfect and re-bed pens between kiddings, using generous amounts of straw.
- Snatch kids at birth if practical (see CAE control, Chapter 6), which will also help control CAE and *Mycoplasma* spp. Otherwise remove kids from their dams as soon after birth as possible.

5. Kid rearing

- Do not feed pooled colostrum or milk.
- Feed cows' colostrum or goats' colostrum from a CAE and Johne's seronegative animal. Colostrum can be collected and frozen in small feeding size portions for later use.
- Feed pasteurised milk (see 'Pasteurisation of milk', Chapter 23) or milk replacer.
- Provide young kids with access to good quality hay and clean straw to discourage them from eating the straw bedding.
- Rear kids in small groups for the first 6 months in an area isolated from the adults.
- Record the identity of the kids in each rearing group.
- Vaccinate the kids:
  ○ A killed vaccine, Gudair (Virbac), is available in the United Kingdom and Australia, although not in the United States. The vaccine is manufactured in Spain and can be imported and administered under the prescribing cascade provisions in the United Kingdom.
    ◆ Vaccinate kids between 2–3 weeks and 6 months of age, and then rear kids separately.

- Adult goats should also be vaccinated in infected herds.
  ◆ Dose: 1 ml, s.c. or i.m.; the brisket is generally the recommended site for s.c. injection.
  ○ When all goats on the unit have been vaccinated as kids, continue for a further 2 years.
  ○ Vaccination will reduce the number of animals with clinical disease, decrease the number of excretors and the level of excretion and therefore the number of animals with detectable intestinal infection, but animals may still become infected and shed bacteria without ever developing the disease, although shedding will be delayed.
  ○ Clinical disease can occur for several years after the start of vaccination on a farm, but vaccination will greatly reduce or eliminate mortality, reduce the number of clinically ill animals, produce regression of lesions with a reduction in shedding, extend the productive lives of the goats and improve milk yields.
  ○ Within 7 to 15 days an inflammatory nodule is produced at the injection site. The nodule gradually evolves to a persistent, cold, fibrous and permanent one. A more intense reaction occurs when infected animals are vaccinated (secondary antigenic impact).
  ○ Vaccinated kids develop cross-reactivity to *M. tuberculosis* and the use of the vaccine may influence Johne's complement fixation tests and intradermal tests for Johne's disease and tuberculosis.
  ○ There is no simple way to differentiate serologically between vaccinated and infected animals.

Public health considerations

There is continued debate on the connection between Johne's disease and Crohn's disease in humans. *Mycobacterium* species have been detected in humans with Crohn's disease. There is a possibility of the disease being transmitted in raw or inadequately pasteurised milk.

Liver disease

See also Chapter 15.

Chronic fascioliasis

Goats are highly susceptible to *Fasciola hepatica* infestation and appear unable to develop an effective immunity to subsequent challenge.

Aetiology

■ The liver fluke, *Fasciola hepatica*, has an indirect life cycle with the water snail, *Galba (Lymnaea) truncatula*, acting as the intermediate host in the United Kingdom. Other genera of Lymnaeid snails act as intermediate hosts in other parts of the world, including *G. fossaria* and *G. pseudosuccinea* in the United States.

Fluke can cause acute, subacute or chronic disease, according to the numbers and stage of development of the parasite in the liver. Acute fascioliasis occurs when large numbers of immature fluke cause massive destruction of liver tissue, resulting in liver failure and haemorrhage. Subacute fascioliasis occurs when large numbers of fluke are ingested over a longer period, so that, as well as immature fluke in the liver parenchyma, there are adult fluke in the major bile ducts, resulting in weight loss and poor condition, despite adequate food supplies. Chronic fascioliasis is the result of liver damage caused by migrating fluke and blood loss caused by adult flukes in the bile ducts. The browsing habits of goats mean that large numbers of infective metacercariae are unlikely to be ingested over a short period so that although acute and subacute disease does occur, the chronic form is more common. There is no immunity to reinfection with *F. hepatica*.

Clinical signs

■ See Table 9.3, Fascioliasis.
■ The main period for chronic infection is late winter, January to March, from summer infection of snails, or June to July, from winter infection of snails producing metacercariae in the spring.

Laboratory tests

■ Anaemia is initially regenerative but it becomes non-regenerative as iron stores are depleted.
■ Hypoalbuminaemia is a consistent finding due to the loss of albumin together with blood through damaged bile ducts and impaired hepatic synthesis in severe cases.
■ Liver enzymes are of limited diagnostic value and may be normal even in severe cases.

Diagnosis

■ Clinical signs of severe loss of body condition, anaemia and subcutaneous oedema.
■ Faecal egg counts.
■ Coproantigen ELISA detects proteins from the gut of the liver fluke in the faeces of the host animal, but information on sensitivity and specificity is conflicting.
■ Liver fluke DNA can be detected in faecal samples from ~2 weeks post-infection. A DNA- based method, loop-mediated isothermal amplification (LAMP),

Table 9.3 Fascioliasis.

Type		Clinical signs	Fluke number	Eggs/g faeces	Clinical pathology	Post-mortem
Chronic	January–April June–July	Progressive weight loss Anaemia Oedema, ascites	250+ (adults)	100+	Hypochromic macrocytic anaemia Eosinophilia Hypoalbuminaemia AST^ (other liver enzymes normal)	Hepatic fibrosis Hyperplastic cholangitis
Acute	October–January	Sudden death Abdominal pain Dyspnoea, ascites	1000+ (mainly immature)	0	Normochromic normocytic anaemia Eosinophilia Hypoalbuminaemia AST, GGT, SDH, LDH[a]	Liver enlarged and haemorrhagic Tracts of migrating fluke
Subacute	October–January	Rapid weight loss Anaemia Submandibular oedema ascites	500–1500 (adults + immature)	<100	Hypochromic macrocytic anaemia Eosinophilia Hypoalbuminaemia	Fibrinous peritonitis As acute + bile ducts distended by adult fluke

[a]AST, aspartate aminotransferase; GGT, gamma-glutamyltransferase; SDH, sorbitol dehydrogenase; LDH, lactate dehydrogenase.

gives a rapid (<1 h), visual readout without any specialised equipment. LAMP assays have been developed that are specific to liver fluke and rumen fluke, respectively.

- Post-mortem signs of ascites and liver fibrosis, with low to moderate numbers of adult fluke.

Treatment

- In cool temperature climates, fluke transmission generally ceases around December because by then temperatures have been too low (<10 °C) for parasite development for several weeks and snails aestivate for winter.

  Since most fluke transmission occurs from August to November, a single treatment using a fasciolicide with adult-only activity in April or May will prevent early summer contamination of pasture with eggs.
- Treat the whole herd/flock (see 'Drugs for flukes', Appendix).

Chronic fascioliasis drugs

- *Albendazole, 10 mg/kg orally*; efficacy against adult fluke variable (76–92%). At higher doses (15–20 mg/kg) efficacy approaches that of clorsulon but even higher doses will not kill juvenile stages. Fasting animals for 24 hours prior to treatment will increase the efficacy. Also effective against intestinal worms and tapeworms.
- *Clorsulon, 2 mg/kg s.c.* (combination product with ivermectin 200 mg/kg); 97–99% efficacy against adult flukes; not very effective against immature stages.
- *Closantel, 10 mg/kg orally*; moderately effective against fluke from 3 to 4 weeks old and highly effective against adult fluke (97–100%). Also effective against *Haemonchus contortus* and *Oestrus ovis* larvae.
- *Nitroxynil, 10 mg/kg s.c.*; highly effective against mature fluke. Also effective against *Haemonchus contortus*.
- *Oxyclozanide, 15 mg/kg orally*; effective against adult fluke present in the bile ducts of the liver (combination product with levamisole).
- *Triclabendazole, 10 mg/kg orally*; effective against all stages of fluke.

Acute and subacute fascioliasis

The products that control immature fluke are limited and there may be cross-resistance between closantel and nitroxynil.

- *Triclabendazole, 10 mg/kg orally*, is active against all stages of fluke from 2 days old immature forms to adults. Triclabendazole is effective at killing all stages of fluke and is the treatment of choice for acute and subacute fascioliasis *in the absence of resistance*. Drenched goats should be moved to clean pasture or retreated every 3 weeks for the next 3 months at least.
- *Closantel, 10 mg/kg orally*; kills 23–73% of 3–4 week and >90% of 6–8 week immature fluke. Closantel has residual activity for 42 days following treatment. Early immature fluke that survive treatment will be stunted and shed significantly less eggs. *Closantel toxicity* has been reported to cause irreversible blindness in goats as a result of overdosing. Affected animals had dilated pupils and often walked in circles. In most cases doses of 2 to 4 times the sheep label dosage was given but in others the group was given a dosage based on the heaviest animal in the group so that lighter animals received the toxic dose.
- *Nitroxynil, 10 mg/kg s.c.*, is moderately effective against fluke from 8 to 9 weeks old.

Drug resistance

Resistance to fasciolicides, particularly triclabendazole, has been reported in sheep in the United Kingdom. Losses associated with resistant strains of fluke in sheep flocks treated with triclabendazole have been significant. Failure of any fasciolicide to stop eggs in the faeces indicates resistance, unless severe damage to the liver has affected the pharmacokinetics in the animal. The situation in goats is unknown, but because goats are generally treated much less frequently than sheep the pressure on the fluke is much less and resistance is less likely to develop. However, it would be sensible to take precautions to avoid resistance developing on farms.

- Avoid unnecessary use of fasciolicides. Use only if grazing is known to be infected.
- Avoid too frequent dosing:
  o Use a fasciolicide with adult-only activity in April or May. By eliminating flukes from the animals at this time, early summer contamination of pasture with eggs will be minimal when snail populations become active. A temperature of >10 °C is required for parasite development and snails aestivate for winter. Few infected snails, metacercariae or eggs survive the winter unless it is mild.

o Use a product with immature activity during the autumn to early winter to reduce fluke burdens before the spring treatment.

■ Do not buy animals with resistant fluke. Animals (sheep, cattle and goats) purchased from farms with fluke should be treated with closantel to prevent the introduction of triclabendazole-resistant fluke. If possible keep these animals on dry pastures or housed for 4 weeks.

Control

■ Reduce availability of snail populations by drainage, fencing, molluscicides.
■ Prophylactic use of fluke anthelmintics; in non-lactating animals use of a fasciolicide with adult activity in March and May will prevent pasture contamination with fluke eggs.
■ Avoid grazing wet areas if possible during risk periods from late summer.

DEFRA produce annual fluke forecasts based on the temperature and rainfall in the spring and early summer, so that specific control measures can be varied according to the predicted incidence of disease. The disease is commonest in wetter, western areas of the UK, with levels of infection linked to rainfall from May to October.

Dicrocelium dentricum

Dicrocoelium dentricum, the *lancet fluke*, is generally found in the United Kingdom only on islands off the west coast of Scotland, although it has been found at post-mortem in two goats in Devon. It is common in North America and parts of Europe, Asia, North Africa and the Middle East. This fluke is less pathogenic than *F. hepatica*, because it remains in the bile ducts, rather than migrating through the liver parenchyma, and very large numbers of fluke can be carried by individual animals. Goats may have subclinical or chronic infections, with a history of weight loss, lethargy and possibly signs of anaemia and hypoproteinaemia. There are two intermediate hosts: eggs are ingested by various species of land snail (*Zebrina detrita* in the United Kingdom) and ants (*Formica* spp.) eat the slime balls, containing cercariae, expelled by the snails. Because the intermediate hosts are widespread and do not depend on water, control measures adopted for *F. hepatica* are not applicable and the only practicable control measure is the strategic use of anthelmintics, such as netobomin, 20 mg/kg, praziquantel, 50 mg/kg, and albendazole, 15 mg/kg.

Fascioloides magna (the large American liver fluke) is an important cause of morbidity in certain parts of North America and Europe. In goats it generally presents clinically as sudden death (see Chapter 19). The life cycle of *F. magna* is similar to that of *F. hepatica* with snail intermediate hosts belonging to the family Lymnaeidae, such as Stagnicola (Lymnaea) caperata and Galba (Fossaria) bulimoides techella. In North America, in areas where *F. magna* is enzootic in deer, it is found in cattle, sheep and goats. In the areas of central Europe where it occurs, domestic ruminants are rarely infected. Goats are considered an aberrant host and usually die within 6 months from acute peritonitis or extensive haemorrhage caused by migrating juvenile fluke, without previously showing clinical signs. In aberrant hosts, flukes migrate until the host dies and do not mature, so that eggs are not normally passed. Diagnosis depends on the identification of *F. gigantica* at post-mortem examination.

Liver abscess

In adult goats, liver abscesses are an occasional finding at slaughter, generally associated with a variety of other concurrent diseases, such as septicaemia or caseous lymphadenitis (see Chapter 10). Liver abscesses may arise in kids following a navel infection.

Liver tumour

Primary tumours of the liver are rare; secondary tumours occasionally occur.

Ragwort poisoning

See Chapter 21.

Visceral cysticercosis

Cystercus tenuicollis is the metacestode of the carnivore tapeworm *Taenia hydatigena*. After ingestion, migrating cysts pass through the liver. Infection with small numbers is unapparent, but large numbers of cysts will cause widespread damage to the liver parenchyma (hepatitis cysticercosa) and result in depression, anorexia, pyrexia, weight loss, abdominal discomfort and occasionally death in kids. Acute disease is rarely seen in animals over 6 months of age.

The migrating cysts may lead to infection with *Clostridium novyi* (*Clostridium oedematiens* type B, 'black disease'; see Chapter 19).

Hydatid disease

Hydatid cysts are the metacestode stage of the carnivore tapeworm *Echinococcus granulosus*. The cysts initially develop in the liver and in high numbers may cause vascular or biliary obstruction. A local host response may lead to necrosis and infection of the liver. However, clinical disease is uncommon, large numbers of cysts being carried by apparently healthy animals. A proportion of cysts reach the lungs and may produce respiratory signs, particularly if a secondary infection, such as pasteurellosis, occurs.

Public health considerations

Hydatid cysts can also infect man. Although the goat is not a direct source of human infection, an infected animal would indicate environmental contamination, and control of tapeworm infection in dogs should be instigated.

Aflatoxicosis

Goats are relatively resistant to aflatoxins. The clinical signs are similar to those caused by other hepatotoxins such as pyrrolizidone alkaloids, for example ragwort.

Diabetes mellitus

There are occasional reports of diabetes mellitus in a goat, which showed chronic weight loss, polydipsia and polyuria. One goat was maintained satisfactorily for four years on twice daily subcutaneous injections of insulin.

Interference with rumen/intestinal mobility

- Chronic rumen impaction (see Chapter 15).
- Ascites: chronic fascioliasis (see this chapter); passive congestion of the liver.
- Ruminoreticular ulceration.
- Adhesions following surgery (e.g. caesarian section).
- Tumour: carcinomas (rare, older goats).
- Cestode infection? (see Chapter 14); if present in sufficient numbers could occlude the intestinal lumen; otherwise unlikely to cause weight loss.
- Left-sided displacement of the abomasum; see Chapter 15 and 'Periparturient toxaemia'.

- *Foreign body* (*bezoar, trichobezoar*):
  - Despite the fact that many foreign objects are found as incidental findings in the rumen of goats at post-mortem examination, reports of foreign bodies causing physical obstruction in the gastrointestinal tract are remarkably rare.
  - Ingested foreign bodies occasionally obstruct a portion of the intestines, resulting in clinical signs of colic.
  - Trichobezoars (hairballs) have been reported in Angora goats that had clinical signs of anorexia and weight loss. Hard balls of goat hair enclosed in a leathery outer shell occupied large parts of the rumen, leaving little space for food.

Presence of chronic disorders

Recurrent bouts of pyrexia, toxaemia and lethargy or painful conditions will lead to progressive weight loss.
- Chronic pneumonia
  - Pasteurella
  - CAE
  - Lungworm infection
  - Viruses
  - Caseous lymphadenitis
  - Mycoplasma.
- Chronic peritonitis.
- Chronic enteritis
  - Salmonella
  - Chronic enterotoxaemia?
- Chronic mastitis (see Chapter 12).
- Metritis.
- Tuberculosis.

Tuberculosis

Tuberculosis is rare and notifiable. Tuberculosis is discussed more fully in Chapter 17.
- Goats are generally infected with *Mycobacterium bovis* but are also susceptible to infection with *M. tuberculosis* and *M. avium* subsp. *avium*.
- Tuberculosis occurs as a disseminated disease involving the thorax (mediastinal lymph nodes, lungs, pleura) and abdomen (peritoneum, liver, spleen, mesenteric lymph nodes); occasionally superficial lymph nodes are enlarged and palpable. Goats may have extensive lesions without obvious clinical signs, but can present with:
  - Chronic cough due to bronchopneumonia
  - Chronic weight loss ± diarrhoea.

Pruritic conditions

- Lice (see Chapter 11); often present in large numbers in chronically wasted goats, either:
  - as secondary opportunists when a goat is in poor condition from any other cause,
  - very occasionally as a primary cause of weight loss through pruritis and anaemia when there is a heavy infestation.
- *Sarcoptic mange* (see Chapter 11).
- *Scrapie* (see Chapter 12).

Further reading

General

Buchan, G.A.G. (1988) The wasting goat. *Goat Vet. Soc. J.*, **10** (2), 58–63.

East, N.E. (1982) Chronic weight loss in adult dairy goats. *Comp. Cont. Ed. Pract. Vet.*, **4** (10), S419–424.

Owen, N.L. (1977) *The Illustrated Standard of the Dairy Goat*. Dairy Goat Journal Publishing Corporation, Scottsdale, Arizona.

Sherman, D.M. (1983) Unexplained weight loss in sheep and goats. *Vet. Clin. North Amer.: Large Anim. Pract.*, **5** (3), November 1983, 571–590.

Condition scoring

Morand-Fehr, P., Hervieu, J. and Santucci, P. (1989) Notation de létat corporel: à vos stylos. *La Chévre*, **175**, 39–42.

Dentition

McGregor, B. and Butler, K. (2011) Determinants of permanent first incisor eruption in grazing Australian Angora goats. *Australian Veterinary Journal*, **89** (12), 490–495.

Foreign body

Baillie, S. and Anzuino, K. (2006) Hairballs as a cause of anorexia in Angora goats. *Goat Vet. Soc. J.*, **22**, 53–55.

Johne's disease

Johne's Information Center, University of Wisconsin. Available at: www.johnes.org/goats.

Alinovi, C.A., Wu, C.C. and Lin, T.L. (2009) *In utero Mycobacterium avium* subspecies *paratuberculosis* infection of a pygmy goat. *Vet. Rec.*, **164** (9), 275.

Baxendell, S.A. (1984) Johne's disease in goats. *Proc. Univ. Sydney Post Grad. Comm. Vet. Sci.*, **73**, 508–510.

Coad, M. *et al.* (2013) Consequences of vaccination with Johne's disease vaccine, Gudair, for diagnosis of bovine tuberculosis. *Vet. Rec.*, **172**, 266.

Corpa, J.M. *et al.* (2000) Control of paratuberculosis (Johne's disease) in goats by vaccination of adult animals. *Vet. Rec.*, **146**, 195–196.

Eisenberg, S. *et al.* (2011) *Mycobacterium avium* subspecies *paratuberculosis* in bioaerosols after depopulation and cleaning of two cattle barns. *Vet. Rec.*, **168** (22), 587.

Greig, A. (2000) Johne's disease in sheep and goats. *In Pract.*, **22** (3), 146–151.

Juste, R.A. and Perez, V. (2011) Control of paratuberculosis in sheep and goats. *Vet. Clin. North Amer.: Food Anim. Pract.*, **27** (1), 127–138.

Lybeck, K.R. *et al.* (2011) Faecal shedding detected earlier than immune response in goats naturally infected with *Mycobacterium avium* subspecies *paratuberculosis*. *Res. Vet. Sci.*, **91**, 32–39.

Manning, E.J.B. *et al.* (2003) Diagnostic testing patterns of natural *Mycobacterium paratuberculosis* infection in pygmy goats. *Can. J. Vet. Res.*, **67** (3), 213–218.

Neilsen, S.S. (2009) Use of diagnostics for risk-based control of paratuberculosis in dairy herds. *In Pract.*, **31**, 150–154.

Robbe-Austerman, S. (2011) Control of paratuberculosis in small ruminants. *Vet. Clin. North Amer.: Food Anim. Pract.*, **27** (3), 609–620.

Rossiter, C.A. and Burhans, W.S. (1996) Farm-specific approach to paratuberculosis (Johne's disease) control. *Vet. Clin. North Amer.: Food Anim. Pract.*, **12** (2), 383–415.

Saxegaard, F. and Fodstad, F.H. (1985) Control of paratuberculosis (Johne's disease) in goats by vaccination. *Vet. Rec.*, **116**, 439–441.

Stehman, S.M. (1996) Paratuberculosis in small ruminants, deer and South American camelids. *Vet. Clin. North Amer.: Food Anim. Pract.*, **12** (2), 441–455.

Sweeney, R.W. *et al.* (2012) Paratuberculosis (Johne's disease) in cattle and other susceptible species. *J. Vet. Internal Med.*, **26**, 1239–1250.

Tharwat, M. *et al.* (2012) Transabdominal ultrasonographic findings in goats with paratuberculosis. *Canadian Vet. J.*, **53**, 1063–1070.

Thomas, G.W. (1983) Paratuberculosis in a large goat herd. *Vet. Rec.*, **113**, 464–466.

Whitaker, K. (2005) Diagnosis of Johne's disease in goats. *Goat Vet. Soc. J.*, **21**, 16–20.

Whittington, R. *et al.* (2003) Specificity of absorbed ELISA and agar gel immunodiffusion tests for paratuberculosis in goats with observations about use of these tests in infected goats. *Australian Vet. J.*, **81** (1/2), 71–75.

Windsor, P.A. (2015) Challenges of managing paratuberculosis: Australian perspectives. *Conference Paper 28th World Buiatrics Congress*, Cairns, Australia. Available at: http://www.researchgate.net/publication/273204083.

Liver fluke

Cranwell, M.P. *et al.* (2010) *Dicrocoelium dendriticum* in Devon. *Vet. Rec.*, **167**, 263.

Crilly, J.P. and Sargison, N. (2015) Ruminant coprological examination: beyond the McMaster slide. *In Pract.*, **37**, 68–76.

Reddington, J.J., Leid, R.W. and Westcott, R.B. (1986) The susceptibility of the goat to *Fasciola hepatica* infections. *Vet. Parasitol.*, **19**, 145–150.

Sargison, N. (2008) Fluke diseases of UK ruminant livestock. Part 1: Life cycles, economic consequences and diagnosis. *UK Vet.*, **13** (5), 59–67.

Sargison, N. (2008) Fluke diseases of UK ruminant livestock. Part 2: Treatment and control. *UK Vet.*, **13** (6), 54–58.

Taylor, M. (1987) Liverfluke treatment. *In Pract.*, **9** (5), 163–166.

Nutrition

AFRC Technical Committee on Responses to Nutrients Report No. 10 (1998) *The Nutrition of Goats*. CAB International, Wallingford, UK.

British Goat Society (1997) *Feeding Goats, A Modern Guide to Healthy Nutrition*. British Goat Society, Bovey Tracey.

Chamberlain A.T. (1999) Dairy Goat Nutrition. *Goat Vet. Soc. J.*, **18**, 19–28.

Committee on the Nutrition Requirements of Small Ruminants, National Research Council (2007) *Nutrition Requirements of Small Ruminants, Sheep, Goats, Cervids and New World Camelids*. The National Academies Press, Washington, DC.

Oldham, J.D. and Mowlem, A. (1981) Feeding goats for milk production. *Goat Vet. Soc. J.*, **2** (1), 13–19.

Orskov, B. (1987) *The Feeding of Ruminants, Principles and Practice*. Chalcombe Publications, Canterbury.

Randall, E.M. (1985) Nutrition in late pregnancy and early lactation. *Goat Vet. Soc. J.*, **6** (2), 51–55.

Randall, E.M. (1988) Caprine nutrition. *Goat Vet. Soc. J.*, **10** (1), 28–33.

Suttle, N.F. (1989) Predicting risks of mineral disorders in goats. *Goat Vet. Soc. J.*, **10** (1), 19–27.

Webster, A.J.F. (1988) Goat nutrition. *Goat Vet. Soc. J.*, **10**, 46–49.

Periparturient toxaemia

Andrews, A.M. (1985) Some metabolic conditions in the doe. *Goat Vet. Soc. J.*, **6**, 70–72.

Baxendell, S.A. (1984) Pregnancy toxaemia. *Proc. Univ. Sydney Post. Grad. Comm. Vet. Sci.*, **73**, 548–556.

Merrall, M. (1985) Nutritional and metabolic diseases. In: *Proceedings of the Course in Goat Husbandry and Medicine*, Massey University, November, pp. 126–151.

Pinsent, J. and Cottom, D.S. (1987) Metabolic diseases of goats. *Goat Vet. Soc. J.*, **8** (1), 40–42.

CHAPTER 10

External swellings

Throat swellings

The differential diagnosis for throat swellings should include the following.

Thymus enlargement

1. Thymic hyperplasia/non-regression of the thymus

Thymic hyperplasia is a common condition in kids, resulting in soft swellings in the ventral neck region. It is probably a normal developmental occurrence – often confused by owners with 'goitre' (see later in this chapter and Chapter 5). It occurs as early as 2 weeks of age and regresses spontaneously by about 6 months.

2. Thymoma

Thymoma is a relatively common tumour in adult, generally older, goats. It is operable if relatively small and situated externally at the thoracic inlet, but many tumours extend into the chest cavity or are entirely contained within it. Most thymomas remain subclinical and may be an incidental finding on post-mortem examination, but larger masses can prevent swallowing and regurgitation by pressure on the oesophagus at the thoracic inlet, leading to bloating episodes, or produce respiratory or cardiac dysfunction, leading to congestive heart failure.

Extrathoracic tumours produce a subcutaneous swelling at the base of the neck, often of quite significant size, without necessarily producing any clinical signs (Plate 10.1). Intrathoracic tumours usually form a well-defined mass in the cranial thoracic cavity and can be visualised by radiography or as a multiloculated to solid soft tissue mass by ultrasonography. Auscultation of the thorax may reveal a very loud heart on the left side, often displaced caudally, with muffled sounds on the right side.

Biopsy of tumours external to the thorax will confirm the diagnosis. Biopsy of intrathoracic tumours under ultrasound guidance is also possible but the tumour often lies very close to the ventricular wall and so should be undertaken with care. The principal neoplastic cells are polymorphic epithelial cells. Lymphocytes are also present and may predominate, but do not generally undergo neoplastic transformation.

Inoperable tumours may respond temporarily to long-term steroid administration and a rumenostomy may relieve the problem of bloat for a time.

3. Multicentric lymphosarcoma

Thymic tumours may form part of a multicentric lymphosarcoma complex.

Wattles

Wattles are specialised skin appendages, with no apparent function, found in the neck region of goats. Their presence or absence is controlled by an autosomal dominant gene with complete penetrance but variable expression regarding size and location, so that although they are usually bilaterally symmetrical, they occasionally occur singly and in various positions, including the face and ear. They consist of a central cartilaginous core, covered with smooth muscle and connective tissue.

Wattles are rarely traumatised, but removal may be requested on cosmetic grounds in potential show goats, particularly when the wattles are not a matched pair or in an aberrant position like an ear. They are easily removed with a pair of curved scissors at the same time as disbudding. Any bleeding can be controlled with an artery forcep.

Wattle cysts (branchial cleft cysts)

Wattle cysts are an inherited fault resulting in a swelling at the base of one or both wattles, varying from peasize

---

Diseases of the Goat, Fourth Edition. John Matthews.
© 2016 John Wiley & Sons, Ltd. Published 2016 by John Wiley & Sons, Ltd.

to several centimetres in diameter. They occur occasionally in all breeds of goat that have wattles, although they are more prevalent in certain family lines, so that in the United Kingdom they occur particularly in British Alpine and Anglo-Nubian goats. They are usually present at birth, but may enlarge with time and become more noticeable. Surgical removal may be requested if the cyst is unsightly, particularly in show goats. Aspiration is pointless as they will soon refill and there is a risk of abscessation.

Aetiology

■ Wattle cysts are the result of a failure of the branchial clefts to fuse during embryonic development.

Diagnosis

■ The position of the cyst is diagnostic.
■ Wattle cysts can occur in goats without wattles!
■ Histopathology is confirmatory, revealing walls of stratified squamous epithelium with mature hair follicles.

Note: *Dermal inclusion cysts* can sometimes be mistaken for wattle cysts.

Salivary cysts (salivary mucocoele)

Salivary cysts are relatively common, as developmental abnormalities of the parotid salivary gland, resulting in large painless fluid-filled swellings in the submandibular region or side of the face (Plate 10.2). The fluid is alkaline, clear and mucoid, occasionally blood-tinged, unlike the purulent fluid of an abscess. Anglo-Nubian goats are particularly prone to their development. A salivary mucocoele will enlarge and regress in association with feeding.

Damage to the submandibular or parotid salivary glands or their ducts can also lead to the formation of a mucocoele containing saliva.

Treatment

■ Drainage or lancing of the cysts is unsatisfactory. The cysts refill very quickly and there is the danger of creating a permanent fistula, which can result in the loss of large quantities of saliva daily.
■ Surgical excision is straightforward, provided the salivary duct is occluded by ligation; excision of the gland itself is not necessary. Infusion of new methylene blue makes finding the ducts easier. Once the mass is removed, any residual 'blue' indicates the

likelihood of residual tissue that may allow the cyst to reform.

Thyroid enlargement

Thyroid enlargement presents as swellings either side of the trachea.

1. Goitre

See Chapter 5.
■ Enlarged thyroid glands in kids will be part of a syndrome including abortions and/or still births. Thyroid enlargement alone is extremely unlikely.
■ Owners commonly associate any throat swelling with ''goitre', treat with iodine and risk iodine overdose. Genuine goitre is rare in the United Kingdom, except in known areas of iodine deficiency or animals fed large amounts of goitrogenic feeds.
■ Thymic hyperplasia/non-regression (see above) is commonly mistaken for goitre by owners and inappropriately treated.

2. Iodine excess

See Chapter 5.
Iodine overdosage will in itself produce enlarged thyroid glands.

Tumours

1. Lymphosarcoma

Multicentric lymphosarcomas usually involve generalised enlargement of the lymph nodes, particularly in the face and shoulder region, with lesions in the spleen, liver, kidney or intestines. Occasionally the disease is more localised, with the jaw region a predilection site.

2. Malignant melanoma

Malignant melanomas (see later in this chapter) often spread rapidly via the lymphatic system to involve the lymph nodes of the neck.

Other swellings around the head and neck

Abscess

■ Abscessation or cellulitis may arise occasionally as the result of penetrating wounds. A variety of bacteria, including *Streptococcus* spp., *Staphylococcus* spp.,

Trueperella (*Arcanobacterium, Actinomyces*) *pyogenes* and *Moraxella* spp., have been isolated. These present as an individual problem in individual animals.

- An injection abscess may arise at the site of vaccination or other injection because of faulty injection techniques (but most swellings produced by vaccination are sterile – see below).
- *Actinobacillosis lignieresi*, which is normally present in the mouth of ruminants, is occasionally isolated from abscesses around the face and neck of goats. It responds to prolonged (>30 day) daily treatment with procaine penicillin G. Alternatively, sodium iodide, 70 mg/kg as 10–20% solution i.v., can be given twice at weekly intervals.
- Infections with *Yersinia pseudotuberculosis* and *Mycobacterium* species occasionally produce lesions similar to caseous lymphadentitis.

> Because of the risk of spreading caseous lymphadentis, abscesses should be handled carefully and not lanced in situations that could lead to spread of the disease.

Caseous lymphadenitis

Caseous lymphadenitis (CLA) is now a common disease in the United Kingdom, particularly in commercial herds.

Aetiology

- *Corynebacterium pseudotuberculosis*, a gram-positive rod-shaped bacterium. The major secreted toxin is phospholipase D (PLD), which is responsible for causing the abscesses.

Incidence

- Occurs in many countries on all continents and was introduced into the United Kingdom with an importation of Boer goats in 1987.

Transmission

- Contamination of open wounds is the main cause of infection; inhalation is also possible, the tonsils can be infected after ingestion of the organism and kids can be infected by bacteria in milk. Flies can spread the disease.
- Following discharge from an abscess, the organism survives in the environment for many months.

- Spread between farms occurs by purchase of infected animals, by use of equipment (shearing, tattooing, ear-tagging) or by sharing facilities (handling, dipping).
- Spread between animals occurs when the skin is broken by any method, including castration, vaccination, fighting, head butting and browsing, allowing bacteria to enter.
- The incubation period until abscesses are visible in superficial lymph nodes is 2 to 6 months or longer. After introduction into a clean herd, disease prevalance increases steadily, if uncontrolled with a high incidence of disease in the herd developing within 2 to 3 years.

Clinical signs

- Enlarged and abscessed peripheral lymph nodes, particularly of the head and neck (parotid, mandibular and prescapular nodes) (Plates 10.3 and 10.4), but occasionally other sites such as popliteal nodes, depending where the organism gained entry to the body.
- The generalised (visceral) form of the disease causes abscessation of almost any organ and internal lymph nodes following haematogenous spread, but is less common in goats than sheep. Goats with internal abscesses do not always have enlarged peripheral nodes.
- Although goats with external abscesses often show no other clinical signs of disease, goats with internal abscesses may become progressively emaciated and involvement of the thoracic lymph nodes can lead to respiratory signs.

Diagnosis

- Clinical examination: encapsulated abscesses, primarily at lymph nodes.
- Culture of aspirated abscess contents: use a sterile needle through shaved, disinfected skin, avoiding contamination of the environment.
- In goats, the pus is more commonly creamy white or yellow, rather than green as in sheep, and, although there may be caseation and a greenish tinge in older lesions, calcification is rare and the concentric 'onion ring' appearance, seen in sheep, is generally absent. The pus is thick and clinging. If the pus is freely flowing, it is unlikely to be caused by *C. pseudotuberculosis*.

- Serology: a variety of serological tests have been used in eradication and control programmes. Although of value in detecting infected herds, they have limited value in detecting individual infected animals. Most tests are accurate during the period of active abscess formation, but false negatives occur during the early stages of the disease and after abscess rupture, although the animals remain carriers. The synergistic haemolysis inhibition (SHI) test, which measures antibodies to phospholipase D (PLD) exotoxins produced by the organism, is a reliable diagnostic test used in the United States with a sensitivity of 98% for goats, but does not have a high specificity for identifying individual animals with CLA and is not a good predictor of future clinical disease in an infected herd.
- An indirect ELISA test, which detects antiphospholipase D antibodies in ovine and caprine serum, plasma and milk is available in the United Kingdom. The test is indicated for the diagnosis of CLA in animals where external clinical lesions are not present but disease is suspected, or in cases where external lesions are present but bacteriology has proven inconclusive or cannot be undertaken. The test is highly specific (specificity is 99.17%), so there is a very low risk of false positive results. However, test sensitivity is poor (sensitivity 84.79%) and this may lead to false negatives. This makes it most effective when used for screening a group of animals. Due to the relatively low sensitivity of the test, a negative ELISA result on a single animal, for example prior to purchase, should be treated with some caution. Additional assurance may be gained by re-testing ELISA negative animals, at least one month later. It is advisable that the purchased animals should be kept in quarantine during this period.
- Post-mortem examination may reveal internal abscesses.

Treatment

- Consider culling an infected animal to limit the spread of the infection within the herd.
- Surgical drainage, or removal of superficial nodes, will remove visible abscessation but will not necessarily prevent abscesses appearing elsewhere. Submandibular, popliteal, prefemoral and prescapular nodes are relatively easy to remove surgically; supramammary and parotid nodes are more difficult.

- Care should be taken to avoid contamination of the environment with pus; the abscess cavity should be flushed with a strong povidone iodine solution, all pus collected and burnt and the animal isolated until the lesion is completely healed. Gloves should be worn as the disease is potentially zoonotic.
- Pus has been aspirated using a large-gauge needle and 60 ml syringe, containing 25 ml of 10% formalin, with repeat aspirations and flushing allowing all the pus to be removed, but formalin is not licensed for use in food-producing animals and is known to be carcinogenic.
- *In vitro C. pseudotuberculosis* is susceptible to nearly all common antibiotics, but the efficacy of antibiotic therapy *in vivo* is very variable, because of the intracellular nature of the organism and the thick walls of the abscesses. Once abscess formation has occurred, treatment with commonly used antibiotics is unsuccessful. Rifampicin, 10–20 mg/kg orally once daily, has been used in conjunction with erythromycin, 4 mg/kg once daily i.m. or s.c., penicillin, 22 000 IU/kg every 12 hours i.m. or s.c., or long-acting oxytetracycline, 20 mg/kg every 3 days i.m. or s.c. for up to 6 weeks. Erythromycin is highly irritating. Rifampicin is not licensed for use in food-producing animals, has established problems of toxicity and bacterial resistance to it develops quickly. Tulathromycin, 2.5 mg/kg once subcutaneously, has also been used after lancing and lavaging abscesses with saline. It remains to be established by long-term studies, including post-mortem examinations, if antibiotic therapy has a practical role in the treatment of the disease.

Eradication

- Control of CLA in infected herds is outlined in Table 10.1.
- Regularly examine the herd for visible abscesses at least every 3 months, concentrating on the lymph nodes of the head and neck.
- In a herd with bacteriologically confirmed CLA, the detection of a lesion at the site of a lymph node is diagnostic.
- Cull or isolate all infected goats.

If space permits and there is no crossover of use of equipment and with scrupulous hygiene, it may be possible to run separate 'clean' and 'dirty' herds, but on most farms culling is the most sensible option.

Table 10.1 Control of caseous lymphadentitis in an infected herd.

- Identify and cull any animals with obvious disease
- Regularly palpate lymph nodes and isolate any animal with enlarged nodes
- Do not allow abscesses to spontaneously rupture
- Test all suspect or in contact animals >6 months of age every 4–6 months (ELISA)
- Remove any goat testing positive from the seronegative group
- Quarantine any goat with an inconclusive test and re-test >1 month
- Quarantine new herd additions for at least 60 days and until tested clear
- All new herd additions should be inspected for external abscesses or scars where abscesses have been removed and rejected if any are found
- Monitor dead animals at the abattoir or by post-mortem examination

- Disinfect any housing and equipment used by infected animals
- Disinfect regularly all equipment used on animals, e.g. foot shears, tattoo numbers
- Remove environmental hazards such as fencing or troughs with sharp edges or protruding nails
- Control biting and sucking insects, such as lice, with pour-on or injectable drugs

- Remove kids from the adult herd at birth
- Feed heat-treated colostrum, cow colostrum or colostrum substitute, then milk replacer
- Rear kids separately from other animals

- Vaccinate kids at 4 and 8 weeks of age
- Vaccinate all other goats twice, 3–4 weeks apart
- Vaccinate all goats with annual booster, 4 to 6 weeks before kidding

---

A goat infected with CLA is infected for life.

- Never allow abscesses to spontaneously rupture.
- Remove kids from the adult herd at birth and feed heat-treated colostrum, cow colostrum or colostrum substitute, and then milk replacer.
- Rear kids separately from other animals.
- *Vaccination* should be used in conjunction with the culling of infected animals.

Vaccines are available in the United States, Canada, Australia and parts of Europe. The data supporting the efficacy of some of the available vaccines is not very robust. Some available vaccines are combined with clostridial antigens. It is not clear if vaccines licensed outwith the United Kingdom will work in this country, but the Australian CLA vaccine, Glanvac™, is available provided permission has been obtained from the Veterinary Medicines Directorate. Available vaccines mainly activate humeral responses and are more useful at limiting the spread of infection than eliminating an established infection.

An *autogenous CLA vaccine* could be produced under an Emergency Licence issued by the Veterinary Medicines Directorate, but no data are available on the efficacy of these vaccines and anecdotal reports are mixed. The Moredun Institute in Scotland is currently developing a novel CLA vaccine, which should give a greater level of protection than existing vaccines.

Vaccination should be given before exposure to the organism and aims to prevent the establishment of infection in the vaccinated animals. Vaccination interferes with serological testing for CLA and is reported to cause severe reactions in some animals that are already infected. *The use of vaccines will decrease the level of abscesses in a herd, but will not eradicate the disease.*

Kids are vaccinated at 4 and 8 weeks of age and all other animals twice 3–4 weeks apart, with an annual booster 4 to 6 weeks before kidding. Six-monthly boosters should be given if combination vaccines like Glanvac are used.

- If abscess contents contaminate the environment, the whole area, including walls, floors, troughs, water bowls and gates, should be thoroughly cleaned to remove organic material and then disinfected. This is particularly important for any feeders that have slats or keyholes that the goats put their heads through. Most commercial disinfectants are effective.

- ELISA tests may be used as a tool in the control and eradication of CLA in affected herds. Once a bacteriological diagnosis of CLA has been made in a herd, all suspect animals over six months of age are tested on a four- to six-monthly basis. The specificity of the test is high; therefore a positive titre may be regarded as diagnostic of exposure to *Corynebacterium pseudotuberculosis*. Any goat testing positive should be removed from the seronegative group. An animal giving an inconclusive result should be re-tested at least one month later and kept isolated from the seronegative group until after the second test.

Public health considerations

- The disease is rarely transmissible to man. Most cases have involved shearers or abattoir workers. Milk from infected animals should be considered a possible risk.

Vaccination reaction

Sterile swellings commonly occur as a reaction to the clostridial vaccine adjuvant (particularly if oil-based) and may range in size from small nodules to several centimetres in diameter. Some animals seem particularly sensitive to any clostridial vaccine; others will react to only one particular product. In show animals vaccination on the sternum may be preferable to the neck or scapular regions.

Tooth root abscess

Tooth root abscesses present as a lump on the upper or lower jaw, often closely associated with the bone, sometimes with an associated cellulitis. An abscess of the lower jaw may track to the outside on the mandible; an abscess of the upper jaw may discharge into the mouth or sinuses of the skull.

Dentigerous cysts

Dentigerous cysts are sterile fluid-filled spaces surrounding the crown of an unerupted incisor tooth, or sometimes the whole tooth, causing localised enlargement of the mandible with varying degrees of bone destruction or remodelling.

Bottle jaw

'Bottle jaw' is a soft fluid-filled swelling under the jaw as a result of anaemia, particularly haemonchosis (Chapter 18). Other signs of anaemia will also be present.

Impacted cud

Dental abnormalities, such as worn or poorly aligned molars in older goats, may result in retention and impaction of cud in the mouth, producing swollen cheeks. Cud retention can also occur with facial nerve paralysis in listeriosis (see Chapter 11), otitis media or trauma to the facial nerve.

Osteodystrophia fibrosa

Osteodystrophia fibrosa (see Chapter 8) in growing kids causes marked bilateral enlargement of the mandibles.

'Big head'

Clostridial infections (*Cl. novyi* or *Cl. oedematiens*) in bucks that have been fighting produce a swollen head ('big head') as part of an acute illness associated with lethargy, anorexia and pyrexia.

Skin tumours

The incidence of skin tumours is very low in the United Kingdom. The major tumours – papillomas, squamous cell carcinomas and malignant melanomas – occur most commonly in white dairy or Angora goats with non-pigmented skin exposed to strong sunlight, so the incidence is likely to remain low unless the greenhouse effect produces a dramatic climate change! Selecting for pigmented skin, particularly on the udder, reduces the incidence of tumours.

1. Cutaneous papillomas (warts)

Papillomatosis in sheep is caused by a virus of the papovirus group, but a viral cause has not been confirmed in goats. Three types of papillomas have been described in the goat:

- Mammary.
- Cutaneous.
- Genital.

Cutaneous papillomas occur particularly on the head, neck and thoracic limb and are flat, circumscribed with a crusty surface and ring-wormlike in appearance. Generally, a spontaneous resolution occurs in a few months. Occasionally, surgical removal or the use of autogenous vaccines is indicated.

Tumours of the udder of white goats often persist without the regression normally associated with viral papillomas, although some totally or partially regress during the non-lactation period only to recur the following year during lactation. Animals with persistent lesions may develop squamous cell carcinomas in subsequent years.

2. Squamous cell carcinomas

Squamous cell carcinomas occur particularly perianally, around the vulva and udder and on the eyelid and nictitating membrane in areas of non-pigmented skin in response to stimulation by ultraviolet irradiation. In the early stages the tumours appear as thickened areas of skin, enlarging rapidly and becoming ulcerated and often coalescing to form large masses.

Tumours of the udder can eventually erode through the wall of the teat, leading to mastitis and may metastasise to the supramammary lymph node.

3. Malignant melanoma

Malignant melanomas commonly occur on the head and ears, and occasionally on the vulva or perianally, arising as small firm nodules from black pigmented areas and enlarging rapidly to form a black mass. Rapid spread via the lymphatic system may occur to involve the regional lymph nodes. Some melanomas may be unpigmented and resemble squamous cell carcinomas.

Mouth tumours

1. Lymphosarcoma

The goat appears unique in that lymphosarcoma commonly involves bony tissues of the face, with the mandible and maxilla being predilection sites (Plates 10.5 and 10.6). Affected animals present with varying degrees of mouth pain, dysphagia, inability to graze and weight loss. Most affected animals are between 2 and 4 years of age.

2. Fibromatous or periodontal epulis

A periodontal epulis similar to that seen in the dog has been reported on the mandible of a pygmy goat.

3. Other tumours

A variety of other tumours – sarcoma, adenocarcinoma, osteoma, fibrosarcoma, fibroma, giant cell tumour (Plate 10.7) – are occasionally found in the mouths of goats and cause localised swelling.

Orf (contagious ecthyma; contagious pustular dermatitis (CPD))

Orf is a pox virus infection causing pustules and then crusty, scabby lesions on the commissures of the lips (Plates 10.8 and 10.9), gums, nostrils, buccal mucosa and occasionally the udder, feet or tail. Unlike papillomas, which are firmly attached to the skin, orf scabs can be picked off, revealing inflamed, granulating areas.

In does, lesions are usually found on the udder and teats, making milking and suckling difficult and bacterial mastitis may follow. In suckling kids, lesions are largely confined to the mouth and nostrils, but may extend further into the mouth and throat, where secondary bacterial infection may occur. Excess salivation may be obvious and debilitation and even death may occur if the painful lesions prevent feeding.

It can often be difficult to differentiate between orf and other conditions causing dermatitis around the mouth and nose (Plate 10.10). Artificially reared kids can develop crusty lesions when their noses and mouths become immersed in milk and weaned kids may also develop facial lesions, particularly if they are on rough grazing, such as thistles or gorse, which causes abrasions to the skin.

Initial lesions take 4 to 6 weeks to heal. Reinfection may occur, but lesions are usually milder and resolve faster. After recovery, animals are usually immune for 2 to 3 years, although individual animals may show clinical signs the following year.

The disease is easily transmitted and the virus can remain viable in crusts for months. Colostrum does not contain protective antibodies, so kids are susceptible to infection, even if their dams are immune.

Diagnosis
- The virus can be demonstrated in fresh scabs by electron microscopy. Submit scabs from fresh lesions to the laboratory in a screw-topped container.

Treatment
- Secondary bacterial infection can be controlled with antibiotic sprays and/or long-acting parenteral antibiotic injections.
- Proprietary antacids like Pepto-Bismol or Gaviscon are reported to dry out the orf lesions and sooth intraoral lesions.
- WD-40 is also reported to help the healing process, so that treated lesions heal in a shorter time. When spraying around the nares, the nose should be kept shut to avoid inhalation. Pox viruses have a high percentage of lipid in their cell walls so it is likely that WD40 inactivates the virus by solubilizing the lipid content of the cell wall.

Prevention

- In infected herds, *vaccination* can be considered. Orf vaccine is administered by scarification of the skin, using a special applicator, and not by injection. Vaccinated animals develop mild lesions of orf at the site of vaccination, which is usually the inside of the ear or the underside of the tail, and live virus will be shed for 3 or 4 weeks, so the vaccine should only be used on farms where there is an existing problem. The scabs that form at the vaccination site contain live virus. Virus can live on the ground in shed scabs for months or even years in a dry environment.

   Adults and kids should be vaccinated 3 to 4 weeks before the period of disease risk, with revaccination every 5 to 12 months. Kids can be vaccinated from 1 to 2 days of age. The vaccine should not be used during the last 2 months of pregnancy.

   The live vaccine is susceptible to heat and sunlight and must be handled carefully as it contains live vaccine that can infect people.

Public health considerations

- Orf is a frequently recognized zoonosis among people working with infected animals, generally causing localised lesions on the hands or forearms, so gloves should be worn when handling or treating infected animals or in-contact utensils.

Bluetongue virus (BTV)

Bluetongue is a notifiable disease in the UK, but there is no slaughter policy and infected animals can be treated.

Aetiology

- Acute viral disease caused by an RNA orbivirus affecting domestic and wild ruminants. There are at least 24 recognised serotypes of BTV, differentiated on the basis of the specificity of reactions between the outer coat proteins of the virus and neutralising antibodies. There is also considerable variation within each serotype. Virulence between serotypes varies. Serotype 8 is currently present in the United Kingdom and Northern Europe, serotypes 1, 2, 4, 9 and 16 have been identified in the Mediterranean Basin in recent years, with serotype 1 extending its range in Southern France; in the United States, serotypes 2, 10, 11, 13 and 17 are endemic.
- Cross-protective immunity against heterologous serotypes is poor.

- Some serotypes can adapt better to different midge hosts than others, in particular serotypes 1 and 8.
- A serotype new to a given ruminant population can cause very serious economic damage.
- Embryos can be transferred from infected does to recipient does without transfer of disease to recipient or kids.

Vector

- Ruminants cannot directly infect one another.
- Bluetongue is transmitted by midges of the genus *Culicoides*: in Northern Europe *by Culicoides dewulfi*, a subspecies of *Culicoides obsoletus* (other *C. obsoletus* subspecies or *Culicoides pulicaris* may also be involved); in the United States by *C. variipennis*. Other, but not all, *Culicoides* spp. are capable of virus transmission.
- Inoculation of the virus takes place during feeding on the host animal.
- A period of capitance is necessary after midges have ingested infected blood before they can pass on infection and ambient temperatures above 10 °C are required.
- Larvae inhabit the top layer of permanently non-submerged humid environments. *C. dewulfi* is known to breed in cattle and horse dung and *C. obsoletus* species are abundant in maize silage.
- *C. dewulfii* does not travel far from larval breeding areas, so unless goats are near horse or cattle dung, they are at less risk than in warmer countries.
- Unlike some species of midge, *C. dewulfii* enters animal housing so housing animals at times of midge activity is not protective.

Epidemiology

- Climatic conditions and vector biology are critical to the spread of the disease, with the season of maximum infection, June to December, correlating with increases in insect vector populations. Midge populations are decimated by frost and cold weather, but mild winters allow populations to survive, so that the disease can re-emerge the following summer.
- Climatic circumstances, such as temperature and wind, play an important role in the distribution of the midge and thus the spread of the disease.
- The incubation period in sheep is 7 to 10 days.

Clinical signs

Bluetongue in goats is generally subclinical, but it is possible that they act as symptomless carriers of the virus. Clinical signs were seen in a small number of goats during the recent outbreak in Northern Europe:

- Mild depression.
- Slight loss of appetite.
- Transient pyrexia (40.5 °C).
- Hyperaemia of the oral and nasal mucosa.
- A drop in milk production may be the first clinical sign in lactating animals.
- Disease may be more severe when previous exposure has occurred (sensitization).

More severe clinical signs have been reported from Asia:

- Pyrexia and anorexia lasting 3 to 4 days.
- Hyperaemia of the buccal and nasal mucosae, progressing to congestion and swelling, with petechiae and ulceration, particularly of the dental pad and commissures of the mouth.
- Excessive salivation.
- Nasal discharge, clear initially, becoming purulent and blood stained.
- Coronitis with lameness in one or more legs.
- Diarrhoea.
- Abortion.

> Single or multiple lesions in the mouth may be mistaken for foot and mouth disease (FMD), but the classic sign of bluetongue is a swollen face (oedema of the face, muzzle and ears), which does not occur in FMD.

When severe clinical signs are present as in sheep, the differential diagnosis for bluetongue includes: orf (contagious pustular dermatitis), acute photosensitisation, foot and mouth disease, lameness due to footrot, foot abscess and other foot conditions, acute haemonchosis (with depression and submandibular oedema), facial eczema, *Oestrus ovis* infestation, pneumonia, plant poisoning, Akabane disease and, exotically, peste des petits ruminants/rinderpest.

Diagnosis

- Bluetongue is generally identified in goats only when the disease is occurring simultaneously in cattle or sheep.
- A definitive diagnosis of bluetongue requires virus isolation from blood or tissue from acutely affected animals or detection of RNA specific to BTV by a polymerase chain reaction.
- Viraemia can last for up to 21 days after infection and measurable antibody responses occur during viraemia.
- As antibodies can persist for years after exposure and cross-reactivity with other orbi viruses can occur, serum antibody tests (AGID or ELISA) are not definitive in endemic areas.
- Novel diagnostic techniques have recently been developed for BTV, including real time and conventional RT-PCR assays, which are useful for the detection of circulating virus before the peak of viraemia, seroconversion and the development of clinical signs.

Prevention

- Because even a single bite from an infected midge can produce disease, preventing disease in the presence of infected midges is very difficult.
- Although housing will reduce exposure to midges, species like *C. dewulfi* enter livestock buildings, so that housing in Northern Europe is of limited value in preventing animals being bitten.
- Insecticides are of very limited value, if any at all, under European epidemiological conditions. Frequent applications of synthetic pyrethroid pour-ons, containing deltamethrin, may reduce midge activity, thus reducing the chance of infection spreading within the herd, but will not stop individual animals being bitten.

In warm climates, where the vector midge is *Culicoides immicola,* the use of insecticides has proved useful as an aid in controlling bluetongue. *C. immicola* bites on the back, neck and head, and will not go indoors, so housing is also a benefit in those areas. In Europe, *C. dewulfii* behaves differently; it goes indoors and prefers to bite on the abdomen. The persistence of insecticides on the skin is probably at best a few hours, and, as the insecticide does not reach the biting area unless you spray the animal from underneath, it is of no value at all against this midge. An exception is that misting lorries with insecticide before a journey of any length may help limit spread by killing midges that might travel to an unaffected area. There are no insecticides licensed for use in goats, so standard meat and milk withdrawal periods apply after their use.

- Animals that have recovered from BTV are resistant to infection by the same serotype for months and may have *some* partial cross-protection to other serotypes.
- *Vaccination*
  o Vaccines must contain the serotype(s) present in a particular location as the various serotypes confer little cross-immunity. Vaccines should be administered before the insect season so that maximum protection occurs during high risk periods.
  o Kids younger than 3 months may have passively acquired maternal antibodies that prevent effective vaccination.
  o An inactivated BTV-8 bluetongue vaccine is available in the United Kingdom and Northern Europe. Cattle require 2 injections and sheep and goats 1 injection.
  o Modified live tissue culture vaccines given in the first 5 to 10 weeks of pregnancy can be teratogenic or cause early embryonic death; abortion can occur in late pregnancy and infertility has been reported in breeding rams.

Foot and mouth disease
See Chapter 7.

In goats, the disease is usually relatively mild or subclinical. Many infected goats have such mild symptoms that they are easily missed on clinical examination. However, they are still infectious to other livestock. Lesions in the mouth and around the foot tend to heal very quickly and can easily be missed in goats, which are otherwise well.

Clinical signs
- Mouth vesicles consistently form, but are much smaller than in cattle, and much less painful, so the characteristic drooling of saliva associated with FMD in cattle is absent, although a slight to moderately noticeable bubbling of saliva round the mouth may occur.
- Healing mouth lesions tend to be seen mainly as white dots on the tongue, about 1 to 2 mm across, and are only visible if the animals are 'mouthed', that is examined by opening the mouth and looking.
- In the 2001 outbreak in the United Kingdom, great confusion was caused in sheep and goats by an unknown viral disease, which caused erosions in the front of the dental pad. FMD *never* causes erosions on the front of the dental pad unless there are erosions elsewhere in the mouth.

Herpes virus
Caprine herpesvirus 1 (CpHV-1) has been identified as causing wart-like lesions on the eyelid and proliferative lesions around the mouth and hard palate as well as vulvovaginitis, abortion, ulcerative enteritis and pneumonia (not confirmed but possibly present in the United Kingdom).

Diagnosis
- Culture of virus; serology.

Mycotic dermatitis (dermatophilosis)
See Chapter 7.

Ringworm
See Chapter 11.

Actinomycosis ('lumpy jaw')
Actinomycosis occurs rarely in goats, mimicking the bovine disease and producing hard painful swellings on the mandible and maxilla.

Diagnosis
- Direct smears, culture in anaerobic conditions or biopsy show the Gram-positive filamentous organism *Actinomyces bovis*.

Treatment
- Intramuscular/local antibiotics; surgical excision and drainage.

Body swellings

Abscess

Haematoma/seroma

Tumour
Reported tumours include squamous cell carcinoma, melanoma, lymphosarcoma, papilloma, haemangioma and histiocytoma.

Hernia
- **Umbilical.** Incomplete closure of the umbilical ring results in an umbilical hernia, with a hernial sac consisting of an inner peritoneal layer and outer skin, which is reducible by digital pressure. No genetic predisposition has been confirmed in goats and some hernias will occur as sequel to umbilical remnant

infection, but a genetic component should always be suspected and affected animals bred from with caution.

Small hernias (< than one finger size) may be encouraged to close if detected and reduced shortly after birth by wrapping the abdomen in conforming bandage and/or adhesive tape, but most hernias will not spontaneously close without intervention (see 'Umbilical repair', Chapter 26).

If an umbilical swelling is irreducible and no umbilical ring is detectable on palpation, *umbilical infection* should be suspected and investigated. Infection results in umbilical swelling, pain, abscessation and possible discharge from the umbilicus. In the absence of external signs of infection, ultrasonography may help to distinguish between a hernia and thickened or abscessed tissue. *Umbilical abscesses* should be drained, the area treated locally and parenteral antibiotics administered. Umbilical infection usually results from a failure to correctly treat the navel of newborn lambs at birth with strong veterinary iodine within the first 30 minutes of life. Iodine solutions are preferred to antibiotic aerosol sprays and are cheaper.

Ascending infection from an infected navel can result in peritonitis, joint-ill or more general infection.

A *patent urachus* is occasionally reported and results in dribbling of urine, urine scalding of the ventral abdomen and dermatitis. In the absence of infection and gross inflammation, daily cauterisation with iodine or silver nitrate may result in closure. Surgical closure will be necessary if the urachus remains patent for more than a few days (see Chapter 26).

Herniation of the intestines through the umbilicus occurs occasionally in newborn kids due to overzealous licking by the doe.

- **Inguinal/scrotal.** Inguinal/scrotal hernias are uncommon in the goat. They present as a soft reducible swelling below the inguinal ring. Strangulation is rare.
- **Ventral.** Rupture of the ventral abdominal muscles caudal to the umbilicus occurs spontaneously, usually in multiparous does or occasionally following trauma and results in swelling of the ventral abdominal wall and dropping of the udder (see Chapter 16).

Prolapse

- Rectal (see Chapter 4).
- Vaginal (see Chapter 4).

Ectopic mammary tissue

May result in a bilateral enlargement of the vulva lips in late pregnancy.

Ticks

The sheep tick, *Ixodes ricinus*, is sometimes found on goats grazing sheep pastures. The hedgehog tick, *I. hexagonus*, is also occasionally identified.

Keds

The sheep ked, *Melophagus ovinus*, occasionally infects goats.

Coenurus cyst of *Taenia multiceps*

Can occur as a subcutaneous cyst.

Warble flies

Typical swellings under the skin on the back have been reported, although not from the United Kingdom.

Leg swellings

- **Orf.** See 'Other swellings around the head and neck'.
- **Chorioptic mange.** See Chapter 11.
- **Mycotic dermatitis (strawberry footrot)**. See Chapter 11.

Further reading

General

Fubini, S.L. and Campbell, S.G. (1983) External lumps on sheep and goats. *Vet. Clin. North Amer.: Large Anim. Pract.*, **5** (3), November 1983, 457–476.

Bluetongue

Backx, A. *et al.* (2007) Clinical signs of bluetongue virus serotype 8 infection in sheep and goats. *Vet. Rec.*, **161** (17), 591–593.

Derksen, D. and Lewis, C. (2007) Bluetongue virus serotype 8 in sheep and cattle: a clinical update. *In Pract.*, **29** (6), June 2007, 314–318.

Elliott, H. (2007) Bluetongue disease: background to the outbreak in NW Europe. *Goat Vet. Soc. J.*, **23**, 31–39.

Caseous lymphadenitis

Baird, G. (2005) Caseous lymphadenitis in goats. *Goat Vet. Soc. J.*, **21**, 21–23.

Brown, C.C. and Olander, H.J. (1987) Caseous lymphadenitis of goats and sheep, a review. *Vet. Bull.*, **57** (1), 1–12.

Debien, E. *et al.* (2013) Proportional mortality: a study of 152 goats submitted for necropsy from 13 goat herds in Quebec, with a special focus on caseous lymphadenitis. *Canadian Vet. J.*, **54**, 581–587.

Lloyd, S., Lindsay, H.J., Slater, J.D. and Jackson, P.G.G. (1990) *Corynebacterium pseudotuberculosis* infection (caseous lymphadenitis) in goats. *Goat Vet. Soc. J.*, **11** (2), 55–65.

Washburn, K.E. *et al.* (2009) Comparison of three treatment regimens for sheep and goats with caseous lymphadenitis. *JAVMA*, **234** (9), 1162–1166.

Washburn, K.E. *et al.* (2013) Serologic and bacteriologic culture prevalence of *Corynebacterium pseudotuberculosis* infection in goats and sheep and use of Bayesian analysis to determine value of assay results for prediction of future infection. *JAVMA*, **242** (7), 997–1002.

Williams, C.S.F. (1980) Differential diagnosis of caseous lymphadenitis in the goat. *Vet. Med. Small Animal Clin.*, **75**, 1165.

Williamson, L.H. (2001) Caseous lymphadenitis in small ruminants. *Vet. Clin. North Amer.: Food Anim. Pract.*, **17** (2), 359–371.

Windsor, P.A. (2011) Control of caseous lymphadenitis. *Vet. Clin. North Amer.: Food Anim. Pract.*, **27** (1), 193–202.

Dentigerous cyst

Miller, C.C., Selcer, B.A., Williamson, L.H. and Mahaffey, E.A. (1997) Surgical treatment of a septic dentigerous cyst in a goat. *Vet. Rec.*, **140**, 528–230.

Developmental cysts

Brown, P.J. *et al.* (1989) Developmental cysts in the upper neck of Anglo-Nubian goats. *Vet. Rec.*, **125**, 256–258.

Hypothyroidism

Rijnberk, A., *et al.* (1977) Congenital defect in iodothyronine synthesis; clinical aspects of iodine metabolism in goats with congenital goitre and hypothyroidism. *Br. Vet. J.*, **133**, 495–503.

Lymphosarcoma

Guedes, R.M.C., Facury Filho, E.J. and Lago, L.A. (1998) Mandibular lymphosarcoma in a goat. *Vet. Rec.*, **143**, 51–52.

Orf

Spyrou, V. and Valiakos, G. (2015) Orf virus infection in sheep or goats. *Vet. Microbiol.*, **181** (1–2), 178–182.

Thymic hyperplasia

Pritchard, G.C. (1988) Throat swellings in goats. *Goat Vet. Soc. J.*, **10** (1), 34–37.

Thymoma

Parish, S.M., Middleton, J.R. and Baldwin, T.J. (1996) Clinical megaoesophagus in a goat with thymoma. *Vet. Rec.*, **139**, 94.

Rostkowski, C.M., Stirtzinger, T. and Baird, J.D. (1985) Congestive heart failure associated with thymoma in two Nubian goats. *Can. Vet. J.*, **26** (9), 267–269.

CHAPTER 11

Skin disease

Initial assessment

The preliminary history should consider:
- Clinical signs observed by owner and how long present.
- Individual or herd problem.
- Contact with goats and other animals.
- General health of affected goat and of herd.
- Response to any treatment given.
- Management (feeding, worming, etc.).

Clinical examination

The goat should be carefully examined:
- For ectoparasites.
- For signs of intercurrent disease, for example Helminthiasis.
- To assess its behaviour (rubbing, nibbling, pruritis, etc.); study the goat, preferably in its own surroundings.
- To assess the general condition of the animal – weight, etc.; evidence of malnutrition. Malnourished goats will have a dry scaly skin, often with a heavy lice burden.

Examination of skin
- Head/neck, particularly the periorbital area and pinnae; mouth and mucocutaneous junction of the lips.
- Thorax/abdomen, particularly the axillae, udder and inguinal regions.
- Perineal region.
- Legs and feet.

Table 11.1 shows the common distribution of lesions in skin diseases while Table 11.2 lists the external parasites that cause skin disease, together with their effects and treatment.

Record
- Distribution of lesions (use sketches if indicated).
- Type and size of lesions.
- Quality of skin: colour, elasticity, odour, temperature.
- Response of animal to palpation of lesions.
- Hair loss or damage to follicles.
- Skin secretions.
- Self-inflicted damage.

Laboratory investigation

Hair sample: pluck with tweezers from the edge of the active lesion.
- Direct microscopy: identification of ringworm.
  Note: Wood's lamp is normally negative in goats with ringworm.
- Culture
  - Fungal media (ringworm)
  - Blood agar (*Dermatophilus congolensis*).

Skin swab: from active lesion near the scaly or scabby area.
- Culture on blood agar. *Staphylococcus aureus* in pure culture is generally significant, but may be a secondary infection.

Impression smear: of pus under a crust.
- Stain with Dip Quick, Giemsa or new methylene blue.
- Useful for *Dermatophilus congolensis* and candidiasis.

Skin scrapings: essential for diagnosis of some manges. Scraping taken from each of a number of *active* lesions, collected and covered with potassium hydroxide before being warmed in a waterbath overnight.

Diseases of the Goat, Fourth Edition. John Matthews.
© 2016 John Wiley & Sons, Ltd. Published 2016 by John Wiley & Sons, Ltd.

Table 11.1 Distribution of lesions.

Legs, face and neck	Ears	Feet
■ Staphyloccocal dermatitis	■ Sarcoptic mange	■ Chorioptic mange
■ Ringworm	■ Dermatophilosis	■ Staphylococcal dermatitis
■ Sarcoptic mange	■ Ringworm	■ Fly worry
■ Dermatophilosis	■ Ear mites	■ Dermatophilosis
■ Orf	■ Photodermatitis	■ Sarcoptic mange
■ Zinc deficiency	■ Frostbite	■ Orf
■ *Pemphigus foliaceus*	■ *Pemphigus foliaceus*	■ Zinc deficiency
		■ Contact dermatitis
		■ *Pemphigus foliaceus*
		■ Foot and mouth disease

Udder	Perineum
■ Staphylococcal dermatitis	■ Orf
■ Fly worry	■ Staphylococcal dermatitis
■ Orf	■ Tumours
■ Zinc deficiency	■ Ectopic mammary gland
■ Sunburn	■ Caprine herpes virus
■ Tumours	

o Sarcoptic mange: mites difficult to find; diagnosis difficult from scrape; repeated deep scrapings required.

o Demodectic mange: many mites found when the nodule is expressed.

o Chorioptic and psoroptic mange: mites easily found in scrapes from legs and ears respectively.

Skin biopsy: whole thickness skin strips taken under local anaesthesia; preferably from normal, marginal and abnormal areas; fix in formol saline. A 6 or 8 mm biopsy punch is suitable for goats. Multiple skin biopsies enable bacterial and fungal cultures to be performed as necessary.

Electron microscopy: useful in diagnosis of orf; scabs fixed in buffered gluteraldehyde.

Blood sample

o Anaemia (lice infestation, etc.).

o Neutrophilia (bacterial infection).

o Eosinophilia (allergic, parasitic infestation).

Treatment of external parasites

There are no drugs licensed for the treatment of ectoparasites in goats in the United Kingdom and very few licensed for use on cattle or sheep producing milk for human consumption.

Rational treatment involves extrapolation from products licensed for use in cattle and sheep, preferably, or, outwith the EU, from dogs and cats where no other suitable products exist, if permitted by regulatory authorities. All of these preparations have a mandatory withholding time for milk of *at least* 7 days and for meat of 28 days, which can cause major difficulties in formulating control strategies for milking herds and may lead to welfare problems. Wherever possible, the opportunity should be taken to treat young stock and dry goats. Table 11.3 lists the treatments available.

There are significant differences between the skin/fibre lipid content of sheep and goats so that non-systemic preparations, such as pour-ons, which are formulated for sheep, are much less efficacious in the goat. These preparations bind and move with skin or hair fibre lipid. The skin/fibre lipid content of the goat is more similar to that of cattle. Cattle non-systemic products are likely to be more effective, but even in cattle the bioavailability of the avermectin/milbemycin drugs is greatly reduced in the pour-on form as compared to the parenteral route.

Pour-on preparations formulated for cattle should be selected rather those formulated for sheep

Table 11.2 External parasites causing skin disease.

	Causal agent	Incidence	Distribution of lesions	Clinical signs	Pruritus	Diagnosis	Treatment
Lice	*Bovicola (Damalinia) caprae, B. limbata, B. crassiceps* (biting) *Linognathus stenopsis* (sucking)	+++	Head, neck, back	Hair loss Broken hairs Moth-eaten coat	++	Naked eye	Amitraz Pyrethrins and synthetic pyrethroids Avermectins, Moxidectin Fipronil, dips
Sarcoptic mange	*Sarcoptes scabiei*	+	Head, ears,body Lymph nodes	Alopecia Crusting lesions Self-inflicted damage Weight loss	+++	Skin biopsy (skin scraping)	Doramectin Ivermectin Moxidectin Amitraz
Cheyletiella Forage mites Harvest mites	*Cheyletiella* species *Tyroglyphidae* species *Trombicula autumnalis* species	Rare	Legs, face, lower body	Exudative patches	++	Naked eye	As for lice
Psoroptic mange	*Psoroptes cuniculi*	Rare	Ear (head, body)	Head shaking Excoriation of pinnae	++	Skin scraping	Canine ear preparations Doramectin, Ivermectin Moxidectin, Amitraz
Chorioptic mange	*Chorioptes caprae*	+++	Lower caudal limbs Occasionally ventral abdomen/sternum	Hair loss Broken hairs Moth-eaten coat	–	Skin scraping	Avermectins, Moxidectin Lime sulphur Amitraz, Fipronil
Demodectic mange	*Demodex caprae*	++	Head, neck, body	Hard nodules with yellow caseous material	–	Microscopy on expressed material	Amitraz
Pustular dermatitis	*Staphylococcus aureus*[a]	+++	Udder, teats, ventral Abdomen, groin, body	Pustular scabs Dry, scaley coat	–	Culture	Local/parenteral antibiotics, udder washes
Ringworm	*Trichophyton verrucosum Microsporum canis Trichophyton mentagrophytes*	Rare	Head, body	Raised circular crusty lesions	–	Microscopy Culture	Topical preparations *Griseofulvin in feed* (not legal in EU)

[a] *Staphylococcus aureus* is often a secondary invader in other skin conditions, e.g. mange.

Avermectins and milbemycins

The avermectins (ivermectin and doramectin) and the milbemycins (moxidectin) have a wide range of activity against immature and mature arthropods and nematodes. Use of these products for louse and mite control exposes the animal's nematode population to the drugs and could contribute to anthelmintic resistance buildup in the population at a time of year when treatment of nematodes may not be needed. It is important to use these products sensibly and at the correct dose for goats.

Doramectin and moxidectin have residual action for mite control, but ivermectin has no residual action and two or three weekly injections are needed to control mites.

Pyrethrins and synthetic pyrethroids

Cypermethrin, deltamethrin, flumethrin and permethrin pour-on and spot-on preparations are used for treating lice, ticks and mites and for fly control.

Plunge dips

Plunge dips can be used in fibre goats for the treatment of lice and mange conditions, using synthetic pyrethroid (cypermethrin and flumethrin) or organophophorus compounds (diampylate (diazinon) and propetamphos).

Table 11.3 Treatment of external parasites.

| | Lice | | Chorioptic mange | Sarcoptic mange | Demodectic mange | Psoroptic mange | Ticks/keds |
	Sucking	Biting					
Amitraz	+	+	+	+	+	+	+
Cypermethrin		+				+	+
Alphacypermethrin	+	+				+	+
Deltamethrin	+	+					+
Permethrin	+	+	+	+		+	
Pyrethrin/piperonyl peroxide	+	+					
Doramectin	+	+	+	+		+	
Eprinomectin	+	+		+		+	
Ivermectin	+	+−	+−	+		+	
Moxidectin		+	+	+		+	
Fipronil	+	+	+	+			
Flumethrin	+	+				+	+
Lime sulphur			+	+		+	

+ = effective; +− = part control

Note: none of these products is licensed for goats in the UK and not all (e.g. Fipronil) are licensed for use in food-producing animals in the EC. Particular care should be taken when treating goats producing milk for human consumption.

Cypermethrin is effective against many ectoparasites; animals should be dipped twice at intervals of 14 days. Flumethrin has residual action and is effective against lice, ticks, keds and mange mites. Diazinon also has residual action. Only diazinon-containing sheep dips are currently available in the United Kingdom and are authorised for control of mites. A Certificate of Competence is required for their purchase and use.

Shower applications and jetting races, using diazinon-based plunge dipping formulations, have been used to control Angora goat ectoparasites, but wetting of animals with high-volume sprays in cold, windy weather may predispose them to pneumonia.

Lime sulphur

Lime sulphur sprays and dips are labelled for use against sarcoptic, psoroptic and chorioptic mites in sheep in the United States. A lime sulphur equine dip is available in the United Kingdom.

Supportive treatment

Animals may require antibiotics to treat secondary infection, particularly with *Staph. aureus* and corticosteroids to reduce anaphylactic reactions, even when the primary cause of the disease, for example mite infection, has been identified and treated.

Pruritic skin disease

Lice

The biting louse *Bovicola* (*Damalinia*) *caprae* and the blood-sucking louse *Linognathus stenopsis* (Plates 11.1 and 11.2), affect dairy goats in the United Kingdom, producing pruritus and hair loss, particularly on the head, neck and back (Plate 11.3). Most dairy goats with lice have biting rather than blood-sucking lice. The biting lice *Bovicola limbata* and *Bovicola crassiceps* have been reported from Angora goats in the United Kingdom and can cause significant damage to the fleece. *B. caprae* is host specific for short-coated dairy goats and *B. limbata* is host specific for Angora goats; although individual lice can be found on dairy goats in close contact, they do not establish permanent colonies. Mixed infections of biting and sucking lice are common. *Linognathus africanus* infest Angoras and other breeds of goats and have been reported from Australia and the United States.

Cross-infestations between sheep and goats with biting lice have occasionally been reported. The sheep louse, *Bovicola ovis*, can persist and reproduce on goats, which act as possible reservoirs of infection. Goat lice appear to be host specific. Blood-sucking and biting goat lice were shown experimentally to survive on sheep for 5 to 7 days but not reproduce.

Lice are very common and in particular will multiply where animals are debilitated for any reason and may complicate the problem by producing anaemia (see Chapter 18). The damage to fleece can cause financial loss in Angora goats. The whole life cycle of the louse is spent on the goat.

Treatments (both topical and injectable) should be repeated in 10 to 14 days to kill any lice that have emerged from eggs. All animals (of the same species) in contact with the infested animal should also be treated.

Diagnosis

- Lice are visible to the naked eye. Under magnification, biting lice are seen to have broad heads with wide mouth parts, whereas sucking lice have pointed heads to enable them to pierce the skin and suck blood.

Treatment

- As lice dislike warm weather and ultraviolet light, lice numbers decrease in summer and rise in winter. The best time for treatment is thus late summer or autumn when lice numbers are lowest. The whole herd should preferably be treated at the same time.
- Sucking lice can be treated with injectable ivermectin or dormectin, or topical treatments, but only topical treatments are totally effective against biting lice. As mixed infections are common, topical treatments may be preferable if the species of louse has not been identified.
- Most treatments are not effective against nits, so treatment should be repeated after 10 to 14 days to kill young lice before they mature.
- Shearing Angora goats will remove many lice and expose the remaining population to dessication and rain, further reducing numbers. Insecticidal treatments are usually more effective after shearing. Showers and jetting races have been used for controlling Angora goat ectoparasites, but wetting of animals with high-volume sprays in cold, windy weather may predispose them to pneumonia.
- Bathing and grooming dairy goats will also remove large numbers of lice.
- The pharmokinetics of pour-on formulations, which bind and move with skin or hair fibre lipid, may be different on goats with short hair as opposed to Angora goats with long fibres, resulting in treatment failures.

Amidines

Biting and sucking lice:

Amitraz, 0.025% solution, by spray or wash.

Pyrethrins and synthetic pyrethroids

Sucking and biting lice:

Permethrins:

Cypermethrin 1.25% solution, 0.25 ml/kg (maximum 20 ml) by pour-on.

Deltamethrin 1%, 'spot-on'.

Permethrin 4%, 'pour-on'.

There are also many preparations containing products marketed for use in dogs and cats as shampoos and powders that can be used on pet and pygmy goats, if regulations permit.

Cypermethrin resistance is a concern in Angora goats in the United Kingdom.

Pyrethrins:

As with permethrin, dog and cat sprays and powders containing pyrethrins and piperonyl butoxide can be used on pet and Pygmy goats, where regulations permit.

Pyrethroid preparations can take up to 6 weeks before they are fully dispersed across the coat.

Avermectins and milbemycin

Sucking lice and partial control of biting lice:

Doramectin, 400 mcg/kg, 2 ml/50 kg s.c.

Eprinomectin, 0.5 mg/kg, 5 ml/50 kg 'pour-on'

Ivermectin, 400 mcg/kg, 2 ml/50 kg s.c.

Moxidectin, 400 mcg/kg, 2 ml/50 kg s.c.

Note: Use of these products for lice control exposes the animal's nematode population to avermectin chemistry and could contribute to anthelmintic resistance buildup in the population at a time of year when treatment of nematodes may not be needed. Although pour-on preparations are not generally recommended for the control of endoparasites, eprinomectin pour-on has been shown to be effective for the targeted treatment of ectoparasites.

Fipronil

Biting and sucking lice:

Suitable for pygmy goats or individual pet goats as it is expensive! Is not licensed in the United Kingdom for food-producing animals.

Dips

Fibre goats can be dipped, using products approved for sheep, such as synthetic pyrethroid (cypermethrin) or organophosphorus preparations (diazinon). The body should be immersed for at least 30 seconds, until the coat is completely saturated. The head should be immersed once or twice, allowing the animal to breathe between immersions.

Other treatments

Anecdotal reports indicate that detergents, boric acid, diatomaceous earths and citrus-based products control lice, but there is no scientific data to support or refute this.

Prevention and control

■ Maintaining a closed herd or isolating and treating incoming animals for 3 weeks with regular inspection will prevent the introduction of louse infestations.

Sarcoptic mange

Sarcoptic mange is a relatively common disease affecting goats of all ages. It is transmitted primarily by direct contact but also by indirect contact such as milking, handling, etc.

Clinical signs

■ Lesions start around the eyes and ears with erythema and small nodules, progressing to hair loss, thickening and wrinkling of the skin, in response to intense pruritus and scratching over the head, neck and body (Plates 11.4 and 11.5). Secondary infection with *Staphylococcus aureus* is common.
■ Affected goats often lose condition and the milk yield falls because of the intensity of the irritation.

Diagnosis

■ Demonstration of the mite, *Sarcoptes scabiei*, in deep skin scrapings may be extremely difficult as very few mites can be found even with severe lesions; skin biopsy may demonstrate mites.

Treatment

1 **Avermectins and milbemycin**
   Doramectin, 400 mcg/kg, 2 ml/33 kg s.c.
   Ivermectin, 400 mcg/kg, 2 ml/50 kg s.c.
   Moxidectin, 400 mcg/kg, 2 ml/50 kg s.c.
   Moxidectin and dorametlin are more persistent than ivermectin. Treatment with ivermectin should be repeated after 7 days.
2 **Amidines**
   Amitraz 0.025% solution, by spray or wash
   Use of soap and water or antiseborrhoeic shampoo to remove crusts before using amitraz will ensure better penetration of the drug. Washes can be repeated after 7 to 14 days as necessary.
3 **Lime sulphur**. At least four treatments with 5% lime sulphur washes at 7 day intervals are required. Disadvantages of lime sulphur are that it has a foul smell, stains white hairs yellow and is potentially irritating in concentrations in excess of 5%.

Fly worry

Many fly species are irritant to goats, resulting in reduced weight gain, reduced feed efficiency and decreased milk yields. They include *Musca domestica* (house fly), *Musca autumnalis* (face fly), *Morellia simplex*, *Lyerosia irritans* (horn fly), *Hydrotea irritans* (head fly), *Stomoxys calcitrans* (stable fly), *Tabunus* species (horse flies) and *Chrysops* species (deer flies). Biting flies are particularly worrying to housed goats in the summer, producing quite severe lesions superficially resembling staphylococcal dermatitis on the udder but generally more pruritic. Under typical UK climatic conditions, up to 15 generations of flies can be produced in one year. Flies can also transmit diseases, including infectious keratoconjunctivitis.

Topical creams and washes will ease the lesions. Control of flies in the goat house will help prevent the problem.

Myiasis (blowfly strike) is much less common than in sheep, but may occur around the head following fights, in wounds in soiled areas around the tail, breech and penis, or on the feet of animals with footrot/scald. Myiasis flies include *Lucilia sericata* (green bottle), *Protophormia terraenovae* (blue bottle) and *Wohlfahrtia magnifica* (flesh fly).

The insect growth regulator, cyromazine, can be used in animals at risk and will give up to 10 weeks protection against fly strike after topical application. Dicyclanil, available as a pour-on formulation containing 5% w/v dicyclanil, prevents larval development and affords 16 weeks protection.

Organophosphates (diazinon), pyrethrins and synthetic pyrethroids (high *cis*-cypermethrin, alpha-cypermethrin, deltamethrin and permethrin) and amidines (amitraz) are effective against myiasis flies.

Black flies (*Simulium* species), mosquitoes (*Anopheles* and *Culex* species) and midges (*Culicoides* species) will all feed on goats and may cause allergic reactions. *Culicoides* species are particularly significant as they transmit bluetongue and other viruses (see Chapter 10). Because even a single bite from an infected midge can produce disease, preventing disease in the presence of infected midges is very difficult. Although housing will reduce exposure to midges, some species, for example *C. dewulfi*, will enter livestock buildings.

Frequent applications of synthetic pyrethroid pour-ons (deltamethrin) may reduce midge activity, thus reducing the chance of infection spreading within the herd, but will not stop individual animals being bitten. Monthly applications have been recommended when the midges are active.

Efficient manure management, good drainage and drain management will help limit fly problems by reducing fly breeding sites. Larvacides are available for environmental control of flies in fly breeding areas and residual adulticides can be used on posts, milking pipes, etc. The early deployment of fly traps will help reduce breeding numbers.

Other external parasites

Harvest mites are the reddish or orange larvae of the free-living trombiculid mite, *Trombicula autumnalis*, which attaches to the pasterns, muzzle, ears or ventral abdomen when goats are exposed to infested fields or woods or contaminated fodder in the late summer. The mites produce severe localised pruritis and exudative patches and even anorexia in severe cases. Other mites such as *Cheyletiella* and *poultry mites* (*Dermanyssus gallinae*) are also occasionally reported. The small red poultry mites are nocturnal feeders and so are rarely actually seen on the goat, but the combination of a pruritic goat housed with poultry or roosting birds, particularly in the late summer months, would suggest a provisional diagnosis of infestation. *Forage mites* (*Tyroglyphidae* spp.) are chance contaminants from

bedding, food, etc., which are occasionally associated with a dermatitis. Most lice treatments will also kill mites.

Flea infestations are uncommon in temperate climates, although cat, dog (*Ctenophalides* spp.) and human (*Pulex irritans*) fleas are found occasionally on goats. Infestations can cause significant pruritus and hair loss. The cat flea adapted to sheep, goats and cattle in Israel in the early 1980s and human flea infestations of farm animals have been reported from France, Italy and Greece. Lice treatments are suitable for the control of fleas, but environmental control and biosecurity are as important as the treatment of individual animals.

Scrapie
See Chapter 12.

Scrapie causes pruritus and self-mutilation but is not as pruritic in goats as in sheep.

Psoroptic mange
Psoroptes cuniculi parasitises the ear, generally without clinical signs, occasionally producing head shaking and ear scratching with the hind feet. Infestations are usually confined to the ears with scaly lesions found on the inside of the pinnae. Lesions are occasionally found on the head, neck, withers, back, abdomen, pasterns and interdigital spaces, with younger animals generally shower milder symptoms and older or debilitated animals having body lesions. Kids are infected by their dams and may show clinical signs by 10 days of age. Severe vestibular disease and facial nerve paralysis may occur if the tympanic membrane ruptures.

Psoroptes ear mites are thought to act as vectors for mycoplasma organisms (Chapter 17). The host specificity of *Psoroptes* in the ears of sheep and goats is equivocal. It is possible that they may transfer between the ears of sheep and goats under certain circumstances of shared habitat.

Railettia caprae is a mite affecting the ears of goats in Australia, Mexico and the United States, but not in the United Kingdom.

Sheep scab mites (*P. ovis*) cannot infest the bodies of short haired dairy goats but sheep scab-like lesions have been recorded on the bodies of Angora goats.

Diagnosis
- Identification of mite: larger than Chorioptes with long jointed pedicel and trumpet-shaped suckers.

Treatment

- Canine ear mite preparations can be used where the mites are confined to the ears, but removal of wax plugs and crusting is necessary to allow penetration of the drug. Several weekly treatments are necessary.
- Subcutaneous injections of doramectin, ivermectin or moxidectin (see treatment of lice) will kill the mites but cannot be used in lactating goats.
- Body mange can be treated with avermectin or moxidectin injection or by amitraz or lime sulphur washes.

Nematode infections

1. Strongyloidiasis

A localised dermatitis can occur as part of the immune response to the larvae of *Strongyloides papillosus*, the threadworm of the small intestine. Strongyloidiasis affects the lower limbs, causing pruritus, with stamping and nibbling.

2. Onchocerciasis

The adult worms of *Onchocerca* species can live in the connective tissues of goats producing fine skin nodules, particularly in the neck and shoulder region, with mild pruritus. The microfilaria migrate into the dermis and are ingested by *Culicoides* spp. and *Simulium* spp. in which the larvae develop into an infective stage. Other goats are infected when the midges feed.

3. *Parelaphostrongylus tenuis* infection

P. tenuis causes subclinical infection in whitetail deer in North America. In aberrant hosts like the goats, it produces clinical signs of focal myelitis or encephalomyelitis (see Chapter 12).

Migrating *P. tenuis* larvae occasionally produce oozing sores along the back of infected goats, with or without associated neurological signs. Treatment is with fenbendazole 25 mg/kg and dexamethasone for 5 days.

Autoimmune skin disease

Pemphigus foliaceus is an autoimmune disease in which the animal develops autoantibodies that are attached to intercellular desmosomal antigens, possibly desmoglens, in the upper layers of the dermis. The triggers for autoantibody production in the goat are not understood.

Transient pustules rapidly progress to crusty pruritic lesions with multifocal alopecia. Much of the body may be involved, especially the skin in the perineal and scrotal regions and on the ventral abdomen and face.

Diagnosis

- Cytology using a Tzanck preparation: pustular material from the undersurface of a fresh pustule is applied to a microscope slide for staining to show large numbers of acantholytic keratinocytes mixed with neutrophils and sometimes eosinophils. Because the pustules are sterile, there should be no cocci or other bacteria associated with polmorphonuclear cells, although secondary bacterial infection can be a complication.
- Pustules should be swabbed for microbial culture and hairs and crust collected for dermatophyte culture to help eliminate other diseases.
- A skin biopsy is required for a definitive diagnosis. The presence of acantholytic keratinocytes within vesicles in the granular or upper spinous cell layers is a diagnostic feature.

Treatment

- Remission has been achieved with an immunosuppressive induction dose of prednisolone, 1 mg/kg i.m. every 12 hours followed by a maintenance dose of 1 mg/kg i.m. every 48 hours. Long-acting methylprednisolone acetate injections can then be given every 4 to 6 weeks as necessary. Gold salts (gold sodium thiomalate) 1 mg/kg i.m. every 7 days have been used in conjunction with dexamethasone sodium phosphate injections.

Malignant catarrhal fever (MCF)

A generalized erythemic, alopecic condition with marked accumulation of keratinous debris around the nares has been described in an 18 month old goat. The condition was similar to the condition seen in sika deer due to ovine herpes type 2 virus (Ov-VH2) infection. Histopathological findings included a marked mural folliculitis and virus was detected in the peripheral circulation and in the skin by PCR.

Photosensitisation

Photosensitisation is caused by the accumulation of photodynamic chemicals in the skin, which become stimulated by sunlight on exposed, non-pigmented areas.

- Primary: due to ingestion of plants such as St. John's wort (*Hypericum perforatum*) or buckwheat (*Fagopyrum esculentum*) (see Chapter 21).
- Secondary: in animals with hepatic dysfunction due to accumulation of phylloerythrin, a breakdown derivative of chlorophyll. Normally the liver degrades phylloerythrin, keeping serum levels negligible. Any liver damage affecting bile excretion may be implicated – liver disease, hepatotoxic drugs, chemicals, mycotoxins or plant toxins, for example bog asphodel (*Northecium ossifragum*).

Clinical signs

- Pruritus, erythema, oedema and swelling of the skin, with blistering and scab formation, particularly of non-pigmented areas of the face, eyelids, muzzle, ear and tail.
- Head shaking and rubbing of the face and head.
- Affected areas may ooze serum with development of secondary bacterial infection.
- Necrosis of ear tips.

Treatment

- Prevent access to any photosensitising plant.
- Protect from sunlight.
- Symptomatic and supportive therapy; corticosteroids during the early stages will help reduce oedema; antibiotics because of secondary bacterial infection.
- Treatment of primary disease if liver damage is present.

Non-pruritic skin disease

A wide variety of non-specific lesions can occur in dairy goats kept commercially. Some of these are due to poor environmental conditions, such as standing or lying in wet conditions with inadequate bedding (Plate 11.6). Hair loss can occur from rubbing on the bars of mangers, racks or dividers (Plate 11.7). Other lesions may have no obvious aetiology (Plates 11.8 and 11.9), but a common feature is often a secondary Staphylococcal infection.

Chorioptic mange

Chorioptic mange is a very common infection of goats in the United Kingdom, particularly in housed goats in the winter but occurring throughout the year. Legs should always be checked for chorioptic mange during routine foot trimming.

Aetiology

- The surface dwelling mite, *Chorioptes caprae*, feeds on epidermal debris, causing exudative dermatitis and skin lesions, which are associated with a hypersensitivity reaction. Morphologically the mite resembles those seen on cattle and may in fact be *Chorioptes bovis*. Some goats are particularly susceptible to infection, or react more strongly to infection, and there appears to be a familial tendency to develop lesions, so that only individual animals within a herd have clinical signs and these are often related animals.
- The mites can survive off the host for many weeks in the environment and many infested animals are not severely affected and so act as a major reservoir.
- The life cycle takes 3 weeks, with the lifetime reproductive output of each mite being 20 eggs.

Clinical signs

- These white/brown scabby lesions are generally at the back of the pasterns (Plate 11.10, 11.11), but occasionally extend as far as the knee or hock in severe infections. Very occasionally lesions may be found on the ventral abdomen, sternum or even upper body. Lesions may be complicated with a *Staphylococcus aureus* infection.
- Similar lesions are produced in goats standing in wet conditions (Plate 11.12) and these need to be distinguished from mite lesions.

Diagnosis

- Microscopical identification of the non-burrowing surface dwelling mite, *Chorioptes caprae*. The mites are generally easily found; short pedicel with flask-shaped suckers on legs.
- Take clear packing tape and touch it repeatedly to the lesions on the animal. The interdigital space is often a good source of mites. Put the tape into a disposable petri dish until it can be examined under the microscope.
- Skin biopsies are of no use because the mite lives on the surface.
- Mites are not found in the crusts, but should be looked for in adjacent areas, clipping the hair as necessary.

Treatment

Treatment of chorioptic mange is extremely frustrating because of lack of effective drugs and the necessity to treat milking animals with drugs with long withholding times.

- Success of treatment with injectable avermectins and moxidectin (see treatment of lice) is variable because of the superficial location and the feeding habits of the mites, so repeat injections at 7 to 10 day intervals are necessary, particularly with less persistent drugs like ivermectin.
- Eprinomectin pour-on, twice, at two weekly intervals.
- Before topical treatments are used, the skin should be thoroughly washed to remove crusts and scabs. Topical treatments include amitraz, phosmet, ivermectin, moxidectin and fipronil (see treatment of lice). At least two treatments at 10 to 14 day intervals will be required and fortnightly treatments to cover two life cycles, that is up to 6 weeks, may be necessary.
- 5% lime sulphur has been used for its fungicidal, bactericidal, keratolytic and antipruritic properties. Its ability to penetrate lesions due to its keratolytic action, as well as its antiparasitic and antipruritic action, makes sulphur an excellent potential topical medication to treat chorioptic mange. At least four treatments at 7 days intervals are required. Disadvantages of lime sulphur are that it has a foul smell, stains white hairs yellow and is potentially irritating in concentrations in excess of 5%.
- Secondary bacterial infections should be treated with systemic antibiotics.

Demodectic mange (*Demodex caprae*)

Demodectic mange is relatively common. Goatlings most commonly show clinical disease following infection as a kid. It is usually an individual rather than a herd problem.

Clinical signs

- Small nodules (generally about 1 to 2 cm) in the skin of the head, neck and body due to multiplication of the mite in individual sebaceous glands. Yellow caseous material, containing numerous mites, can be expressed from the nodules.

Diagnosis

- Microscopical identification of mites in caseous material from nodules. Very easy to find in smears. Cigar-shaped body with bluntly pointed abdomen.

Treatment

- Where the lesions are widespread or generalised, topical treatment with 0.05% amitraz is necessary. No other treatments have been shown to be consistently effective. Nodules will persist for a considerable time after the mites have died, so it is difficult to know when a clinical cure is achieved.
- If there are only a small number of lesions, they can be treated by lancing each nodule and squeezing out the contents. The area can be washed with amitraz after the nodules have been expressed.

Staphylococcal dermatitis (pustular dermatitis)

Staphylococcus aureus infection is very common, causing pustules of variable size up to 4 cm, especially on the udder, teats and groin (Plates 13.5 and 13.6), but also on the ventral abdomen and occasionally any part of the body (Plate 11.9). First kidders are particularly affected soon after parturition. Pustules are easily broken and spread, healing as a scabby or impetigo-like lesion, and infection may be spread between goats at milking by hands, cloths or milking dusters. The lesions are generally non-painful and milk yield is not affected.

The disease is colloquially known as 'goat pox' but true 'goat pox' caused by capripoxvirus does not occur in the United Kingdom (see below).

Note: *Staphylococcus aureus* is a common secondary invader of other skin lesions.

Treatment

- Topical antiseptics, such as chlorhexidine, and antimicrobial ointments will help if only a limited number of lesions are present.
- Systemic antibiotic therapy, based on culture and sensitivity tests wherever possible, may be required in more severe cases. Empirical therapy includes procaine penicillin, amoxycillin or clavulanic acid/amoxycillin.

Goat pox

Suspect goat pox when an acute disease of goats is accompanied by pyrexia, pox-like skin lesions and high mortality.

The disease could be introduced by importation of live animals (or genetic material?) from endemically infected countries. The viruses can also be transported on clothing, equipment and unprocessed wool products. Outbreaks have occurred previously in Europe, including Greece, Italy and Bulgaria, having spread from illegal imports from Turkey. Therefore there is potential for further spread of these capripoxviruses to and/or within Europe. This, together with the fact that the United Kingdom currently imports cattle hides, sheep skins and wool from European countries without the requirement for treatment prior to export, raises concern that capripoxviruses could be introduced into the United Kingdom.

Present distribution

Endemic in Northern Africa, the Mediterranean basin/Middle East, central Asia (including south Russia and western China) and the Indian subcontinent as far east as Myanmar.

Aetiology

- Sheep pox and goat pox are considered to be a single disease by OIE. The viruses causing these diseases are members of the *Capripoxvirus g*enus of pox viruses (family *Poxviridae)* and arc clinically indistinguishable. Strains of sheep pox virus (SPPV), goat pox virus (GTPV) and lumpy skin disease virus (LSDV) cannot be differentiated serologically.
- The virus replicates in the cells of the dermis and other tissues and disseminates around the body in macrophages. There are many strains that vary in virulence depending on whether sheep or goats are affected. Sheep pox and goat pox viruses are generally considered host-specific, but different strains show different host preferences and it is not unknown for both sheep and goats to be infected by the same strain of virus. Goat breeds vary in susceptibility.

Transmission

- Direct contact with infected animals: aerosols, nasal secretions, saliva.
- Pox lesions may become walled off by the immune response but not resorb ('sitfasts') and act as an infective source for several months.
- Indirect contact with abraded material. The virus can remain viable for up to 6 months in animal pens out of direct sunlight and for at least 3 months in dry scabs on the fleece, skin and hair from infected animals.
- Contaminated objects such as farm equipment, vehicles, bedding and fodder.

- Insects, including stable flies, can act as mechanical vectors.

Clinical signs

The disease is characterised by fever, lethargy and an oculo-nasal discharge with typical pox-like lesions that appear over the body surface.

- Sudden onset pyrexia.
- Oculonasal discharges and excess salivation.
- Necrotic plaques may develop on the mucosa of the oral cavity.
- Inappetance.
- Reluctance to move.
- Skin lesions appear in 1–2 days, initially areas of erythema, developing over the next 2 weeks to a papule, vesicle, pustule with exudation and scab formation. Lesions extend over the entire skin, particularly the head and ears, perineum and tail. The mucous membranes of the nostrils, mouth and vulva and the tongue may also be affected.
- Acute respiratory distress.
- In a severe outbreak, affecting a naive population, morbidity and mortality can reach 100%. Mortality peaks about two weeks after the onset of the skin lesions.
- The disease is more severe in kids than adults.

Post-mortem findings

- Characteristic epidermal and mucosal lesions.
- Ulceration in the lining of the trachea and gastrointestinal tract.
- Lung lesions with pale grey nodules may be present.

Differential diagnosis

- Contagious pustular dermatitis (orf).
- Bluetongue.
- Mycotic dermatitis.
- Mange.
- Photosensitisation.

Laboratory examination

- Serology on paired blood samples from animals with pyrexia.
- Virus identification on sera, vesicular fluid, scabs and skin scrapings of lesions and lesions in the respiratory and gastrointestinal tract. Fresh samples should be taken within the first week of the disease appearing.

o Cell inoculation and identification by immunofluorescence.

o Staining of intracytoplasmic inclusion bodies.

o Inhibition of cytopathic effect using positive serum.

o ELISA.

Control

- Diseased sheep or goats should be destroyed and their carcases burnt or buried.
- Movement controls for animals and vehicles.
- Vaccination of in-contact animals:

o Live attenuated vaccines give good immunity and are used in emergency situations.

o Cell-cultured attenuated and inactivated vaccines have been used to prevent disease. Inactivated vaccines provide about five months protection but there is no ready commercial source.

Orf

See Chapter 10.

Zinc deficiency

Zinc deficiency is probably more common than generally recognised. Zinc deficiency is not regarded as a clinical problem of grazing animals in the United Kingdom, but has been reported to occur under natural conditions in areas around the Mediterranean, North Africa and North America.

Diets should usually be adequate in zinc, but:

- An excess of copper will interfere with zinc uptake as will a high calcium intake (e.g. lucerne).
- Individual goats may not absorb adequate amounts.
- Some male goats may have higher requirements.

Clinical signs

- Hair loss and hyperkeratosis and parakeratosis with thickened, wrinkled skin, particularly on the hind limbs, scrotum, neck and head.
- Hair loss on the ears of Anglo-Nubian kids has also responded empirically to zinc supplements.

Note: zinc deficiency may also result in infertility with low conception rates.

Laboratory tests

- Zinc blood levels can be estimated using a sample taken into a sodium citrate vacutainer, but correlation between serum and dietary zinc levels may be poor.

Treatment

Response to zinc supplementation should be rapid.

- Zinc sulphate drench 1% or zinc sulphate tablets, 250 mg to 1 g daily, orally for 2 to 4 weeks; zinc methionine may be absorbed better from the abomasum and small intestine.
- Slow-release boluses containing zinc, cobalt and selenium are available.

Urine scald

Male goats urinate on themselves during the breeding season, particularly down the back of the forelegs, face and beard, which will result in staining, hair loss and possibly scalding of the skin.

Similarly, staining will occur on goats that are recumbent or housed in dirty conditions. Urine scald can also be a problem after urethrostomy and marsupialization surgery to treat urolithiasis.

Alopecia/skin thickening in older male goats

Older male goats (particularly British Toggenburg and British Alpine) commonly have thickened scaly skin, especially over the head and back, possibly due in part to urine scald, nutritional deficiency during the breeding season (zinc related?) and as a response to rubbing, although the exact aetiology is unknown.

Treatment with baby oils or olive oil thinned with surgical spirit has been suggested as suitable for removing excess scaling to allow new hair to grow, following thorough shampooing. Zinc sulphate supplements should also be considered (see zinc deficiency, above).

Labial dermatitis in artificially reared kids

Kids reared artificially may develop erythema and hair loss around the face and mouth due to wetting. Occasionally, a secondary infection with *Staphylococcus aureus* occurs (see Staphylococcal dermatitis). Labial dermatitis needs to be distinguished from the early stages of orf (see Chapter 10) and from dermatophilosis (see Chapter 7).

Ringworm (dermatophytosis)

Ringworm is an uncommon infection acquired from other hosts. *Trichophyton verrucosum* from cattle is seen most frequently, occasionally *T. mentagrophytes* from rodents and *Microsporum canis* from dogs or cats. Lesions are initially circular, crusty and raised, later irregular in shape, often occurring on the head, ears and neck (Plate 11.12). The course of the disease is 4 to 5 weeks in animals with competent immune systems.

Diagnosis
- Microscopy and culture.
- *Trichophyton* species do not fluoresce under a Wood's lamp.

Treatment
- Topical fungicides.
- Copper naphthenate spray.
- Eniliconazole, 0.2% solution by wash or spray, every 3 days for three or four applications.
- Natamycin, 0.01% solution locally, repeat after 4 or 5 days and again after 14 days if required.
- *Griseofulvin, 7.5 mg/kg orally for 7 days.* Under present EU legislation, griseofulvin cannot be used in food-producing animals as no official residue limits have been set.

Pygmy goat syndrome (seborrhoeic dermatitis)
Certain families of pygmy goats develop non-pruritic crusty lesions around the eyes, ears, nose and head and in the axilla, groin and perineal region. The aetiology of the condition is unknown.

Treatment
- Topical treatment with combination corticosteroid and antibiotic ointments will ease smaller lesions.
- Parenteral treatment with corticosteroids and antibiotics produces complete resolution for up to 4 weeks, but the lesions recur. Although oral therapies for ruminants are generally discouraged, oral prednisolone, with the dose tapered to effect, daily or every other day, can be used to control the condition long-term or long-acting methylprednisolone acetate injections can then be given every 4 to 6 weeks as necessary.

Malassezia infection
Clinical disease associated with *Malassezia* infections of goats, including *M. pachydermatis* and *M. sloofiae*, have been reported by dermatologists in recent years in goats with scaling, alopecia and crusting lesions. As in other species, the organisms are probably opportunistic pathogens. The diagnosis of *Malassezia* dermatitis in goats is most likely to be made by cytological examination of skin impressions or by examination of skin biopsy samples. Miconazole, chlorhexidine, selenium sulphide or enilconazole shampoos can be used for treatment, soaking animals for 10 minutes, twice weekly for 3 weeks. Any predisposing or underlying disease will also need treating.

Golden Guernsey goat syndrome ('sticky kid')
Golden Guensey goat syndrome is an hereditary disease caused by an autosomal recessive gene. Affected kids are born with sticky, greasy, matted coats that remain abnormal throughout life (Plate 11.13).

Mycotic dermatitis (dermatophilosis)
See Chapter 7.

Dermatophilus congolense causes 'lumpy wool' and 'strawberry footrot' in sheep and goats.

Iodine deficiency
See Chapter 6.

Iodine deficiency may result in weak kids born with thin sparse hair coats, as part of a syndrome of abortion, weak kids and stillbirths. Older goats may show poor growth rate and dry scabby skin as a result of general malnutrition.

Selenium/vitamin E deficiency
A deficiency of selenium/vitamin E may produce a dry coat and dandruff.

Skin disease presenting as swellings

Neoplasia
- Papilloma
- Melanoma
- Squamous cell carcinoma
- Haemangioma
- Haemangiolipoma
- Sebaceous gland tumours.

Orf
See Chapter 10.

Ticks

Several species of ticks have been reported from goats in the United Kingdom. *Ixodes ricinus*, the castor bean tick, occurs widely throughout the country and the hedgehog tick, *Ixodes hexaganus*, is also occasionally found. Other ticks include *Haemaphysalis punctata* in southern England and *Dermacentor reticulatus* in Wales. Ixodes is a three-host tick, with all three stages – larva, nymph and adult – feeding on a different mammalian host. Heavy tick burdens will cause loss of condition, but the most important consequence of tick infestation is the transmission of bacterial, viral or protozoal diseases in endemic areas. These include *tickborne fever* (see Chapter 2) and *tick pyaemia* (see Chapter 8).

Keds

Melophagus ovinus is a wingless bloodsucking fly that infests both sheep and goats, with the whole life cycle completed on the host. Heavy infestation may cause anaemia and irritation, but keds are generally of limited pathological significance. Keds are often present with lice and are controlled by routine lice treatments.

Abscess

See Chapter 10.

Further reading

General

Foster, A. (2011) Goats with skin disease – anything new? *Goat Vet. Soc. J.*, **27**, 7–11.

Jackson, P. (1982) Skin diseases in goats. *Goat Vet. Soc. J.*, **3** (1), 7–11.

Jackson, P. (1986) Skin diseases in goats. *In Pract.*, **8** (1), 5–10.

Scott, D.W., Smith, M.C. and Manning, T.O. (1984) Caprine dermatology. Part I. Normal skin and bacterial and fungal disorders. *Cont. Ed. Pract. Vet.*, **6** (4), S190–211.

Scott, D.W., Smith, M.C. and Manning, T.O. (1984) Caprine dermatology. Part II. Viral, nutritional, environmental and congenitohereditary disorders. *Cont. Ed. Pract. Vet.*, **6** (8), S473–485.

Scott, D.W., Smith, M.C. and Manning, T.O. (1984) Caprine dermatology. Part III. Parasitic, allergic, hormonal and neoplastic disorders. *Cont. Ed. Pract. Vet.*, **7** (8), 5437–5452.

Smith, M.C. (1981) Caprine dermatologic problems: a review. *J. Am. Vet. Med. Assoc.*, **178**, 724.

Smith, M.C. (1983) Dermatologic diseases of goats. *Vet. Clin. North Amer.: Large Anim. Pract.*, **5** (3), 449–456.

Walton, G.S. (1980) Skin lesions and goats. *Goat Vet. Soc. J.*, **1** (2), 15–16.

Wright, A.I. (1989) Dermatology. *Goat Vet. Soc. J.*, **10** (2), 64–66.

Blowfly strike

Wall, R. and Lovatt, F. (2015) Blowfly strike: biology, epidemiology and control. *In Pract.*, **37** (4), 181–199.

Ectoparasites

Bates, P. (2004) Therapies for ectoparasiticism in sheep. *In Pract.*, **26**, 538–547.

Bates, P. (2009) The host specificity of Psoroptes mites and lice infesting sheep and goats. *Goat Vet. Soc. J.*, **25**, 77–81.

Bates, P. (2013) Goat ectoparasites in the UK: an update. *Goat Vet. Soc. J.*, **29**, 4–8.

Bates, P. (2013) Control of goat ectoparasites in the UK: an update. *Goat Vet. Soc. J.*, **29**, 38–46.

Bates, P., Rankin, M. Cooley W. and Groves, B. (2001). Observations on the biology and control of the chewing louse (*Bovicola limbata*) of Angora goats in Great Britain. *Vet. Rec.*, **149** (22), 675–676.

Cornall, K. and Wall, R. (2015) Ectoparasites of goats in the UK. *Vet. Parasitol.*, **207** (1–2), 176–179.

Gnad, D.P. and Mock, D.E. (2001) Ectoparasite control in small ruminants. *Vet. Clin. North Amer.: Food Anim. Pract.*, **17**, 245–263.

Jackson, P., Richards, H.W. and Lloyds, S. (1983) Sarcoptic mange in goats. *Vet. Rec.*, **112**, 330.

Taylor, M (2002) Parasites of goats: a guide to diagnosis and control. *In Pract.*, **24**, 76–89.

Malignant catarrhal fever

Foster, A.P. *et al.* (2010) Generalized alopecia and mural folliculitis in a goat. *Vet. Path.*, **47** (4), 760–763.

Malassezia

Eguchi-Coe, Y., Valentine, B.A., Gorman, E. and Villarroel, A. (2011) Putative *Malassezia* dermatitis in six goats. *Vet. Dermatol.*, **22** (6), 497–501.

Pin, D. (2004) Seborrhoeic dermatitis in a goat due to *Malassezia pachydermatis*. *Vet. Dermatol.*, **15** (1), 53–56.

Pemphigus foliaceus

Cornish, J. and Highland, M. (2010) Successful treatment of juvenile pemphigus foliaceus in a Nigerian Dwarf goat. *J. Amer. Vet. Med. Assoc.*, **236**, 674–676.

Janzen, A.M. *et al.* (2011) Pemphigus foliaceus in a juvenile cashmere goat and outcome after prednisolone and methylprednisolone therapy. *Canadian Vet. J.*, **52**, 1345–1349.

Targino, J. *et al.* (2008) *Pemphigus foliaceous* in a Boer goat. *Ciencia Rural, Santa Maria*, **38**, 2633–2635.

Valdez, A., Gelberg, H.B., Morin, E.L. and Zuckermann, F.A. (1995) Use of corticosteroids and aurothioglucose in a pygmy goat with *Pemphigus foliaceus. J. Amer. Vet. Med. Assoc.*, **207** (6), 761–765.

Pygmy goat dermatitis

Jefferies, A.R., Casas, F.C., Hall, S.J.G. and Jackson, P.G.G. (1991) Seborrhoeic dermatitis in pygmy goats. *Vet. Dermatol.*, **2** (3/4), 109–117.

CHAPTER 12

Nervous diseases

Animals with severe anaemia, liver, kidney, lung or myocardial disease may present with apparent nervous dysfunction.

Initial assessment

The preliminary history should consider:
- Herd/flock or individual problem.
- Age.
- Sex.
- Stage of pregnancy/lactation.
- Diet/dietary changes.
  Specific management practices should be discussed:
- Disbudding, castration, dipping.
- Prophylactic therapies – coccidiostats, anthelmintics.
- Feeding/grazing routine; changes in the routine
  A careful study of the environment should be made:
- Feed sources – silage, grazing.
- Water sources.
- Fertilisers/weedkillers.
- Trace element availability.
- Possible sources of poison.

Clinical examination

- Examine the animal(s) undisturbed in their usual surroundings – are they bright, alert, responsive or dull and depressed?
- Response to approach – apprehension, trembling, etc.
- Head carriage
  o Hyperaesthesia
  o Defective vision
  o Head tilt
  o Tremors
  o Head pressing
  o Lateral deviation
  o Circling movements.
- Ability to rise – signs of weakness, opisthotonus, coma, semicoma.
- Locomotion – move animal slowly at first, then faster. Watch for knuckling, circling, incoordination, ataxia, aimless wandering.
- Physical examination – general examination plus specific features referable to neurological disorders, for example drooping of ear or eyelid, facial paralysis, retention of cud, blindness, nystagmus, size of pupils, visual and acoustic reactions.
- Examine eye with ophthalmoscope.
- Specific neurological examination – refer to appropriate textbook; techniques applicable to dog or cat can be used in goats. Examination of neurological reflexes may help localise the problem area.
  o Menace reflex: retina, optic tract, posterior cerebrum, cranial nerve VII.
  o Pupillary reflex: retina, optic tract, brain stem.
  o Nictitating reflex: rostral brain stem, cranial nerves III and IV.
  o Fixation reflex: retina, optic tract, posterior cerebrum, cranial nerves II, IV and VI and cranial cervical nerves.
  o Pedal reflex: spinal reflex arcs.
  o Cutaneous reflex: spinal reflex arcs.
  o Oculocardiac reflex: brain stem, cranial nerves V and X.
  Table 12.1 gives some indication of how clinical signs relate to sites of lesions and possible aetiologies.

Diseases of the Goat, Fourth Edition. John Matthews.
© 2016 John Wiley & Sons, Ltd. Published 2016 by John Wiley & Sons, Ltd.

Table 12.1 Nervous diseases.

Convulsions			Site of lesion: cerebrum	
Infectious	**Metabolic**	**Toxic**	**Parasitic**	**Epilepsy**
Meningioencephalitis	Cerebrocortical necrosis	Organophosphates	Coenurosis (gid)	
Enterotoxaemia	Periparturient toxaemia	Lead	*Oestrus ovis*	
Tetanus	Hypomagnesaemia	Levamisole		
Pseudorabies	Hypoglycaemia	overdose		
	Hepatoencephalopathy			

Muscle tremors		Site of lesion: cerebrum
Infectious	**Metabolic**	**Poisoning**
Meningoencephalitis	Hypoglycaemia	*Prunus* (cyanide)
Scrapie	Cerebrocortical necrosis	Laburnum
Louping ill	Hypocalcaemia	Hemlock
Border disease	Hypomagnesaemia	Nitrate, nitrite
CAE	Hepatoencephalopathy	Oxalate
Rabies	Enzootic ataxia	Urea
		Organophosphates
		Levamisole overdose

Coma		Site of lesion: cerebrum, midbrain
Infection	**Metabolic**	**Poisoning**
Meningoencephalitis	Cerebrocortical necrosis	Organophosphates
Enterotoxaemia	Periparturient toxaemia	Salt poisoning
Pseudorabies	Hypocalcaemia	Oxalate
	Hepatoencephalopathy	
	Uraemia	

Excitability, hyperaesthesia, constant chewing	Aimless wandering, head pressing, fear or aggression	Site of lesion: cerebrum	
Infection	**Metabolic**	**Poisoning**	**Parasitic**
Meningioencephalitis	Cerebrocortical necrosis	Organophosphates	Coenurosis (gid)
Pseudorabies	Periparturient toxaemia	*Prunus* (cyanide)	*Oestrus ovis*
Rabies	Hypomagnesaemia	Nitrates (rape, beet tops)	
	Hepatoencephalopathy		

Opisthotonus		Site of lesion: cerebrum, cerebellum, midbrain, pons
Infectious	**Metabolic**	**Any cause of convulsions**
Enterotoxaemia	Cerebrocortical necrosis	
Tetanus meningoencephalitis	Hypomagnesaemia	
Brain abscess		
CAE		
Rabies		

Table 12.1 (*Continued*)

Circling	Site of lesion: cerebrum	
Infectious Listeriosis Brain abscess CAE Rabies	**Metabolic** Cerebrocortical necrosis	**Parasitic** Coenurosis (gid) *Oestrus ovis*

Circling	Site of lesion: vestibular system
Infectious **Otitis media/interna**	

Hypermetria	Site of lesion: cerebellum
Parasitic Coenurosis (gid) *Oestrus ovis*	**Metabolic** Enzootic ataxia

Ataxia	Site of lesion: spinal cord lesions vestibular system, cerebellum, cerebrum	
Infectious Listeriosis Meningoencephalitis Brain abscess Scrapie CAE Rabies *Rhodococcus* spp. **Parasitic** Tick pyaemia Cerebrospinal nematodiasis *Oestrus ovis*	**Metabolic** Hypocalcaemia Hypomagnesaemia Cerebrocortical necrosis Enzootic ataxia **Neoplasia**	**Poisoning** Oxalate *Prunus* (cyanide) Fool's parsley **Congenital vertebral or spinal deformities**

Head tilt	Site of lesion: vestibular system	
Infectious Listeriosis Otitis media/interna Brain abscess CAE	**Parasitic** Ear mites Cerebral nematodiasis	

Laboratory investigation

- Complete blood count.
- Specific tests as indicated.
- Cerebrospinal fluid analysis and culture.

Cerebrospinal fluid collection
Lumbosacral space

Restrain animal in lateral recumbency with hind legs pulled forward to flex the spine; prepare the site surgically and block with local anaesthetic. Insert a 0.9 mm ×

38 mm spinal or disposable needle into the depression between the last lumbar and first sacrodorsal spinous process, advancing the needle slowly until a slight pop is felt when the dura mater is penetrated. Approximately 1 ml of CSF per 5 kg of body weight can be collected.

Atlanto-occipital site

Samples obtained from the atlanto-occipital site are more likely to represent accurately intracranial lesions, but sedation or general anaesthesia is necessary. Use the lumbosacral space if the animal is too ill to risk sedation.

Prepare the site surgically and place the animal in lateral recumbency with the head at right angles to the neck and horizontal to the ground. Insert a 0.9 mm × 38 or 63 mm spinal needle or 0.9 mm × 38 mm disposable needle with the needle pointing towards the lower jaw and advance slowly until the dura mater is penetrated.

Note: trauma to the brain stem may cause death.

Cerebrospinal fluid analysis and culture

Collect CSF in an EDTA tube for cytological examination and a plain tube for biochemical analysis and bacteriological culture. Table 12.2 gives normal values.

- Colour – should be clear and colourless. Turbidity indicates a viral, bacterial, fungal or parasitic infection. Yellowish discoloration (xanthochromia) indicates presence of blood pigments from trauma or vascular damage.
- Protein level – normal goats have a level of 0 to 0.39 g/litre; can be measured with urinary reagent strips; > 1 + is abnormal. Protein levels are increased in infective conditions, may be slightly elevated in traumatic conditions and remain normal in degenerative congenital or toxic conditions.
- Cell counts – use undiluted fluid in a haemocytometer; allow cells to settle for 5 to 10 minutes before counting. Normal goats have counts of 0 to 4 white cells/µl. Elevated white cell counts may be found in

Table 12.2 Normal values for cerebrospinal fluid.

Specific gravity	1.005
Colour	Colourless
Total protein	0–0.39 g/litre
Glucose	3.0–4.0 mmol/litre
White blood cells	0—4/µl
Red blood cells	None

viral conditions (mononuclear cells), parasitic conditions (neutrophils, occasionally many eosinophils), and bacterial or fungal infections (usually neutrophils; with listeriosis half neutrophils, half mononuclear cells). Red cells may be found following trauma.
- Glucose levels – use urinary reagent strip. Normal levels are about 80% the blood glucose level, that is about 3.0 to 4.0 mmol/litre.
- Blood content – use urinary reagent strip.
- Gram stain of CSF smear following sedimentation.
- Bacterial culture.

Post-mortem examination

Many neurological disorders are likely to be fatal or even present as sudden death. Animals should be chemically euthanised, rather than shooting or stunning, to avoid damage to the brain.

All organ systems in the body should be routinely examined before examination of the brain. The spinal cord, middle ears and peripheral nerves should be examined as necessary, depending on the clinical presentation.

Often no gross pathology is found and samples should be taken for laboratory testing. Central nervous tissue is best preserved by fixing in a minimum of 10 times their volume of 10% formol saline. Gentle agitation in a warm environment encourages rapid fixation.

Treatment

> Early aggressive treatment may mean the difference between recovery and death.

Specific treatment should be instigated as soon as a diagnosis is made. Until such time, general supportive therapy is indicated.
- *Sterilise the CSF* with broad-spectrum antibiotics, intravenously for the first 4 days.

Trimethoprim/sulphonamide, 15–24 mg combined/kg every 6 to 12 hours
Oxytetracycline, 3–10 mg/kg every 12 to 24 hours
Benzylpenicillin, 2 vials of crystalline penicillin (each vial contains 5 megaunits (3 g) of benzylpenicillin)

intravenously + 20 ml procaine penicillin (300 000 i.u./ml) intramuscularly divided between 2 sites, then 5 ml procaine penicillin every 24 hours for the next 5 days

Ceftiofur, 1 mg/kg every 24 hours

Ampicillin, 3 mg/kg every 8 hours

Gentamicin, 3 mg/kg every 8 hours, alone or in combination with trimethoprim/ sulphonamide combinations

Chloramphenicol, 5–10 mg/kg, every 12 to 24 hours (prohibited in food-producing animals in the EU)

Doses required to penetrate into the CSF are often higher than recommended by the manufacturers: trimethoprim/sulphonamide combinations penetrate well, ampicillin penetrates well if the CNS is inflamed, gentamicin and tetracyclines penetrate relatively poorly. Treatment should be continued for at least 48 hours after the goat seems normal and may be required for as long as 10 to 14 days.

■ *Stop convulsions.*

Diazepam, 0.25–0.5 mg/kg, 2–4 ml/40 kg i.v. to effect

Phenobarbitone, 24 mg/kg *slowly* i.v. to effect, then 12 mg/kg i.v. every 8–12 hours as required

■ *Correct fluid and electrolyte imbalances*, with intravenous fluids, in animals that are not drinking or have collapsed (or subcutaneous fluids if handling stresses the goat). Most animals will be acidotic. If in doubt, use lactated Ringer's solution.

Electrolytes can be given orally by stomach tube – up to 8 litres daily will be required.

> A goat may survive the neurological challenge only to die of dehydration.

■ *Resolve CNS inflammation.*

Flunixin meglumine, 2 mg/kg, i.v. or i.m. every 12 or 24 hours for up to 5 days

Carprofen, 1.4 mg/kg, s.c. or i.v. every 36 to 48 hours

Ketoprofen, 3 mg/kg, i.v. or i.m. daily for up to 3 days

Meloxicam, 0.5 mg/kg, i.v. or s.c. every 36 to 48 hours

Methylprednisolone, 10–30 mg/kg i.v. every 4 to 6 hours for 24 to 48 hours

Dexamethasone, 1.1 mg/kg i.v. once

Dimethyl sulphoxide (DMSO), 1g/kg as 10% solution in i.v. drip over 30 minutes every 24 hours for 3 or 4 days (50 ml DMSO in 500 ml saline/50 kg)

Phenylbutazone, 4 mg/kg, i.v. (banned from use in food-producing animals in the EU)

■ *Reduce cerebral oedema.*

Dexamethasone, 0.1 mg/kg i.v.

Mannitol, 1.5 g/kg slowly i.v.

Neonatal kids (Table 12.3; see also Chapter 5)

■ Congenital infections.
■ Hypoglycaemia.
■ Birth trauma.
■ Enzootic ataxia (swayback).

Kids up to 1 month old (Table 12.3)

Kid mentally alert

Spinal abscess and vertebral osteomyelitis

Spinal abscesses and vertebral osteomyelitis occur sporadically in kids, generally following a bacteraemia subsequent to a navel infection.

Aetiology

■ A number of bacteria including *Staphylococcal* spp., *T. pyogenes* (*C. pyogenes*), *Pasteurella* spp. and *Fusobacterium necrophorum* have been implicated.

Clinical signs

■ A gradual onset of clinical signs may occur where abscessation results in increasing compression of the spinal cord, with signs progressing from slight hind limb ataxia to complete hind limb paralysis (Table 12.4), and in these cases long-term broad-spectrum antibiotic therapy or more specific therapy based on CSF culture and sensitivity may be satisfactory. In other cases, acute clinical signs, with paraparesis or tetraparesis and pain around the spinal lesion, may occur some time after the original infection when there is a sudden collapse of a vertebra and spinal cord compression.

Table 12.3 Nervous disease in kids.

Neonatal	<1 month	2–7 months
Congenital infections	**Kid mentally alert**	Trauma
Hypoglycaemia	Spinal abscess	Delayed swayback
Birth trauma	Trauma	Spinal abscess
Enzootic ataxia (swayback)	Floppy kid syndrome	Coccidiosis
	Congenital vertebral lesions	Tetanus
	Tick pyaemia	CAE
	Kid mentally impaired	Louping ill
	Bacterial meningitis	Hepatic encephalopathy
	Focal symmetrical encephalomalacia	
	Tetanus	
	Disbudding meningoencephalitis	
	Louping ill	

Table 12.4 Localisation of spinal cord lesions.

Site of lesion	Clinical signs
C1–C6	Tetraparesis
	Hyperactive reflexes
	Cervical pain
	Cutaneous sensation loss
C6–T2	Fore and hind limbs weak and ataxic
	Thoracic limbs – reduced reflexes and flaccid paralysis
	Pelvic limbs – increased reflexes and spastic paralysis
	Horner's syndrome
	Myotic pupils
T2–L3	'Dog sitting', hopping
	Thoracic limbs – normal function
	Pelvic limbs – increased reflexes and spastic paralysis
	Polyuria
	Loss of cutaneous sensation in innervated area
L4–S2	'Dog sitting'
	Thoracic limbs – normal function
	Pelvic limbs – reduced or absent reflexes and flaccid paralysis
	Loss of cutaneous sensation in innervated area
S1–S3	Flaccid tail and anus – no anal tone, tail does not move
	Flaccid bladder – urine dribbling

Diagnosis

- Radiography may demonstrate a collapsed vertebra, but can prove very difficult.
- CSF may appear normal or show increased numbers of neutrophils.

Floppy kid syndrome

Floppy kid syndrome (FKS) is a metabolic acidosis without dehydration affecting kids between 3 and 10 days of age. Affected kids are normal at birth, but develop sudden onset of profound muscular weakness (flaccid paresis or paralysis or ataxia). Kids show decreased muscle tone, anorexia, and lethargy. The kids cannot use their tongues to suckle but can swallow. Affected kids show no signs of diarrhoea, respiratory disease or other signs referable to a specific organ system (see Chapter 5).

Trauma

In all age groups, trauma to the head or spinal cord may cause neurological signs. Kids are particularly prone to spinal cord and vertebral injuries because of their inquisitive active nature.

Haynets should be avoided and the spacing on hayracks or gates should be chosen carefully. Trauma can also arise from kicks or bites from other species of animals and from fighting, and neck injuries can also occur in tethered goats.

Pathological vertebral fractures can occur in malnourished animals with diets deficient in calcium and vitamin D. Exostosis may develop over incomplete fractures of a vertebral body and subsequently produce neurological signs.

Congenital vertebral lesions

Congenital vertebral lesions ran result in compression of the spinal cord with resulting neurological clinical signs, which may not become apparent for several weeks after birth.

Tick pyaemia (enzootic staphylococcal infection)

See Chapter 7.

Kid mentally impaired

Bacterial meningitis
Aetiology
- Generally secondary to septicaemia, with infection from the navel or intestine; enterotoxigenic *E. coli* is generally the causal organism, but also *Staphylococci*, *Streptococci*, *Pasteurellae*, *Klebsiella* and *Haemophilus* species.

Clinical signs
- Variable neurological signs.
- Lethargy, drowsiness or hyperaesthesia, pyrexia.
- Failure to suck.
- Compulsive wandering; head pressing.
- Nystagmus, apparent blindness.
- Convulsions, coma.
- Death.
- Often the history of diarrhoea or diarrhoea present concurrently.

Treatment
- Antibiotic therapy. *E. coli* meningitis is difficult to treat because most bactericidal antibiotics do not penetrate well into the CSF. Trimethoprim-sulphonamide preparations given intravenously at a level of 16 to 24 mg of the combined drugs/kg three times daily alone or in combination with gentamicin 3 mg/kg intramuscularly or intravenously (dilute in equal volumes of saline) have been recommended.
- General supportive therapy with fluids, anticonvulsants and anti-inflammatory drugs.

Focal symmetrical encephalomalacia (enterotoxaemia)
Aetiology
- The epsilon toxin produced by *Clostridium perfringens* type D (see Chapter 15) affects the cerebral vasculature, producing haemorrhage and oedema.

Clinical signs
- Generally affects kids, occasionally adult animals.
- Lethargy.
- Head pressing, apparent blindness, trembling.
- Ataxia.
- Opisthotonos, convulsions, coma.
- Death.

  Note: (1) A similar condition in calves is produced by a labile *coccidial toxin*. It has been suggested that coccidial infections (q.v.) may be implicated in the condition in kids.

  (2) *Enterotoxigenic E. coli* can also produce similar neurological signs; see 'Bacterial meningitis'.

Tetanus
Aetiology
- Gram-positive bacillus *Clostridium tetani* produces a neurotoxin responsible for the clinical syndrome.

Epidemiology
- *Clostridium tetani* spores enter through wounds following disbudding, castration, shearing, kidding, ear tagging, etc., resulting in clinical signs 4 to 21 days later.

Clinical signs
- Variable neurological signs – erect ears, elevated tail, extended neck, rocking horse stance, rigidity and hyperaesthesia on stimulation.
- Prolapsed third eyelid.
- Dysphagia, difficulty in opening mouth.
- Lateral recumbency, death.

Diagnosis
- Clinical signs.
- Isolation and identification of *Cl. tetani*.

Treatment
- Clean any obvious wound, expose to the air, debride, flush with hydrogen peroxide and apply penicillin locally.
- Tetanus antitoxin, 10 000–15 000 units i.v. every 12 hours for at least 24 hours.
- Diazepam, 0.5 mg/kg i.v., 5 ml/50 kg to effect, or
- Acepromazine (ACP), 0.05–0.1 mg/kg, i.v.
- Benzylpenicillin, 2 vials of crystalline penicillin (each vial contains 5 megaunits (3 g) of benzylpenicillin) intravenously + 20 ml procaine penicillin (300 000 i.u./ml) intramuscularly divided between 2 sites, then

5 ml procaine penicillin every 24 hours for the next 5 days.

- Supportive therapy: intravenous fluids, nasogastric tube to relieve bloat and for food and fluids, enema, deep bed with regular changes in position.

Prevention

- Routine vaccination with a multivalent clostridial vaccine (see enterotoxaemia, Chapter 15).

Disbudding meningoencephalitis

Prolonged or excessive pressure with a disbudding iron can cause heat necrosis to bone, meninges and brain.

Clinical signs

- Sudden death – sometimes within hours but often several days or even weeks after disbudding.
- Depression, anorexia, pyrexia, fits.

Post-mortem findings

- Focal meningoencephalitis.
- Meningeal and superficial cerebrocortical necrosis with infiltration by neutrophils and mononuclear cells.

Treatment

As for bacterial meningitis.

Louping ill
Aetiology

- Acute encephalomyelitis caused by flavivirus transmitted by the tick vector, *Ixodes ricinus*.

Epidemiology

- Louping ill is transmitted exclusively by the nymph and adult tick. Virus titres that are high enough for tick infection are only obtained in sheep; infection in the goat is thully secondary to septicaemias irrelevant to the maintenance of the viral cycle.
- Strong colostral immunity is imparted to kids so that young animals in endemic areas will be susceptible in their second year of exposure. This is in contrast to tickborne fever (see Chapter 2) where no colostral protection is conferred, resulting in kids being susceptible during their first season. In endemic areas, tickborne fever and louping ill do not simultaneously affect the same animals. However, when goats are moved into endemic areas, all ages of goats could be at risk.

Clinical signs

- In adult goats the disease is generally subclinical. Within 24 to 48 hours of infection, a febrile reaction occurs and the temperature may remain elevated for several days before returning to normal. Clinical signs are not usually recognised during this period and neurological signs only develop if the virus gains entry to nervous tissue. In other animals, recovery is rapid and the animals remain immune to subsequent infection. Susceptibility to clinical disease is increased by stress factors such as age, cold, nutrition and transportation and, in particular, by concurrent infection such as toxoplasmosis and tickborne fever.
- Severe clinical infection can be produced in kids that drink infected milk.
- Lethargy, excessive salivation.
- Intermittent head shaking, twitching of lips, nostrils and ears.
- Muscle tremors, particularly neck and limbs, followed by muscular rigidity.
- Jerky, stiff movement, with progressive incoordination, loss of balance with frequent falling.
- Apparent blindness, head pressing.
- Convulsions, paralysis, recumbency and death.

Post-mortem findings

Non-suppurative encephalomyelitis.

Diagnosis

- Serology – detection of IgM antibody is diagnostic, but animals have little antibody while clinically ill.

Treatment

- None.

Control

- Prevent exposure to ticks:
  ○ Improve hill grazing to remove tick habitat.
  ○ Pyrethroid dips.
- Vaccination, 1 ml s.c. (louping ill vaccine, MSD) at least 4 weeks before exposure to infection; repeat every 2 years. Lambs from vaccinated dams have passive immunity for 2 to 3 months after birth.

Public health considerations

The high titres of virus excreted in goats' milk provide a potential zoonotic risk. Goats in tick areas should be vaccinated to reduce the possible risk to the public.

Kids 2 to 7 months old (Table 12.3)

Trauma

See earlier this chapter.

Delayed swayback

See Chapter 5.

Spinal abscess

See earlier this chapter.

Coccidiosis

See Chapter 13.

Kids with severe coccidiosis sometimes show nervous signs – dullness, depression, head pressing, opisthotonos and death.

Caprine arthritis encephalitis

See Chapter 6.

CAE virus can produce neurological signs in the kid (caprine leucoencephalitis) and the adult goat, although neurological signs are much less commonly reported than the other forms of the disease.

Juvenile form: kids 2 to 4 months old

Consistent with upper motor neurone disease involving an ascending infection of the spinal cord. Spinal reflexes frequently remain intact (cf. swayback).

Clinical signs

- Pyrexia or fluctuating high temperature (not always).
- Bright and alert, good appetite until recumbent.
- Tremor.
- Initial lameness and ataxia, progressing over a number of days to hemiplegia or tetraplegia, circling, hyperaesthesia, blindness and recumbency with torticollis (indicates disease involving higher centres, particularly the midbrain).

Treatment

- None.

Adult form

Neurological signs are often preceded by other clinical signs of CAE (arthritis, pneumonia, mastitis) and may be complicated by painful arthritic lesions. In the absence of arthritis, it may resemble listeriosis.

Clinical signs

- Knuckling of fetlocks, circling, progressing to paresis and paralysis.

Laboratory tests

- Serology: kids are often seronegative at this age, although passive maternal antibodies may be detected. Test kid's dam and any goat used to supply the kid with milk.
- CSF analysis: generally elevated white cell count (many mononuclear cells) and protein level.

Post-mortem findings

- Perivascular mononuclear cell infiltration and perivascular demyelination in the white matter.
- Gross lesions may be visible in the spinal cord as swollen brownish areas of malacia that are usually unilateral.

Hepatic encephalopathy

Stunted kids with intermittent neurological signs may have a *portosystemic shunt*. Hepatic encephalopathy occurs because ammonia absorbed from digesting food in the intestine is not converted to urea by the liver, but instead increases the permeability of the blood–brain barrier and leads to vasogenic oedema. Possible clinical signs include lethargy, inappetence, failure to thrive and neurological signs such as ataxia, head pressing, blindness, head bobbing, seizures, stargazing, tremors, circling, drooling, opistotonus and paddling.

Older kids, goatlings and adult (Table 12.5)

Infectious disease

Listeriosis
Aetiology

- *Listeria monocytogenes*, a Gram-positive, ß-haemolytic bacillus.

Table 12.5 Causes of nervous disease in older kids, goatlings and adults.

Infectious disease	Metabolic disease	Space-occupying lesions
Listeriosis	Cerebrocortical necrosis	**Brain**
Scrapie	Hypocalcaemia	■ Cerebral abscess
Louping ill	Hypomagnesaemia	■ Coenuriasis
CAE	Transit tetany	■ Pituitary abscess syndrome
Pseudorabies	Pregnancy toxaemia	■ *Oestrus ovis*
Rabies	Acetonaemia	■ Tumour
Tetanus		
Botulism	**Poisoning**	**Spinal cord**
Malignant catarrhal fever	■ Lead, arsenic, mercury	■ Spinal meningitis
Trauma	■ Plants	■ Spinal abscess
	■ Organophosphates	■ Vertebral osteomyelitis
Vestibular disease	■ Urea	■ Tumours
	■ Rafoxanide	■ *Coenurus cerebralis*
■ Otitis media/externa		■ Cerebrospinal nematodiasis
■ Psoroptic mange	**Epilepsy**	
Hepatic encephalopathy		

Transmission

■ By ingestion of the organism, which is resistant in the environment, surviving in the soil and water for several months and in silage for over 5 years.

■ Direct contact with the products of abortion by ingestion or via the conjunctivae.

■ Venereal transmission may occur.

■ Latent carriers exist and when stressed may excrete the organism.

■ The incubation period at 10 to 15 days is generally shorter than in sheep.

Clinical signs

1 **Encephalitis**

o Depression, anorexia, pyrexia.

o Facial paralysis, drooping of ears and eyelids (often asymmetrical), protruding of tongue, drooling of saliva.

o Dysphagia – cud remains in mouth.

o Head tilt, nystagmus, circling, head pressing.

A recumbent animal with its head turned to one side almost certainly has listeria if, when it is turned over on to its other side, it immediately flips back to the original position.

o Progressively uncoordinated movement – knuckling, rigidity, paresis.

o Recumbency, opisthotonos, convulsions.

o Death (mortality rate 3 to 30%).

Note: (1) Very acute encephalitis does not always present as the 'circling disease' more typical of sheep. Goats may be presented as dull and uncoordinated, with death occurring in as little as 6 hours. The disease may be mistaken for hypocalcaemia or even pneumonia.

(2) Abortion and encephalitis occur in the same goat more commonly than is the case for sheep.

2 **Sudden death**

o Because the disease in goats may be very acute – goats are much more susceptible to listerial encephalitis than sheep – listeriosis should be considered in a differential diagnosis of sudden death (see Chapter 18).

3 **Septicaemia**

o Lethargy, pyrexia (41 °C) and bloody diarrhoea in young animals, with signs lasting from a few days to several weeks.

4 **Abortion**

See Chapter 2.

5 **Keratoconjunctivitis**

See Chapter 20.

6 **Metritis/vaginal discharge**

Diagnosis

■ Physical and neurological examination:

o Clinical signs vary depending on areas of the brain involved but include mostly upper motor neurone signs involving ipsilateral limbs.

- Laboratory tests:
  - o Examination of CSF: elevated protein content (>0.4 g/litre); elevated white cells (>10 cells/μl, mononuclear cells and neutrophils – a predominantly mononuclear cell population is characteristic of listeriosis).
  - o Examination of urine: glucosuria, ketonuria.
  - o Examination of paired serum samples.
  - o Culture and identification of *L. monocytogenes* from brain, liver, spleen, kidney and heart, fetal stomach, uterine discharges, milk and placenta.
- Post-mortem examination:
  - o Gross brain lesions may be minimal, possibly congested meninges and oedema.
  - o Suppurative meningoencephalitis of the pons and medulla oblongata. Microabscesses in the brain stem are usually unilateral; vasomeningeal cellular infiltration.

Treatment

- See 'Treatment' earlier in this chapter.
- Early treatment is essential. The initiation of treatment in the early stages of the disease appears as important as the choice of antibiotics.
- High doses of antibiotics (ampicillin or trimethoprim/sulphonamides or gentamicin, in combination with trimethoprim/sulphonamides or benzylpenicillin/procaine penicillin), intravenous where possible, and with maintenance doses for at least 7 days.
- Supportive therapy:
  - o Fluid therapy to correct dehydration (with sodium bicarbonate to correct acidosis where necessary), either intravenously or by stomach tube.
  - o Flunixin meglumine.
  - o B vitamins, particularly B1, because rumen activity is depressed and there is little production of vitamin B1 by ruminal microorganisms.
  - o Nutritional supplements and slurries of lucerne pellets can be fed by stomach tube.
  - o Recumbent animals should be kept on thick bedding and turned regularly.
- It may be advantageous to treat all animals in an affected group with long-acting ampicillin.
- Nutritional support will need to be continued during the animal's recovery because chewing and swallowing may be difficult for some time. Soft food such as

soaked sugar beet pulp may be useful and it is important to ensure that the water intake is maintained.
- Rumen stimulants administered by stomach tube and the transfer of rumen contents from a healthy animal will help to restore normal rumen function.

Control

- Difficult.
- Avoid soil-contaminated feed, particularly silage, but animals grazing low-lying swampy/boggy areas or being fed on the ground are also at risk.
- Ensure good-quality silage is made. Reject silage from damaged or punctured bales. Do not feed:
  - o Mouldy silage.
  - o Silage with a pH content >5.
  - o Silage with an ash content >70 mg/kg DM.

  Use of additives when making grass silage will produce more acid conditions that discourage listerial growth.

  The pH of silage can be checked by making a 1:10 dilution of the silage in water (preferably distilled) and measuring the pH with paper or a pH meter. Several silage samples should be taken from different locations inside the bale and mixed thoroughly in a ziploc bag with the water for at least 2 minutes.
  - o Remove any silage not eaten within 24 hours.
- Feed dry hay – avoid big bales of hay in wet conditions.
- Keep food and water containers clean: avoid faecal contamination.
- Vaccination – experimental studies have yielded variable results. Sheep vaccine is available in parts of Europe.

Public health considerations

- Carrier goats may excrete the organism under stress. Milk may be infected and unpasteurised milk and milk products should not be consumed. Pasteurised cheese has also been implicated in outbreaks, where low-temperature pasteurisation has been used.

Transmissible spongiform encephalopathies (TSEs)

The transmissible spongiform encephalopathies (TSEs) are a group of diseases occurring in man and animals that are characterised by a degeneration of brain tissue, giving a sponge-like appearance. They include scrapie in goats and sheep, bovine spongiform encephalopathy (BSE), transmissible mink encephalopathy, chronic wasting disease of deer and elk and variant Creutzfeldt–Jakob disease (vCJD) and Kuru in man.

Scrapie

Scrapie is a transmissible spongiform encephalopathy (TSE) of sheep, goats and mouflons that is characterized by progressive neurodegeneration, spongiform changes and deposition of partially proteinase K-resistant prion protein in the central nervous system. In most parts of the world, scrapie is a notifiable disease. There is no evidence that scrapie is harmful to people. Natural scrapie in goats is rare although potentially underreported. There are active surveillance systems in place in many parts of the world, including a harmonized active surveillance scheme throughout the EU, which includes the examination of fallen stock and healthy slaughtered animals. Only Australia and New Zealand are recognised as being free of classical scrapie, although an atypical scrapie case was detected in New Zealand.

Aetiology

- Scrapie is observed as two types, classical and atypical scrapie. The susceptibility to both types is modulated by polymorphisms of the prion gene.
- Scrapie is associated with modification of a normal host encoded prion protein (PrP^c) to a misfolded abnormal isoform protein (PrP^{Sc}), which accumulates in amyloid plaques in lymphoreticular and nervous tissues, leading to progressive neurodegeneration and death. Prions are small proteinaceous particles that resist inactivation by procedures known to modify nucleic acids. The abnormal prion protein that forms in animals with scrapie is resistant to denaturing detergents, heat and proteinase K digestion.
- More than 20 separate strains of scrapie exist and development of the clinical disease depends on the scrapie strain and on host genetic factors.
- In sheep, the susceptibility to scrapie has been shown to be genetically controlled. Variations in the PrP gene result in differing susceptibilities or resistance to the prion and thus to natural and experimental scrapie. Different allelic forms of PrP are known to affect many characteristics of TSE disease (age at onset, incubation period, disease phenotype) in man, cattle, sheep and mice. Different strains of scrapie target different alleles

of the PrP gene. In sheep, all except one of the 15 known PrP genotypes are known to have some susceptibility to classical scrapie and some are known to be also susceptible to BSE. The only exception is the homozygous ARR genotype (ARR/ ARR).

- The situation in goats appears different in that no genetic influence is apparent in experimental infection, with goats being almost completely susceptible. However, goats show a similar variation in the length of disease incubation to that described in sheep, suggesting a variation in susceptibility to the disease. Goat PrP is expressed from a single gene (Prnp), which appears >99% homologous to that of the sheep, but goats do not share the scrapie modulation polymorphisms present in sheep. Analysis of the caprine PrP gene has revealed several different alleles. In goats, 29 polymorphisms of the caprine Prnp have been found in different countries and breeds and at least 5 of these seem to be associated with TSE susceptibility (I/M$_{142}$, N/D$_{146}$, S/D$_{146}$, R/Q$_{211}$ and Q/K$_{222}$. Experimental results suggest that, like the ARR allele in sheep, the K$_{222}$ allele is associated with a high, but not absolute, resistance to scrapie. The haplotype 146S/D is also considered a candidate for breeding resistance into the goat population. However, there is a low frequency of these alleles in goat populations and, at present, there is insufficient data about the level of resistance to scrapie of these different Prnp gene mutations to develop large-scale genetic selection against scrapie in goats.
- An age-related susceptibility means that maximum opportunity for disease spread is from dam to kid between birth and 9 months of age.

Transmission

Exact transmission routes are not entirely resolved. Scrapie can transmit laterally between animals under natural conditions, either via direct contact or through contamination of the environment. The oral route is the most efficient and the main source of infection is the infectious placenta. Scrapie in goats is often found in herds mixed with sheep, but spread also occurs from goat to goat. Possible routes of transmission are:

- Doe to kid.
  - Prenatal?
    - Scrapie does not appear to be transmitted transplacentally, as lambs and kids delivered by caesarian section from susceptible dams remain

scrapie free and there is some evidence that snatching kids at birth stops transmission. The abnormal prion protein is found in placenta and allantoic fluid, but not in the amnionic fluid. Ingestion of placenta or allantoic fluids by other goats and newborn kids will transmit the disease.

♦ Infection of egg: embryo transplant studies suggest egg transmission is unlikely.

o Post-natal:

♦ Licking or sucking.

■ Lateral:

o Oral. Prion diseases can be highly transmissible between individuals by direct contact and through highly stable environmental reservoirs that are refractory to decontamination.

♦ By ingestion of fetal membranes (known to be heavily infected).

♦ Contamination of pasture, troughs, buildings, etc. (but very low levels of infection in body fluids). Prions remain active for many years adsorbed to clay in soil and even extensive cleaning, disinfection, repainting and regalvanising of pens and equipment is unlikely to successfully decontaminate buildings, leading potentially to reinfection after depopulation and repopulation of a farm.

♦ By ingestion of milk.

♦ By goat feed containing scrapie-infected meat and bone meal as with BSE in cattle.

♦ Abnormal prion protein is found in the mammary gland of sheep with interstitial mastitis induced by retroviruses (OPP or Maedi-Visna).

o Conjunctival?

o Direct infection via needles, etc.? Instruments must be soaked in 2.5N NaOH for disinfection for at least 24 hours before autoclaving, in order to ensure sterilization.

o A blood transfusion can transmit the disease, but 400 to 500 ml of blood is Required.

o The disease is not transmitted by males.

Clinical signs

■ Scrapie is a progressive fatal degenerative disease of the central nervous system, associated with a number of clinical signs ranging from subtle behavioural abnormalities to more severe neurological signs. The incubation time depends on the route of infection, the animal's age at infection, its genotype, the strain of scrapie involved and the infectious dose. Because of the long incubation period, the disease is rarely seen in goats less than 2 years old. Animals infected close to parturition often first show clinical signs at around 3 or 4 years of age, but cases have been reported up to 10 years of age.

■ Two forms of scrapie, pruritic and nervous, have been described in the goat, but there is considerable overlap between the two forms and many naturally infected animals show a combination of pruritic and neurological signs.

■ Initially, clinical signs may be very non-specific. Behavioural changes, increased excitability, lethargy or apprehension, weight loss despite a good appetite, reduced milk yield and, in some animals, more specific signs may not become apparent, at least for a considerable period. Most goats, however, progressively show more obvious signs.

> Scrapie should be considered in any neurological disease of uncertain aetiology.

o *Pruritic signs*:

♦ Scratching with hind feet.

♦ Rubbing poll, withers and back (Plate 12.1).

♦ Nibbling abdomen, sides or udder when touched.

♦ Biting at limbs.

o *Neurological signs.* Neurological signs can be classified into three categories: changes in mental status, abnormalities of movement and changes in sensation.

♦ Behavioural changes.

♦ Hyperaesthesia.

♦ Tremor of the head and neck or whole body.

♦ Incoordination, particularly of hind limbs.

♦ Postural and gait changes, for example high-stepping fore limbs.

♦ Ataxia.

♦ Ears pricked, tail cocked and carried over back (Plate 12.1).

♦ Excessive salivation with strings of saliva at mouth (Plate 12.2).

♦ Cud dropping.

♦ Ocular changes: nystagmus; apparent blindness.

♦ Death in weeks or months.

To help identify clinical cases, a short examination protocol has been produced to aid the assessment of the specific clinical signs associated with pruritic and non-pruritic forms of TSEs in sheep, which could also be applied to goats. This includes assessment of behaviour, vision (by testing the menace response), pruritus (by testing the response to scratching) and movement (with and without blindfolding). The protocol is described at: http://www.ncbi.nlm.nih.gov/pmc/articles/PMC4089440/.

Diagnosis

- The clinical signs are not pathognomonic for scrapie, so the diagnosis needs to be confirmed by the demonstration of pathognomonic spongiform lesions and the immunodetection of pathological prion protein (PrP^{Sc}) depositions in the CNS. PrP^{Sc} depositions can be detected by immunohistological and biochemical methods.
- Histological lesions of the central nervous system – bilaterally symmetrical vacuolation of the neurons in the brainstem and spinal cord. In cases where an animal is in either a preclinical or a subclinical phase of the disease, the characteristic neuropathological changes associated with clinical scrapie may be absent or extremely limited and identification of scrapie infection relies on immunochemical demonstration of brain PrP^{Sc}.
- Immunohistochemistry (IHC) of brain (the gold standard) and lymphoid tissue (lymph nodes, tonsil, spleen, third eyelid, rectal mucosa) to detect PrP^{Sc}.
- EU TSE screening testing involves sampling the obex and screening with a rapid screening method (BioRad ELISA) – uses specific antibodies and colour indicators to detect abnormal prion protein (PrP^{Sc}). Positives are confirmed using Western blot (WB) analysis and/or immunohistochemistry (IHC).
- IHC staining of biopsied lymphoid tissue from the third eyelid has been developed as an ante-mortem test for sheep in the United States, but has not been validated in the EU, as 40 to 60% of adult sheep do not have enough lymphoid follicles in the third eyelid to make the sample readable. Other lymphoid tissues, such as the submandibular lymph node and rectal mucosa from within 1 cm of the mucocutaneous junction may also yield positive diagnoses, perhaps as early as 14 months after exposure. In 2008, rectal biopsy was approved by the United States Department of Agriculture's Animal and Plant Health Inspection Service as an effective option for detecting scrapie

in live animals following a large-scale study, which compared the test results from rectal and third eyelid biopsies with test results obtained post-mortem from the same animals on brain-stem, lymph node, tonsil and rectal biopsy. False negative results may occur when the scrapie prion is restricted to brain tissue and is not present in the lymphoid tissue.
- Mouse bioassays involve injecting specially bred mice with suspensions of brain tissue from suspect animals to observe whether or not they produce clinical disease. Factors such as incubation times and the pattern of lesions in the brain can be used to characterise the TSE, for instance to differentiate between scrapie and BSE.

Post-mortem findings

- There are no gross pathological lesions.
- Histologically there is vacuolation of nerve cells in the medulla, pons and midbrain, with interstitial spongy degeneration. The development of clinical signs is not necessarily reflected by the severity of the pathological changes.

Atypical scrapie

Atypical scrapie is distinguished from classical scrapie by clinical and epidemiological as well as by molecular and histological features. Routine active TSE surveillance programmes in Europe and the United States identified cases of atypical scrapie with an unusual distribution of CNS lesions and with Western blot (WB) of the abnormal prion protein different from that found in other known TSE strains. The first of these new scrapie types was called Nor98. Atypical cases of scrapie were first detected because they were ELISA positive but WB and IHC negative. Subsequent modification of the IHC method detected staining, but with a different pattern from classical scrapie. Findings (including WB) differed from those seen with bovine spongiform encephalopathy of sheep or goats. The effect of genotype on disease expression with the Nor98 strain and other abnormal strains remains unclear.

In most flocks/herds only a single case of atypical scrapie is found and the mode of transmission of atypical scrapie under natural conditions is not understood and it is possible that the disease arises spontaneously and this may be associated with a very low or absent natural transmission. Experimental transmission has been shown by intracerebral injection in rodents and sheep and by oral challenge under experimental conditions in newborn lambs.

The frequency of atypical scrapie cases increases with the age of the animals, which are usually over 5 years old. There are limited reports describing clinical signs of atypical scrapie in goats, but these include ataxia, weight loss and behavioural changes, such as nervousness and anxiety. One goat was described with blindness, stiff gait and apathy. Pruritus does not appear to be a feature of the disease, although it has been described in two sheep in the United Kingdom.

TSE surveillance in goats is based on rapid tests using brainstem material. It is recommended that samples of cerebellum should also be included to diagnose atypical scrapie. In atypical scrapie, the vacuolation of the grey matter is most prominent in the cerebellar cortex, neocortex hippocampus, basal nuclei and nucleus accumbens, with the brainstem affected to a much lesser degree.

Bovine spongiform encephalopathy

Bovine spongiform encephalopathy (BSE) has been transmitted experimentally to goats by intracerebral injection and oral dosing with brain homogenate derived from cattle with BSE. The transmission of disease by oral dosing showed the theoretical risk of feeding BSE contaminated feed to goats.

BSE has been confirmed in two goats – one in a healthy goat, which was slaughtered in France during 2002, and one in Scotland, which was killed in 1990 and subsequently identified in 2005 during retrospective examination of tissues from animals previously identified as 'spongiform encephalopathies consistent with scrapie' using an immunohistochemistry method that discriminates between BSE and scrapie. Examination of other stored tissues has failed to identify any further cases in the EU. BSE was not found in the offspring of the Scottish or French goats or in other goats from the farms, suggesting that if the goats did become infected through the feeding of contaminated meat and bone meal, the disease was not maintained naturally. There is no evidence for BSE in the current EU goat herd.

Limited experimental work also supports the supposition that BSE is not transmitted naturally between goats. There is no evidence of maternal transmission to offspring or transmission by contact of sires with BSE-infected dams and no evidence of TSE disease in any of the offspring that developed from embryos from infected donors.

Control programmes for scrapie (and BSE) in goats
Breeding for resistance

- Selection for genotypes in sheep with delayed onset of clinical signs of scrapie forms the basis of many countries' attempts to control the disease (including the UK National Scrapie Plan), but there is no guarantee that these animals are free of the disease and the identification of atypical forms of scrapie has complicated the issue; selecting for genetic resistance to classical scrapie does not offer any protection against atypical scrapie.
- There is insufficient data about the level of resistance to scrapie of different Prnp gene mutations to develop large-scale genetic selection against scrapie in goats. Furthermore, there is a low frequency in goat populations of those alleles that have been identified as conferring possible resistance.

Eradication

- Attempts have been made to eradicate scrapie from sheep flocks by complete depopulation and re-stocking. These have often failed, possibly due to the survival of the agent in the environment or the fact that the sheep used for restocking were themselves infected.
- In goats, slaughter of identified clinical cases, their cohorts and offspring is the only method of control for scrapie as genetic resistance to scrapie is poorly defined. Depending on national policies, identification of a clinical case within a herd may lead to slaughter of the entire herd and/or the herd of origin.
- At present there are no effective methods for on-farm decontamination after scrapie contamination. The presence of prions in buildings means that attempts to restock farms with non-resistant animals, as is necessary with goats, may be doomed to failure.

Louping ill

See this chapter.

Tetanus

See this chapter.

Caprine arthritis encephalitis (CAE)
See this chapter.

Pseudorabies (Aujesky's disease)
Aetiology
- Herpes virus occurring mainly in pigs but occasionally in goats, other ruminants, dogs and cats in contact with pigs.

Clinical signs
- Intense pruritus.
- Mania, ataxia.
- Paralysis, death.

Diagnosis
- Clinical signs.
- History of exposure to pigs.
- Viral isolation; fluorescent antibody test.

Treatment
- None.

Rabies
In areas where rabies is present, it should always be considered in neurological cases.

Aetiology
- Rhabdovirus spread by the bite of an infected animal.

Clinical signs
Rabies in goats can present with a variety of clinical signs. There are two forms:
- *Furious form* – less common. Clinical signs include hyperexcitability, ataxia, sexual excitement, mania, hoarse voice, paralysis, death. Affected animals may attack people and other animals.
- *Dumb form* – clinically similar to listeriosis. Animals are depressed and progress to recumbency. Clinical signs include ataxia, swaying of hindquarters, tenesmus, paralysis of anus, salivation, loss of voice, paralysis, death.

Post-mortem
- Histopathology shows Negri bodies in brain tissue.

Prevention
- Rabies can be prevented through vaccination with products approved for sheep, with vaccination commencing at 3 to 4 months of age.

Malignant catarrhal fever
Malignant catarrhal fever (MCF) is a disease syndrome caused by several herpes viruses and characterised by inflammation, ulceration and exudation of the oral and upper respiratory mucous membranes and sometimes eye lesions and neurological signs. It is of economic importance in the ruminant species it affects, including cattle, bison and deer. In other species, such as sheep and goats, the infection is generally subclinical, but they can act as reservoir hosts for susceptible species. Caprine herpes virus 2 (CpHV-2), which is endemic in goats in some countries, including the United States, can cause clinical MCF in several species of deer including sika deer (*Cervus nippon*), roe deer (*Capreolus capreolus)*, moose *(Alces* alces) and white-tailed deer (*Odocoileus virginianus*). Clinical disease is rarely reported in goats, but has occurred naturally in goats in the United Kingdom and Germany infected with the sheep herpes virus OvHV-2. These animals presented with pyrexia and neurological signs, mainly ataxia and tremors, and one goat had bilateral corneal opacity. Goats thus appear to be clinically susceptible hosts to OvHV-2 and reservoir hosts for CpHV-2.

Botulism
Aetiology
- *Clostridium botulinum*, an anaerobic, Gram-positive spore-forming rod found in soil, vegetation and as a normal inhabitant of the intestines of various livestock, including poultry. Neurotoxins are produced in decomposing carcases and vegetation: types C or D (generally from poultry carcases/litter); type B (from decomposing plant-derived feeds).
- Preformed toxins are ingested, absorbed from the intestine and enter the nervous system via the blood.
- The toxins interfere with the release and function of the neurotransmitter Acetylcholine, producing flaccid paralysis.

Risk factors
- An association between the use of poultry litter as feed or bedding (now illegal) was suggested in the 1970s and has been reported in many different countries. Poultry litter stored or spread some distance from susceptible animals may be transported, possibly by foxes or birds, into areas where ruminants are housed, even on neighbouring farms.
- Feed contaminated by rodent carcases.

- Spoiled feedstuffs – silage, brewer's grains, decaying vegetation.

    Soil and vegetation contaminated by *Cl. botulinum* type B can become incorporated into big bale silage and may use grass protein as a substrate for multiplication under suitable conditions, followed by autolysis and the release of large amounts of toxin.
- Factors that promote pica, for example starvation, that encourage animals to eat sources of the toxin they would otherwise ignore.
- Access to water contaminated by decaying carcases, such as animals drowning in header tanks or troughs.

Clinical signs

- All ages of animal are potentially susceptible to botulism.
- Recumbency, with lack of muscle tone, leading to ataxia, progressive flaccid paralysis commencing with the pelvic limbs and death in most cases, although mildly affected animals may survive.
- Goats, like sheep, characteristically develop an arched back with a drooping tail, head and neck.
- Affected animals may drool saliva, due to flaccidity of the tongue, and have difficulty swallowing, but the muscles of mastication and swallowing are not as obviously affected as in cattle.
- Sudden death if large amounts of toxin are ingested.

Laboratory tests

- The mouse inoculation test, using serum, is the gold standard for the diagnosis of botulism. Using specific antitoxins to protect the mice enables the toxin type to be identified and this may help to identify the source of the outbreak and in determining the possible risk to humans.
- Diagnosis is confirmed by demonstrating toxin in serum or viscera such as the liver.
- The highest concentration of toxin is likely to be in peracutely affected animals.
- Normal gut contents contain low levels of *C. botulinum* organisms, which may multiply after death, so samples should be removed as soon as possible after death and stored frozen.

Prevention

- Avoid feeding of contaminated feedstuffs – feed only well fermented silage; provide adequate rodent control and avoid contact with poultry litter.

- Various vaccines are available worldwide for use in cattle and sheep, although none are licensed for use in the United Kingdom. Cattle vaccines, which protect against *Clostridium botulinum* types C and D, can be obtained under a Special Treatment Certificate by applying to the Veterinary Medicines Directorate.

West Nile fever

- West Nile virus (WNV) is primarily an infection of birds and wild birds are the main reservoir hosts. Passeriformes (perching birds) are important in virus amplification. Among mammals, disease occurs mainly in equids (horses, donkeys and mules). A few clinical cases have been reported in other domesticated mammals, including alpacas, sheep and reindeer. Goats can be infected and antibodies to WNV are commonly detected in areas were the virus is circulating, but the vast majority of animals are asymptomatic.
- WNV has emerged as a significant human and veterinary pathogen in North America, southern Europe, the Middle East, Central and South America and the Caribbean. In some regions, the viruses do not seem to be endemic, but are reintroduced regularly by migratory wild birds. These viruses may either cause outbreaks or circulate asymptomatically. Although antibodies to the virus have been found in birds in the United Kingdom, virus infection has never been identified.

Aetiology

- West Nile virus is an arbovirus in the *Flavivirus* genus of the family Flaviviridae. The two most common genetic lineages of WNV are lineage 1 and lineage 2. Both lineages contain virulent viruses, as well as strains that usually cause asymptomatic infections or mild disease.
- West Nile virus is primarily transmitted by mosquitoes. Members of the genus *Culex* are the main vectors worldwide, although other mosquito genera can also be infected. Transovarial transmission has been demonstrated in some species of mosquitoes, and is likely to be important in overwintering. Dormant mosquitoes that survive the winter may also harbor WNV.

Clinical signs

- The incubation period in horses is 3 to 15 days. Infections in other mammals are uncommon and the incubation period is unknown.
- Clinical cases in ruminants are uncommon and in most cases only a single animal is infected.
- Most affected animals have had neurological signs, which were often the first apparent signs. These include ataxia, muscle twitches, partial paralysis, impaired vision, head pressing, teeth grinding, aimless wandering, convulsions, circling and an inability to swallow.
- Some animals have initially been pyrexic, lethargic and anorexic. Most affected animals have died within 1–2 days.

Diagnosis

- A diagnosis of West Nile fever in a goat with a neurological disease should not be made on the basis of a single positive antibody titre, which merely indicates that the animal has been exposed to the virus.

Treatment

- No specific treatment is available.
- Symptomatic treatment is directed towards treatment reducing CNS inflammation, supporting the animal when recumbent and providing nutrition and fluids either orally by stomach tube or intravenously.

Human infection

- Human infection is usually acquired through mosquito bites.
- Some species of birds, mammals and reptiles can shed the virus in secretions and excretions.
- Tissues from infected animals, especially the brain, are also sources of exposure.

Metabolic disease

Cerebrocortical necrosis (CCN, polioencephalomalacia)
Aetiology

CCN has been associated historically with a thiamine (vitamin B1) deficiency, but it is now recognised that there is also an association with a high sulphur intake.

- Thiamine (vitamin B1) is usually produced in adequate amounts by ruminal microflora. Lower levels of thiamine result in a lower supply of carbohydrates to the neurons in the brain. Deficiency can arise due to:
  - Thiaminase 1 and 2 production by ruminal bacteria, possibly following ingestion of mouldy or fungal contaminated feed or acidosis resulting in changes in rumen microflora. Both enzymes are responsible for degrading thiamine.
  - Prolonged diarrhoea, for example coccidiosis.
  - Drug therapy, for example thiabendazole, levamisole and amprolium.

    Note: take care when treating diarrhoea as treatment may exacerbate CCN.
  - Ingestion of plants containing thiaminase, such as bracken (*Pteridium aquilinum*), Nardoo fern (*Marsilea drummondii*) and rock fern (*Cheilanthes sieberi*). These plants are unpalatable, so field cases are uncommon.
- Microbial reduction of ingested sulphur in the rumen leads to hydrogen sulphide (H_2S) gas accumulating in the rumen gas cap. Although elemental sulphur and sulphates are generally non-toxic, H_2S and its various ionic forms block cellular energy metabolism by interfering with cytochrome oxidases, which particularly affect the CNS with its requirement for a high, continuous energy production. Animals with sulphur-associated CCN have normal thiamine levels. The excess sulphur can come from a variety of sources, including water, high grain diets and forage:
  - Water sources with high sulphur content are likely to be a particular risk during hot weather, when the animals' water intake is increased and evaporation will have led to an increase in water sulphur concentrations.
  - High grain rations that lead to a rumen pH <6.0 encourage the formation of H_2S.
  - Maize, sugar beet and sugar cane by-products can have a high sulphur content if acidifying agents containing sulphur have been added.
  - Ethanol by-products, especially dried distillers grain with solubles (DDGS) may contain a high concentration of sulphur.
  - Lucerne (alfalfa) has a high protein and sulphur-containing amino acid content and can be a significant source of sulphur, if large amounts are fed.
  - Some weeds, including Canada thistle (*Cirsium arvense*), kochia (*Kochia scoparia*), and lambsquarter (*Chenopodium* spp.) can accumulate high concentrations of sulphate.

o Brassicas, including turnips, often contain high levels of sulphur (>0.50% on DM basis) and this, together with their low fibre levels, can result in CCN in grazing animals.

Clinical signs

- Generally young animals are affected, but also older animals.
- Stargazing, ataxia, nystagmus, blindness (normal pupillary light reflexes, dorsomedial strabismus), head pressing, collapse + convulsions and opisthotonus.
- Severe but transient diarrhoea.
- Afebrile (except during convulsions).
- Death 1 to 2 days after the onset of clinical signs.

Laboratory tests

- Estimates of thiamine levels can be made: (1) indirectly by erythrocyte transketolase assay on heparinised blood or (2) directly on samples of frozen brain, liver or heart.
- Thiaminase levels can be estimated in frozen faecal or rumen samples.
- CSF may show slightly elevated protein levels and white cell count (but relatively acellular compared to pituitary abscess syndrome or listeriosis).
- Urine may test positive for glucose due to hyperglycaemia.

Post-mortem findings

- Cerebral oedema produces a swollen brain with disparity in colour between the normal grey of the cerebellar grey matter and the comparatively pale or yellowish grey cerebral cortex.
- Cut surface of cerebral cortex exhibits autofluorescence under ultraviolet light.

Treatment

- Thiamine, 10 mg/kg i.v., every 6 hours for 24 hours.
- Multivitamin preparations can be used if thiamine is not available, but must be given according to the thiamine content (usually 10 or 35 mg/ml).

    The response to thiamine is diagnostic if thiamine deficiency is involved, but will only be successful if treatment is commenced early; in more advanced cases there may be residual brain damage and blindness.

Animals with CCN apparently caused by excess sulphur sometimes show some level of improvement when thiamine is administered, although the response is typically less than with a primary thiamine issue.

- Unaffected animals in a group should be treated as a preventative.
- Support therapy with corticosteroids (dexamethasone, 2 mg/kg i.m. or s.c.), diuretics and hypertonic intravenous drips may aid recovery by reducing the cerebral oedema.

Hypocalcaemia (milk fever)

See Chapter 4.

Hypocalcaemia may occur in late pregnancy, during parturition and at any stage of lactation, particularly in heavy milkers, and in any age of adult goat. The disease is most common in young, high-yielding first kidders in the first few weeks after parturition. Older goats are more likely to suffer from hypocalcaemia around and during parturition. In heavy milking goats, an absolute deficiency of calcium at any stage of lactation will precipitate the disease.

All recumbent or comatose goats should be treated as potentially hypocalcaemic and given calcium.

Many toxic conditions, for example enterotoxaemia and mastitis, may show a temporary response to calcium therapy.

Hypomagnesaemia (grass tetany)
Aetiology

- Heavy milking goats grazing lush heavily fertilised grass may receive a diet deficient in magnesium. The disease usually occurs fairly early in lactation soon after starting to graze rich pasture. Pregnant goats on poor pasture in early spring may also develop the disease.

Incidence

- The disease is of sporadic occurrence in the United Kingdom because most high yielding goats are, at least in part, zero grazed and supplied with hay, browsings and concentrates.

Clinical

- *Acute*: excitement, tremors, twitching of facial muscles; hyperaesthesia, aimless wandering, falling over, frothing at the mouth; convulsions, death; some animals may be found dead (Plate 12.3).

- *Subclinical*: inappetence, apprehension, milk yield decreased, mild ataxia, may convulse in response to noise or handling; may be spontaneous recovery or progression to acute phase.
- *Chronic*: other animals in an affected herd may show poor growth, reduced milk yield and dullness due to low serum magnesium levels.

Diagnosis
- Clinical signs.
- Response to treatment.
- Serum magnesium levels (normal 0.83 to 1.6 mmol/litre).

Treatment
- Calcium borogluconate 20% with magnesium and phosphorus, 80–100 ml i.v. or s.c., plus 100 ml magnesium sulphate 25% s.c.
- Oral maintenance dose of at least 7 g calcinated magnesite or equivalent while dietary imbalances are corrected.

Prevention
- Correct diet: good quality fibre, adequate energy plus adequate magnesium (supplement where necessary, for example magnesium sheep bullets).
- Avoid grazing heavily fertilised pastures.

Transit tetany
Aetiology
- Combined hypocalcaemia/ hypomagnesaemia brought on by stress, particularly transport, but also by late pregnancy, fear, etc.
- May occur in castrated males.

Clinical signs
- As for acute hypomagnesaemia.

Treatment
- As for acute hypomagnesaemia.

Periparturient toxaemia
See Chapter 4.

Does with *pregnancy toxaemia* and *acetonaemia* occasionally show nervous signs – ataxia, tremors around the head and ears, reduced vision or blindness, head pressing, stargazing and eventually recumbency, coma and death.

Does with *post-parturient toxaemia (fatty liver syndrome)* generally only show nervous signs terminally when starvation results in recumbency and coma.

Space-occupying lesions of the brain

Cerebral abscess
Aetiology
- Pyogranuloma or abscess resulting from a bacterial infection often with *Corynebacterium* species, *Staphylococcus aureus, Fusobacterium necrophorum* or *Trueperella pyogenes (Arcanbacterium pyogenes, C. pyogenes)*; often follows fight wounds in male goats or following a middle ear infection that progresses to the inner ear, meninges and brain.

Clinical signs
- Variable; may be associated with meningitis or act as a space-occupying lesion with head tilt, visual defects, circling (with head turned towards the side of the lesion), etc. Brain stem compression may cause ataxia, weakness or asymmetric pupil size.
- CSF changes variable – often increased white cell count (neutrophils).

Coenuriasis (gid)
Aetiology
- The central nervous system of the goat is invaded by *Coenurus cerebralis*, the cystic larval stage, or metacestode, of the tapeworm *Taenia multiceps*.
- The life cycle of *T. multiceps* depends on the ingestion of the larval stage by a carnivore, including the dog. This only occurs when the carnivore ingests raw, infected sheep or goat brain or offal contaminated by a ruptured cyst. *Taenia multiceps* then lives in the small intestine of the carnivore. The goat becomes infected by consuming herbage contaminated with onchospores or *Taenia* eggs. The embryos then pass via the blood to the brain. Intracranial pressure from the cyst produces the clinical signs.

Clinical signs
- Clinical signs depend on the location of the cyst and the pressure it exerts on the surrounding brain tissue. Pressure on the cerebral hemispheres results in

incoordination, blindness, head tilt, head pressing, circling and stargazing. Gait abnormalities occur when the cerebellum is involved. Skull softening as a result of bone rarefaction may occur when the cyst is superficial.

Diagnosis

- Intradermal gid test: 0.l ml cyst fluid injected into the caudal fold beneath the tail or shaved area of skin on the neck; 0.1 ml sterile water used as control. Skin thickening at this site within 24 hours classified as positive. Not very reliable.
- Serology and haemalology of no diagnostic use; CSF – increased white cell count particularly eosinophils and mononuclear cells.
- Surgery or post-mortem examination.

Treatment

- Surgical removal of the cyst, when it can be located by skull softening, under sedation and local anaesthesia or general anaesthetic. Skin incised and bone removed with trephine or scalpel blade. After the dura mater is penetrated, the cyst will often bulge through and can be removed by applying negative suction pressure by syringe or pipette.
- Where there is no skull softening but the cyst site can be approximately located by detailed neurological examination, ultrasound examination via a trephine site may aid localisation.
- Radiography can also be used, but interpretation of the results is difficult.

Control

- Regular treatment of all dogs on the farm for tapeworm.
- Dogs should be prevented from consuming raw goat or sheep brain and offal.

Pituitary abscess syndrome
Aetiology

- Abscessation of the pituitary gland following lymphatic or blood-borne infection often with *Trueperella pyogenes (Arcanbacterium pyogenes, C. pyogenes)*, but also many other Gram-positive (*Streptococcus, Staphylococcus, Actinomyces*) and Gram-negative (*Fusobacterium, Bacteroides, Pasteurella, Pseudomonas, Actinobacillus*) bacteria from another infected focus in the body,

for example mastitis, arthritis, lung abscess, sinusitis or intracranial damage with secondary sepsis after fighting.

Pressure by the enlarging abscess acts as a space-occupying lesion affecting the adjacent areas of the brain and brain stem and producing various neurological signs depending on the extent of the abscess. Cranial nerve functions are progressively affected, usually asymmetrically.

Incidence

- Generally adult animals; more commonly males.

Clinical signs

Varying clinical signs but commonly:
- Anorexia, depression.
- Bradycardia (see below).
- Dysphagia.
- Head pressing.
- Blindness (pupillary light reflexes often absent; ventrolaleral strabismus, cf. cerebrocortical necrosis).
- Nystagmus.
- Ataxia, opisthotonus, recumbency.
- Death.

Note: (1) The progressive nature of the neurological signs means that repeat neurological examinations and assessment of cranial nerve function are important for diagnosis.

(2) Bradycardia is an uncommon finding in the goat but occurs in the pituitary abscess syndrome and other space-occupying lesions of the brain because pressure on the hypothalamus causes increased vagal tone. Bradycardia may also occur in severe milk fever, hypothermia, hypoglycaemia, botulism and trauma to the head.

Laboratory findings

- CSF – elevated white cell count (mostly neutrophils), elevated protein level.
- Haematology – not diagnostic; fibrinogen and globulin often elevated.

Post-mortem findings

- Pituitary abscess – generally evident grossly, occasionally only on histopathological examination.
- Generally a chronic infection elsewhere in the body.
- Histopathology shows coagulative and liquefactive necrosis of the pituitary gland, particularly

the adenohypophysis with neutrophil and some mononuclear cell infiltration.

- Culture of abscess sample yields pure or mixed culture of aerobic bacteria.

Treatment

- None.

Oestrus ovis

Aetiology

- *Oestrus ovis*, the sheep and goat nasal fly, deposits L1 larvae around the nostrils. The larvae normally migrate to the nasal passages and then the frontal sinuses where they develop to the third instar. Third stage larvae are sneezed on to the pasture after 35–40 days, where they pupate and emerge as adults 2–10 weeks later. In the United Kingdom, *O. ovis* is most prevalent in the southern counties of England and Wales.

Clinical signs

- Usually limited to panic when the flies are laying and a mucopurulent discharge when the larvae are in the nasal passages and sinuses.
- More severely affected animals can have a haemorrhagic discharge, sneezing, wheezing breath, snorting and head shaking.
- Larvae may rarely migrate via the ethmoid bones to the brain, producing clinical signs as for *Coenurus cerebralis*.
- Larvae may also occasionally enter the eye or nasolacrimal system, causing conjunctivitis

Diagnosis

- Post-mortem examination of the nasal turbinates or sinuses, confirming the presence of active larvae.
- An ELISA test has been validated in the United Kingdom.

Treatment

- Ivemectin in the autumn to eliminate larval stages from the nasal cavity.

Tumour

Brain neoplasms are very rare. There is a single report of a glioma.

Space-occupying lesions of the spinal cord

Although more common in kids (q.v.), *spinal meningitis*, *abscessation* and *vertebral osteomyelitis* may occur in adult animals, producing varying degrees of paraparesis or tetraparesis. Vertebral abscesses may be a component of caseous lymphadenitis.

Tumours, for example lymphosarcoma and meningioma, *Coenurus cerebralis cysts* (see earlier in this chapter) and *vascular hamartoma* may rarely act as space-occupying lesions of the spinal cord.

The clinical signs depend on the location and degree of damage to the spinal cord, although signs are usually bilaterally symmetrical, varying from paresis and stiffness to paralysis.

Cerebrospinal fluid (CSF) is variable, often showing an increased white cell count (neutrophils). Treatment should be based where possible on culture and sensitivity of the CSF or use long-term broad-spectrum antibiotic therapy.

Rhodococcus equi

- Infections in individual goats have sporadically been reported from the United Kingdom, India, the United States, Australia, Botswana, Trinidad, the Netherlands, Canada, Spain and South Africa. In most cases the goats have been less than 1 year old. Infection produces abscesses in multiorgan systems including the liver and lungs. Abscesses can cause vertebral osteomyelitis and compression of the spinal cord resulting in ataxia and limb paresis. *R. equi* is an important cause of pneumonia in foals and has also been reported as a cause of pneumonia in immunosuppressed people.

Cerebrospinal nematodiasis

- Aberrant spinal cord migration of any nematode may occasionally cause neurological signs, generally referrable to spinal cord disease. Neurological signs are produced as the result of tissue destruction and inflammation caused by randomly wandering L3 larvae. CSF shows elevated white cells (mainly eosinophils and mononuclear cells) and protein levels. Treatment with ivermectin and dexamethasone may be successful if combined with adequate supportive care.

- In the United States, aberrant migration of the *meningeal worm* (*Parelaphospostrongylus tenuis*) in susceptible hosts like the goat causes damage to the central nervous system and may result in death. The definitive host is the white tailed deer where meningeal worms reside in the meninges of the deer, rarely causing clinical disease.
- The natural hosts of *Elaphostrongylus cervi* are cervids such as red, roe, maral and sika deer in Eurasian countries and in these species pathogenicity is low. When non-specific hosts like sheep and goats are infected, neurological signs occur.

Clinical signs
- Affected animals are depressed and gradually lose weight.
- Clinical signs generally reflect asymmetrical, focal spinal cord lesions, including hypermetria, ataxia, stiffness, muscular weakness, posterior paresis, paralysis, head tilt, arching neck, circling, blindness, seizures and death.
- Hind limbs are generally affected first with progression to the fore limbs.
- The course of the disease ranges from acute, with death within days, to chronic, with ataxia lasting months or years.

Control
- Deer proof fencing.
- Reduce the availability of snails and slugs that act as the intermediate hosts.

   Eliminate organic matter (leaves, compost, wood piles, etc.) from pastures and around livestock buildings; avoid grazing low-lying wet fields; drain and fence wet areas; use molluscicides where appropriate; use chickens or game birds to reduce the numbers of molluscs; vegetation-free buffer zones (e.g. gravel or limestone) around fencelines will reduce the migration of snails and slugs.
- Remove thick undergrowth to expose grazing to fluctuations in temperature (dessication and freezing will reduce the numbers of infective larvae on pasture).

Treatment
- Prophylactic treatment against migrating larvae may be achieved with administration of ivermectin, 0.2 mg/kg every 30 days or doramectin every 45 days during periods of risk.

Although anthelmintic resistance is unlikely to develop in the meningeal worm because the infections do not become patent, repeated anthelmintic treatments will increase the likelihood of resistance developing in other nematode worms.

Trauma

Trauma (q.v.) to the head and neck should always be considered, particularly in male goats running together or tethered animals.

Vestibular disease

Otitis media/interna
Otitis media/interna occur as sequelae to otitis externa or following rhinitis and pharyngitis, or via haematogenous spread.

Clinical signs
- Head tilt, circling towards side of affected ear, nystagmus with the fast component directed away from the affected ear.
- Eye drop on the affected side.
- Facial paralysis.

Ear mite infection (psoroptic mange)
See Chapter 10.

Hepatic encephalopathy

Hepatic encephalopathy is uncommon; severe hepatic insufficiency may result in lethargy, depression and neurological signs such as behavioural changes, ataxia, tremors, fits, convulsions and coma.

Halothane-induced acute hepatic necrosis has been described as producing depression, lethargy, salivation, head pressing, chewing motions, icterus and recumbency. Hepatotoxicity occurred after prolonged (3 to 9 hours duration) anaesthesia. Studies using halothane anaesthesia of shorter duration have not produced evidence of hepatic damage.

Poisonings

A variety of drugs, plants and chemicals can be neurotoxic.

Lead

Although lead poisoning has been produced experimentally in goats, cases of accidental poisoning are rarely reported, despite the propensity of goats for chewing painted wood. Goats appear resistant to lead poisoning compared to cattle and dogs, either through innate resistance or disinclination to ingest lead.

Aetiology
- Lead from old painted wood (check partitions, doors, etc.), car batteries, motor oil, etc.

Clinical signs
- Abdominal pain, anorexia, weight loss.
- Diarrhoea, tenesmus.
- Abortion.
- Depression, incoordination, head pressing, ataxia.
- Blindness does not appear to be a prominent feature of poisoning in goats compared with other species and cerebrocortical necrosis should be considered a more likely diagnosis in animals presenting with neurological signs and blindness.

Laboratory tests
- Blood lead estimation.
- Basophilic stippling of erythrocytes stained with Wright's stain.
- Kidney or liver lead levels: > 4 ppm.
- CSF – acellular.

Post-mortem findings
- Cerebral oedema.
- Mucoid enterocolitis.

Treatment
- Sodium calciumedetate, 75 mg/kg, daily in four divided doses, slowly i.v. or s.c. for 2 to 5 days. Dilute 1 ml in 4 ml glucose or sodium chloride 0.9%.

Other heavy metals

Poisoning with other heavy metals such as *arsenic* and *mercury* may occasionally occur, giving neurological signs such as incoordination, blindness, muscle tremors and convulsions, together with abdominal pain and diarrhoea.

Plants

See Chapter 21.

Plant poisoning is unlikely to produce nervous signs in goats in the United Kingdom.
- Rape (*Brassica rapus*) can produce blindness, head pressing and violent excitement.
- Bracken (*Pteridium aquilinum*), although unlikely to induce a thiamine deficiency under normal conditions where ruminal synthesis of thiamine is adequate, might exacerbate or precipitate cerebrocortical necrosis.
- Oxalate poisoning, which can produce ataxia, muscle tremor, paralysis and death, might be produced by eating large amounts of rhubarb or common sorrel.
- Fool's parsley (*Aethusa cynapium*) can cause indigestion, panting and ataxia.
- Cherry laurel (*Prunus laurocerasus*) causes cyanide poisoning, with animals often being found dead. Less severe cases show dyspnoea, staggering gait, jerky movements and convulsions.
- Laburnum (*L. anagyroides*) and hemlock (*Corium maculatum*) contain nicotine-like alkaloids resulting in rapid respiration, salivation, excitement and muscle tremors followed by depression, incoordination, convulsions and death.
- Ragwort (*Senecio jacobaea*) produces an hepatic neurotoxicity.

Organophosphates
Aetiology
- Exposure to organophosphates, for example dips or drenches.

Clinical signs
- Abdominal pain, inappetence, incoordination, diarrhoea, muscular tremors, dyspnoea, paralysis, convulsions, coma and death.

Treatment
- Atropine, 0.6–1 mg/kg, 1–1.5 ml/kg, one quarter i.v,, the rest s.c. or i.m., every 4 to 6 hours for up to 24 hours.

Rafoxanide

The flukicide rafoxanide has a much lower safety margin in goats (4 to 6 times) than sheep (20 times). Overdosage may cause degeneration and oedema of the retina, optic tract and related areas of the CNS, and death. Rafoxanide is no longer available in the United Kingdom.

Urea (hyperammonaemia)

Aetiology

- Overfeeding of urea in rations.

Clinical signs

- Abdominal pain, muscle tremor, ataxia, hyperaesthesia.
- Mydriasis, convulsions and death.

Treatment

- Vinegar 0.5 to 1.0 l orally, as an acidifying agent.

Epilepsy

A single case of partial epilepsy in a Nubian goat has been properly documented. However, the incidence of 'fits' is much higher. Because they are usually not fully investigated, the aetiologies of these fits are unknown. Most owners cull goats that have repetitive fits without resorting to medication. Kids that recover from disbudding meningoencephalitis may continue to have fits into adult life.

Further reading

General

Allen, A.L., Goupil, B.A. and Valentine, B.A. (2012) A retrospective study of spinal cord lesions in goats submitted to 3 veterinary diagnostic laboratories. *Can. Vet. J.*, **53** (6), 639–642.

Barlow, R.M. (1987) Differential diagnosis of nervous diseases of goats. *Goat Vet. Soc. J.*, **8**, 73–76.

Baxendell, S.A. (1984) Caprine nervous diseases. *Proc. Univ. Sydney, Post Grad. Comm. Vet. Sci.*, **73**, 333–342.

Brewer, B.D. (1983) Neurologic disease of sheep and goats. *Vet. Clin. North Amer.: Large Anim. Pract.*, **5** (3), 677–700.

Callan, R.J., Van Metre, D.C. (2004) Viral diseases of the ruminant nervous system. *Vet. Clin. North Amer.: Food Anim. Pract.*, **20**, 327–362.

Finnie, J., Windsor, P. and Kessell, A. (2011) Neurological diseases of ruminant livestock in Australia. I: general neurological examination, necropsy procedures and neurological manifestations of systemic disease, trauma and neoplasia. *Australian Vet. J.*, **89** (7), 243–246.

Finnie, J., Windsor, P. and Kessell, A. (2011) Neurological diseases of ruminant livestock in Australia. II: toxic disorders and nutritional deficiencies. *Australian Vet. J.*, **89** (7), 247–253.

Kessell, A., Finnie, J. and Windsor, P. (2011) Neurological diseases of ruminant livestock in Australia. III: bacterial and protozoal infections. *Australian Vet. J.*, **89** (8), 289–296.

Kessell, A., Finnie, J. and Windsor, P. (2011) Neurological diseases of ruminant livestock in Australia. IV: viral infections. *Australian Vet. J.*, **89** (9), 331–337.

Nietfeld, J.C. (2012) Neuropathology and diagnostics in food animals. *Vet. Clin. North Amer.: Food Anim. Pract.*, **28** (3), 515–534.

Thompson, K.G. (1985) Nervous diseases of goats. *Proceedings of the Course in Goat Husbandry and Medicine*, Massey University, November 1985, pp. 152–161.

Windsor, P., Kessell, A. and Finnie, J. (2011) Review of neurological diseases of ruminant livestock in Australia. VI: postnatal bovine, and ovine and caprine, neurogenetic disorders. *Australian Vet. J.*, **89** (11), 432–438.

ß-Mannosidosis

Kumar, K., Jones, M.Z., Cunningham, J.G., Kelly, J.A. and Lovell, K.L. (1986) Caprine ß-mannosidosis: phenotypic features. *Vet. Rec.*, **118**, 325–327.

Botulism

Hogg, R., Livesey, C. and Payne, J. (2008) Diagnosis and implications of botulism. *In Pract.*, **30**, 392–397.

Caprine arthritis encephalitis

Adams, D.S., Klevjer-Anderson, P., Carlson, J.L., McGuire, T.C. and Gorham, J.R. (983) Transmission and control of CAE virus. *Amer. J. Vet. Res.*, **44** (9), 1070–1075.

Dawson, M. (1987) Caprine arthritis encephalitis. *In Pract.*, 8–11.

DeVilbiss, B. *et al.* (2013) Computed tomography findings in a 5 year old Australian cashmere goat (*Capra hircus*) suffering leukoencephalomyelitis due to caprine arthritis encephalitis virus. *Canadian Vet. J.*, **54** (10), 960–964.

Knight, A.P. and Jokinen, M.P. (1982) Caprine arthritis encephalitis. *Comp. Cont. Ed. Pract. Vet.*, **4** (6), S263–S269.

Cerebrocortical necrosis

Baxendell, S.A. (1984) Cerebrocortical necrosis. *Proc. Univ. Sydney Post Grad. Comm. Vet. Sci.*, **73**, 503–507.

Smith, M.C. (1979) Polioencephalomalacia in goats. *J. Am. Vet. Med. Assoc.*, **174** (12), 1328–1332.

Cerebrospinal fluid

Mueller, K. (2010) Clinical procedures in goats. *Goat Vet. Soc. J.*, **26**, 15–18.

Scott, P. (1993) Collection and interpretation of cerebrospinal fluid in ruminants. *In Pract.*, **15** (6), 298–300.

Scott, P. (1994) Cerebrospinal fluid analysis in the differential diagnosis of spinal cord lesions in ruminants. *In Pract.*, **16** (6), 301–303.

Coenuriasis

Gascoigne, E. and Critty, J.P. (2014) Control of tapeworms in sheep: a risk-based approach. *In Pract.*, **36**, 285–293.
Harwood, D.G. (1986) Metacestode disease in goats. *Goat Vet. Soc. J.*, **7** (2), 35–38.
Welchman, D. de B. and Bekh-Ochir, G. (2006) Spinal coenurosis causing posterior paralysis in a goat in Mongolia. *Vet. Rec.*, **158**, 238–239.

Disbudding meningoencephalitis

Wright, H.J., Adams, D.S. and Trigo, F.J. (1983) Meningoencephalitis after hot iron disbudding of goat kids. *Vet. Med./Small Animal Clin.*, **78** (4), 599–601.

Ear mites

Littlejohn, A.I. (1968) Psoroptic mange in the goat. *Vet. Rec.*, **82**, 148–155.
Williams, J.F. and Williams, S.F. (1978) Psoroptic ear mites in dairy goats. *J. Am. Vet. Med. Assoc.*, **173** (12), 1582–1583.

Enzootic ataxia

Inglis, D.M., Gilmour, J.S. and Murray, I.S. (1986) A farm investigation into swayback in a herd of goats and the result of administration of copper needles. *Vet. Rec.*, **118**, 657–660.
Whitelaw, A. (1985) Copper deficiency in cattle and sheep. *In Pract.*, **7** (3), 98–100.

Focal symmetrical encephalomalacia

Oliveira, D.M. *et al.* (2010) Focal symmetrical encephalomalacia in a goat. *J. Vet. Diagn. Invest.*, **22**, 793–796.

Hepatic encephalopathy

Kinde, H. *et al.* (2014) Congenital portosystemic shunts and hepatic encephalopathy in goat kids in California. *J. Vet. Diag. Invest.*, **26** (1), 173–177.
McEwen, M. *et al.* (2000) Hepatic effects of halothane and isofluorane anaesthesia in goats. *J. Am. Vet. Med. Assoc.*, **217**, 1697–1700.
Morris, D.D. and Henry, M.M. (1991) Hepatic encephalopathy. *Comp. Cont. Ed. Pract. Vet.*, **13** (7), 1153–1161.

Listeriosis

Braum, U., Stehle, C. and Ehrensperger, F. (2002) Clinical findings and treatment of listeriosis in 67 sheep and goats. *Vet. Rec.*, **150**, 38–42.
Harwood, D.G. (1988) Listeriosis in goats. *Goat Vet. Soc. J.*, **10** (1), 1–4.

Louping ill

Balseiro, A. *et al.* (2012) Louping ill in goats, Spain 2011. *Emerg. Infect. Dis.*, **18** (6), 976–978.
Reid, H. (1991) Louping-ill. *In Pract.*, **13** (4), 157–160.

Malignant catarral fever

Twomey, D.F. *et al.* (2006) Multisystemic necrotising vasculitis in a pygmy goat (*Capra hircus*). *Vet. Rec.*, **158** (25), 867–869.

Meningitis

Jamison, J.M. and Prescott, J.F. (1987) Bacterial meningitis in large animals. Part I. *Comp. Cont. Ed. Pract. Vet.*, **9** (12), F399–406.
Jamison, J.M. and Prescott, J.F. (1988) Bacterial meningitis in large animals. Part II. *Comp. Cont. Ed. Pract. Vet.*, **10** (2), 225–231.

Metabolic and nutritional diseases

Andrews, A.H. (1985) Some metabolic conditions in the doe. *Goat Vet. Soc. J.*, **6** (2), 70–72.
Finnie, J. *et al.* (2011) Neurological diseases of ruminant live stock in Australia. II: toxic disorders and nutritional deficiencies. *Australian Vet. J.*, **89**, 247–253.
Merrall, M. (1985) Nutritional and metabolic diseases. *Proceedings of the Course in Goat Husbandry and Medicine*, Massey University, November, pp. 126–131.
Pinsent, J. and Cottom, D.S. (1987) Metabolic diseases of goats. *Goat Vet. Soc. J.*, **8** (1), 40–42.
Rook, J.S. (2000) Pregnancy toxaemia of ewes, does and beef cows. *Vet. Clin. North Amer.: Food Anim. Pract.*, **16** (2), 293–318.

Oestrus ovis

Bates, P. (2007) Sheep nasal bot fly and differential diagnosis of bluetongue. *Vet. Rec.*, **160**, 671.
Dorchies, P., Duranton, C. and Jacquiet, P. (1998) Pathophysiology of *Oestrus ovis* infection in sheep and goats: a review. *Vet. Rec.*, **142**, 487–489.

Parasitic disease

Nagy, D.W. (2004) *Parelaphostrongylus tenuis* and other parasitic diseases of the ruminant nervous system. *Vet. Clin. North Amer.: Food Anim. Pract.*, **20**, 393–412.

Pituitary abscess syndrome

Perdrizet, J. and Dinsmore, P. (1986) *Comp. Cont. Ed. Pract. Vet.*, **8** (6), 5311–5318.

Rhodococcus equi infection

Jeckel, S. *et al.* (2011) Disseminated *Rhodococus equi* infection in goats in the UK. *Vet. Rec.*, **169** (2), 56.

Transmissable spongiform encephalopathies

Acin, C. (2015) Scrapie: a particularly persistent pathogen. *Vet. Rec.*, **176** (4), 97–98.

Andrews, A.H., Laven, R. and Matthews, J.G. (1992) Clinical observations on four cases of scrapie in goats. *Vet. Rec.*, **130**, 101.

Fast, C. and Groschup, M.H. (2013) Classical and atypical scrapie in sheep and goats. In: *Prions and Diseases:* Volume 2, *Animals, Humans and the Environment* (eds Zou, W.-Q. and Gambetti, P.), Chapter 2, pp. 15–44. Springer, New York.

Foster, J.D., Hope, J. and Fraser, H. (1993) Transmission of bovine spongiform encephalopathy to sheep and goats. *Vet. Rec.*, **133**, 339–341.

Foster, J.D. *et al.* (2001) Clinical signs, histopathology and genetics of experimental transmission of BSE and natural scrapie to sheep and goats. *Vet. Rec.*, **148**, 165–171.

Gonzàlez, L. *et al.* (2005) Diagnosis of preclinical scrapie in samples of rectal mucosa. *Vet. Rec.*, **25**, 846–847.

Hawkins, S.A.C., Simmons, H.A., Gough, K.C. and Maddison, B.C. (2015) Persistence of ovine scrapie infectivity in a farm environment following cleaning and decontamination. *Vet. Rec.*, **176** (4), 99.

Konold, T., Bone, G.E., Phelan, L.J. *et al.* (2010) Monitoring of clinical signs in goats with transmissible spongiform encephalopathies. *BMC Vet. Res.*, **6**, 13. Available at: http://www.biomedicalcentral.com/1746-6148/6/13.

Konold, T. and Phelan, L. (2014) Clinical examination protocol for the detection of scrapie. *J. Vis. Exp.*, (83), 51101. Available at: http://www.ncbi.nlm.nih.gov/pmc/articles/PMC4089440/.

Konold, T., Simmons, H.A., Webb, P.R. *et al.* (2013) Transmission of classical scrapie by goat milk. *Vet. Rec.*, **172** (17), 455.

Lacroux, C., Perrin-Chauvineau, C., Corbiere, F. *et al.* (2014) Genetic resistance to scrapie infection in experimentally challenged goats. *J. Virol.*, **88** (5), 2406–2413.

Maddison , B.C. and Gough, K.C. (2012) Scrapie dissemination and environmental persistence. *Goat Vet. Soc. J.*, **28**, 25–34.

Sargison, N. (1995) Scrapie in sheep and goats. *In Pract.*, **17** (10), 467–469.

Seuberlich, T. *et al.* (2007) Atypical scrapie in a Swiss goat and implications for transmissable spongifrom encephalopathy. *J. Vet. Diagn. Invest.*, **19**, 2–8.

Vaccari, G., Panagogiotidis, C.H., Acin, C. *et al.* (2009) State-of-the-art review of goat TSE in the European Union, with special emphasis on PRNP genetics and epidemiology. *Vet. Res.*, **40**, 48–66.

Wood, J.L.N. and Done, S.H. (1992) Natural scrapie in goats: neuropathology. *Vet. Rec.*, **131**, 93–96.

Wood, J.L.N., Done, S.H., Pritchard, G.C. and Wooldridge, M.J.A. (1992) Natural scrapie in goats; case histories and clinical signs *Vet. Rec.*, **131**, 66–68.

Tickborne diseases

Reid, H.W. (1986) Tick and tickborne diseases. *Goat Vet. Soc. J.*, **7** (2), 21–25.

Tumour

Marshall, C.L., Weinstock, D., Kramer, R.W. and Bagley, R.S. (1995) Glioma in a goat. *J. Am. Vet. Med. Assoc.*, **206** (10), 1572–1574.

West Nile virus

West Nile Virus Infection, The Center for Food Security and Public Health, Iowa State University (August 2013). Available at: www.cfsph.iastate.edu/Factsheets/pdfs/west_nile_fever.pdf.

CHAPTER 13

Diseases of the mammary gland

Mastitis

Mastitis is the inflammation of the mammary gland, regardless of cause, characterised by physiological, chemical and generally bacteriological changes in milk and by pathological changes in glandular tissue.

Investigation of mastitis
General clinical examination
- Assess the severity of systemic infection, degree of pyrexia, etc.

Specific udder examination
- Visually and by palpation.
- Compare the two halves.
  - Heat.
  - Swelling.
  - Lumps.
  - Extent of fibrosis.
  - Injuries to teats or body of udder.
- Superficial inguinal lymph nodes. The most obvious mammary lymph nodes lie above each half at the base of the udder between the hind limbs in the perineal region. They are usually inapparent, but will enlarge and feel nodular with infection.
- Udder palpation. Palpate the udder immediately after milking when it is flaccid; check for discernible abnormalities such as abscesses, scar tissue and irregular nodules.
  - Grasp the udder skin between the forefinger and thumb; it should be pliable and easily separated from the underlying tissue.
  - Palpate each half with both hands by placing one hand on the medial side and the other on the lateral side. Deep-palpate by pressing the fingertips towards each other and gradually work the hands towards the bottom of each half. The udder tissue should have a

fine grain. A coarse grain that still feels soft should respond to treatment. Harder udders or those with lumps or nodules are less likely to respond.

Milk sample examination

> In subclinical mastitis the milk may appear grossly normal.

- Use strip cup.
- Compare the two halves.
- Pus.
- Blood.
- Clots.
- Colour.

Laboratory tests
Somatic cell counts

> Somatic cell counts are useful as a herd test to monitor subclinical mastitis.

The somatic cells are neutrophils that migrate into mammary tissue to provide the first immunological line of defence against bacteria that penetrate the physical barrier of the teat canal. The number of somatic cells is directly related to the infection status of the udder, so that a high somatic cell count (SCC) is indicative of mastitis. For dairy cows, regular monitoring of somatic cell counts has become a useful tool for identifying cows with subclinical mastitis. Increasingly, regulatory authorities are attempting to introduce legal limits on the upper bulk milk cell count for goats' milk. However, the additional causal factors for high counts in goats

Diseases of the Goat, Fourth Edition. John Matthews.
© 2016 John Wiley & Sons, Ltd. Published 2016 by John Wiley & Sons, Ltd.

(see Table 13.1) produce much greater variation, meaning that extrapolating cow standards to goats' milk discriminates against wholesome milk.

Unlike the bovine mammary gland, where milk is produced by merocrine secretion, that of the goat produces milk by apocrine secretion, which results in portions of cytoplasm from epithelial cells being pinched off and appearing in milk as DNA-free particles, similar in size to white blood cells. Intact epithelial cells from acini and ducts also appear in the milk (see Table 13.2).

Only those counting methods that are specific for DNA can distinguish cell-like cytoplasmic particles

from somatic cells and thereby give reliable estimates of somatic cell numbers in goat milk. There is poor correlation for goat milk between somatic cell counts obtained by particle counting machines (Coulter counters) and machines that count cell nuclei (Fossomatic counters) as the former cannot differentiate between particulate non-cellular debris and white blood cells. Coulter counters tend to give approximately double the apparent cell counts in goats' milk compared with the Fossomatic method. Counts from Fossomatic counters are themselves consistently higher than direct microscopic cell counts using DNA specific stains, such as Pyronin Y Methyl Green. Microscopic cell counts are the most accurate method but are time consuming and expensive. Direct microscopy with stains, which are non-differential for nucleated particles, such as methylene blue, are inappropriate for goats. On-farm screening tests such as the PortaSCC goat milk test (Portacheck) have been specially developed for goats and validated against Pyronin Y Methyl Green.

Because goats are seasonal breeders, milk bulk tank somatic cell counts show a distinct seasonal variation, with the lowest in April and the highest in September or October. Counts begin to rise about 4 months after kidding and with the onset of oestrus cycles. As in cow's milk, mastitis due to bacterial infection causes a rise in the cell count of milk from the affected half, that is raised somatic cell counts are indicators of impaired udder health. However, as goats consistently have higher cell counts than cattle, particularly towards the end of lactation, results need careful interpretation. Variations in yield, feed intake and stage of lactation, as well as infection, are likely to affect cell counts. Cell counts generally increase with each lactation. Other diseases such as infection with caprine arthritis encephalitis virus (CAE) can cause an increase in somatic cell counts. Anecdotally, some commercial herds report increases in cell counts after vaccination. Variations in bulk cell counts are likely to be much greater in smaller herds, where individual animals can exert a greater influence on the average value, and where the majority of animals are at the same stage of lactation. The influence of factors other than infection is also greater when milk production is low, for example at the end of lactation.

An isolated SCC is not a very important piece of information, though it does give an idea – an SCC of 300 000 is suggestive of healthy animals, a figure of 1 500 000 is

Table 13.1 Factors affecting the somatic cell count.

Bacterial infection (clinical or subclinical mastitis)	Single most important contributer to SCC
Season	Seasonal changes linked to stage of lactation, yield and oestrus cycle
Stage of lactation	Increased SCC in early and late lactation Highest in 'running through' goats
Frequency of milking	More frequent milking increases the migration of neutrophils from blood into the mammary gland
Parity	Increased SCC with each lactation
Oestrus	Increased SCC around oestrus
Infection with other diseases	CAE
Vaccination	May cause an increase in SCC after vaccination
Feeding	High grain feeding + acidosis
Genetics	SCC are heritable (0.12–0.25)

Table 13.2 Difference in milk secretion and somatic cells between the goat and the cow.

Goat	Cow
Apocrine secretion	Merocrine secretion
Nucleated and non-nucleated particles shed	
Neutrophils make up 50–70% of SCC	Neutrophils make up 5–20% of SCC

indicative of mastitis problems and an SCC of 750 000 indicates a farm with an acceptable level of subclinical mastitis. Among goat farmers and veterinarians, it is accepted that high SCCs of above 1 000 000 cells/ml may occur in apparently healthy lactating goats. At a cell count threshold of 1.5 million/ml, 80.5% of bacteriologically negative samples will be correctly classified, but 19.5% of negative samples will be diagnosed as infected and only 41.4% of bacteriologically positive samples diagnosed. Lowering the threshold results in more false positive, but fewer false negative results. At a 1 million/ml cell count threshold, 71.8% of bacteriologically negative samples are correctly classified, 28.2% of negative samples would be diagnosed as infected and 56.5% of bacteriologically positive samples correctly identified.

Differential cell counts may be a better indication of mastitis than the total SCC, with an increase in the percentage of polymorphonuclear leucocytes relative to lymphocytes and macrophages indicating mastitis.

Serial, for example monthly, monitoring of *individual* animals may help establish the presence of subclinical infection. It has been suggested that serial cell counts < 750 000 cells/ml indicate a healthy mammary gland, that 2 or more counts > 750 000 cell/ml indicates infection by a minor pathogen such as coagulase negative *Staphylococci* and that 3 results >1 750 000 indicates infection by a major pathogen such as *Staphylococcus aureus*. *Staphylococci* cause cyclic shedding so infection may not always be detected on culture.

Suggested alternative methods for identifying intramammary infections include *monitoring milk conductivity, blood serum albumin changes* or *measuring alpha-1 acid glycoprotein* in milk. Milk conductivity testing is carried out in some commercial herds either automatically or using hand-held meters for testing individual goats.

Somatic cell count in goats is heritable. In dairy goats in New Zealand the heritability is reported to be 0.12 to 0.15 (cf. cattle 0.05 to 0.12 and dairy sheep 0.054 to 0.18). Selecting for lower SCC may select for reduced susceptibility to mammary infection, reduced duration of infection or reduced SCC in uninfected animals. Estimated breeding values (EBVs) can be determined for individual animals and possibly used in selecting which bucks to use for breeding and kids to retain as replacements, or for which animals to cull. Does with a high EBV SCC were found to have a higher prevalence of any intramammary infections and were more likely to have an infection due to a major pathogen than does with a low EBV SCC. Thus selection for EBV SCC is likely to result in a lower SCC and also lower prevalence of intramammary infection.

California mastitis test

The California mastitis test (CMT) is a simple semiquantitative goat-side test for determining the number of nucleated cells, measuring both neutrophils and epithelial cells. The CMT will only show changes in cell counts above 300 000. High scores can occur, in the absence of mastitis, when there are large numbers of epithelial cells present, such as towards the end of lactation or in systemically ill goats with a low milk yield.

The benefits of the CMT include:
- Can be carried out by the milker.
- Instant result.
- Gives an indication of the infection in each half.
- Cheap test.

The test is carried out in following way:
- Stimulate milk let-down and discard the foremilk.
- Draw one or two squirts of milk from each half into the paddle dish.
- Tip the paddle so that most of the milk is discarded.
- Add an equal volume of reagent to the remaining milk.
- Swirl the milk using a circular movement and examine for the presence of a gel or slime reaction.
- Record the result by half.
- Rinse out the paddle before testing the next goat.

There are a number of ways to score the CMT, but dividing the result into four categories is one of the easiest. A negative result is seen when the milk remains watery. A score of 3, the highest, is when the solution almost solidifies. The CMT is very subjective and the results can vary as a result of who is carrying out the test (Table 13.3).

Table 13.3 California mastitis test.

Score	Gelling
Negative	None
1	Mild
2	Moderate
3	Heavy, almost solidifies

In goats, the California mastitis test is more suitable for excluding a diagnosis of mastitis than showing its presence, that is a low score means that mastitis is unlikely to be present, although a high score may produce false positive results. It is also useful for checking the cell counts of individual halves after mastitis treatment (and possibly discarding this milk until it returns to normal), comparing milk from the two halves of the same goat and identifying halves with high cell counts for bacteriology sampling.

Bacteriology on a sterile milk sample

In some types of mastitis excretion of bacteria is only intermittent, for example *Pseudomonas* spp. and chronic *Staphylococcus aureus*. Coagulase-positive *Staph. aureus* is the most common cause of caprine mastitis.

Collect a sample. Clean the teats thoroughly with 70% ethanol, discard foremilk, collect 20 ml of milk from each udder half in sterile containers. If not tested immediately store at 4 °C (the sample can be frozen for several weeks if necessary).

It is only necessary to use standard bacterial media in the United Kingdom, as *Mycoplasma* spp. are not implicated in mastitis. In areas of the world with *Mycoplasma* mastitis, special techniques are required. The bacteria present should be identified and antibiotic sensitivity tests carried out. Coagulase positive *Staph. aureus* is the commonest cause of caprine mastitis, causing gangrenous, non-gangrenous or subclinical mastitis. Coagulase negative *Staphylococci* are the most frequently isolated organisms, but are of uncertain significance and probably commensals rather than primary pathogens.

Environmental mastitis caused by organisms such as *E. coli*, *Pseudomonas* spp. and *Klebsiella* spp. is rare and most frequently seen as subclinical mastitis.

Many other bacteria, including *Streptococcus* spp. and *Pasteurella haemolytica* occasionally cause mastitis. *Yersinia pseudotuberculosis* has been isolated from the milk of an aborting goat. Fungi and yeasts such as *Candida albicans* are occasionally isolated.

Mycoplasma spp. have not been reported as causing mastitis in the United Kingdom, but they are an important problem in many other countries including a number of EU members (see later in this chapter)

Acute phase proteins

Acute phase proteins are inflammatory proteins released specifically in response to infection or tissue injury. They include haptoglobin, fibrinogen, C-reactive protein, alpha-1 acid glycoprotein and serum amyloid A. *Milk amyloid A*, which is produced by mammary epithelial cells, and *haptoglobin* are being investigated as indicators of mastitis.

Ultrasonography

A 5 MHz linear array or sector scanner can be used to examine the udder and identify deep-seated pathology that is not readily palpable. The normal udder displays a uniform mixture of hyperechogenic and hypoechogenic material. Abscesses, tumours, haematomas and fibrotic tissue are hyperechogenic and milk is hypoechogenic.

Clinical mastitis

Peracute or gangrenous mastitis
Aetiology
- Commonly *Staphylococcus aureus* infection following a slight injury to the teat at any stage of lactation; occasionally *E. coli* and *Bacillus* species.

Clinical signs
- Marked pyrexia in early stages, often progressing to a toxaemia with subnormal temperature and death; may present as sudden death.
- Udder hard, hot, swollen and painful; minimal thin, bloody serous fluid from teat.
- Pain syndrome – teeth grinding, rapid pulse.

Prognosis
- Guarded; if the animal survives, the affected half becomes gangrenous, cold and clammy, turning blue through purple to black and eventually sloughing.

Treatment
- Economically, treatment is often not worthwhile. In a pet goat or where the goat is to be kept for breeding, treatment is aimed at controlling toxaemia, rather than saving the udder.
- Intensive intravenous antibiotic therapy.

Ampicillin, 3 mg/kg, every 8 hours
Oxytetracycline, 3–10 mg/kg, every 12–24 hours
Fluoroquinalones, 1.25–2.5 mg/kg every 24 hours

- Non-steroidal anti-inflammatory drugs will help reduce the systemic and local udder temperature, decrease the production of inflammatory mediators and improve the clinical demeanour of the animal.

Carprofen, 1.4 mg/kg, i.v.
Flunixin meglumine, 2 mg/kg, i.v.
Ketoprofen, 3 mg/kg, i.v.
Meloxicam, 2 mg/kg initial dose then 0.5 mg/kg every 36–48 hours, i.v.

- Intravenous fluid therapy, 100–200 ml/kg over 4–5 hours.
- Good nursing – rugs, heat and human company.

As the udder sloughs and the teat is lost, milk may still be produced by the dorsal portion and mastectomy (see Chapter 23) may be necessary. Mastectomy can also be considered in male goats. Partial mastectomies under local or general anaesthetic may also be necessary to remove unsightly or necrotic tissue.

- As an alternative to mastectomy, infusions of Lugol's iodine or 100–120 ml of acriflavine or 60 ml of 10% formalin under local anaesthetic can be used to dry up the affected half where this is legal.

Acute mastitis
Aetiology
- A number of different bacteria.

Clinical signs
- Pyrexia, anorexia, lethargy.
- Udder hard, swollen and painful.
- Milk yield decreased; milk consistency changed.
- Milk often thin and watery with clots.

Prognosis
- Clinical recovery may result in subclinical disease or fibrosis and atrophy of the half.

Treatment
- Broad-spectrum antibiotics – parenteral and intramammary. *Staphylococcus aureus* is the most frequent cause of mastitis, so initial treatment should be aimed at this organism, which is frequently penicillin resistant. Use cephalosporins, cloxacillin or amoxycillin/clavulanic acid preparations. Better results are achieved by using parenteral and intramammary antibiotics together, as some drugs, for example cephalosporins, do not pass easily from blood to milk. Use a specific antibiotic once the results of laboratory tests are known.

At the present time, there are no intramammary preparations specifically licensed for goats available in the United Kingdom. Experimental work shows clearly that clearance times of antibiotic preparations from the mammary gland of goats may differ markedly from those from bovine mammary glands. In some cases, for example oxytetracycline and erythromycin, rapid elimination of the drug may occur to the extent that therapeutic efficiency may be compromised. With other preparations, for example amoxycillin trihydrate/potassium clavulanate, prednisolone (Synulox, Zoetis) a withholding time approximately double that for cows is required. With all preparations used out-with data sheet recommendations a minimum 7 day withdrawal period should be imposed for milk.

In addition, the nozzles of some intramammary preparations are too large to be inserted easily into goat teats, with the resultant risk of introducing infection or traumatising the teat. Long-acting preparations, for example cefoperazone (Pathocef, Zoetis), may thus be useful in that only a single tube need be inserted and prolonged action can be obtained within a 7 day withholding period.

Note: when one half is treated, antibiotic may infuse into the milk in the other half.

Always thoroughly clean the teat with spirit before insertion of nozzles and use a teat dip after insertion.
- Oxytocin, 20 U, 2 ml i.m. or s.c. initial dose, then 10 U, 1 ml, prior to each stripping out 2 or 3 times daily. Given immediately before the use of intramammary treatment, oxytocin causes contraction of the smooth muscle in udder ducts, maximising the stripping of the udder, removing infective and toxic material and allowing greater penetration of the intramammary infusion. Higher doses are given than those employed for milk letdown in normal goats.
- Supportive therapy, as for peracute mastitis, if necessary – intravenous fluids and non-steroidal anti-inflammatory drugs.

Mild clinical mastitis

Aetiology

- A number of different bacteria.

Clinical signs

- Only very mild or no systemic signs.
- Local udder reaction, possibly with slightly swollen half, small clots or pus in milk; milk often thinner than usual. Most milk samples presented for testing are from goats that are not clinically ill but where there are a few clots or crystals in the milk, poor keeping quality of milk, milk taint or curdling on boiling milk.
- Prebiotics and probiotics are reported to reduce somatic cell counts and eliminate clinical mastitis by supporting the immune system.

Terminal fibrosis and atrophy

The endpoint of most forms of mastitis is fibrosis and atrophy of the affected mammary tissue as healing takes place. Lesions may be confined to localised areas or may involve the greater part of the half. Fibrosis produces palpable induration and decreased milk yield. Contraction of the fibrous tissue produces visible and palpable atrophy (Plate 13.1). Pockets of infection may remain and form abscesses (Plate 13.2).

Subclinical mastitis

Udder and milk secretions are clinically normal with subclinical mastitis, although fibrosis and atrophy may be present from a previous clinical infection. There is usually some reduction in milk yield which may be economically significant. There may also be a reduction in the levels of butterfat and no fat solids and a decreased keepability.

The true level of subclinical mastitis is unknown, although surveys have suggested a prevalence of between 17 and 36% in commercial herds in the United Kingdom.

Even without incurring direct losses due to discarded milk and the purchase of antibiotics, subclinical mastitis will still cause economic loss through reduction in milk yields. Changes in compositional quality will also affect the production of dairy products such as cheese.

Subclinical intramammary infections contribute to the total bulk milk cell count. There are also legal limits on the total bacterial levels in milk and the level of *Staphylococcus aureus*.

Bacteria implicated in subclinical intramammary infections

Various bacteria are implicated in subclinical mastitis, varying from herd to herd.

- *Coagulase negative staphylococci* are the most common organisms isolated from udder halves and many strains are reported. They are primarily skin commensals and, although their pathogenicity varies, may result in decreased milk yields and increased cell counts. One of the commonest, *Staphylococcus caprae*, can cause clinical and subclinical mastitis and will persist during the dry goat period if not treated.
- *Staphylococcus aureus* is more important as a cause of peracute and acute mastitis and generally only has a low prevalance, but if present subclinically causes a marked increase in cell counts and is economically important. Only a limited spread occurs between goats.
- *Corynebacterium* spp., Gram-positive rods originating from skin flora, can cause subclinical mastitis and raised cell counts. Their presence often indicates inadequate hygiene at milking. The slow growth of these organisms in culture means that they are easily missed after 24 or even 48 hours' incubation, so they may be more prevalent than previously realised.
- *Streptococci*, commensals of the oropharyngeal cavity, are isolated from udders less commonly in goats than cattle, but both *Streptococcus dysgalactiae* and *Streptococcus uberis* are occasionally isolated. They are of low pathogenicity but their presence in the udder is associated with significantly higher SCCs.
- *Pseudomonas aeruginosa*.
- Other organisms such as *Listeria monocytogenes*, *Nocardia farcinica* and *Streptococcus zooepidemicus* are occasionally isolated and are important because they are potentially zoonotic.
- *Mycoplasma* spp. should be considered out-with the United Kingdom or in imported goats, particularly from the Mediterranean area.

Treatment

- Subclinical infections are much easier to treat when the goat is dry.
- Bovine staphylococcal vaccines have been used to help control coagulase negative *Staphylococcus* spp. in herds with high somatic cell counts.

Investigating high somatic cell counts

See Table 13.5 later, which investigates a mastitis problem or high somatic cell count.

Mycoplasmal mastitis

Contagious agalactia

Suspect contagious agalactia when goats and sheep have agalactia, arthritis and keratoconjunctivitis.

The disease is most likely to be introduced through the importation of inapparent carriers, although contaminated fomites can transmit the disease between premises.

Incidence

- Contagious agalactia affects sheep and goats mainly in the Mediterranean region, including southern Europe and the Middle East and occasionally the United States, where it is a federally reportable disease. It is absent from the United Kingdom, Australia and New Zealand.

Aetiology

- *Mycoplasma agalactiae* is the recognised cause of contagious agalactia, but for regulatory purposes the OIE also recognises *M. capricolum* subsp. *capricolum, M. putrifaciens* and *M. mycoides* subsp. *capri* (*M. mycoides* subsp. *mycoides* (large colony type)) as causes of contagious agalactia. Only *M. putrefaciens* has been reported from Australia.

Transmission

- *Mycoplasma agalactiae* is shed for months via milk, urine, faeces and ocular and nasal discharges, contaminating the environment.
- Infection is by ingestion or inhalation.

Clinical signs

Septicaemia occurs in infected animals and the organism then localizes in the udder, joints and eyes.

- Pyrexia.
- Inappetence and depression.
- Mastitis, acute or chronic; swelling of mammary lymph nodes.
- Agalactia – milk production ceases in about 2 to 3 days. Agalactia is followed by udder atrophy, but fibrosis is

uncommon, so normal lactation may occur after the next kidding.

- Keratoconjunctivitis, with epiphora and blepharospasm, and arthrtitis, with marked lameness, may occur in the infected goats and in kids drinking their milk.
- Abortion.
- Mortality can be high in kids, in adults usually <20%.

Diagnosis

- Isolation of the organism from mammary secretions or arthrocentesis samples, using appropriate culture techniques for mycoplasma. Long-term surveillance by culturing milk is necessary to detect infected does.
- Serological tests – complement fixation or ELISA – do not permit specification of the mycoplasma.
- PCR testing is available for the detection and differentiation of mycoplasma species. However, some closely related species may be misdiagnosed.

Treatment

- Treatment is ineffective and, as animals are likely to become carriers, culling of all infected animals is recommended.

Control

- Vaccines appear to offer little protection and carrier animals are likely to persist.
- Identifying and culling infected animals.

Other *Mycoplasma*

Out-with the United Kingdom, *Mycoplasma* species are increasingly recognised as significant udder pathogens where special culture techniques are used to identify them. Infection should be suspected when clinical signs support a diagnosis of mastitis but routine bacterial culture fails to identify a causal organism. *M. argini, M. putrefaciens, M. mycoides* subspecies *capri, M. mycoides* subspecies *mycoides* and *M. capricolum* have all been associated with mastitis in goats. Milk production decreases rapidly and the udder atrophies. Both mammary glands may be involved and the supramammary lymph nodes enlarged. Mycoplasmal mastitis may be part of clinical syndromes including agalactia and abortion and polyarthritis, keratoconjunctivitis and pneumonia in nursing kids with variable kid mortality.

Control of Mycoplasma

- Antibiotics such as Tylosin 20 mg/kg i.m. twice daily have been used but treatment is rarely successful in clearing disease, a carrier state may persist and culling of infected animals is important in controlling disease.
- Vertical transmission can be minimised by snatching kids (see 'CAE control', Chapter 23) and using pasteurised or artificial colostrum + pastereurised milk or milk powder (also helps control CAE, Q-fever and Johnes disease). Pasteurisation at 65.5 °C for 1 hour eliminates *Mycoplasma*.
- Scrupulous hygiene at milking will limit horizontal transmission.
- Vaccination with strain-specific vaccines has been tried with variable reported success but vaccinated animals may remain persistent carriers.

Dry-goat therapy

Dry-goat therapy with long-acting intramammary antibiotic treatments should be used whenever there has been clinical mastitis or evidence of subclinical mastitis during the lactation; many infections, for example *Staph. aureus*, are easier to treat during the dry period.

There are pros and cons to using dry-goat therapy routinely; there is a danger of introducing infection when inserting tubes (especially with an inexperienced goatkeeper or a goat with a small teat orifice). In commercial herds, some veterinarians routinely recommend the use of dry goat therapy when the bulk milk somatic cell count level is > 1 million.

Always thoroughly clean the teat with spirit before insertion and use a teat dip after insertion. Always use a separate tube for each half.

> It is the veterinary surgeon's responsibility to advise the goatkeeper that milk withdrawal times in goats after using dry-cow therapy can be substantially different from that recommended for cows. The antibiotic screening tests in common use by dairies (see below) are extremely sensitive and antibiotic residues have been detected in goats' milk many months after treatment with some products, resulting in major loss of income from discarded milk.

Drying off

An 8 week dry period before parturition as with cows is generally recommended, although some research works indicates that this is not necessary. Goats should be fit but not fat – a condition score of 3 is ideal. Many high-yielding goats will still be giving substantial quantities of milk (4.5+ litres daily) at this stage. Milking should preferably be stopped abruptly – stopping milking stops production of prolactin, so naturally reducing milk secretion. In high yielders, the udder may become quite large until the pressure stops milk production, but within a few days the udder will shrink and become softer. Pressure of milk causes an inflammatory response so leucocytes collect in the udder, helping to prevent infection. Reducing concentrates for a few days before drying off may help reduce milk production in very high yielders. Milking only once daily for 1 week before drying off will also help. Udders should *never* be partially milked out as this increases the susceptibility to infection. Teat dipping for a week after stopping milking will help prevent infection during drying off.

The somatic cell counts of goats contain 40–87% polymorphonuclear leucocytes, unlike cows and sheep, where macrophages predominate. Goats have 10 times more cytoplasmic particles in their milk than ewes and so may be more resistant to infection during early involution. Neutrophils infiltrate the udder at drying-off, but have a short life span, unlike macrophages, which contain fat globules and cellular debris.

The milking machine and mastitis

The milking machine can affect the incidence of mastitis in three ways:
1. Bacteria can be spread from goat to goat on contaminated liners.
2. Teat-end damage allows bacteria to enter the udder. Teat-end damage can result from a number of factors, including vacuum levels being too high, defective pulsation and overmilking (Plate 13.3). Teats should be routinely monitored at every milking.
3. Machine faults that lead to rapid fluctuations in vacuum will cause milk droplets to be driven back up against the teat-ends. Milk may penetrate the teat sphincter and enter the teat sinus, spreading disease if the milk contains pathogens.

Table 13.4 Milking machine settings.

Vacuum level	37–52 kPa measured at the claw
Pulsation rate	90 ppm (80–120)
Pulsation ratio	60:40 (50:50)

The milking vacuum used varies according to the dimensions of the plant and the need to lift milk or not. The manual will give the correct vacuum level. Vacuum levels should be checked on the gauge at the start of every milking session and pulsation rates assessed on a weekly basis by inserting a thumb into an activated teat cup and counting the number of times the liner collapses every 60 seconds (Table 13.4).

Rubber liners require changing after milking 2500 animals. Silicone liners require changing after approximately 5000 milkings. Liners that go beyond their normal life expectancy will slip more, milk slower and increase discoloured teats.

Maintenance of the milking machine is a specialist job. Most milking plants require some service input from a dairy engineer every 750 operating hours.

Preventing and controlling mastitis

- Keep goats in a clean, dry environment, on a well balanced diet.
- Ensure bedding is kept clean and dry at all times.
- Goats are generally cleaner than cows, so it may not be necessary to wash udders before milking. However, udders should be washed if they are obviously dirty or if there is a problem with high bacterial cell counts in milk. Udder washing must avoid possible transfer of pathogens from goat to goat or from teat to teat:
  o Use a disinfectant solution; washing with plain water will probably cause more problems than not washing at all.
  o Use a spray system or wash and wipe with a single service paper towel soaked in disinfectant solution.
  o Dry teats and udder thoroughly with separate disposable paper towels. Water running down the teats will drip into the bucket or be drawn into the liner during milking, carrying bacteria into the milk. Wet udders during milking easily transmit infection.
- Routinely examine animals for mastitis at each milking; use a strip cup or filter in the long milk tube to detect milk clots. During milking the udders should be examined for cleanliness, teat lesions and teat orifice abnormalities and changes in the udder tissue.
- Selective foremilk either a certain proportion of goats on a regular basis and/or any animals giving cause for concern.
- Use a post-milking teat disinfectant:
  o To remove mastitis bacteria that could be transmitted from goat to goat by the milker or milking machine, for example coagulase negative *Staphylococci* and *Corynebacterium* spp.
  o To remove general bacteria from cut or sore teats (generally less of a problem in goats than cows).

The dip should be applied straight after milking has finished, whilst the teat canal is still open, so that a small quantity of dip disinfects the epithelium of the teat canal. Unused dip should be discarded at the end of milking or as soon as it becomes grossly contaminated. Individual animals may occasionally have a skin reaction to the dip or disinfection solution (Plate 13.4).

- Treat mastitis cases promptly, using the full course of treatment. Treatment failures are usually due to:
  o Using the wrong antibiotic.
  o Waiting too long before treatment.
  o Using too low a dosage.
  o Stopping treatment too soon.
  o Presence of microorganisms that have become resistant to treatment.
  o Failure of treatment to reach walled off sites of infection.
  o Chronic cases with poor recovery chances.
- Segregate known infected goats from the others:
  o At milking, milk infected animals last.
  o Do not allow cross-suckling by kids.
  o Do not feed potentially infected milk to young stock.
- Cull chronic or incurable cases.
- Use preventative treatment at drying off (dry-goat therapy) where necessary (but see above). dry-goat treatments have at least twice the cure rates of treatments during lactation.
- Keep records.
- Maintain equipment in clean conditions; milking machines should be tested regularly.
- Vaccines are available against *Staphylococcus aureus* and may be useful in herds with a known high incidence

Table 13.5 Investigating a mastitis problem or high somatic cell count.

Study available data:	■ Somatic cell counts
	■ Bacterial counts
	■ Bacteriology
	■ Milking machine service records
Examine housing	■ Space
	■ Bedding
	■ Cleanliness
Inspect milking machine	■ Cleanliness
	■ Teat cup and liner conditions
	■ Condition of vacuum pump
Palpate udders	■ Compare halves
	■ Heat
	■ Swelling
	■ Lumps
	■ Extent of fibrosis
	■ Injuries to teats or body of udder
	■ Superficial lymph nodes
Collect milk samples for bacteriology from	■ Animals with high positive California milk test
	■ Animals with udder abnormalities
	■ First lactation animals – infections will have been recently acquired and thus indicative of current herd situation

of the organism or gangrenous mastitis. The efficacy of vaccination is reported as variable.

■ Table 13.5 gives a rational approach for investigating a mastitis problem or high somatic cell count.

Antibiotic screening tests

Antibiotic screening tests are used routinely both on the farm to identify when milk is fit to be allowed in the bulk tank and by dairies to identify if milk is free of contamination. There is no single test that detects all antibiotics at the maximum residue limit (MRL) and tests may be oversensitive, that is they detect much lower levels of antibiotic than the MRL, so that milk which is legally fit for human consumption may be condemned.

Two residue tests are commonly used in the United Kingdom. *Delvo SP* (Gist-Brocades BV, the Netherlands) is currently the industry standard. It detects B-lactam antibiotics, penicillins, sulphonamides, tetracyclines, macrolides and aminoglycosides and is used as an on-farm test kit and by dairies to test individual farm samples. *Beta Star* (Neogen), which detects B-lactam antibiotics and penicillins, has the advantage that it provides a result in five minutes, compared to two and

Table 13.6 Sensitivities of antibiotic tests to EU MRLs.

	MRL	Beta Star	Delvo SP
Penicillin	4	2–4	2
Cloxacillin	30	5–10	15

half hours for Delvo SP. This means that it can be used as a rapid test before milk is unloaded at the dairy.

Both these tests are oversensitive to some of the B-lactams and penicllins (Table 13.6) and some false positives can be anticipated.

Table 13.7 suggests a protocol for investigating problems with antibiotic residues in milk and Table 13.8 ways of avoiding residues in milk.

High bacteria counts in milk

The bacterial level in raw milk is a significant concern for both producers and dairies. High bacterial counts will result in milk being condemned and producers suffering financial loss.

Bacteria numbers in milk are determined by testing the bulk tank samples that are collected by milk hauliers

Table 13.7 Investigating antibiotic residues in milk.

Causes	Solutions
Milk from treated goats entered the bulk tank before the end of the recommended withdrawal time	
■ Failure to observe withdrawal time	■ Provide ongoing farmer and milker training Ensure dispensed medicines are clearly labelled with the correct withdrawal period
■ Poor identification of doe	■ Visually mark (spray, leg band, etc.) all treated does
■ Forgetting doe was treated	■ Record all treatments in the medicine book so there is a permanent written record of all antibiotic treatments and withhold times
■ Poor communication between person who treated and person who milks	■ Wipe-board in parlour identifying treated does and milk withdrawal time Separate recently dried and treated goats from lactating goats
■ Keeping milk from untreated half	■ Discard milk from treated and untreated halves
■ Contaminated milk inadvertently enters tank	■ Milk treated does last or with separate equipment Thoroughly clean equipment after milking treated does
■ Purchased goat has been unknowingly treated (e.g. dry-goat therapy)	■ Test milk from purchased goats to ensure it is free of residues before milk is put in the tank
■ Pregnant does that have received dry-goat treatment kid earlier than expected	■ Check expected kidding dates and date of treatment to ensure that the milk withdrawal period has ended Whenever a goat kids early or aborts strictly follow the recommended length for the dry period Use appropriate antibiotic tests before milk is allowed into the bulk tank Consult with veterinarian and/or manufacturer
Prolonged persistence of drug in milk	
■ Cow withdrawal times applied to antibiotics not specifically licensed for goats	■ Use drugs licensed for goats wherever possible Apply minimum statutory withhold time of 7 days after all other antibiotic treatments Check with drug manufacturer for recommended withhold times (particularly important with dry-goat therapy) Consult FARAD[a] Avoid dry-cow products with prolonged action
■ Antibiotics used that are not approved for use in lactating animals	■ Only use drugs licensed for use in lactating farm animals
■ Antibiotics used at a higher dose or more frequently than instructed by veterinarian	■ Use drugs in accordance with label instructions, according to veterinarian's prescription
■ Drug administered by different route from label recommendations	■ Use drugs in accordance with label instructions, according to veterinarian's prescription
Antibiotic inadvertently contaminated milk	
■ Udder contaminated with antibiotic ointment	■ Use only products approved for lactating animals, according to instructions Follow a recommended practice of udder preparation
■ Medicated feed	■ Any medicated feed not intended for lactating animals should be kept separate from the milkers' food Use separate storage and handling equipment Store all drugs correctly; ideally drugs for lactating and non-lactating animals should be kept separately

[a]FARAD: Food Animal Residue Avoidance Databank, www.farad.org.

prior to transferring the farm bulk tank contents to the tanker. Sampling is mandatory and the bacteria count is determined using a standard test format, such as the standard plate count (SPC) or plate loop count (PLC).

Test results provide an estimate of the total number of bacteria present in the sample. The number, expressed as bacteria per ml, does not identify species of bacteria present, just the estimated total number. This value represents the number of bacteria that have entered the tank from all possible sources. It includes bacteria in milk from infected udders, bacteria normally present on teat skin and bacteria found in dirt on the outside of the teats and udder. It also includes bacteria in dirt, water and manure that may have entered the cluster

Table 13.8 Avoiding residues in milk.

- Use veterinary medicines licensed for farm animals
- Label all dispensed medicines with the recommended withdrawal time
- Ensure that the farmer understands that the drug is being used off-label and that, although the withdrawal recommendations are the best available, they will not be supported by the pharmaceutical company if residue problems occur
- Ensure all goats are correctly identified
- Maintain a separate treatment group and milk these animals last
- Take particular care if animals have been treated with intramammary tubes – very prolonged persistence has been reported with some products
- Discard all the milk from treated goats, not just milk from treated halves
- Observe the correct withdrawal period
- Use antibiotic screening kits as recommended by the manufacturer
- Test the milk from bought-in goats, particularly if they may have received dry-cow treatment

during fall-offs, liner slips or when components are rinsed off with water and contamination is carried into the system. Finally, it may be from bacteria buildup on inadequately cleaned milk contact surfaces anywhere in the system. Milk cooling problems may also contribute to elevated bacteria counts because warm temperatures accelerate bacterial growth. The objective is to keep raw milk bacteria counts as low as possible and when problems occur each of these issues has to be considered (Table 13.9). Additional test procedures, for example for coliforms and *Staphylococcus*, will help to identify possible sources of contamination.

'Hard udder'

'Hard udder' is indicated by a firm, swollen udder in freshly kidded goats (often first kidders), little milk production with poor milk letdown, and non-responsiveness to treatments for oedematous udders, for example diuretics. The milk appears normal with no evidence of bacterial mastitis. Increased milk production and softening of the udder occurs after about a week, but milk production remains suboptimal throughout the lactation because of the indurative changes in the udder tissue.

In the United Kingdom, at least, the condition appears to be part of the CAE complex. All goats seen by the author with this condition have been CAE seropositive and since the widespread introduction of CAEV control measures the incidence has fallen to zero.

Udder oedema

Occasionally, the normal physiological oedema of the udder, which occurs prior to parturition, is excessive, resulting in an udder that is hard and swollen. Unlike the 'hard udder' syndrome, milk production is not severely affected. In the United Kingdom, although some goats may need milking before kidding to ease the udder, it is extremely rare to have to resort to any further treatment. In contrast, the condition is reported to be common in British Alpines, particularly first kidders, in Australia, suggesting that some factor other than a normal physiological process is involved. In severe cases of oedema, hot compresses, liniments and frequent stripping may be necessary together with injections of a diuretic:

- Frusemide, 5 ml i.m. or i.v. every 12 hours for 3 days.

Trauma to the udder

Traumatic injury to the teats and udder associated with butting and being trodden on are common and may result in large painful swellings, possibly accompanied by mastitis. Any wounds should be carefully treated and antibiotic cover given to prevent the occurrence of mastitis. Gangrenous mastitis commonly results from quite small abrasions near the teat tip.

Teat damage can also result from incorrectly set milking machines and overmilking (see earlier in this chapter).

Abscesses

Abscesses in the udder may arise from mastitic episodes or from penetrating lesions to the udder. Deep abscesses are not possible to treat; abscesses just below the skin of the udder can be satisfactorily drained.

Fibrous scar tissue

Fibrous lumps arise as a sequel to mastitis or trauma. Because they are an obvious fault in the show ring,

Table 13.9 Investigating high bacteria counts in milk.

Causes	Solutions
Contamination by faecal organisms ■ Dirty goats ■ Dirty udders ■ Units drop off during milking	■ Check faecal indicators, enterobacteriacae and coliform, in bulk raw milk regularly ■ Keep goats in a clean, dry environment, including walkways and collecting areas ■ Restrict goat access to unclean areas ■ Keep animals clean ■ Review udder preparation ■ Do not milk goats that have diarrhoea ■ Regularly service milking machine
Contamination by mastitic organisms or their toxins	■ Establish robust mastitis prevention plan ■ Check bulk milk tank for level of bacteria, particularly Staphylococcus species ■ Use automatic conductivity metering in the parlour ■ Selectively examine foremilk with use of hand held conductivity meter if available ■ Check somatic cell count on regular basis ■ Do not milk goats with visibly traumatised or diseased teats/udders
Improper cooling of milk	■ Bacteria multiply rapidly when milk is stored >4C or cooled too slowly. The faster milk can be cooled down when it leaves the udder the better the quality of the milk ■ Ideal storage 1-2C ■ Cooling range 1-4C; milk should reach temperature within 2 hours and preferably 30 minutes ■ Temperature should never go above 10C when milk added to bulk tank and reach temperature within 1 hour and preferably 30 minutes
Inadequate cleaning of milking system	■ Check wash cycle - temperatures, chemicals, equipment function ■ Check water quality
Machine faults	■ Check service records ■ Check machine settings ■ Check for worn/deteriorated liners/rubbers

owners resort to numerous methods to try to get rid of them. Topical applications of anti-inflammatory creams, herbal remedies, etc., will reduce the size of surface lumps but the most successful treatment is cold laser treatment, initially twice weekly, and then weekly.

Pustular dermatitis of the udder

See 'Staphylococcal dermatitis', Chapter 10 (Plates 13.5 and 13.6).

Fly bites

Biting flies may produce quite severe lesions, superficially resembling staphylococcal dermatitis on the udder. Topical creams and washes will ease the lesions.

Tumours

See Chapter 10.

Orf

See Chapter 10.

Maiden milkers

Many kids and goatlings from heavy milking strains show udder development and milk production, particularly during the summer months (Plate 13.7). Similarly, older females may 'come into milk' every summer and then generally go dry in the winter, although some does may milk steadily for years without ever being mated. The vast majority of these animals do not require milking – milking stimulates production of more milk necessitating more regular milking, possibly predisposing to mastitis and acting as a nutritional drain on a growing animal. In well grown, well fed animals feed reduction may help control milk production. Milking is only necessary if the amount of milk makes the goat uncomfortable – the udder should be completely emptied as partial milking predisposes to infection; teats should be dipped after milking. The milk produced is normal and wholesome unless it becomes mastitic.

Treatment with prolactin secretion inhibitors, such as cabergoline, does not appear to influence milk production in these animals. Mastectomy (see Chapter 26) can be considered in does with large, poorly attached or pendulous udders that physically cause problems for the animal. These are often does in which the teats are poorly defined with large teat cisterns ('bottle teats').

Although a number of hormonal abnormalities, such as pituitary adenomas, have been described under a catch-all heading of *inappropriate lactation syndrome*, hormonal abnormalities appear to be uncommon in maiden milkers, although are more commonly encountered in older animals, possibly as an incidental finding.

'Witch's milk'

Newborn kids occasionally show mammary development and milk production. No treatment is necessary.

Milking males (gynaecomastia)

Many males from high-yielding families, particularly British Saanen and Saanen males, show mammary development and some degree of milk production during the summer months (Plate 13.8). The condition is often unilateral, but may be bilateral. For this reason, and to limit the risk of laminitis, the protein and energy levels of feed should be reduced during the summer. In most males, dietary management will control mammary development without resorting to milking. However, regular checks should be made as gangrenous mastitis is not an uncommon sequel in these animals.

The males are often related to females that are precocious milkers, that is come into milk without being mated, and females that are capable of extended, long lactations over several years without being remated. The karyotype of these males has rarely been investigated but their fertility is not affected, unless the size and proximity of the 'udder' raises the temperature of the testicles. A German Toggenburg goat, which was karyotyped, had no cytogenetic abnormalities and normal plasma concentrations of testosterone and oestradiol. Hyperprolactinaemia was considered the cause of gynaecomastia, leaving the semen quality undisturbed. A Canadian Nubian buck with active lactation with abscessation and mammary gland adenocarcinoma also had a normal karyotype.

Other males with gynaecomastia may have endocrine imbalances due to hypophyseal, testicular or adrenal abnormalities.

Milk problems

Blood in the milk ('pink milk')

'Pink milk' is usually a sign of trauma rather than mastitis.

Haemorrhage into the udder from a damaged blood vessel occurs most commonly in first kidders in the first few days after kidding as the udder adapts to milk production and the stresses of regular milking. It may also occur at other times during lactation, particularly if the goat is milked by someone other than the regular attendant. The degree of haemorrhage determines whether the milk is coloured pink or there is merely a pink sediment after the milk has been allowed to stand. Culture of a sterile milk sample will confirm the absence of infection in these cases – bloody milk is not a common sign of mastitis.

Treatment is usually not necessary, the condition being self-limiting in a few days.

Milk leakage ('weeping teats')

Milk will sometimes leak from a teat, particularly at the junction between the teat and the udder. Some goats have milk-secreting tissue in the wall of the teat and under pressure from milking, milk oozes through pores in the skin to the surface. The problem usually occurs shortly after lactation and first commencement of milking and, if pressure on the area can be avoided at milking, will often resolve itself. Cauterisation of the leaking area with a silver nitrate stick after each milking may help resolve the problem or suturing of severe leaks may be necessary. Milk may collect subcutaneously in the area rather than leaking out, forming a cyst (see 'Cystic dilation of the teat sinuses', below) which may interfere with milking.

Cystic dilation of the teat sinuses

Cystic dilation of the teat sinuses has also been described, with varying numbers of cysts 3 to 8 mm in diameter projecting from the teat surface (Plate 13.9), but without milk leaking to the surface. If the cysts are making milking difficult, they can be drained and then, with the needle still *in situ*, 0.25 to 0.5 ml of tincture of iodine can be infused to kill the aberrant milk secreting cells. Cysts destroyed in this way will not recur during subsequent lactations but new cysts may form elsewhere. The condition can be confused with the thickening and fibrosis of the base of the teat, which may occur as a result of repetitive mild trauma at milking in first-kidders.

Investigation of milk taint (Figure 13.1)

Initial assessment
- Individual or group of animals involved – generally an individual animal problem.
- Recent or persistent problem.
- Machine/hand milking – technique; relief milkers.
- Dairy hygiene and practice.
- Storage of milk.
- Type of taint:
  - 'Goaty' or not.
  - Obvious before tasting or only after tasting.
  - Present as soon as milked or develops over a few hours.

Herd problem
Consider:
- *Feed taint*:
  - Plants such as kale, turnips, swedes, garlic, cow parsley, camomile, etc., can produce an abnormal flavour in milk (see Chapter 21).
  - Certain diets, for example brewer's grains and especially those that are fermented, such as silage and haylage, may change the flavour of milk.
  - Sudden changes of diet to include lucerne or clover may produce a temporary change in milk flavour. Action. Identify possible sources of taint, house animals and zerograze on hay rather than green plants; introduce all changes of diets gradually.
- *Genetic factors*. Certain goats have a high natural lipase enzyme activity causing the release of fatty acids, particularly caproic acid. Action. Identify particular families of goats involved.
- *Vitamin B12 deficiency*:
  - Cobalt deficiency (see Chapter 9).
  - Helminthiasis (see Chapter 14).
Results in accumulation of branch chain and odd chain fatty acids and sweet sickly smell. Action. Worm animals and correct deficiency.
- *Mastitis*. Widespread subclinical mastitis may present as a herd problem. Action. check milking technique, milking machine maintenance.
- *Poor milking technique*. Bacterial contamination of milk.
- *Poor dairy hygiene*. Bacterial contamination of milk, inadequate filtration, cooling, refrigeration and freezing of milk.
- *Agitation of milk*. Releases free fatty acids, particularly caproic acid. Action. Check pumps and length of milk lines, etc.
- *Oxidation*:
  - Exposure to copper or iron (oily/cardboard flavour).
  - Exposure to sunlight or fluorescent light (flat/burnt flavour).
- *Storage taint*. Milk readily picks up strong flavours from other foods, etc.

Individual goat problem
- Identify goat.
- One or both halves of the udder involved? Unilateral generally means mastitis, bilateral may be mastitis.
- Examine udder for lumps, fibrosis, abscess, etc.
- If no bacteria is isolated, consider other causes of taint as discussed under 'Herd problem'.

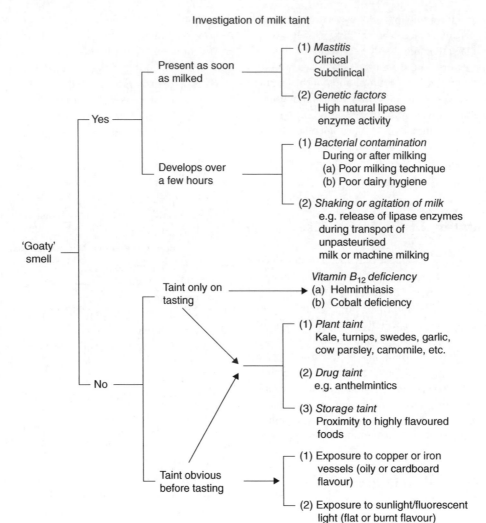

Figure 13.1 Identification of the cause of milk taint (after Mews, 1987).

Self-sucking

Self-sucking is a quite common problem in both commercial herds and small hobby herds, which once started is very difficult to stop. In larger herds, goats have been observed to self-suckle more frequently after milking, whilst high-yielding goats in show herds appear to self-suckle in response to full, tight udder prior to milking. Some of these animals may leak milk when the udder is full.

Feeding management is considered to be a potential factor affecting self-suckling, although studies testing for this hypothesis have found contradictory results. A significant reduction in the frequency of self-suckling was found in animals fed *ad libitum* with straw in addition to their ordinary diet. It has been postulated that this may satisfy the goats' behavioural needs by increasing their ruminating time and oral activity.

A variety of preventative devices can be tried – udder bags, Elizabethan collars, noxious sprays such as Bitter Apple, teat tape (3 m), etc. – but many chronic suckers are culled.

Teat abnormalities

'Pea' in the teat (lacolith; milk stone)

Occasionally a teat obstruction occurs preventing the flow of milk during milking. This is generally a small mineral deposit formed within the teat cistern, which is too big to pass through the teat orifice, but teat lumen granulomas also occur.

Mineral deposits can usually be removed by manipulation and pressure; removal of a granuloma or larger deposit may require teat surgery, with the teat opened along its long axis (see 'Teat lacerations', Chapter 26).

Supernumerary and abnormal teats

Supernumerary and abnormal teats are inherited defects, which result in disqualification in show dairy animals (Plate 13.10). There is thus an ethical consideration before surgical interference is undertaken. All kids, male and female, should be checked for teat abnormalities at disbudding, but many abnormalities will not become apparent until later. Discrete, definite supernumerary teats can be simply removed with scissors at disbudding or later. Double teats and fishtail teats are best left intact. Discrete supernumerary teats are not considered a problem by Boer goat breeders.

Teat tumours

Papillomatous tumours occasionally occur on the teat (Plate 13.11) and can be traumatised by milking.

Teat injuries

Repair of teat injuries is discussed in Chapter 26. Even small superficial injuries can interfere with milking (Plate 13.12).

Teat biting

Teat biting is a behavioural abnormality of adult dairy goats where one or more goats in a group start biting the teats of other goats, although the culprits are rarely identified. It occurs almost exclusively in groups of dairy goats when they are in season, but are not mated in order to delay kidding dates. The breeding season can be either the natural autumn period or an induced breeding season brought on by light control. The condition tends to worsen further into the breeding period, probably associated with greater synchronisation of females at successive heats, leading to a frenzy of activity at each oestrus period. The incidence within a herd appears unrelated to stocking density.

Lesions vary from scrapes and scratches through severe bruising to the tip of the teat being bitten off (Plate 13.13). The main problems result from bruising and the resultant teat occlusion, which makes milking difficult. One or more teats may be bitten, and udder conformation seems to affect the prevalence in some herds. Introduction of infection into the teat canal may result in mastitis.

Morbidity rates vary, are typically 1–2%, but can be up to 15%. Culling rates of affected animals vary from 0 to 50%.

Although male goats have been observed teat biting, running vasectomised males with groups of females is highly effective at preventing the condition, provided the males are sexually active.

In some herds teat biting is also accompanied by *tail biting*, the cause of which is not understood, but may be a behavioural abnormality that develops in one or more goats that have been teat biting. A dietary association causing pica has been suggested as a possible cause of tail biting in calves.

Further reading

Cystic dilation

Yeruham, I., Sharir, B., Friedman, S. and Perl, S. (2005) Cystic dilation of the teat sinuses in doe goats. *Vet. Rec.*, **156** (26), 844.

Gynaecomastia

Janett, F., Stckli, A., Thun, R. and Nett, P. (1996) Gynecomastia in a goat buck. *Schweiz Arch. Tierheilkd.*, **138** (5), 241–244.
Jaszczak, K. *et al.* (2010) Cytogenetic, histological, hormonal and semen studies in male goats with developed udders. *Animal Science Papers and Reports, Institute of Genetics and Animal Breeding, Jastrzębiec, Poland*, **28** (1), 71–80.
Wooldridge, A.A. *et al.* (1999) Gynecomastia and mammary gland adenocarcinoma in a Nubian buck. *Can. Vet. J.*, **40** (9), 663–665.

Machine milking

Edmondson, P. (1993) The milking machine and mastitis. *In Pract.*, **15** (1), 12–17.
Lu, C.D., Potchoiba, M.J. and Loetz, E.R. (1991) Influence of vacuum level, pulsation ratio and rate on milking performance and udder health in dairy goats. *Small Ruminant Research*, **5**, 1–8.

Mollram, T.T., Smith, D.L.O. and Godwin, R.J. (1991) Analysis of parlour design parameters for goat milking. *Small Ruminant Research*, **6**, 1–13.

Ohnstad, I (2006) Milking machine maintenance for dairy goats. *Goat Vet. Soc. J.*, **22**, 43–44.

Roberts, J.R. (1989) The importance of correct maintenance of milking machines in goats. *Goat Vet. Soc. J.*, **10** (2), 89–93.

Mastectomy

Arlt, S. *et al.* (2011) Mastectomy in goats with inappropriate lactation syndrome. *Tierärztliche Praxis (Groß- und Nutztiere)*, **39** (1), 27–32.

Cable, C.S., Peery, K. and Fubini, S.L. (2004) Radical mastectomy in 20 ruminants. *Vet. Surgery*, **33** (3), 263–266.

Kerr, H.J. and Wallace, C.E. (1978) Mastectomy in a goat. *Vet. Med. Small Anim. Clin.*, **73** (9), 1177–1181.

Toniollo, G. *et al.* (2010) Surgical treatment of gynaecomastia in a Saanen goat. *Acta Scientiae Veterinariae*, **38** (2), 201–204.

Mastitis

Anderson, J.C. (1983) Mastitis in goats. *Goat Vet. Soc. J.*, **4** (1), 17–20.

Baxendell, S.A. (1984) Mastitis. *Proc. Univ. Sydney, Post Grad. Comm. Vet. Sci.*, **73**, 473–483.

Bergonier, D. *et al.* (2003) Mastitis of dairy small ruminants. *Vet. Res.*, **34**, 689–716.

Berry, E. (2006) Update on caprine mastitis. *Goat Vet. Soc. J.*, **22**, 40–42.

Contreras, A. *et al.* (2005) Mastitis in small ruminants *International Dairy Federation Conference Proceedings*, pp. 67–74.

Cripps, P. (1986) The prevention and control of mastitis in goats. *Goat Vet. Soc. J.*, **7** (2), 48–51.

Karzis, J., Donkin, E.F. and Petzer, I.M. (2007) The influence of intramammary antibiotic treatment, presence of bacteria, stage of lactation and parity in dairy goats as measured by the California Milk Cell Test and somatic cell counts. *Onderstepoort J. Vet. Res.*, **74** (2), 161–167.

Karzis, J., Donkin, E.F. and Petzer, I.M.(2007) Intramammary antibiotics in dairy goats: withdrawal periods of three intramammary antibiotics compared to recommended withdrawal periods for cows. *Onderstepoort J. Vet. Res.*, **74** (3), 217–222.

Karzis, J., Donkin, E.F. and Petzer, I.M. (2007) Intramammary antibiotics in dairy goats: effect of stage of lactation, parity and milk volume on withdrawal periods, and the effect of treatment on milk compositional quality. *Onderstepoort J. Vet. Res.*, **74** (3), 243–249.

Kautz, F.M. (2014) Use of a staphylococcal vaccine to reduce prevalence of mastitis and lower somatic cell counts in a registered Saanen dairy goat herd. *Res. Vet. Sci.*, **97** (1), 18–19.

Koop, G., Van Wernen, T., Schuiling, H.J. and Nielen, M., (2010) The effect of subclinical mastitis on milk yield in dairy goats. *J. Dairy Sci.*, **93**, 5809–5817.

Manser, P.A. (1986) Prevalance, causes and laboratory diagnosis of subclinical mastitis in goats. *Vet. Rec.* **118**, 552–554.

Mavangira, V. *et al.* (2013) Gangrenous mastitis caused by Bacillus species in six goats *J. Am. Vet. Med. Assoc.*, **22** (6), 836–843.

Mavrogianni, V.S., Menzies, P.I., Fragkou, I.A. and Fthenakis, G.C. (2011) Principles of mastitis treatment in sheep and goats. *Vet. Clin. North Amer.: Food Anim. Pract.*, **27** (1), 115–120.

McDougall, S. *et al.* (2010) Diagnosis and treatment of subclinical mastitis in early lactation in dairy goats. *J. Dairy Sci.*, **93** (10), 4710–4721.

Menzies, P. and Ramanoon, S.Z. (2001) Mastitis of sheep and goats. *Vet. Clin. North Amer.: Food Anim. Pract.*, **17** (2), 333–358.

Milk hygiene

Edmondson, P. (2007) Avoidance of medicines residues in milk: an update. *In Pract.*, **29**, 147–150.

Milk taint

Baxendell, S.A. (1984) Goat milk taints. *Proc. Univ. Sydney Post Grad. Comm. Vet. Sci.*, **73**, 493–494.

Cousins, C.M. (1981) Milk hygiene and milk taints. *Goat Vet. Soc. J.*, **2** (1), 20–24.

Knight, A.P. and Walter, R.G. (eds) (2004) Plants affecting the mammary gland. In: *A Guide to Plant Poisoning of Animals in North America*. Teton New Media, Jackson, Wyoming.

Mews, A. (1987) Goat milk taints. *Goat Vet. Soc. J.*, **8** (1), 29–31.

Probiotics

Baines, D.D.S. *et al.* (2011). Characterization of haemorrhagic enteritis in dairy goats and the effectiveness of probiotic and prebiotic applications in alleviating morbidity and production losses. *Fungal Genomics and Biology*, **1** (1), 1000102.

Self-suckling

Martinez-de la Puente, J. *et al.* (2011) Effects of feeding management and time of day on the occurrence of self-suckling in dairy goats. *Vet. Rec.*, **168** (14), 378.

Somatic cell counts

Bagnicka, E. *et al.* (2011) Relationship between somatic cell count and bacteria pathogens in goat milk. *Small Ruminant Res.*, **100**, 72–77.

Barth, K., Aulrich, K., Müller, U. and Knappstein, K. (2010) Somatic cell count, lactoferrin and NAGase activity in milk of infected and non-infected udder halves of dairy goats. *Small Ruminant Res.*, **94**, 161–166.

Boulaaba, A., Grabowski, N. and Klein, G. (2011) Differential cell count of caprine milk by flow cytometry and microscopy. *Small Ruminant Res.*, **97**, 117–123.

Hall, S.M. and Rycroft, A.N. (2007) Causative organisms and somatic cell counts in subclinical intramammary infections in milking goats in the UK. *Vet. Rec.*, **161** (1), 19–22.

Koop, G., Van Wernen, T., Toft, N. and Nielen, M. (2011) Estimating test characteristics of somatic cell count to detect *Staphylococcus aureus*-infected dairy goats using latent class analysis. *J. Dairy Sci.*, **94**, 2902–2911.

McDougall, S., Lopez-Villalobos, N. and Prosser, C.G. (2011) Relationship between estimated breeding value for somatic cell count and prevalence of intramammary infection in dairy goats. *New Zealand Vet. J.*, **59** (6), 300–304.

Min, B.R., Tomita, G. and Hart, S.P. (2007) Effects of subclinical intramammary infection on somatic cell counts and chemical composition of goats' milk. *J. Dairy Res.*, **74** (2), 204–210.

Paape, M.J. and Capuco, A.V. (1997) Cellular defense mechanisms in the udder and lactation of goats. *J. Anim. Sci.*, **75**, 556–565.

Park, Y.W. (1991) Interrelationships between somatic cell counts, electrical conductivity, bacteria counts, percent fat and protein in goat milk. *Small Ruminant Research*, **5**, 367–375.

Persson, Y. and Olofsson, I. (2011) Direct and indirect measurement of somatic cell count as indicator of intramammary infection in dairy goats. *Acta Vet. Scand.*, **53**, 15.

Souza, E.N. *et al.* (2012) Somatic cell count in small ruminants: friend or foe? *Small Ruminant Res.*, **107** (2–3), 65–75.

Teat biting

Coleshaw, P.R. (2004) Teat biting in goats. *Goat Vet. Soc. J.*, **20**, 8.

Udder conditions

Baxendell, S.A. (1984) Other udder conditions of goats. *Proc. Univ. Sydney Post Grad. Comm. Vet. Sci.*, **73**, 484–489.

Karzis, J., Donkin, E.F. and Petzer, I.M. (2007) Withdrawal periods and tissue tolerance after intramammary antibiotic treatment of dairy goats with clinical mastitis. *Onderstepoort J. Vet. Res.*, **74** (4), 282–288.

Yeruham, I. *et al.* (2005) Cystic dilation of the teat sinuses in doe goats. *Vet. Rec.*, **156** (26), 844.

Ultrasonography

Fasulkov, I.R. (2012) Ultrasonography of the mammary gland in ruminants: A review. *Bulgarian J. Vet. Med.*, **15** (1), 1–12.

Fasulkov, I.R., Georgiev, P.I.A., Antonov, A.L. and Atanasov, A.S. (2010) B mode ultra-sonography of mammary glands in goats during the lactation period. *Bulgarian J. Vet. Med.*, **13**, 245–251.

Fasulkov, I., Yotov, S., Atanasov, A. and Antonov, A. (2013). Evaluation of different techniques of teat ultrasonography in goats. *J. Fac. Vet. Med. Istanbul Univ.*, **39** (1), 33–39.

Santos, V.J.C. *et al.* (2014) Conventional and Doppler ultrasonography on a goat with gangrenous mastitis *Arq. Bras. Med. Vet. Zootec.* (online), **66** (6) [cited 2015-08-30], 1931–1935. Available at: http://www.scielo.br/scielo.php?script=sci_arttext&pid=S0102-09352014000601931&lng=en&nrm=iso. ISSN 0102-0935. http://dx.doi.org/10.1590/1678-7062.

Slosarz, P. *et al.* (2010) Machine induced changes of caprine teats diagnosed by ultrasonography. *African J. Biotech.*, **9** (50), 8698–8703.

Wojtowski, J. *et al.* (2006) Application of ultrasound technique for cistern size measurement in dairy goats. *Archiv Tierzucht, Dummerstorf*, **49** (4), 382–388.

CHAPTER 14

Diarrhoea

Diarrhoea may be produced by a number of pathogens, toxic substances and nutritional causes.

Initial assessment

The preliminary history should consider:
- Individual or group problem.
- Age of animal(s).
- Weaned or unweaned.
- Acute or chronic problem.
- Nutrition:
  - Basic diet.
  - Change in diet.
  - Level of concentrate feed (change in batch, excessive amount).
  - Possible mineral deficiencies.
- If unweaned kids, consider:
  - On dam or artificially reared.
  - Whole milk or milk replacer.
  - Ad lib or restricted feed.
  - Bottle, bowl or machine fed.
  - Type of milk powder, concentration fed and temperature.
  - One person or number of people responsible for feeding.
- Housing:
  - Individual or group.
  - Deep litter or slats.
  - Mixing of age groups.
- Grazing:
  - Zero grazed.
  - Access to pasture.
  - Pasture rotation.
- Access to toxic materials or plants.
- Preventative medications.
- Clostridial vaccinations.

- Anthelmintics (frequency, dose rate, accurate assessments of weight? class of anthelmintics).

Clinical examination

A full detailed clinical examination is essential to reach an accurate diagnosis.
- Diarrhoeic animals may be hypoproteinaemic with signs of oedema, for example bottle jaw, and/or anaemia (see Chapter 18).
- Examine mucous membranes.
- The diarrhoea may be a secondary problem, for example in severe toxaemias such as acute mastitis.
- Animals may be bright, afebrile and eager to feed or dull, lethargic, pyrexic and anorexic.
- Note type and consistency of faeces – colour, mucus, blood.
- Presence or absence of abdominal pain (see also Chapter 15).
- Signs of dehydration.

Laboratory investigation

- Fresh material is essential for diagnosis. Submission of a live, acutely ill animal may make a definitive diagnosis easier.
- A *faeces sample* (20 to 30 ml) should be collected early in the course of the disease. The submission of a good faeces sample enables the laboratory to perform a range of different tests appropriate to the age of the animal from which the sample was taken, including bacterial smears and cultures, virology and examinations for roundworms and fluke eggs and protozoan parasites. A faecal swab does not permit diagnosis of anything other than a bacterial infection.

Diseases of the Goat, Fourth Edition. John Matthews.
© 2016 John Wiley & Sons, Ltd. Published 2016 by John Wiley & Sons, Ltd.

The sample should be as fresh as possible, ideally collected directly from the rectum or from the ground immediately after defaecation. It should be placed in an airtight container and stored at 4 °C if there is any delay its submission to the laboratory.

- A complete range of samples for investigation from a live animal includes:

  o Fresh faeces; air-dried smears of fresh faeces.

  o Blood samples: EDTA, serum and air-dried blood films.

- At post-mortem, freshly fixed sections from all levels of the small and large intestine and unopened loops of intestine.

- The antibody status of kids can be assessed by the use of the *zinc sulphate turbidity test* on serum.

Treatment of kids

Specific treatments should be instigated where the cause of the diarrhoea is known. In other cases or before a laboratory diagnosis is reached, symptomatic treatments may be of value.

- Keep the kid warm and dry.
- Isolate infected kid(s). If infectious disease is suspected, wherever possible move healthy kids to a clean pen.
- *Kids with diarrhoea should continue to receive milk,* but if nutritional scour is suspected where milk replacer is being fed, feeding practices should be investigated and

corrected as necessary (see below). Feeding milk:

  o Maintains the kid's energy input. Prolonged feeding of oral hydration solutions alone will result in energy starvation, as only about 30% of the kid's daily energy requirements will be met.

  o Maintains lactose levels, stimulating lactase activity and reducing the risk of diarrhoea relapses.

  o Provides antimicrobial, lactoferrines, lactoperoxidases and lysozymes

  o Maintains the correct abomasal pH.

- *Avoid diluting milk with water or oral replacement fluids* containing bicarbonate and citrate as it inhibits milk clotting.

- *Dehydrated kids will additionally require fluid therapy to replace fluid loss and correct the electrolyte imbalance,* either with oral rehydration therapy or intravenous fluids in valuable animals.

  o Rehydration gels containing propionate and formate to maintain the acid/base balance (rather than bicarbonate or citrate) can be added to milk as they do not prevent milk clotting.

  o Oral rehydration therapy with electrolyte solutions, 250–500 ml (50 ml/kg) every 6 hours.

  o Healthy diarrhoeic kids will generally drink from a bottle.

  o Intravenous balanced electrolyte solutions, 20–120 ml/kg, given over a period of 4 to 5 hours, depending on the degree of dehydration.

The amount of replacement fluid required can be estimated from the percentage fluid loss based on body weight (see Table 14.1). A dehydrated kid requires

Table 14.1 Fluid loss and associated clinical signs of diarrhoea.

Percentage fluid loss based on body weight	Clinical signs
0–5	Mild, barely detectable, increased thirst
	Capillary refill ~ 2 seconds
5—10	Moderate, mouth dry, skin remains erect when pinched, tacky mucous membranes
	Capillary refill 3–4 seconds
10	Severe, body cold, eyes shrunken, comatose
	Capillary refill > 4 seconds

Table 14.2 Amount of fluid required for 5 kg with 5% fluid loss.

5% of 5 kg to replace lost fluid = 0.25 kg + 10% of 5 kg for maintenance = 0.50 kg
Total fluid required is 0.75 kg = 0.751 = 750 ml

a weight of fluid equal to the estimated loss due to dehydration, plus a weight of fluid equal to 10% of body weight for daily maintenance. For practical purposes, 1 kg = 1 litre of fluid. Table 14.2 gives a typical estimation of the amount of fluid required.

Additional bicarbonate is required to combat acidosis in cases of severe diarrhoea, that is 150 to 650 mg sodium bicarbonate depending on the degree of dehydration (1 teaspoonful = 5 g).

- Use non-specific oral antidiarrhoeal treatments such as *kaolin* or *kaolin/pectin* mixtures. They are commonly used empirically, with apparently beneficial effect in young kids.

Note: gelling agents like pectin may lengthen the duration of scouring if toxins are present.

- Use *spasmolytics* to relieve pain and intestinal spasm:

  Metamizole, hyoscine butylbromide (Buscopan Compositum, Boehringer Ingelheim), 1 ml/10 kg i.v., s.c. or i.m.

- Use *non-steroidal anti-inflammatory drugs* for analgesia and to limit the cytokine cascade following release of endotoxin:

  Flunixin meglumine, 2.2 mg/kg

- Use *oral or parenteral antibiotics* if a bacterial cause is strongly suspected or confirmed, but do not use them indiscriminately. Some antibiotics may prolong the diarrhoea by delaying regeneration of the intestinal mucosa. In ruminating animals, antibiotic therapy may have deleterious effects on the rumen micoflora. Parenteral antibiotics are essential if the kid is septicaemic.
- Once antibiotic treatment has ceased, re-establishment of a beneficial intestinal flora can be aided by the use of live yoghurt or probiotics.

Treatment of older goats

Specific treatments, such as *anthelmintics*, should be instigated where the cause of the diarrhoea is known or strongly suspected. All diarrhoeic goats at grass should be assumed to be harbouring gastrointesinal parasites until proven otherwise. In other cases or before a laboratory diagnosis is reached, symptomatic

treatments may be of value. *Pain relief, spasmolytics* and *fluid therapy* are the cornerstone of treatment (see earlier in the chapter).

Treatment of individual animals with a non-specific diarrhoea can be frustrating. In practice, diarrhoeic goats fall into two categories, either acutely ill severely depressed anorexic animals that require analgesia and fluid therapy or less severely affected animals in which the diarrhoea is probably self-limiting even without treatment.

- *Restrict concentrates* for 24 hours, gradually increasing to the normal ration as the diarrhoea is controlled and correcting any obvious dietary excess. Continue to feed roughages such as hay.
- *Fluid intake* should be encouraged by taking water to the goat and/or offering warm water. If necessary electrolyte solutions can be supplied by stomach tube and dehydration corrected with intravenous fluids, via a jugular catheter:

  Percentage of dehydration can be estimated from Table 14.1 and then fluid deficit estimated:
  Fluid deficit (litres) = % dehydration × body weight (kg)
  After correcting fluid deficits and dehydration:
  Maintenance needs are approximately 5% of body weight/day (1 litre of fluid = 1 kg), i.e. 50 ml/kg/day or 2 ml/kg/hour
  Diarrhoeic animals should be given 2 × maintenance

The physical condition of the animals should be assessed daily and the fluid rate adjusted accordingly. Monitoring the *packed cell volume* (*PCV*) and *total protein* (*TP*) levels are useful in assessing the progress of fluid therapy.

- Use spasmolytics to relieve pain and intestinal spasm:

  Metamizole, hyoscine butylbromide (Buscopan Compositum, Boehringer Ingelheim) 1 ml/20 kg i.v., s.c. or i.m.

- Use non-steroidal anti-inflammatory drugs for analgesia and to limit the cytokine cascade following release of endotoxin:

  Flunixin meglumine, 2 mg/kg, 0.2 ml/4.5 kg

■ The value of non-specific *oral antidiarrhoeal medicines*, such as kaolin or kaolin/pectin mixtures, etc., is debatable because of the dilution effect in the rumen, but they are not contraindicated.

■ Human drugs to reduce intestinal intestinal motility have been used empirically, but are not licensed for food-producing animals:

> *Loperamide hydrochloride, 100–200 ug/kg, 0.5–1 ml/kg orally* (syrup), every 8 or 12 hours or *1–2 capsules/20 kg orally* (capsules), dissolving contents in small amount of water, every 8 to 12 hours

■ Use parenteral *antibiotics* if a bacterial cause is strongly suspected or confirmed, but do not use them indiscriminately. Some antibiotics may prolong the diarrhoea by delaying regeneration of the intestinal mucosa. In ruminating animals, antibiotic therapy may have deleterious effects on the rumen micoflora.

■ Once antibiotic treatment has ceased, re-establishment of a beneficial intestinal flora can be aided by the use of live yoghurt or *probiotics* or ground-up fresh faecal pellets from an adult goat. Probiotics are reported to improve milk production and rumen function in goats with greater benefits being derived when there are environmental or pathogen challenges present.

Table 14.3 lists causes of diarrhoea in different ages of goats.

Birth to 4 weeks

> Adequate intake of **colostrum** is important for preventing all neonatal diseases.

Preventing diarrhoea in kids

Environment

■ Kids should be born in a clean, draught-free environment.

■ Keep in small groups of a similar age.

■ Avoid overcrowding.

■ Provide clean, dry, well strawed pens for each batch of kids (Plate 14.1). Do not mix kids of different age groups.

■ Do not 'hold back' kids that have failed to reach target weight and mix with younger kids.

Table 14.3 Causes of diarrhoea.

<4 weeks	4–12 weeks	Older kids and adult goats
Dietary/nutritional mismanagement	**Nutritional mismanagement**	**Gastrointestinal parasites**
Bacteria	**Gastrointestinal parasites**	■ *Teladorsagia*
■ *Enterotoxigenic E.coli* (ETEC)	■ *Teladorsagia*	■ *Trichostrongylus*
■ *Salmonella*	■ *Trichostrongylus*	■ Rumen fluke
■ *Clostridium perfringens* types B and C	**Protozoa**	**Nutrition**
■ *Campylobacter*	■ Coccidia	■ Inappropriate feeding
Viruses	■ Giardia	■ Overfeeding
■ *Rotavirus*	**Bacteria**	**Stress**
■ *Coronavirus*	■ *Clostridium perfringens* type D	**Coccidiosis**
■ *Adenovirus*	■ *Salmonella*	**Bacteria**
Protozoa	■ *Yersinia*	■ *Clostridium perfringens* type D
■ *Cryptosporidium*		■ *Salmonella*
■ *Giardia*		**Toxic agents**
Gastrointestinal parasites		■ Poisonous plants
■ *Strongyloides papillosa*		■ Mycotoxins
		■ Poisonous minerals
		■ Drugs
		Hepatic and renal disease
		Copper deficiency

- Raise food and water containers above the floor to avoid faecal contamination.
- Clean deep litter pens every 3 weeks.

Feeding
- Ensure adequate colostrum within 3 hours of birth.
- Offer hay soon after birth and creep feed or goat mix by the 2nd week of life.
- Maintain scrupulous cleanliness of feeding bottles, teats, milk machines, etc.
- Feed milk at the correct temperature and concentration.
- Use the same dedicated person to rear the kids as far as possible.

Dam
- *Clostridium perfringens* type D vaccination 4 to 6 weeks before kidding; *E.coli* vaccine if a problem is identified on the premises.

Dietary scour

> Nutritional mismanagement is the major cause of diarrhoea in kids under 4 weeks.

The majority of cases of diarrhoea in artificially reared kids between 2 and 12 weeks of age are related to nutrition, either directly through sudden changes in concentration or type of milk replacer, changing between goat's milk and milk replacer, overfeeding or varying the temperature at which the milk is fed, or indirectly through dirty utensils or contamination of feed. Correction of feeding practices and symptomatic treatment will result in the rapid resolution of uncomplicated nutritional diarrhoea, but where secondary infection is involved the treatment may need to be more prolonged. Nutritional upsets may also predispose to or coexist with bloat, colic and mesenteric torsion (Chapter 16), all of which are potentially life threatening.

The role of infectious agents in diarrhoea in young kids

> The role of infectious agents in diarrhoea of young kids is unclear.

In kids under 4 weeks, the specific aetiology of the diarrhoea will often remain unknown. Viruses, such as rota virus and coronovirus, are commonly isolated from diarrhoeic kids but are also identified in non-diarrhoeic kids. Enterogenic *E. coli* can also be isolated from both diarrhoeic and non-diarrhoeic kids. In contrast, the identification of *Cryptosporidium* spp. is always significant.

E. coli
Coliform bacteria are commensals of the alimentary tract and can readily be identified on faecal culture. Enterotoxigenic *E. coli* (ETEC) are probably significant as a cause of diarrhoea in newborn kids and may complicate infections caused by cryptosporidia, rotavirus and coronavirus in kids up to 2 to 3 weeks of age. Other strains of *E. coli* cause septicaemia and chronic arthritis.

Aetiology
- Enterotoxigenic strains of *E. coli* (e.g. K99 and F41) produce an enterotoxin that causes the release of electrolytes and water from the cells lining the small intestine, resulting in diarrhoea. The enterotoxin is non-antigenic, but ETEC have antigenic fimbriae that enable the bacteria to adhere to the intestinal epithelium.

Clinical signs
- Acute, profuse, watery yellow diarrhoea in very young kids.
- Dehydration and death.

Laboratory diagnosis
- Isolation of the organism on faecal culture.
- Detection of the K99 and F41 antigen by isolation on special media and slide testing for the antigen with specific antisera.
- Immunofluorescence of frozen sections of small intestine.

Treatment
- Antibiotics – orally. Enterotoxigenic strains of *E. coli* are generally sensitive to the commonly used oral antibiotics, such as neomycin or spectinomycin. As ETEC do not invade the intestinal wall, affected kids do not develop bacteraemia, so parenteral antibiotics are not necessary.

- General supportive therapy (see earlier in this chapter).

Control

- Vaccination – multivalent *E. coli* sheep vaccines (K99 and F41 serotypes) are available (although not licensed for goats) and can be used in herds with a known problem. Does should be vaccinated eight and four weeks before kiddings.

Public health implications

Goat kids are important carriers of verotoxin-producing (VTEC) *E.coli* 0157, particularly kids. Although it does not cause disease in the goat, it is a potential zoonotic risk on farms open to the public. The bacteria are often present intermittently in faeces and remain for a variable time.

Salmonella

Salmonellosis causes peracute septicaemia and sudden death in neonatal kids and an acute diarrhoea in kids and older goats, often following stress, and abortion in later gestation (Chapter 2). Outbreaks of diarrhoea and abortion may occur concurrently.

Aetiology

- *Salmonella typhimurium* and *S. dublin* are most common, but several other serotypes have been associated with disease.

Transmission

- Infection is most often acquired from other goats that are excreting the organism and are either clinical or pre-clinical cases of the disease or symptomless carriers. However, other sources of infection may occasionally be significant.
- Infection from food and water.
- Infection from other domestic animals or man.
- Infection from wild animals or birds.

Clinical signs

- Lethargy, pyrexia.
- Diarrhoea, often profusely watery and yellow ± dysentery. Blood in the faeces is not a typical feature of salmonellosis in goats, in contrast to other ruminants (Plate 14.2).
- Abdominal pain.
- Dehydration.

- Death in severe cases.
- Sudden death in very young kids.

Post-mortem findings

- Enteritis, abomasitis, septicaemia, enlarged mesenteric lymph nodes.

Laboratory diagnosis

- Culture of faeces – rectal swabs or faeces using selective media.
- Isolation of organism from mesenteric lymph nodes, hepatic lymph nodes, heart, blood, spleen, lungs, etc.
- The organism may be excreted in milk.

Treatment

- Antibiotics – orally or parenterally. Antibiotics should be selected following sensitvity testing, particularly when dealing with *S. typhimurium*.
- General supportive therapy (see earlier in this chapter).

Clostridium perfringens types A, B and C

Clostridium perfringens type C, producing α and β toxins, has occasionally been associated with an acute haemorrhagic enteritis, particularly in kids under 3 weeks of age. *Clostridium perfringens* type B, producing α, β, and ε toxins, rarely contributes to disease in goats, but has been reported as causing an acute enteritis in kids.

Clostridium perfringens type A, producing α toxin, is a common isolate from cases of caprine enterotoxemia, but its pathological role is equivocal, as it is a normal commensal of the gastrointestinal tract and its presence is generally of no clinical significance. Enteric disease associated with type A is generally mild, with minimal damage noted in the intestinal mucosa, but it in the United States it has been implicated in causing hemorrhagic abomasitis in young ruminants, often accompanied by severe diarrhoea. *Clostridium perfringens* type A, producing β2 toxin as well as α toxin, has been implicated in disease in 5 week old kids.

Aetiology

- Clostridia produce β toxin in the small intestine causing local necrosis with resultant haemorrhagic diarrhoea.

Clinical signs

- Acute, profuse haemorrhagic diarrhoea.

- Abdominal pain.
- Death.

Post-mortem findings
- Severe haemorrhagic enteritis affecting part or most of the ileum. The mucosa is congested and dark red and large deep ulcers are often present.

Laboratory investigation
Confirmation of the disease at post-mortem is generally only possible in a freshly dead animal as β toxin is very unstable.

- Collect 20 to 30 ml of intestine contents, to which 2 to 3 drops of chloroform have been added, in a universal container and submit to the laboratory.
- Gram-stained impression smears from the small intestine show Gram-positive rods.
- β toxin can be demonstrated using mice protection tests with specific antisera or by an ELISA test.
- *Clostridium perfringens* is a normal inhabitant of the intestine and its isolation at post-mortem is not necessarily significant.

Prevention
- Vaccination of the dam in late gestation to confer protection on the kids via the colostrum (see *Clostridium perfringens* type D in 'Colic in kids', Chapter 15).

Treatment
- Administration of clostridial antitoxins if available.
- General supportive therapy (see 'Treatment' section in this chapter).

Campylobacter
Campylobacter spp., largely *Campylobacter jejuni*, have occasionally been isolated from diarrhoeic kids and are a potential zoonotic hazard.

Viral diarrhoea

Rotavirus, coronavirus and adenovirus have been reported to cause diarrhoea in kids. Mixed infections with enterotoxigenic *E. coli* or *Cryptosporidia* may occur. Other viruses such as caprine herpes virus (CpHv-1) have also been implicated in diarrhoea in neonatal kids, but the clinical significance of these isolates is unclear. *Rotavirus* is the most common enteric virus of goats.

Aetiology
- Three *rotavirus* groups have been detected in kids: group A (cattle), group B (sheep) and group C, but only group B rotavirus has been found in association with enteritis.
- Rotavirus infects and destroys the epithelial cells of villi in the small intestine, producing malabsorption and diarrhoea.
- At least two serotypes of caprine *adenovirus* (GAdV) have been described and adenovirus has been implicated in causing diarrhoea and dyspnoea in young kids in the United States. There are no reports of adenovirus infection from the United Kingdom.

Clinical signs
- Acute, profuse watery diarrhoea, dehydration and death.
- Many kids will carry inapparent infections.

Laboratory investigation
- Demonstration of viral particles in faeces by electron microscopy.
- Demonstration of viral antigen in faeces by an ELISA test.
- Immunofluorescence on frozen intestinal section.

Cryptosporidiosis
Aetiology
- *Cryptosporidium parvum* is a small protozoan parasite related to enteric coccidia, which parasitises the distal small intestine, caecum and colon, resulting in villous atrophy, blunting and fusion, reducing the mucosal surface area, causing malabsorption and deficiencies in mucosal enzymes, particularly lactose. The life cycle is direct and closely resembles that of other Eimerian coccidia, although it is as short as 3 or 4 days, so environmental contamination can reach high levels very rapidly.

Transmission
- Cryptosporidium lacks host specificity so one domestic species may spread infection to another.
- Purchased infected animals will introduce the disease into a herd.
- Mice and rats may act as a reservoir of infection.
- Infective oocysts are highly resistant and will persist in paddocks or in pens for over a year.

- Oocysts sporulate in the intestine and are immediately infective when passed in the faeces, so rapid transmission occurs.
- Kids are usually infected within the first week of life and are fairly resistant by 4 weeks of age. Infection may be contracted from grooming.

Clinical signs

- Watery diarrhoea in kids 1 to 4 weeks of age.
- Dehydration.
- Anorexia.
- High morbidity (up to 100%).
- Mortality may be high because of dehydration.

Post-mortem examination

- Post-mortem lesions resemble those due to other causes of diarrhoea.

Laboratory investigation

> The isolation of *Cryptosporidium* is always significant.

- Faecal smears air dried, fixed in methanol and stained with Giemsa will show the oocysts as blue circular structures with reddish granules.
- Oocysts can be concentrated by flotation in saturated salt or sugar solutions and examined by phase contrast microscopy or after staining.
- Cryptosporidium can be demonstrated in histological sections of small and large intestines provided the post-mortem material is very fresh.
- Fluorescent antibody on faecal smears; ELISA for faecal antigen/oocysts.

Treatment

- There are no licensed antiprotozoal drugs or antibiotics for the treatment of cryptosporidiosis in kids. Halofuginone, paromomycin and decoquinate are reported to reduce oocyst shedding (and thus environmental contamination) and to reduce episodes of diarrhoea in experimentally infected kids.

  Halofuginone lactate, 2 ml/10 kg body weight, can be given orally for the treatment and prevention of cryptosporidiosis. It is cryptosporidostatic, acting on the free-living sporozoite and merozoite stages of the parasite's life cycle, so that signs of the disease are reduced while the kid itself becomes more immunologically competent against cryptosporidium. It also suppresses the output of oocysts, reducing environmental contamination. Treatment should be given within 24 hours of diarrhoea starting to help individual kids and reduce oocyst secretion. Once diagnosed on the holding, all kids should be treated daily after feeding for 7 consecutive days, commencing at 24–48 hours of age.

  Decoquinate, 2.5 mg/kg/day (Deccox, Zoetis), can be dissolved in milk and fed to kids for 21 days. It has also been used to medicate the feed of pregnant goats for 21 days before kidding at the same dose rate.
- Symptomatic treatment, including correction of dehydration (see earlier in this chapter).

Control

- Improve hygiene.
  o Clean dry bedding.
  o Keep utensils and feeding apparatus clean.
  o Regular weekly cleaning of pens with high-pressure water; allow to dry thoroughly before restocking.
- Reduce infection.
  o Separate kids at birth and feed colostrum from bottle.
  o House kids in small groups, or individually, away from the adult herd.
  o Immediately isolate any kid with diarrhoea.
  o Use all-in, all-out system.

Prevention

- Ammonia-based disinfectants are effective. Once the disease is established on the premises, high-temperature pressure washing with detergent and hot water (>60 °C) kills infective oocysts.

Public health considerations

- Cryptosporidium is potentially zoonotic, causing no or only mild disease in adults, but possibly severe disease in children or the immunosuppressed.

Giardiasis

Although *Giardia* are commonly present in domestic ruminants, there is often only a limited pathogenic effect and there are few reports of clinical disease in kids.

Aetiology

- A protozoan parasite, *Giardia* inhabits the microvilli of the duodenum and proximal jejunum, causing villous atrophy and blunting.

Transmission

- Faecal contamination of water, food or environment by an infected animal.

Clinical signs

- Chronic but sometimes intermittent watery diarrhoea.

Laboratory investigation

- Demonstration of motile flagellates in wet faecal smears stained with Giemsa to show the flagellae, pear-shaped central bodies and binucleate appearance.
- Cysts can be concentrated by flotation in zinc sulphate.

Treatment

- Fenbendazole, 7.5 mg/kg orally for 5 days.
- *Metronidazole, 20 mg/kg, 0.5 ml/10 kg orally or s.c. daily.*

  Note: metronidazole is banned from use in food-producing animals in the EU.

Public health considerations

- *Giardia* is a possible zoonosis by direct contact with sick animals or through faecal contamination.

Strongyloides papillosus

Strongyloidosis is a relatively common infection, occasionally producing diarrhoea in suckling kids. Kids are initially infected via the dam's milk so feeding of pooled milk or milk replacer will reduce the number of larvae transmitted. Subsequently, infection is by ingestion or skin penetration and heavy infections may result in a localised dermatitis (see Chapter 11).

Diagnosis

- Faecal examination for typical embryonated eggs.

Treatment

- Any broad-spectrum anthelmintics.

From 4 to 12 weeks

> The common causes of diarrhoea in older kids are **coccidiosis** in housed animals and **gastrointestinal parasitism** in grazed animals.

Nutrition

Until weaning, many cases of diarrhoea in artificially reared kids continue to be related to feeding practices (see Chapter 6) and may be complicated by secondary infection. It is often difficult clinically to distinguish between diarrhoea caused by a nutritional upset and coccidiosis. Correction of feeding practices and symptomatic treatment will result in the rapid resolution of uncomplicated nutritional diarrhoea, whereas coccidiosis will require specific medication. Diarrhoeic episodes will cause kids to suffer a growth check and may be associated with bloat, colic and mesenteric torsion (see Chapter 16), all of which are potentially life threatening.

In older kids, as in adults, overfeeding of concentrates without adequate roughage either through bad management or stealing food (see Chapters 15 and 16) will cause diarrhoea.

Gastrointestinal parasitism

Gastrointestinal parasitism is the major differential diagnosis in older kids or adult goats showing diarrhoea, unthriftiness, poor growth rates, anaemia or hypoproteinaemia.

Unlike most other domestic ruminants, goats are browsers rather than grazers, preferentially ranging over a large area, often consuming as many as twenty-five different plant species. Many of the 'weed' species consumed by goats have a higher mineral and protein content than grasses, because of their greater root depth. In extensive grazing systems, goats will reject any plants contaminated with the scent of their own species urine or faeces, thus limiting parasite infestation. However, this means that, conversely, goats have not evolved with the ability to develop an acquired immunity to gastrointestinal parasites and adults remain susceptible to infection with gastrointestinal nematodes throughout their lives in intensive grazing systems and often have levels of infection high enough to cause clinical or subclinical disease. Because goats do not become fully immune to nematodes, they can develop and sustain much higher nematode burdens than sheep if exposed to the same level of challenge. However, because the severity of clinical disease is related to the host's immune response, the severity of disease in the goat may be less than in sheep with the same worm burden.

Teladorsagia is the most important parasite in cool climates. Worms develop in the gastric glands of the abomasum. As worms develop they destroy the glands, leading to increased abomasal pH and leakage of pepsinogen into the plasma, affecting appetite, digestion and nutrient utilisation and resulting in diarrhoea. Table 14.4 lists the helminth parasites found in goats in the United Kingdom.

Infection with intestinal nematodes produces villous atrophy and crypt hyperplasia, with loss of fluid and plasma proteins into the intestinal lumen, resulting in a protein-losing enteropathy. Loss of brush border enzymes affects nutrient absorption.Affected kids suffer a setback in growth or weight loss. In adult goats, subclinical parasitic gastroenteritis may produce decreased milk production, while more severely affected animals may lose weight.

Epidemiology

- The epidemiology of gastrointestinal nematodes in goats and sheep is similar, despite the apparent differences in the susceptibility of goats and sheep to infection.

Table 14.4 Helminth parasites of goats in the UK (after Taylor, 2006).

Helminth species	Comments
Abomasum	
Haemonchus contortus	Sporadic blood feeding nematode causing anaemia
Telodorsagia circumcincta	'Ostertagian'parasites. Common infection of goats (and sheep) causing diarrhoea and weight loss
Ostertagia trifurcata	
Telodorsagia davtiani	
Ostertagia leptospicularis	Ostertagian parasites of deer affecting domestic ruminants
Skrjabinagia kolchida	
Trichostrongylus axei	Common parasite of ruminants and equids
Small intestine	
Bunostomum trigonocephalum	Potentially pathogenic hookworm – relatively uncommon in goats (and sheep)
Capillaria longipes	Common infection of no clinical significance
Cooperia curticei	Common infection of goats (and sheep) and significant cause of disease
Cooperia oncophora	Parasite of cattle also affecting goats (and sheep)
Moniezia expansa	Common tapeworm of goats (and sheep)
Nematodirus battus	Can cause disease in goats occasionally, more common and significant in sheep
Nematodirus filicollis	Common infection and occasionally significant cause of disease in goats (and sheep)
Nematodirus spathiger	Common and occasionally significant cause of disease in goats (and sheep)
Strongyloides papillosus	May cause clinical disease in 2–6 week old kids
	Common infections of goats (and sheep) and significant causes of disease
Large intestine	
Oesophagostomum venulosum	Common infection but low pathogenicity
Trichuris ovis	Common but usually of no clinical significance
Chabertia ovis	Usually moderate and insignificant infection
Skrjabinema ovis	Very common oxyurid parasite in goats
Liver	
Fasciola hepatica	Occurs in goats in endemic areas causing disease syndromes similar to sheep
Dicrocoelium dendriticum	Rare in UK; confined to a few localised areas
Cysticercus tenuicollis	Metacestode stage of *Taenia hydatigena*, tapeworm of dog, fox and mustelids
Lungs	
Dictyocaulus filaria	Occasional cause of disease in first season kids
Protostrongylus rufescens	Occur in the small bronchi where they rarely cause disease
Cystocaulus ocreatus	*Trichostrongylus colubriformis, Trichostrongylus vitrinus* – pr<run onesent in the lung parenchyma
Muellerius capillaris	forming nodules. Mild infections, usually inapparent. Heavy infections may cause bronchopneumonia
Neostrongylus linearis	and emphysema
CNS	
Coenurus cerebralis	Metacestode of *Taenia multiceps*, tapeworm of dogs and foxes

- Larvae and eggs overwinter on pasture. Ingestion of overwintered larvae produces clinical or subclinical disease in late spring/early summer.
- A periparturient rise in egg production by goats kidding in spring gives a midsummer rise in pasture larvae – clinical or subclinical disease develops from mid to late summer onwards.
- Overt clinical disease or subclinical parasitism is occasionally seen in the autumn and winter months.
- The occurrence of disease depends on:
  o The degree of contamination of the pasture with nematode eggs by the adults and kids in the spring and early summer.
  o The subsequent grazing management.
  o Climate (rainfall and temperature).
  o Stocking densities.

Investigation of suspected gastrointestinal parasitism

- History.
- Clinical examination. Any of the following may indicate worm infestation, particularly in the kid or young goat, but all ages are potentially susceptible as only limited protective immune response develops with age:
  o Reduced growth rate/weight loss (see Chapter 9).
  o Reduced fibre growth.
  o Reduced milk production.
  o Diarrhoea.
  o Anaemia (see Chapter 18).
  o Sudden death (see Chapter 19).

Note: (1) Subclinical levels of infection may cause significant losses in production (weight gain, milk production, etc.) without other overt clinical signs.

(2) Combinations of clinical signs may be seen as animals are usually parasitised by more than one species.

(3) Trace element deficiencies can act synergistically with parasitism to cause poor growth.

As in sheep, the main species involved in producing scouring are *Teladorsagia* spp. and *Trichostrongylus* spp. *Haemonchus contortus* infection causes severe anaemia, oedema and lethargy.

Clinical signs and history may be diagnostic; if not, laboratory diagnosis is necessary.

Laboratory diagnosis
Faecal egg counts

1 **Kids**. Generally good correlation between egg counts, worm burden and disease:

> 500 to 2000 eggs/g faeces = subclinical infection
> >2000 eggs/g faeces = clinical infection

One to two weeks after treating with anthelmintics counts should approach zero. If not, suspect anthelmintic resistance or a drenching procedure.

Confusion may occur if kids are given anthelmintic treatment shortly before a faecal sample is taken as clinical signs may persist due to chronic intestinal damage even though egg counts are low.

2 **Adults**
  o Correlation is less exact and counts may be misleading:
    ♦ Depressed egg production as a result of partial host immunity: worm burden and therefore damage is greater than the count suggests.
    ♦ Worm burden required to produce clinical disease depends on other factors such as nutrition and milk production level.
    ♦ Larvae may produce disease before egg production.
    ♦ Diurnal and seasonal variations in egg production occur.

Note: significant worm burdens can occasionally develop in deep litter systems given suitable conditions of temperature and humidity.

Ten samples are generally recommended from a group of animals. Fresh (warm) faeces samples are collected from the ground, ideally 5 g (i.e. 10–15 pellets), and sent to the laboratory in an airtight container or bag to arrive within 48 hours, as any eggs that hatch into larvae would not be counted. Worm egg counts are carried out on two subsamples from the pooled faeces.

Kids at risk of infection should be monitored every 4 weeks or more frequently if mean egg counts are rising.

Worm egg counts are suitable for monitoring Trichostrongyle-type and *Haemonchus contortus*. When Trichostrongyle-type eggs/g reach 300–400 eggs in kids, treatment is probably indicated, but this will depend on the type of husbandry and pasture available. When egg counts reach 150–300 epg, it would be advisable to monitor frequently if worming is not carried out, rather than risk clinical disease occurring.

A *post-drenching efficacy check* can be carried out which involves carrying out a worm egg count on 6–10 animals 10 days after treatment. If eggs are present then further investigation is required to determine if resistance is present. It takes about 3 days for all the eggs in the gastrointestinal tract to pass out, so if treatment is 100% effective there will be virtually no eggs present at this time. However, because the drugs can shock the worms without killing them, but preventing egg production, it is necessary to wait about 10–14 days before sampling to ensure that non-egg-producing worms are not still present. This is most often seen with avermectins/milbemycin, although it can happen with benzimidazole drugs for a shorter period. Worms acquired after treatment will not produce eggs in the faeces for at least 18–21 days.

Plasma pepsinogen levels

- Levels > 3 U may indicate severe ostertagiasis.

Haematology

- Anaemia and hypoproteinaemia are consistent with Haemonchosis and Trichostrongylosis.

Post-mortem examination

- Identify various worms present. Goats are infected with the same parasites that affect sheep and also some of the parasites that affect cattle:

  Abomasum: *Haemonchus contortus, Teladorsagia* spp., *Trichostrongylus axei*

  Small intestine: *Trichostrongylus* spp., *Nematodirus* spp., *Bunostomum trigonocephalum, Cooperia curticei, Strongyloides papillosus*

  Large intestine: *Oesophagostomum columbianum, Chabertia ovina, Trichuris ovis*

- Estimate the number of worms present. The significance of numbers depends on other factors such as overall herd health, clinical signs, etc. As a rough guide:

Trichostrongylus colubriformis	4000 = subclinical infection
	8000 = diarrhoea in young goats
	20 000 = death in young goats
Haemonchus contortus	500 = subclinical infection
	1000 = anaemia in young goats
	2500 = death in young goats

Treatment and control

> Goats only develop limited immunity to nematodes. Control is necessary in all ages.

Adult goats are susceptible to infection with gastrointestinal nematodes and often have levels of infection high enough to cause clinical or subclinical disease. Newly kidded goats, kids and debilitated animals are most susceptible and control is most important in these groups.

Establish an optimum worm control strategy for each holding

Parasitic nematode infections occur in the same wide range of environmental conditions under which livestock are raised. Animal management and the seasonal patterns of parasite infections and species distribution vary considerably. Each holding is different and control must be adapted to the individual holding, as no single control system is suitable for all goat systems. The aims of nematode control are to *reduce the larval challenge to the goats to a level that does not inhibit performance or welfare*. Aim to *minimise the use of anthelmintic treatment*, using anthelmintics only when necessary, to *reduce the rate of selection for resistance* and to preserve drug efficacy for as long as possible by *selective treatment* and *increased refugia*.

Many pet goats, particularly those acquired as young kids, will never have acquired a worm burden and will not need treating; neither will animals not exposed to infection through routine grazing.

Monitoring faecal egg counts before treatment provides information about the worm status of individual goats and the herd and allows decisions to be made as to whether anthelmintic use is necessary. Faecal egg counts after anthelmintic treatment show the efficacy or otherwise of treatment. It takes about 3 days for all the eggs in the gastrointestinal tract to pass out, so if treatment is 100% effective there will be virtually no eggs present at this time. However, because the drugs can shock the worms without killing them, but preventing egg production, it is necessary to wait about 2 weeks before sampling to ensure that non-egg-producing worms are not still present. This is most often seen with avermectins/milbemycin, although it can happen with benzimidazole drugs for a shorter period. Worms acquired after treatment will not produce eggs in the faeces for at least 18–21 days.

All control strategies rely on a combination of:

- *Pasture management to avoid infection*. Controlled grazing methods allow pastures to rest, reducing contamination. Soil organisms – earthworms, dung beetles and nematophagous fungi – destroy parasite eggs and larvae.

  o *Extensive husbandry* allows goats to follow their preferred browsing habits, without close cropping of grass. Lower stocking densities in organic systems will help to reduce worm burdens.

  o *Rotation of grazing* adopts a 3 year rotation of paddocks, growing crops such as kale or lucerne. If pasture remains ungrazed for more than twelve months, it can be considered clean pasture, although a three year rest period is required for complete elimination of parasite contamination.

  o *Sharing grazing* with horses or cattle (not sheep) helps control, because:

    ♦ Various species of worms affect the different species of animals.

    ♦ The animals prefer different lengths of forage and therefore do not compete for the same part of the pasture.

    ♦ Transmission is dependent on ingesting the parasite larvae on certain parts of the forage.

  o *Preventing close cropping* of the pasture sward. The majority of larvae crawl only about 2.5 cm from the ground on to plants, so preventing grazing below this level will reduce infestation.

  o *Making hay* is fairly effective at reducing pasture contamination.

  o *Zero grazing* is the only financially practical solution for large milking herds because of the necessity to withhold milk from human consumption after drug administration.

Generally, only very low levels of infection, if any, develop in deep litter systems.

- *Limiting infection by grazing management, together with minimal anthelmintic treatment*.

  o *Maintain safe pasture*, particularly for kids. Safe pasture is pasture not grazed in the second half of the previous year or pasture left ungrazed until mid-July when overwintered larvae have died off.

  o *Kid early*, *indoors*, to prevent the a periparturient rise in faecal egg counts.

  o *Delay turnout* until mid-July when overwintered larvae on the pasture have died off.

- *Do not treat and move animals immediately on to clean pasture*. Traditional pasture management practices relying solely on anthelmintic treatment to kill the parasites introduce a heavy selection pressure for worm resistance. Since only the survivors of treatment form the next generation of worms, without dilution from L3 larvae on pasture, resistance rapidly evolves.

Pasture management practices that should be avoided include:

- Treatment and turnout to 'clean' pasture in the spring.
- Dose and immediately move to clean pasture during the grazing season.
- Poor man's clean grazing (2 or 3 strategic doses or treatment every 3 weeks from turnout to mid-June).

The importance of refugia

After any anthelmintic treatment, there will be some surviving nematodes in the goat. These will be the resistant worms. In situations where the offspring of these worms provide the majority of larvae for grazing animals, resistance will rapidly develop. To prevent resistance developing, a substantial number of worms needs to be left untreated each time anthelmintics are used so that these non-resistant worms essentially provide the next generation. The exact percentage that needs to be left untreated to ensure that resistance does not develop or only develops very slowly has not yet been demonstrated, but the proportion of the parasite population exposed to drug treatment is thought to be crucial in the drug resistance selection process.

Worms are *in refugia* (i.e. not selected by anthelmintic treatment) if they are:

- Larvae on pasture.
- In untreated animals.

- Stages in animals that are not affected by treatment (e.g. immature Teladorsagia with levamisole treatment).

In general, the larger the *in refugia* population in comparison to the exposed population, the more slowly resistance will develop. In a situation where animals are continually exposed to a nematode burden, a few worms are good for the goat by providing a source of susceptible worms, thus maintaining the effectiveness of the available anthelmintics for a longer period. The selective treatment of animals significantly increases the percentage of the worms *in refugia*, slowing the rate with which resistance develops.

Targeted treatments

The entire group of animals is treated at a time when there are significant numbers of parasites *in refugia*.

Before targeted treatments can be used successfully, it is necessary to understand:

- The parasite species present on the farm and their prevalence on pasture.
- The disease risk periods for the parasite species.
- The effectiveness on the farm of the various anthelmintic groups.

When the parasite situation on the farm is understood, defined faecal egg count thresholds can be used to trigger targeted treatment in groups of grazing animals when FECs reach the determined level.

The potential of using ELISAs in targeted anthelmintic treatment regimes by detecting antibodies against gastrointestinal parasites in milk and serum is under investigation.

Targeted selective treatments (TSTs)

Individual animals within the group are treated as necessary. *In general, anthelmintics should only be used if the goats actually need worming and have developed typical clinical signs*. Parasites are not equally distributed in groups of animals – 20 to 30% of animals harbour most of the worms and are responsible for most of the egg output.

TSTs are commonly used in areas where *Haemonchus contortus* is the most important parasite using the FAMACHA anaemia score to identify which animals to treat (see Chapter 17). In the United Kingdom, the commonest worms are *Teladorsagia* and *Trichostrongylus*, so, unfortunately, there is no simple means of identifying which animals can be left untreated, although body condition, clinical signs and faecal egg counts are all helpful.

- *High milk production* in grazing dairy goats has been shown to correlate well with high FECs; the increased protein requirements for milk production means the immune response is compromised, decreasing the goat's resistance to parasites. By targeting those animals with the highest milk production, anthelmintic use can be reduced substantially without resulting in lower herd milk yields.
- *Liveweight gain* in growing animals has been used to determine which animals to treat. If an animal is performing efficiently there is no need to treat, but any animal not reaching a determined target weight is performing inefficiently and so will benefit from treatment.
- *Improved nutrition* in grazing animals, particularly an increase in protein intake, together with the provision of an adequate level of minerals and trace elements, will enable animals to maintain condition despite carrying a worm burden.

If it essential to treat all the animals in a group, it is better to move the animals about 2 days before treating them. This allows the animals to seed the pasture with refugia before treatment, but only 2 days of egg shedding should not make the pasture highly contaminated.

Broad-spectrum anthelmintics

There are only four basic classes of anthelmintics available for treating goats (see Table 14.5). A novel drug, derquantel, is also available in combination with abamectin for the treatment of sheep, but there is no published information on its efficacy on goats and there is no intention to register it for use in goats. It does not have a marketing authority in Australia, New Zealand or the United Kingdom, where it is licensed for use in sheep and its use is proscribed in female sheep that are producing, or may in the future produce, milk or milk products for human consumption.

In the United Kingdom, there are no licensed products for treating goats. Products licensed for use in lactating cattle and sheep can be used in goats under the 'cascade' system, but milk should not be used for at least 7 days after treatment. Ivermectin is not suitable for milking goats as the withholding time for milk is 14 days if treated during lactation and 28 days if treatment occurs before lactation commences. Moxidectin is not licensed for use in lactating goats, sheep or cattle. Out-with

Table 14.5 Groups of broadspectrum anthelmintics.

Group 1	**Benzimidazoles**	**Probenzimidazoles**
1 – BZ White	Albendazole	Netobimin
	Fenbendazole	Febantel
	Mebendazole	Thiophanate
	Oxfendazole	
Group 2	**Imidazothiazoles/Tetrahydropyrimidines**	
2 – LV Yellow	Levamisole	
	Morantel	
	Pyrantel	
Group 3	**Macrocytic lactones (Avermectins)**	**Macrocytic lactones (Milbemycin)**
3 – ML Clear	Abamectin	Moxidectin
	Doramectin	
	Eprinomectin	
	Ivermectin	
Group 4	**Monepantel**	
4 – AD Orange	**(Zolix, Elanco AH)**	
Group 5	**Derquantel**	
5 – SI Purple	Available only in combination with Abamectin	
	(Derquantel, 5-SI + Abamectin, 3-ML; Startect,	
	Zoetis)	
	No market authorization for use in goats	

the United Kingdom, withholding times have been determined for drugs used 'off-licence' and drug manufacturers should be consulted. In the USA, FARAD (Food Animal Residue Avoidance Databank) provides a searchable repository of comprehensive residue avoidance information (www.farad.org).

What dose of anthelmintic?

> Underdosing increases the rate of selection for anthelmintic resistance by exposing nematodes to sublethal concentrations of anthelmintic.

Dose rates for sheep cannot be directly extrapolated to goats. Higher dose rates are often required in goats. The half-life of some drugs that are eliminated mainly by metabolism in the liver is, in goats, about half that for sheep. In addition, goats may also show a higher incidence of rumino-reticulum bypass, which reduces the effective drug concentration. Therefore, in general, a dose 1.5 to 2.0 times the ovine anthelmintic dose is recommended for goats. However, idiosyncratic reactions to levamisole have been noted in individual fibre-producing goats.

Benzamidazoles: >2 times sheep dose rate

Albendazole, Febental, Fenbendazole, Oxfendazole, 7.5–10 mg/kg orally (*20 mg/kg* has been recommended as a quarantine drench)

Mebendazole, *22.5 mg/kg* orally

Netobimin, *11.25 mg/kg* orally

Albendazole has a better efficacy than Fenbendazole.
Albendazole should not be used in the first 3 weeks of pregnancy (teratogenic).

There is substantial gut recycling in ruminants that increase the available drug so a lower dose is needed than in dogs and cats. However, as in small animals, there is a substantial improvement in efficacy by *dosing a second time* 12 hours after the first dose, as the contact time between the drug and the parasite is increased. It is unlikely that a 3 day regime will substantially improve efficacy over a 2 dose regime.

Withholding food (not water) for 24 hours prior to treatment will also improve efficacy by slowing the transit of digesta and increasing the contact time of the drug with the parasite. This is not recommended for dairy or pregnant animals.

Benzimidazole anthelmintics are ovicidal. If they are still effective against the adults, they will also kill the eggs.

Levamisole: 1.5 times sheep dose rate, 12 mg/kg orally

(Do not exceed this rate as levamisole is toxic in goats at dose rates approaching20 mg/kg; do not use injectable preparations; do not use during the last 3 weeks ofpregnancy because it may have some effect on uterine contractions; do not use indebilitated animals.)

Although levamisole and morantel are chemically different, their mode of action is similar. However, there may be some degree of difference in the level of resistance to them and levamisole *may* kill worms resistant to morantel and pyrantel. They are only active against metabolising worms in the gastrointestinal tract and have a short duration of effect.

Avermectins: use 2 times sheep dose rate, 400 micrograms/kg, 20 mg/50 kg, 1 ml/25 kg orally or s.c.

Note: there are conflicting reports in the literature as to the most effective dose rate of avermectins for goats, with some authors reporting that the sheep dose rate is equally effective in goats. However, in the face of increasing reported resistance, it seems safer to recommend the higher dose rate.

Moxidectin is not licensed for use in lactating goats, sheep or cattle and should not be used in goats producing milk for human consumption. Prolonged withholding times are required for other macrocyclic lactones.

Ivermectin is not suitable for milking goats as the withholding time for milk is 14 days if treated during lactation and 28 days if treatment occurs before lactation commences.

Ivermectin is excreted in the faeces with the highest levels occurring about 24 hours after treatment, so larvae hatching out of eggs will be killed.

Parasites resistant to ivermectin will still be killed by moxidectin for a time. The reverse is not true – if resistance to moxidectin develops, there will be resistance to all macrocytic lactones.

Monepantel (Zolvix, Elanco AH): *use 2 times sheep dose rate, i.e. 5 mg/kg, 2 ml/10 kg*

In New Zealand, there is a 35 day milk withdrawal period when it is used in lactating ewes.

Haemonchus contortus worms resistant to Monepantel have been identified in sheep in Australia, but no resistance to *Trichostrongylus* or *Teladorsagia* had been identified by 2015.

Authorised combinations of two different anthelmintic classes are available commercially, either:

- With different spectrums of activity to treat roundworms and flukes or roundworms and tapeworms. These products should only be used when animals are at risk from both types of helminth. When mixed infections are not a risk, narrow-spectrum formulations should be used

  or

- With similar spectrums of activity but distinct mechanisms of action fewer resistant worms survive treatment, possibly enabling continued nematode control in the presence of multiple drug resistance. The intention is to delay resistance by reducing the number of resistant genotypes that survive treatment because multiple mutations conferring resistance to each of the anthelmintic classes must occur for the parasite to survive. It remains important that there are sufficient parasites *in refugia*, so that selection for resistance to multiple anthelmintic classes does not occur. These products should only be used as part of an overall worm control strategy for the particular holding.

What route of administration?

In general, the *oral* route is recommended for all groups of anthelmintics. The use of topical anthelmintics ('pour-ons') in goats is not well documented and there is very little data available concerning efficacy and drug dosages in goats. Because goats carry less subcutaneous fat than cattle, the absorption of pour-on preparations and hence their bioavailability and efficacy is likely to be reduced. Even in cattle, the bioavailability of the avermectin/milbemycin drugs is greatly reduced in the pour-on form as compared to oral or parenteral routes. Pour-ons are absorbed relatively slowly and excreted even more slowly, leaving a long tail of subtherapeutic blood levels. *The pharmokinetics of these drugs as 'pour-ons' in goats means that regular use is likely to promote the development of resistance and should thus be avoided*.

Although a number of studies consistently demonstrate a high therapeutic efficacy of topical eprinomectin at 1 mg/kg bodyweight against a broad range of gastrointestinal and pulmonary nematode parasites of goats, it should be used only as a targeted treatment for ectoparasites (see Chapter 11) to avoid promoting anthelmintic resistance in gastrointestinal parasites. Widespread resistance to eprinomectin has been demonstrated in goats in Switzerland where it is widely used because it is licensed with a zero withhold time for milk.

Approved oral preparations for food-producing animals should be used whenever possible. In the absence of oral preparations, eprinomectin and moxadectin 'pour-ons' have been used orally off-label in the United States at the cattle dose. Alcohol-based ivermectin and doramectin 'pour-ons' should not be administered orally, although the equine water-based solutions can be diluted with tap water to produce a suitable volume for drenching. Diluting injectable solutions produces smaller volumes, which are easier to drench, than the oral preparations, so that the likelihood of the goat receiving the correct dose is increased.

Injectable formulations of avermectin/milbemycins tend to have a higher bioavailability than the oral forms, but different tissues have different concentrations of the drug available. For abomasal parasites, concentrations tend to be higher with the injectable forms, but for intestinal worms, the concentration is higher with the oral form.

However, given by the injectable route, levels of ivermectin persist that will produce selection for resistance. Thus for ivermectin, oral is probably better if the goal is to preserve its efficacy for as long as possible. Once resistance is present, it may be possible to get better results in the short term with the injectable form. For moxidectin, the injection is probably better for abomasal worms (*Teladorsagia*, *Haemonchus*), but the oral route is better for intestinal worms. Moxidectin persistence is prolonged with either route.

Note: Nematodirus battus has a different life cycle to other nematode worms as the L3 larva develops inside the egg. Treatment with anthelmintics is effective, except for injectable ivermectins or injectable moxidectin. Doramectin requires an increased dose.

Benzimidazoles are highly effective and there is no reported resistance in goats in theUnited Kingdom, so these are the drugs of choice. No anthelmintic has a persistent effect against *N. battus* so several treatments may be necessary over the period of risk.

Preventing the spread of anthelmintic resistance

Anthelmintic resistance is forever.

Table 14.6 Smart drenching programme.

Know the resistance status of the herd or flock
Sound pasture management
Keep resistant worms off the farm
Administer the correct dose of anthelmintics
Utilise host physiology wherever possible
Use selective anthelmintic treatments

Adopt a sensible control programme (Table 14.6)

There is a significantly higher selection pressure for anthelmintic resistance in goats than sheep because:
- Goats develop and sustain much higher nematode parasite burdens than sheep exposed to the same level of challenge. This means that a larger proportion of the parasite population is exposed to anthelmintic at the time of treatment.
- Anthelmintic efficacy is lower in goats than sheep.
- The contribution of host immunity is much less in goats.

Globally, resistance to each class of anthelmintic drugs in individual nematode species has been reported much earlier in goats than sheep. In the United Kingdom and worldwide, anthelmintic resistance has been reported in all the major gastrointestinal nematodes of goats, in particular *Haemonchus*, *Teladorsagia* and *Trichostrongylus*, but also *Nematodirus* and *Cooperia* spp. Resistance has occurred to all three main groups of anthelmintics. Resistance to one drug in a group confers resistance to all others in the group, because they have the same mechanism of action. Exceptions to this within the group are due to differences in potency and are only temporary.

The various species of worms in a herd may have different levels of anthelmintic resistance, so that, for instance, although *Haemonchus* may have high levels of resistance to benzimidazoles, the same anthelmintic may still be effective against *Trichostrongylus* and *Teladorsagia* and could be used to control these worms at certain times of the year when *Haemonchus* is not a problem. Similarly, some herds may have resistant *Teladorsagia* but susceptible *Trichostrongylus*.

Most studies have looked at fibre and meat goats. The situation in dairy goats in the United Kingdom is largely unknown and it is likely that in populations of dairy animals and pet animals that have never been cross-grazed with fibre goats or sheep, nematodes may remain susceptible to treatment with all of the three main groups of anthelmintics, although herds should be carefully monitored for the presence of anthelmintic resistance.

What causes resistance?

- Frequent treatment – 3 or more treatments/year.
- Treating and moving to clean pasture – no 'dilution' of resistant larvae by susceptible larvae.
- Underdosing – worms with low-level resistance survive.
- Treating when few larvae are on the pasture.
- Treating all animals at the same time – no refugia.

Detection of resistant nematodes

- The *faecal egg count reduction test* provides an estimation of anthelmintic efficacy by comparing faecal worm egg counts of the same identified animals before and after treatment. It is suitable for the detection of resistance at levels >25% in most gastrointestinal nematodes and can be used to detect resistance to all types of anthelmintics. Groups of 10 animals with, preferably, at least 200 e.p.g. each are individually weighed and ear tag numbers recorded. *Individual* rectal faecal samples are collected and an accurate rate of anthelmintic given. Faecal samples are collected again from the same animals 3–7 days after administering levamisole, 10–14 days after giving a benzimidazole and 14–18 days after a macrocyclic lactone. The longer period for benzimidazoles and macrocyclic lactones is due to the temporary sterilising action that these anthelmintics can have on female worms. Efficacies < 95% are indicative of the presence of resistant strains. A 95% reduction indicates that 1 in 20 of the parasites treated is resistant to the drug, compared to a 'native' nematode population never previously exposed to the drug, which might have < 1 in 100 000 parasites resistant to the drug. However, no reduction in the clinical efficacy of the drug will be obvious at 90–95% FEC reduction.

  False negative results can occur as egg production does not always correlate well with actual worm numbers and the test only measures the effects on egg production by mature worms.
- The *larval development test* is suitable for the detection of benzimidazole, levamisole and avermectin/milbemycin resistance. Samples with positive egg counts are submitted from any affected animal or representative sample from a herd (at least 6 animals). Two full universal containers (>50 g) should be submitted. The sample should be kept at room temperature. Nematode eggs are isolated from faeces and placed in the wells of a microtitre plate containing growth media and anthelmintic. The concentration of anthelmintic required to block the development of nematode larvae is related to the effectiveness of the drug in the animal. The mean faecal egg count in the sample should be >350 eggs/g but samples with >500 are preferred.
- Other *in vitro* tests include the *egg hatch test*, which determines the ability of eggs to survive in different concentrations of anthelmintic.

If resistance is diagnosed

- Stop using the group of anthelmintics to which resistance has been diagnosed.
- Alternate annually between the remaining two anthelmintic families.
- Check annually to ensure that these groups are still effective.
- Minimise anthelmintic use by strategic control methods.
1 Avoid introducing resistance on to the holding
   o For *any* incoming goats, inquire about the resistance status on the farm of origin. The introduction of susceptible worms on to a farm can be beneficial; the introduction of resistant worms should be avoided.
   o If goats are coming from a farm where there is no levamisole resistance, and preferably no benzimidazole resistance, they should be left untreated for as long as possible, as they will introduce worms with genes for susceptibility.
   o In the absence of reliable information about status, assume all introduced goats (and sheep) to be sources of multiple anthelmintic resistance.
   o Treat with an *effective* anthelmintic on arrival. The aim is to *deworm* the goats not just give an anthelmintic!
      ◆ In those countries where only the three main groups of anthelmintics are available, the best current advice is to treat introduced goats with the correct dose per weight of a *combination of drugs from all three older anthelmintic groups*, **e.**g. albendazole, 20 mg/kg, levamisole HCl, 12 mg/kg,

and ivermectin, 400 μg/kg, or a combination of moxidectin, 400 μg/kg, and levamisole (given as *separate drenches straight after each other;* do not mix drugs together).

◆ Where a group 4 anthelmintic is available, *drench with monepantel (Zolvix, Elanco AH) 5 mg/kg + moxidectin 400 μg/kg* given as separate drenches.

○ Yard or house animals on concrete for 48 hours after treatment to ensure that any viable nematode parasite eggs have been expelled before the animals go on to pasture.

○ Introduce the new animals on to pasture already grazed and contaminated by the holding's original stock, so that any resistant nematodes surviving the anthelmintic treatment will be 'diluted out' by the existing nematodes on pasture, thus ensuring that they make up only a small part of the otherwise susceptible population *in refugia.*

Note: the prolonged protection against reinfection with abomasal worms imparted by moxidectin will reduce the ability of worms already on the farm to establish themselves in the newcomers and thereby reduce this dilution effect.

○ Adopt biosecurity measures to prevent the introduction of sheep or goat faeces on to the farm by straying animals or as manure.

○ In the United Kingdom, fibre and meat goats and sheep are most likely to carry resistant nematodes and should not be grazed with dairy goats unless the effectiveness of anthelmintic treatment has been established.

Moxidectin has a higher potency than other macrocyclic lactones, such as ivermectin. It is concentrated in fat soon after administration, creating a reservoir from which it is slowly released, giving prolonged action against *T. circumcincta* and *Haemonchus.* This persistence of action is reduced in thin goats with little body fat.

Although there is side resistance between the avermectins and milbemycin, resulting in much higher levels of moxidectin being required to kill resistant populations, the high potency of moxidectin means that the recommended dose rate of 200 μg/kg is still effective against ivermectin-resistant populations in the animal at the time of treatment, but the persistence of action is reduced because the amount of drug released from body fat is too low to kill any resistant nematodes that are subsequently acquired by grazing.

2 **Administer the correct dose.** Underdosing increases the rate of selection for anthelmintic resistance by exposing nematodes to sublethal concentrations of anthelmintic.

○ Estimation of the weight of goats is often very imprecise and many goats are underdosed. Wherever possible goats should be weighed, for example while at shows in cattle markets, or weigh bands can be used. With the exception of levamisole, anthelmintics have a wide safety margin so overdosing is not a problem and groups of goats should be dosed at the rate for the largest in the group.

○ Drenching equipment should be well maintained and correctly calibrated.

The drench should be delivered over the tongue into the pharynx/oesophagus; it is essential that the full dose reaches the rumen. If the drench is put in the mouth, the oesophageal groove may be stimulated to close so that the rumen is bypassed and the drug delivered into the abomasum, leading to faster drug absorption and decreased efficiency.

3 **Only treat if necessary**

○ The minimum number of treatments should be used. Increasing the frequency of treating with anthelmintics increases selection pressure and leads to increased prevalence of resistant genotypes.

○ Establishing an effective control programme on each holding prevents unnecessary dosing.

4 **Rotate the anthemintic group used annually (?)**

○ Rapid alternation of drug families exposes a single generation of nematodes to two different drugs and may lead to selection of individuals with dual resistance.

○ *Annual (slow) rotation* between anthelmintic groups minimises the development of both single and multiple resistance when compared to more regular rotation, but it is essential to test the efficacy of each drug being recommended before changing.

○ *The effectiveness of the drugs being used in any rotation system should be determined every 2 years.*

○ *Targeted treatment using different dewormers* in different situations may be preferable to annual rotation on holdings where developing resistance is a problem. Different species of worms may have different resistance to specific anthelmintics in some herds.

o In areas where there are multiresistant worms and few effective drug choices, parasitologists are now advocating *not* to rotate, but rather to use one group of drugs until it is no longer effective and then switch to another drug. Rotation can hide the development of resistance because resistance develops gradually and resistance can develop to all drugs before it is noticed. The progressive nature of drug resistance is better monitored when a single drug is used.

5 **Establish an optimum worm control strategy for each holding.** Worm control strategies should aim to reduce the infection rate at all stages between the egg falling to the ground in the faeces and the goat ingesting the L3 larvae by good pasture management as well as bolstering the immune systems of the host animals by genetic selection, improved nutrition and management rather.than relying on killing worms in goats.

Alternative dewormers

Many studies are being undertaken to find alternatives to anthelmintics, but currently no non-chemical dewormers have been shown to be *practically* effective in controlling worms in livestock. Alternative dewormers include:

- *Botanical dewormers*, such as garlic, wormwood species (*Artemesia vulgaris, Artemesia cina)*, tansy *(Tanacetum vulgare)* and greater birdsfoot trefoil (*Lotus pedunculatus)*, wild ginger, conifers such as common juniper (*Juniperus communis)*, crucifers (mustard family), cucurbits (seeds of squash, pumpkins, etc.), ferns, umbilliferae and many others, which are still to be fully evaluated.
- *Forages* containing condensed tannins, for example *Sericea lespedeza*, birdsfoot trefoil (*Lotus corniculatus, Lotus pedunculatus)* and Sanfoin hay have been shown to have a beneficial effect in reducing parasite loads in small ruminants, either when used as forage crops or when fed as dried products (hay, ground hay, pellets and cubes) or by extracting the condensed tannins to be used as a drench or mixed with feed. Different species produce different condensed tannins and, perhaps, different mixtures of tannins. The levels of these can change with season, plant genetics and possibly other factors like stress. The condensed tannins are different from the tannins in oak leaves and acorns, which can be toxic. Some of the perceived positive effects of tannins may be due to an improved

protein supply to the small intestine from higher levels of forage, which can help to maintain the immune response when protein resources are scarce. *Sericea lespedeza* has been shown to effectively reduce faecal egg counts (affects female worm fecundity), reduces the hatch rate of eggs and appears to impair larval development. Chicory (*Cichorium intybus)* can be readily grown in the United Kingdom and is very palatable, with good nutritional value. A large number of studies in sheep have shown it has good antiparasitic properties, which could be utilized by using chicory in deworming paddocks in rotational grazing.There is speculation that animals may be able to self-medicate when they are parasitised by selecting plants for their tannin content, but there is considerable confusion as to whether this is a real phenomenon or a reflection on the palatability of the plants at certain times of the year and the availability of alternative forage.

- *Nematophagus fungi*, for example *Duddingtonia flagrans*, which parasitise larvae, are endogenous in most faeces. Spores can be intentially fed and there may be management practices that increase their numbers. The development of the fungi depends on environmental factors and temperatures in the United Kingdom are too low to allow sufficiently rapid fungal development to reduce larval numbers on pasture.

- *Copper sulphate*, in 1% aqueous solution, was used as an anthelmintic for many years before the availability of anthelmintic drugs, being reportedly particularly effective against *Haemonchus*, but less so against the small trichostrongyles. It was also used for the expulsion of tapeworms (*Monezia)*. Solutions of copper and nicotine sulphate were a more effective anthelmintic than copper sulphate alone. More recent attempts to verify its usefulness have not been successful and it has a narrower safety margin as the copper is readily absorbed and can lead to copper toxicity.

The use of *copper oxide wire particles (COWPs)* in controlling resistant *Haemonchus* has been investigated and have been shown to be effective in reducing infection levels based on faecal egg counts and PCVs. COWPs are only effective against abomasal worms, leaving small and large intestinal worms unaffected. The copper in a COWP is a form that is poorly absorbed, which makes it safe to administer with less risk of copper toxicity than copper sulphate. Boluses of 2–4 g appear safe in goats, but overuse of copper could result in toxicity, and COWPs should only be used under the supervision of a veterinary surgeon. COWPs pass from the rumen to the abomasum where they are retained. Free copper is released in the abomasum creating an environment that causes expulsion or death of worms.

- *Diatomaceous earth (DE)* fed at 2% of the ration has been claimed to be an effective anthelmintic, but there is considerable research showing that oral DE does *not* reduce faecal egg counts or the worm burden. If DE has any effect, it may be in causing the faecal pellet to dry out faster, reducing the number of eggs that get to the L3 stage.
- *Genetic selection.* A small number of the most suscepti- ble animals in the herd contribute the greatest amount of pasture contamination because they shed the most eggs in their faeces. Conversely, animals with the low- est faecal egg count in the herd may be those with the greatest parasite resistance, so identifying these ani- mals by faecal egg counts can help select for animals with greater parasite resistance. Animals that do well on heavily contaminated pastures with little or no use of anthelmintics should be retained and bred from; infected animals should be culled.
- *Vaccination.* A vaccine, Barbervax, against *Haemonchus contortus*, developed by the Moredun Research Institute, is licensed for sheep in Australia and has been shown to be very effective in goats. The vaccine works against all *Haemonchus*, including anthelmintic-resistant worms and provides between 75 and 95% protection. It is given as a series of 5 subcutaneous injections of 1 ml, at approximately 6-week intervals over the *Haemonchus*-risk season. Following the third vaccination, generally at wean- ing, protection against the development of significant *Haemonchus* burdens lasts for at least 6 weeks. In most cases, an oral anthelmintic is also given at weaning to ensure that the vaccine is not overwhelmed by existing *Haemonchus* burdens and to control other worms such as *Trichostrongylus*. Animals in poor body condition or showing signs of worms may not respond fully to vaccination and may require addi- tional support, but because the number of larvae on the pasture remains low due to the reduced worm egg output in other animals, even the small percentage of animals that do not respond to vaccination have a much reduced larval intake. Faecal egg counts should be used to check that heavy worm burdens are not present when vaccine protection is being established at the second or third injection, and then monitored periodically to ensure low counts are maintained. Breeding for worm-resistant animals and good pasture management to reduce larval intake complement vaccination. In the second year, 4 or 5 booster injections are given at 6-weekly intervals. Some immune memory persists so that the first injection restores the immunity gained from lamb vaccination.

Although the vaccine only targets *Haemonchus con- tortus*, the lower level of anthelmintic use means that resistance is likely to develop more slowly in all species of worms.

The Moredun Institute is also exploring the development of a vaccine to control *Teladorsagia circumcincta*.

Cestode infection

Moniezia spp. commonly affect goats and proglottid segments can be detected in faeces, but clinical, or even subclinical, infection is unlikely to be attributed to tapeworms, unless very large numbers are present in kids. Heavy infestation in kids may produce poor growth rates, a pot-bellied appearance and constipation. Complete occlusion of the intestinal lumen produces colic (see Chapter 15).

Benzimidazole drugs (see Table 14.5), *albendazole*, 10 mg/kg, *febantel*, 7.4 mg/kg, *fenbendazole*, 15 mg/kg, and *oxfendazole*, 10 mg/kg, are effective against *Moniezia* spp. at higher doses than required for nematode control.

Praziquantel, 3.75 mg/kg orally, is licensed for sheep in the United Kingdom in combination with lev- amisole and is effective against adult forms of *Moniezia*. The injectal form of praziquantel is not licensed for food-producing animals in the United Kingdom, but has been used at 5 mg/kg s.c. Some goats are irritated by the injection.

Note: (1) The metacestode stages of *Taenia multiceps* (*Coenurus cerebralis*) cause gid (sturdy) and have been reported in the brain, muscles and subcutaneous tissues of the goat (see Chapter 11).

(2) The metacestode stages of *Taenia hydatigena* (*Cys- ticercus tenuicollis*) rarely cause disease in goats, but acute infections have been reported (see Chapter 9).

(3) Hydatid disease or echinococcosis (see Chapter 9) due to *Echinococcus granulosus* has been rarely reported in goats in the United Kingdom but is more common in the rest of the world.

Rumen flukes

Rumen flukes are trematode parasites that infect cattle, sheep and goats as well as a number of wild ruminants. They are found worldwide, with varying prevalence depending on climatic conditions, but especially in humid regions. In endemic regions prevalence can be very high with up to 80% of the animals in a herd infected.

Aetiology

Rumen flukes are small (<1.5 cm long and 0.5 cm wide) digenean (2-host) trematode parasites, consisting of numerous genera in the family *Paramphistomum*, including *Paramphistomum*, *Cotylophoron*, *Calicophoron* and *Gigantocotyle*. Rumen fluke eggs started to appear in diagnostic samples from cattle in the United Kingdom and Ireland in the late 2000s. Originally thought to be *Paramphistomum cervi*, these have now been identified as *Calicophoron daubneyi*, which is the predominant rumen fluke species in mainland Europe, including France, Spain and Italy.

- The predilection site of adult flukes is the rumen; immature flukes congregate in the small intestine (duodenum and jejunum).
- There is an indirect life cycle, similar to that of *Fasciola hepatica*, with freshwater snails as the intermediate hosts (*Galba (Lymnaea), Bulinus, Planorbis, Stagnicola, etc.*). In Europe, where *C. daubneyi* is dominant, the favoured snail intermediate host is *Galba truncatula*. The two species of stomach fluke that infect ruminants in Australia, *Calicophoron calicophorum* and *Paramphistomum ichikawai*, are transmitted by the snails *Gyraulus scottianus* and *Helicorbis australiensis*, respectively.
- Livestock ingest metacercariae whilst grazing contaminated pastures. Once in the small intestine the young flukes leave the cysts, attach to the intestinal mucosa and continue development. Most of the pathogenic effects are caused by the immature fluke developing in the small intestine, where they cause erosion and petechiation. In goats, the immature flukes may spend a longer time in the intestines than in cattle or sheep and this can result in more severe clinical signs.

- The immature flukes migrate to the rumen, where they complete development to adult flukes and start producing eggs about 2 to 4 months after the metacercariae were first ingested. Adult fluke are well tolerated on the surface of the rumen and can be present in the rumen in large numbers whilst remaining essentially non-pathogenic.
- Cattle develop resistance after exposure to the parasite, which protects against immature fluke infections in subsequent years, but sheep and goats remain susceptible.

Clinical signs

Clinical signs are similar to nematode gastroenteritis and the two diseases commonly occur together. Young and debilitated animals are generally more severely affected than healthy adults.

- Moderate infections with the immature fluke may cause reduced weight gains or milk production, or ill-thrift.
- More severe infections cause profuse, projectile, watery diarrhoea with mucus and traces of blood and a characteristic foetid smell, with weight loss, dehydration, mild to moderate anaemia and submandibular oedema and death in 5 to 10 days.

Diagnosis

- Generally diagnosed by the presence of rumen fluke eggs in faeces and/or rumen fluke parasites at post-mortem.
- The eggs are operculated (~130 × 80 μm), very similar to those of *Fasciola hepatica*, and, although slightly lighter, are easily misidentified visually.
- Faecal antigen ELISAs specific for *F. hepatica* do not cross-react with rumen fluke.
- Liver fluke DNA can be detected in faecal samples from ~2 weeks post-infection. A DNA-based method, loop-mediated isothermal amplification (LAMP), gives a rapid (<1 h) visual readout without any specialised equipment. LAMP assays have been developed that are specific to liver fluke and rumen fluke, respectively.

Treatment

- Only treat if there are clinical signs of paramphistomosis.

- *Oxyclozanide, 15 mg/kg*, has confirmed activity against immature and adult rumen fluke. Activity against adult fluke is >95%, but it is less effective against immature fluke.
- In the United Kingdom, no flukicide containing oxyclozanide has a label claim for rumen fluke.

Control

- Reduce the availability of the snail populations by drainage and fencing off affected areas, providing alternative water sources, molluscicides.
- Encysted metacercariae do not survive dryness, but can survive and remain infective for up to 1 year in a humid and temperate environment and are capable of overwintering.

Coccidiosis

Coccidiosis is the most important cause of diarrhoea in housed kids > 4 weeks.

Aetiology

- Coccidia are protozoan parasites: goats are affected by 12 species of *Eimeria* that are all specific for the goat except *E. caprovina*, which is transmissible between sheep and goats. Coccidia species found in goats in the United Kingdom are listed in Table 14.7. Related protozoa such as *Isospora, Sarcocystis* and *Toxoplasma* do not generally multiply in the intestinal tract of the ruminant. The coccidial species of cattle, poultry or domestic pets do not cause coccidiosis in the goat.

Transmission

- All goats are infected with coccidia.

Table 14.7 Coccidia species found in goats in the UK.

Species	Site of infection	Pathogenicity
Eimeria arloingi	Small intestine	+
Eimeria caprina	Small and large intestine	++
Eimeria christenseni	Small intestine	+
Eimeria hirci	Unknown	++
Eimeria ninakohylakimovae	Small and large intestine	+++++
Eimeria alijevi	Small and large intestine	
Eimeria aspheronica	Unknown	
Eimeria caprovina	Unknown	
Eimeria jolchijevi	Unknown	

- It is probable that all kids are infected during their first few weeks of life and that management standards determine whether or not the levels of infection are sufficient to cause clinical signs of the disease. Kids become infected by ingestion of food, bedding and water contaminated with sporulated oocysts.
- Oocysts are ingested by the kid, rapidly undergo maturation and multiply. The cycling of a single oocyst could result in 1 to 2 million oocysts being passed 3 to 4 weeks later.
- Infection can occur indoors in intensive rearing situations or at pasture when the grass is sufficiently short for ingestion of oocysts lying on the soil surface.
- Oocysts are resistant to low temperature and will overwinter on pasture or indoors to provide a source of infection the following spring.

Epidemiology

- Kids become infected in the first few weeks of life, with the highest incidence of clinical disease between 4 and 7 weeks of age. After this, faecal oocyst excretion decreases as the kids acquire immunity to coccidia.
- Stress factors such as weaning, transport, changes in diet and adverse weather conditions can also predispose to the development of clinical disease, possibly by producing a relaxation of immunity.

Clinical signs

- Depression.
- Anorexia.
- Weight loss.
- Diarrhoea, possibly with blood and/or mucus.
- Dehydration.
- Death.

In severely infected kids massive release of meronts and merozoites from the intestinal cells can produce sudden-onset colic, shock and collapse or kids may be found dead with no signs of diarrhoea.

Recovered kids may show ill-thrift with a reduced growth rate and poor fibre production.

> Helminthiasis can occur concurrently with coccidiosis in kids at grass.

Diagnosis

The diagnosis of clinical coccidiosis must be based on the history, observation of clinical signs, post-mortem findings, faecal oocyst counts and oocyst speciation. Diagnosis based on the number of oocysts in faecal samples poses a number of problems:

- All kids are infected with coccidia.
- A severe challenge and the subsequent asexual reproductions can result in considerable damage to the intestine and clinical signs in the prepatent phase before the sexual cycle occurs with release of oocysts in the faeces. In very heavy infections the damage to the intestinal mucosa may not leave enough epithelial cells in the villi for the sexual cycle to occur.
- The intestines may be so damaged by the infection that clinical signs, that is diarrhoea, persist after the peak of oocyst production.
- Normal kids may have 1000 to 1 000 000 oocysts/g faeces; clinically ill kids may have 100 to 10 000 000 oocysts/g faeces.
- Identification of the species of coccidia present may be helpful. The predominant species in the faeces of the normal goat are *E. arloingi* and *E. hirci*. The most pathogenic species that predominate in kids that are clinically ill are *E. ninakohlyakimovae* and *E. caprina*. They cause severe mucosal destruction in the small and large intestines. *E. christenseni* and *E. hirci* are probably pathogenic. *E. arloingi* causes polyp formation and focal hyperplasia in the small intestine.

Post-mortem findings

- Gross post-mortem finds are often limited.
- Haemorrhage or mucoid enteritis may be obvious in severe infections, but in less severe infections there is generally little haemorrhage into the intestine.
- Small white pinpoint lesions may be present on the mucosal surface of the intestine. Smears taken from these areas show the presence of meronts, gametocytes and oocysts.

Control

Improved hygiene is the cornerstone of coccidiosis control.

The environment
- Avoid overcrowding.

- Provide clean, dry, well strawed pens for each batch of kids.
- Do not mix kids of different age groups.
- Raise food and water containers above the floor to avoid faecal contamination.
- Clean deep litter pens every 3 weeks.
- Slatted floors rather than deep litter may help reduce the oocyst level in some husbandry systems.

The doe
- Feeding a coccidiostat to the does in late pregnancy will reduce oocyst output and thus contamination of the environment, but enough oocysts will remain to infect the kids in intensive housing conditions and the coccidia can rapidly multiply in the non-immune kid.

The kid
- Prophylactic medication may have some success in controlling coccidiosis by reducing the challenge to the kids and allowing them to develop immunity by exposure to a low number of oocysts. However, drug treatment in a contaminated environment will only have a temporary effect. Most drugs are coccidiostats with only a limited coccidiocidal effect.

Treatment

- *Move the kids* from the infected pens as soon as disease becomes apparent.
- No anticoccidial drugs are specifically licensed for goats in the United Kingdom.
- Most anticoccidial drugs are coccidiostats that arrest development of one or more stages in the coccidial life cycle by interfering with cell development but do not totally eliminate the organism. Most drugs act early in the life cycle. Diclazuril has a coccidiocidal effect on the asexual or sexual stages of the development cycle of the parasite, dependent on the coccidia species. Toltrazuril is also coccidiocidal.
- Sulphomamides have traditionally been used to treat coccidiosis because they are cheap and easy to administer. They have a dose-dependent action that is coccidiostatic at lower doses and coccidiocidal at higher doses.
  o *Sulphadimethoxine, 75 mg/kg orally* for 4–5 days.
  o *Sulphamethoxypyridazine, 20 mg/kg, 1 ml/12.5 kg s.c.* once only.
  o *Sulphadimidine, 200 mg/kg, 6 ml/10 kg* initial dose, then *100 mg/kg, 3 ml/10 kg s.c.* or *i.v.* (preferred) daily for up to 5 days total. Sulphadimidine injectable solutions can be given orally in milk or water.

○ *Sulphadiazine, 150 mg/ml*, is included in combination with Neomycin and Kaolin in oral suspension for dosing at 4 ml/10 kg twice daily for up to 5 days. In the United Kingdom, most sulphonamide preparations are no longer available, leaving *potentiated sulphonamides* or the considerably more expensive drugs *decoquinate, diclazuril* and *toltrazuril* available for treatment.

○ *Sulphadiazine + Trimethoprim, 30 mg/kg* daily *s.c.* or slow *i.v.*

○ *Sulphadoxine + Trimethoprim, 15 mg/kg* daily *s.c.* or slow *i.v.*

○ *Diclazuril, 1 mg/kg, 1 ml/2.5 kg orally* as a single dose. Diclazuril has a direct effect on several stages of the life cycle, particularly the first generation meronts. Treatment should be given early before damage to the intestine occurs. Diclazuril has a wide safety margin. Kids can safely be given double the lamb dose at *2 mg/kg.*

○ *Toltrazuril, 20 mg/kg orally, 4 ml/10 kg orally* as a single dose. Toltrazuril persists in the intestine and the lamb dose should not be exceeded.

○ *Decoquinate, 100 g/tonne feed* or *1 mg/kg* for 28 days.

○ *Ponazuril* (Marquis, Bayer Animal Health) is licensed for use in horses in the United States and has been used off-label in goats *5 mg/kg* orally once. All life stages of the parasite are treated. Drug distribution is uneven in the syringe and it is recommended emptying the tube and remixing before use.

○ *Amprolium, 50 mg/kg orally* daily for 3–5 days has been used successfully to control coccidiosis in kids, but is only licensed for use in poultry in the United Kingdom. It can potentially cause polioencephalomalacia at high doses with prolonged administration.

■ Supportive therapy – *fluids, analgesics, intravenous corticosteroids* – is essential in severe cases.

Prophylaxis

> Whenever medicated feed is used, it is important to monitor the feed intake:
>   **Feed intake = Drug intake**
>   Apparent lack of efficacy in small ruminants is often due to inadequate drug intake.

The timing of treatment is critical to prevent disease, but it must also be timed to allow the development of protective immunity.

■ *In feed*

○ *Decoquinate, 100 g/tonne of feed* or *1 mg/kg* for 28 days to kids.

○ *Decoquinate, 50 g/tonne of feed* or *0.5 mg/kg* for 28 days to does.

Monensin is now classified as a growth promoter in the United Kingdom and cannot be used in the control of coccidiosis in goats. Similarly, other growth promoters such as *Lasalocid* and *Salinomycin* are also prohibited. Conversely, in the United States, Monensin is approved for use in non-lactating goats (20 g/ton of feed) and Lasalocid for use in sheep (20–30 g/ton of feed; 0.5–1 mg/kg daily in feed).

■ *In milk*

○ *Sulphadimidine, 200 mg/kg* initially, then *100 mg/kg* for a further 2–4 days every 3 weeks will reduce the level of environmental contamination of oocysts as 3 weeks is close to the prepatent period for many goat *Eimeria*. Sulphadimidine can be given as oral powder or the injectable solution can be added to milk.

■ *Orally*

○ *Diclazuril, 1 mg/kg, 1 ml/2.5 kg orally* at about 4–6 weeks of age when coccidiosis can normally be expected. Under conditions of high infection pressure, a second treatment can be given about 3 weeks after the first dosing.

○ *Toltrazuril, 20 mg/kg, 20 mg/kg, 4 ml/10 kg* every 3–4 weeks. The recommendation for toltrazuril is to treat kids before the expected onset of clinical signs.

Giardiasis (see page 211)

Although more commonly seen in kids < 4 weeks old, it can affect older kids.

Infected animals can continue to shed cysts for many weeks, even though they are clinically normal, so in older diarrhoeic animals identifying Giardia in faeces does not mean it is necessarily the cause of the diarrhoea. Shedding animals remains a source of infection for other kids and for humans.

Bacterial causes
Clostridium perfringens type D (enterotoxaemia, pulpy kidney disease)

Acute disease caused by *Clostridium perfringens* type D presents as diarrhoea, initially yellow-green and soft, later watery with mucus, blood and shreds of intestinal mucosa (see Chapter 16).

Salmonella

See Chapter 2 and this chapter.

Yersiniosis

Aetiology

- *Yersinia enterocolitica* and *Y. pseudotuberculosis*, Gram-negative coccobacilli.

Clinical signs

- *Yersinia pseudotuberculosis* is reported to cause abortion and post-parturient deaths, liver abscesses and granuloma formation and acute and chronic mastitis.
- Both *Y. pseudotuberculosis* and *Y. enterocolitica* cause diarrhoea, with *Y. enterocolitica* being more frequently implicated. All ages can be affected, but generally kids between 1 and 6 months.
- Diarrhoea is watery and non-haemorrhagic.
- Mortality is high and some kids may present as sudden deaths.
- A more chronic illness with dehydration and weight loss may occur.

Diagnosis

- Clinical signs, bacteriology, histopathology.
- Recovery of *Yersinia* spp. from the alimentary tract and internal organs using routine and selective media. Many *Yersinia* spp. inhabit the intestinal tract of clinically healthy animals and a diagnosis of enteric yersiniosis is confirmed by finding typical histological lesions in sections of the intestine and internal tissues.

Treatment

- Tetracyclines will control outbreaks of diarrhoea and abortion.

Public health considerations

- Affected animals and faeces are a potential hazard for humans and *Y. enterocolitica* has been isolated from goats' milk.

Older kids and adult goats

Diarrhoea in older goats can be extremely frustrating as there is often no apparent reason why one goat in a group should suddenly develop diarrhoea.

- *Parasitic gastroenteritis* is the commonest cause of diarrhoea in older goats (at grass), followed by *nutritional factors,* such as *inappropriate feeding or overfeeding,* either deliberately on the part of the keeper, such as overfeeding of concentrates without adequate roughage, or accidentally from stealing food (see Chapters 15 and 16). Similarly, overgrazing on lush grass, excessive feeding of roots, for example mangolds, or kale, excess fruit or bread or mouldy hay will all cause digestive upsets. All changes in diet should be introduced gradually.
- *Stress.* During early lactation, because of movement or mixing, or combinations of these, such as taking recently kidded goats to shows, will also lead to acute diarrhoea without there being any obvious nutritional or infectious cause.
- *Coccidiosis* (see this chapter) can occur in adult goats under stress or in animals with limited immunity because of lack of previous exposure.

Bacteria
Clostridium perfringens type D

See Chapter 16.

Clostridium perfringens type D has been implicated in a chronic form of disease, presenting as herd outbreaks of lethargic, inappetent goats with reduced milk yield and intermittent soft faeces or frank diarrhoea and the deaths of individual goats due to enterotoxaemia. It has been postulated that in intensively housed animals on deep litter there is a gradual build-up of *Cl. perfringens* in the environment, but because Clostridial bacteria are present in the intestines of clinically normal animals, diagnosis is extremely difficult to confirm. Empirically, the disease situation may improve by increasing the frequency of clostridial vaccination to every 3 or 4 months.

Clostridium perfringens type C has also been implicated in outbreaks of haemorrhagic diarrhea in adult goats.

The role of *mycotoxicosis* in these herd outbreaks of diarrhoea requires further elucidation and it is possible that some outbreaks are due to an interaction of mycotoxicosis and bacterial infection (see 'Toxic agents' below).

Salmonella

See Chapter 2 and this chapter.

Campylobacter jejuni

Aborting does usually show no signs of systemic illness but may have diarrhoea (see 'Abortion', Chapter 2).

Escherichia coli

Enteritis caused by attaching and effacing *E. coli* (AEEC) infection has been reported as the cause of death in adult goats. *E. coli* 0145 was identified as the causative organism. Shiga toxin-producing *E. coli* (STEC) have been implicated in outbreaks of haemorrhagic diarrhea in goats.

Toxic agents

A number of toxic agents are capable of causing diarrhoea:

- *Poisonous plants* may be eaten direct or in hay. Plants reported to cause diarrhoea include aconite, bluebell, box, buckthorn, dog's mercury (*Mercurialis perennis*), irises, rhododendron, spurges and wild arum.
- *Mycotoxins*. A number of fungal toxins found in mouldy conserved fodder such as maize (corn) silage, or badly dried cereals, most produced by *Fusarium* species, can potentially cause diarrhoea. Mycotoxicosis has been implicated in outbreaks of *haemorrhagic enteritis* in dairy goats fed mouldy feed during the winter months, together with Shiga toxin-producing *E.coli* (STEC).
- *Poisonous minerals* Copper (footbaths, sprays, etc.); see Chapter 15.

    Basic slag, nitrogenous or other types of fertiliser from recently lop-dressed pasture.

    Industrial waste – fluorides, arsenicals, barium, chromium, mercury, zinc and selenium.

    Fruit sprays.

    Teart pastures – molybdenum.

    Lead – access to old paint or batteries.

- *Drugs* include sulphonamides, carbon tetrachloride, copper sulphate and warfarin.

Hepatic and renal disease

Hepatic and renal disease may cause chronic diarrhoea, but weight loss is a more common presenting sign (see Chapter 9). Hepatic disease and bile duct obstruction lead to a decrease in the level of bile salts in the alimentary tract. This together with general liver distension causes gastrointestinal disturbances of anorexia and constipation, with attacks of diarrhea (see Chapter 15).

Note: (1) *Johne's disease* is not a major cause of diarrhoea in goats and only occurs late on in the course of disease in emaciated animals (see Chapter 9).

(2) Diarrhoea is a component of the clinical syndromes caused by the exotic viral diseases *Peste des Petits Ruminants* and *Rinderpest*.

Copper deficiency

See Chapter 5.

Results in anaemia, illthrift, poor coat, infertility and diarrhoea in growing and adult goats.

Further reading

General

Blackwell, R.E. (1983) Enteritis and diarrhoea. *Vet. Clin. North Amer.: Large Anim. Pract.*, **5** (3), November 1983, 557–570.

Holliman, A. (2009) Neonatal enteritis in goat kids. *Goat Vet. Soc. J.*, **25**, 89–93.

Mitchell, G. (1999) Differential diagnosis of diarrhoea/illthrift in goats at grass. *In Pract.*, **21**, 139–143.

Thompson, K.G. (1985) Enteric diseases of goats. *Proceedings of the Course in Goat Husbandry and Medicine*, Massey University, November, pp. 78–85.

Clostridial disease

Dray, T. (2004) Clostridium perfringens type A and type A and β2 toxin associated with enterotoxemia in a 5-week-old goat. *Can Vet J.*, **45** (3), 251–253.

Uzal, F.A. and Songer, J.G. (2008) Diagnosis of Clostridium perfringens intestinal infections in sheep and goats. *J. Vet. Diagn. Invest.*, **20**, 253–265.

Coccidiosis

Gregory, M. and Norton, C. (1986) *Anticoccidials. In Pract.*, **8**, 33–35.

Gregory, M. and Norton, C. (1986) Caprine coccidiosis. *Goat Vet. Soc. J.*, **7** (2), 32–34.

Howe, P.A. (1984) Coccidiosis. *Proc. Univ. Sydney Post Grad. Comm. Vet. Sci.*, **73**, 468–472.

Lloyd, S. (1987) Endoparasitic disease in goats. *Goat Vet. Soc. J.*, **8** (1), 32–39.

Taylor, M. (2002) Parasites of goats: a guide to diagnosis and control. *In Pract.*, **24**, 76–89.

Taylor, M. (2006) Endoparasites of goats. *Goat Vet. Soc. J.*, **22**, 21–28.

Valentine, B.A., Cebra, C.K. and Taylor, G.H. (2007) Fatal gastrointestinal parasitism in goats: 31 cases (2001–2006). *J. Amer. Vet. Med. Assoc.*, **231** (7), 1098–1103.

Van Veen, T.W.S. (1986) Coccidiosis in ruminants. *Comp. Cont. Ed. Pract. Vet.*, **8** (10), F52–58.

Cryptosporidiosis/giardiasis

Angus, K.W. (1987) Cryptosporidiosis in domestic animals and humans. *In Pract.*, **9** (2), 47–49.

Kirkpatrick, C.E. (1989) Giardiasis in large animals. *Comp. Cont. Ed. Pract. Vet.*, **II** (1), 80–84.

Lloyd, S. (1986) Parasitic zoonoses. *Goat Vet. Soc. J.*, **7** (2), 39–44.

Paul, S. *et al.* (2014) Cryptosporidiosis in goats: a review. *Adv. Anim. Vet. Sci.*, **2** (3S), 49–54.

Rings, D.M. and Rings, M.B. (1996) Managing *Cryptosporidium* and *Giardia* infections in domestic ruminants. *Vet. Med.*, **91** (12), 1125.

Fluid therapy

Jones, M. and Navarre, C. (2014) Fluid therapy in small ruminants and camelids. *Vet. Clin. N. Amer.: Food Anim. Pract.*, **30** (2), 441–453.

Helminthiasis

Abbott, K.A., Taylor, M. and Stubbings, L.A. (2012) *Sustainable Worm Control Strategies for Sheep, A Technical Manual for Veterinary Surgeons and Advisors*, 4th edition (Sustainable Control of Parasites in Sheep – SCOPS). Available at: http://freepdfs.net/scops-technical-manual-4th-edition-june-2012pdf/58e91cac0dbbedd2cc229460e0fbd680/.

American Consortium for Small Ruminant Parasite Control. Available at: http://www.acsrpc.org www.wormx.info.

Anon (2007) *A Review: Alternative Methods of Controlling Internal Parasites in Ruminants*. Available at: www.abdn.ac.uk/organic/organic_14b.php.

Gibbons, L.M. *et al.* The RVC/ FAO Guide to Veterinary Diagnostic Pathology, Sample Collection, Diagnostic tests, Identification. Available at: http://www.rvc.ac.uk/review/Parasitology/Index/Index.htm.

SCOPS – Sustainable Control of Parasites in Sheep. Available at: http://www.scops.org.uk.

The Ohio State University, College of Veterinary Medicine, Veterinary Extension

Sorting Through the Information on Sheep and Goat Parasite Control: A Decision Making Support Tool. Available at: http://vet.osu.edu/extension/decision-tree.

Burke, J.M. *et al.* (2009) Administration of copper oxide wire particles in a capsule or feed for gastrointestinal nematode control in goats. *Vet. Parasitol.*, **168**, 346–350.

Charlier, J. *et al.* (2014) Practices to optimize gastrointestinal nematode control on sheep, goat and cattle farms in Europe using targeted (selective) treatments. *Vet. Rec.*, **174**, 250–255.

Coles, G.C. (2002) Sustainable use of anthelmintics in grazing animals. *Vet. Rec.*, **151**, 165–169.

Cornall, K. and Godber, O. (2014) Endoparasites of goats in the UK. *Goat Vet. Soc. J.*, **30**, 52–59.

Crilly, J.P. and Sargison, N. (2015) Ruminant coprological examination: beyond the McMaster slide. *In Pract.*, **37**, 68–76.

Fleming, S.A. *et al.* (2006) Anthelmintic resistance of gastrointestinal parasites in small ruminants. *J. Vet. Intern. Med.*, **20**, 435–444.

Gokbulut, C. *et al.* (2014) Comparative pharmacokinetics of levamisole-oxyclozanide combination in sheep and goats following *per os* administration. *Canadian J. Vet. Res.*, **78** (4), 316–320.

Greer, A.W. *et al.* (2009) Development and field evaluation of a decision support model for anthelmintic treatments as part of a targeted selective treatment (TST) regime in lambs. *Vet. Parasitol.*, **164** (1), 3–6.

Hamel, D. *et al.* (2015) Anthelmintic efficacy and pharmacokinetics of pour-on eprinomectin (1 mg/kg bodyweight) against gastrointestinal and pulmonary nematode infections in goats. *Small Ruminant Res.*, **127**, 74–79.

Hoste, H. *et al.* (2002) Targeted application of anthelmintics to control trichostrongylosis in dairy goats: result from a 2-year survey in farms. *Vet. Parasitol.*, **110**, 101–108.

Hoste, H., Sotiraki, S. and Torres-Acosta, J.F. (2011) Control of endoparasitic nematode infections in goats. *Vet. Clin. North Amer.: Food Anim. Pract.*, **27** (1), 163–173.

Kenyon, F. *et al.* (2009) The role of targeted selective treatments in the development of refugia-based approaches to the control of gastrointestinal nematodes of small ruminants. *Vet. Parasitol.*, **164**, 3–11.

Malama, E. *et al.* (2014) Development of a milk and serum ELISA test for the detection of *Teladorsagia circumcincta* antibodies in goats using experimentally and naturally infected animals. *Parasitology Research*, **113** (10), 3651–3660.

Mederos, A. *et al.* (2012) A systematic review–meta-analysis of primary research investigating the effect of selected alternative treatments on gastrointestinal nematodes in sheep under field conditions. *Prev. Vet. Med.*, **104** (1–2), 1–14.

Murri, S. *et al.* (2014) Frequency of eprinomectin resistance in gastrointestinal nematodes of goats in canton Berne, *Switzerland. Vet. Parasitol.*, **203** (1–2), 114–119.

Sargison, N. (2011) Responsible use of anthelmintics for nematode control in sheep and cattle. *In Pract.*, **33**, 318–327.

Sargison, N. (2011) The particular problem of anthelmintic resistance in goats. *Goat Vet. Soc. J.*, **28**, 71–79.

Soli, F. *et al.* (2010) Efficacy of copper oxide wire particles against gastrointestinal nematodes in sheep and goats. *Vet. Parasitol.*, **168**, 93–96.

Sutherland, I.A. (2015) Recent developments in the management of anthelmintic resistance in small ruminants – an Australasian perspective. *New Zealand Vet. J.*, **63** (4), 183–187.

Taylor, M. (2002) Parasites of goats: a guide to diagnosis and control. *In Pract.*, **24**, 76–89.

Taylor, M. (2006) Endoparasites of goats. *Goat Vet. Soc. J.*, **22**, 21–28.

Valentine, B.A., Cebra, C.K. and Taylor, G.H. (2007) Fatal gastrointestinal parasitism in goats: 31 cases (2001–2006). *J. Amer. Vet. Med. Assoc.*, **231** (7), 1098–1103.

Zajac, A.M. (2006) Gastrointestinal nematodes of small ruminants: life cycle, anthelmintics, and diagnosis. *Vet. Clin. North Amer.: Food Anim. Pract.*, **22** (3), 529–541.

Rumen fluke

Paraud, C., Gaudin, C., Pors, I. and Chartier, C. (2009) Efficacy of oxyclozanide against the rumen fluke *Calicophoron daubneyi* in experimentally infected goats. *Vet. J.*, **180** (2), 265–267.

CHAPTER 15

Colic

Initial assessment

- Feeding history – overfeeding, change in diet, mouldy feed, etc.
- General physical examination – to determine whether the problem is related to a specific alimentary condition, associated with a more general disease, or not connected with the alimentary tract at all (e.g. urolithiasis).
- Specific examination of the digestive system:
  - Visual inspection: abdominal contour from behind, abdominal distension.
  - Palpation of the left abdominal wall and rumen: filling of the rumen.
  - Percussion: tympanitic sounds, pain.
  - Auscultation: rumen mobility, sounds of left-sided abomasal displacement.

Further investigations

- *Passage of a stomach tube* allows release of accumulated gas and the collection of a sample of ruminal fluid. A simple gag to facilitate stomach tubing can be made by drilling a hole in a piece of wood. Contamination by saliva will increase the pH of the sample.
- Rumen fluid can be collected paracostally by inserting a 14 gauge 38 or 50 mm needle perpendicular to the skin into the rumen in the lower half of the left flank, after preparing the skin with surgical spirit wipes. Fluid is then collected using a syringe.
- *Trocharisation* of the left paralumbar fossa releases accumulated gas.
- *Abdominocentesis*. In adults, use an 18 or 20 gauge needle at the lowest point of the ventral abdomen, 2 to 4 cm to the right of the midline to avoid the rumen. Aseptically prepare the area, use local anaesthetic and

possibly sedation in nervous animals. Fluid should be collected in an EDTA tube for analysis and a sterile plain tube for culture. Normal peritoneal fluid has a clear, slightly yellow appearance, a protein concentration of 10–30 g/litre and a white cell concentration (mainly lymphocytes) of $<1 \times 10^6$ litre.

Examination of rumen contents

- *Measure pH* with indicator papers:
  - In a normal goat, the typical pH is 6.5–7.0.
  - From 2 to 3 hours after a concentrate meal, the pH may drop to 5.5–6.0, returning again to normal within 12 hours after feeding.
  - pH 4.5 to 5.0 suggests a moderate degree of abnormality.
  - pH <4.5 suggests severe acidosis and requires emergency treatment.
- *Methylene blue reduction test* measures the redox potential of the ruminal fluid and reflects the level of activity of aerobic rumen microflora; 20 ml of ruminal fluid is added to 1 ml of 0.03% methylene blue solution in a test tube and the time required for the methylene blue to decolourise is measured. The faster the decolourisation, the more active the microflora – microfloral inactivity will give results of 15 minutes or longer and severe rumen acidosis >5 minutes. A normal goat with a high concentrate ration will have a time of 1 to 3 minutes and a goat on an all-hay diet 3 to 6 minutes.
- *Gram stains* of air-dried smears of normal fluid demonstrate predominantly gram negative flora. Bacterial diversity is greatest in animals on a high forage diet and more uniform in animals on a high concentrate/cereal diet. Lactobacilli (long Gram-positive rods) predominate in animals with acute rumen acidosis.

Diseases of the Goat, Fourth Edition. John Matthews.
© 2016 John Wiley & Sons, Ltd. Published 2016 by John Wiley & Sons, Ltd.

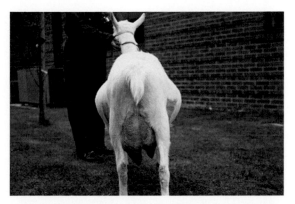

Plate 1.1 Hydrometra – abdominal distension and well developed udder with milk 145 days post-service (Plate provided by Peter Jackson).

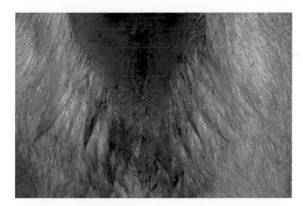

Plate 1.2 Hydrometra – dampness of vulva and perineum after 'cloudburst' (Plate provided by Peter Jackson).

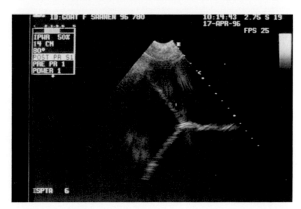

Plate 1.3 Hydrometra – ultrasonographic scan of uterus showing absence of a fetus and echogenic marks caused by superimposition of the fluid-filled uterine horns (Plate provided by Peter Jackson).

Diseases of the Goat, Fourth Edition. John Matthews.
© 2016 John Wiley & Sons, Ltd. Published 2016 by John Wiley & Sons, Ltd.

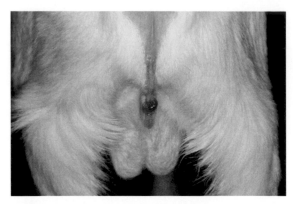

Plate 1.4 Intersex – male pseudohermaphrodite showing perineal urethral orifice, a scrotum containing testes and hypospadia (Plate provided by Peter Jackson).

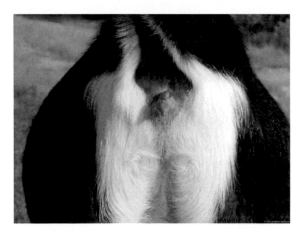

Plate 1.5 Intersex – female pseudohermaphrodite.

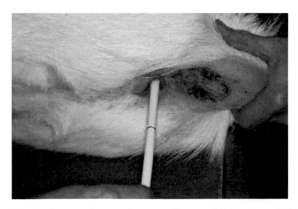

Plate 1.6 Intersex – marked vaginal probe showing shortened vagina (Plate provided by Peter Jackson).

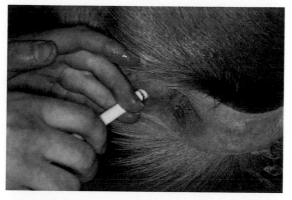

Plate 1.7 Intersex – normal female with marked vaginal probe showing normal vaginal length (Plate provided by Peter Jackson).

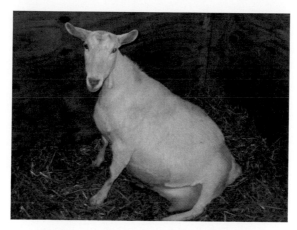

Plate 1.8 Some does will adopt a 'dog-sitting' position during late pregnancy.

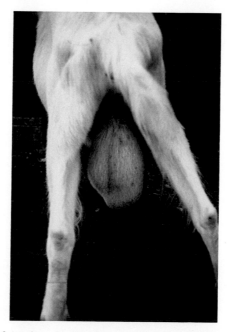

Plate 3.1 Saanen buck with orchitis involving the enlarged right testis (Plate provided by Peter Jackson).

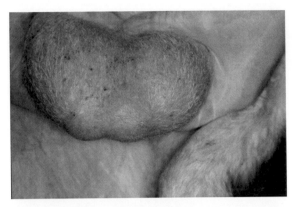

Plate 3.2 Infertile buck showing normal testes with small fibrosed epididymes (Plate provided by Peter Jackson).

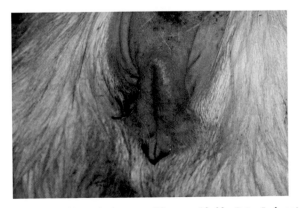

Plate 4.1 Vaginal prolapsed (Plate provided by Peter Jackson).

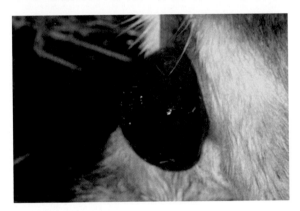

Plate 4.2 Vaginal prolapse replaced and secured by vulval sutures (Plate provided by Peter Jackson).

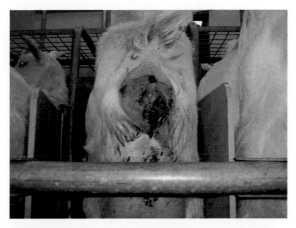

Plate 4.3 Vulval trauma from an assisted kidding (Plate provided by Katherine Anzuino).

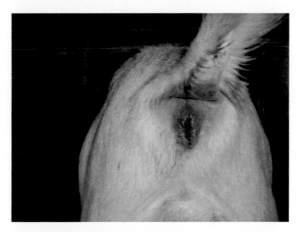

Plate 4.4 Sore vulva post-kidding (Plate provided by Katherine Anzuino).

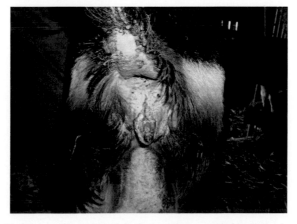

Plate 4.5 Matted hair and dermatitis from purulent vaginal discharge (Plate provided by Katherine Anzuino).

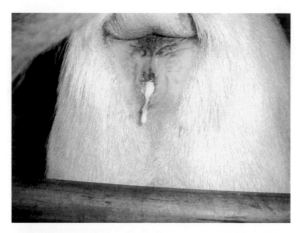

Plate 4.6 Endometritis – white vulval discharge (Plate provided by Katherine Anzuino).

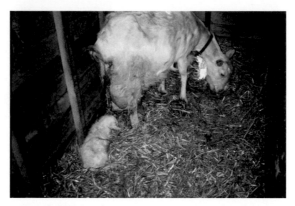

Plate 4.7 Does regularly eat their own (and other goats) placentae; many reportedly 'retained placentae' have, in fact, been eaten by the goat.

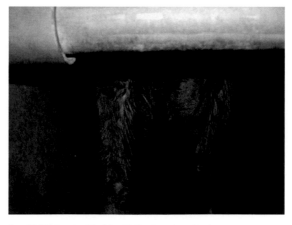

Plate 4.8 Severe urine staining and scald (Plate provided by Katherine Anzuino).

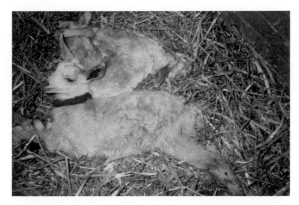

Plate 5.1 Congenital swayback – two kids, one ataxic and paraplegic but able to use its front legs, the other quadriplegic (Plate provided by Tony Andrews).

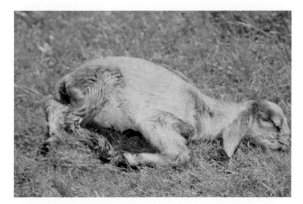

Plate 5.2 Floppy kid syndome – collapsed Anglo-Nubian kid (Plate provided by Peter Jackson).

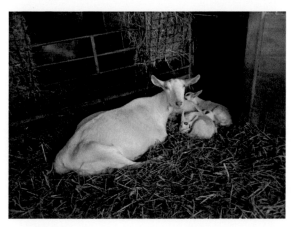

Plate 6.1 Disbudding at 4 days of age allows the kids to stay with the dam for a further 24 hours before being separated for artificial rearing.

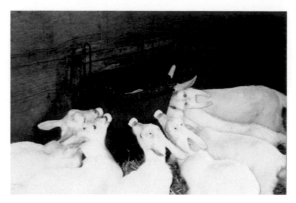

Plate 6.2 With a simple multifeeding unit the quantity of milk fed is restricted to set amounts at set times of the day.

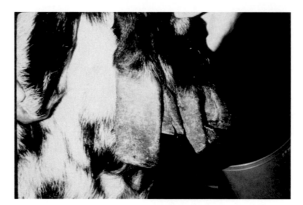

Plate 7.1 Chronic laminitis – showing accentuated depth of claws, 'platform soles'.

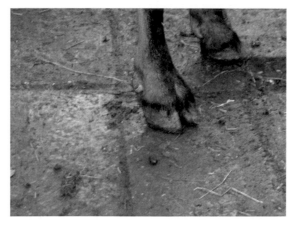

Plate 7.2 Chronic laminitis – depth of claws less pronounced than in Plate 7.1, but still twice normal depth.

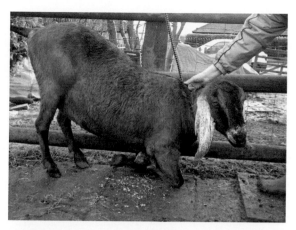

Plate 7.3 Chronic laminitis – affected animals spend a lot of time on their knees because their feet are painful.

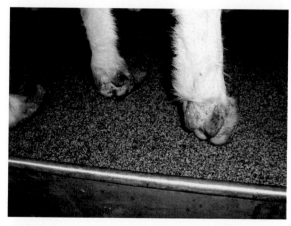

Plate 7.4 Overgrown hooves ('slipper feet'). The pastern dermatitis may be due to wet conditions or chorioptic mange (Plate provided by Katherine Anzuino).

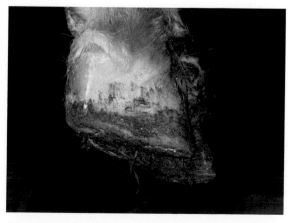

Plate 7.5 Tumours of the foot, involving the interdigital cleft, coronary band and the hoof, are occasionally reported.

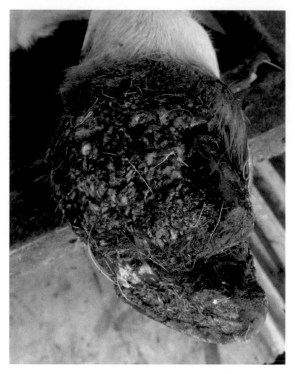

Plate 7.6 CODD type lesion (Plate provided by Leigh Sullivan).

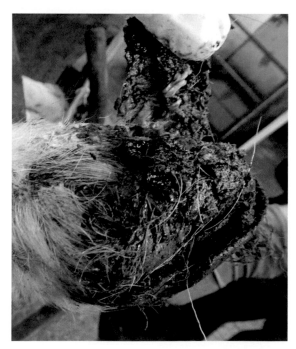

Plate 7.7 CODD type lesion with separated hoof horn removed to show underlying granulomatous and haemorrhagic tissues (Plate provided by Leigh Sullivan).

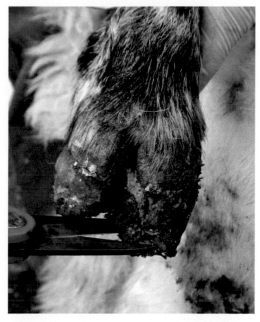

Plate 7.8 CODD type lesion showing separated hoof horn (Plate provided by Leigh Sullivan).

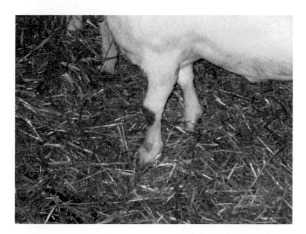

Plate 7.9 Caprine arthritis encephalitis virus (CAE) – doe with distended carpal joints causing lameness.

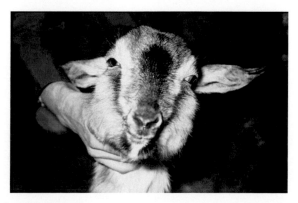

Plate 8.1 Face of goat with osteodystrophia fibrosa.

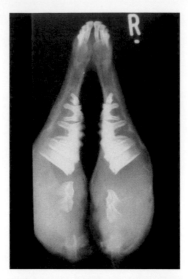

Plate 8.2 Osteodystrophia fibrosa – X-ray of maxillae (Plate provided by Tony Andrews).

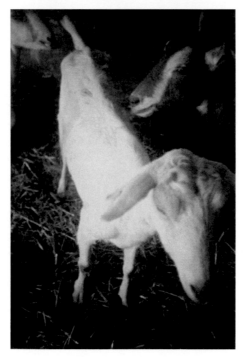

Plate 9.1 Johne's disease – emaciated goat (Plate provided by Tony Andrews).

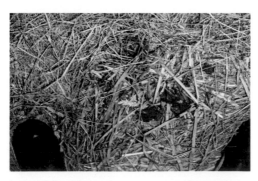

Plate 9.2 Faeces from goat with Johne's disease. Diarrhoea only occurs terminally in goats (Plate provided by Tony Andrews).

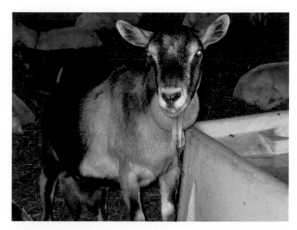

Plate 10.1 Thymoma – a relatively common tumour in adult goats.

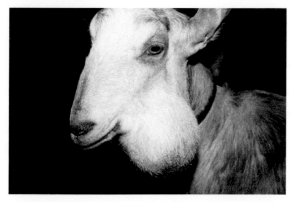

Plate 10.2 Salivary cyst – relatively common as developmental abnormalities, particularly in Anglo-Nubian goats (Plate provided by Peter Jackson).

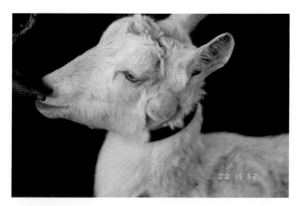

Plate 10.3 Caseous lymphadenitis – abscess. In goats, enlarged and abscessed peripheral lymph nodes, particularly of the head and neck, are the major presenting signs (Plate provided by Peter Jackson).

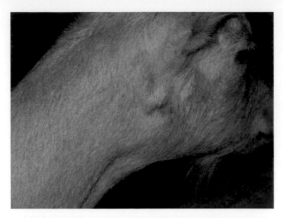

Plate 10.4 Caseous lymphadenitis – ruptured abscess (Plate provided by Peter Jackson).

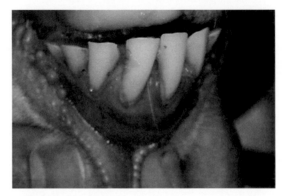

Plate 10.5 Lymphosarcoma – loose incisor teeth preventing prehension of food (Plate provided by Peter Jackson).

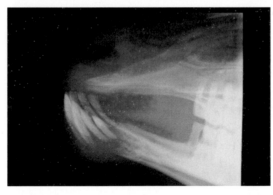

Plate 10.6 Lymphosarcoma – radiograph showing extensive lysis of the mandibular bone (Plate provided by Peter Jackson).

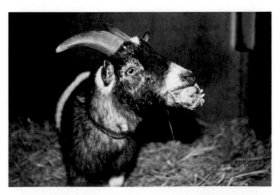

Plate 10.7 Giant cell tumour affecting the mandible and adjacent tissues. A variety of other tumours are occasionally found in the mouths of goats and cause localised swelling (Plate provided by Peter Jackson).

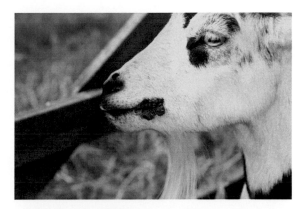

Plate 10.8 Orf lesions on lips (Plate provided by Peter Jackson).

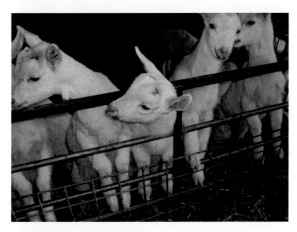

Plate 10.9 Kids with orf (Plate provided by Katherine Anzuino).

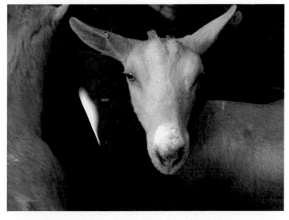

Plate 10.10 Dermatitis nose of unknown aetiology. It can often be difficult to differentiate between orf and other conditions causing dermatitis around the mouth and nose.

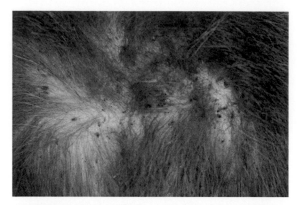

Plate 11.1 Lice infestation (*Linognathus stenopsis*).

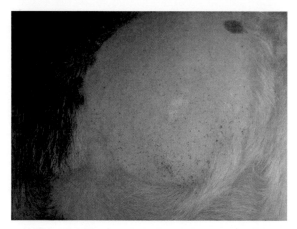

Plate 11.2 Lice infestation (*Bovicola caprae*).

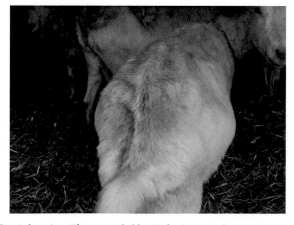

Plate 11.3 Dermatitis back from lice infestation (Plate provided by Katherine Anzuino).

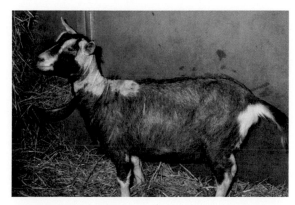

Plate 11.4 Sarcoptic mange (Plate provided by Peter Jackson).

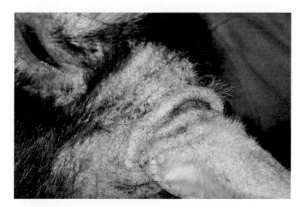

Plate 11.5 Sarcoptic mange, close up view of left ear and eye region (Plate provided by Peter Jackson).

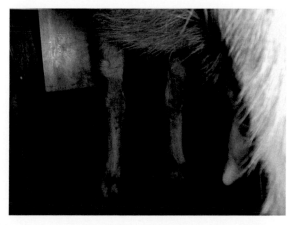

Plate 11.6 Dermatitis legs from lying in wet conditions (Plate provided by Katherine Anzuino).

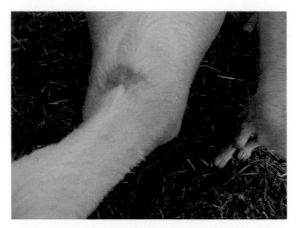

Plate 11.7 Hair loss neck from rubbing on bars of feeders, racks, etc., is common in commercial herds (Plate provided by Katherine Anzuino).

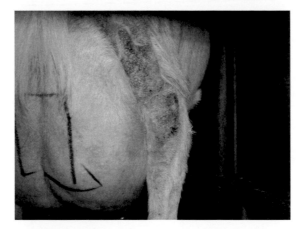

Plate 11.8 Dermatitis leg of unknown aetiology (Plate provided by Katherine Anzuino).

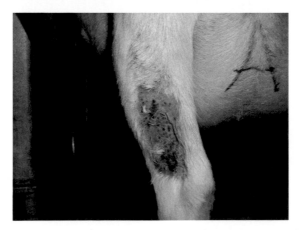

Plate 11.9 Dermatitis leg of unknown aetiology. Secondary bacterial infection frequently occurs with any skin lesions (Plate provided by Katherine Anzuino).

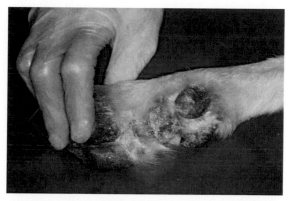

Plate 11.10 Chorioptic mange – caudal view of lower fore limb (Plate provided by Peter Jackson).

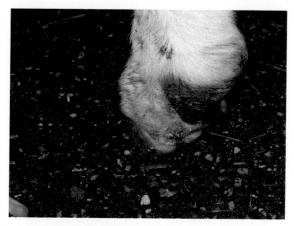

Plate 11.11 Chorioptic mange (Plate provided by Katherine Anzuino).

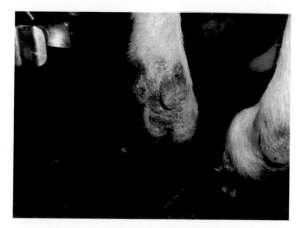

Plate 11.12 Dermatitis caudal lower limb due to wet conditions (Plate provided by Katherine Anzuino).

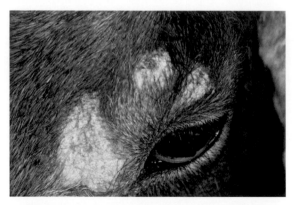

Plate 11.13 Ringworm face (*Trichophyton mentagrophytes*) (Plate provided by Peter Jackson).

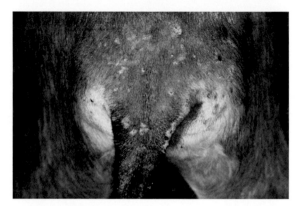

Plate 11.14 Ringworm tail base (*Trichophyton mentagrophytes*) (Plate provided by Peter Jackson).

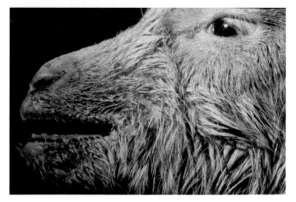

Plate 11.15 Golden Guernsey goat syndrome – 'sticky kid' (Plate provided by Peter Jackson).

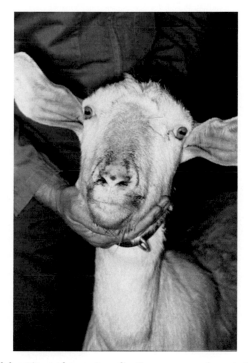

Plate 12.1 Scrapie – regurgitation, cud dropping and excessive salivation may occur in goats (Plate provided by Tony Andrews).

Diseases of the Goat, Fourth Edition. John Matthews.
© 2016 John Wiley & Sons, Ltd. Published 2016 by John Wiley & Sons, Ltd.

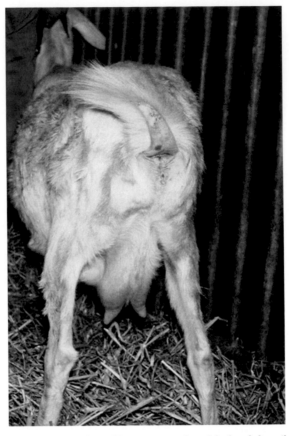

Plate 12.2 Scrapie – scratching and rubbing causes loss of hair; ears may be pricked and the tail cocked and carried over the back (Plate provided by Tony Andrews).

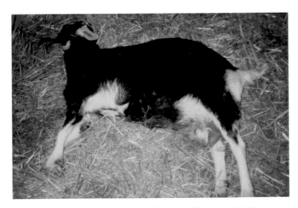

Plate 12.3 Hypomagnesaemia; usually presents acutely, occasionally as 'sudden death' (Plate provided by Tony Andrews).

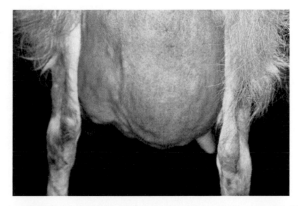

Plate 13.1 Chronic mastitis, showing atrophy of the left half and normal right half (Plate provided by Katherine Anzuino).

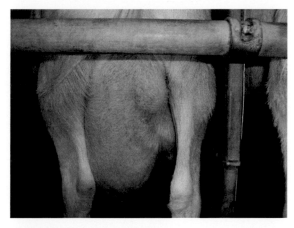

Plate 13.2 Chronic mastitis, showing atrophy of the right half with abscess formation (Plate provided by Katherine Anzuino).

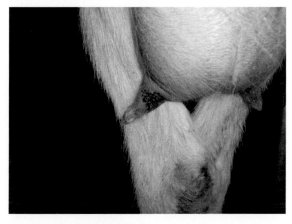

Plate 13.3 Trauma to teat from milking (Plate provided by Katherine Anzuino).

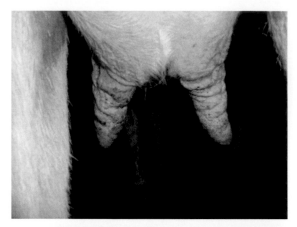

Plate 13.4 Dermatitis udder and teats caused by reaction to disinfection solution or teat dip (Plate provided by Katherine Anzuino).

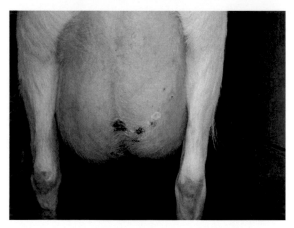

Plate 13.5 Localised Staphylococcal dermatitis udder (Plate provided by Katherine Anzuino).

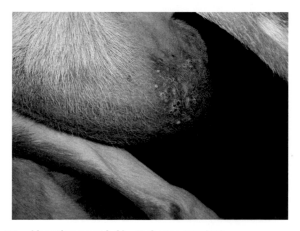

Plate 13.6 Staphylococcal dermatitis udder (Plate provided by Katherine Anzuino).

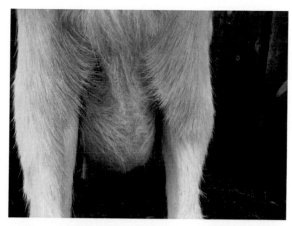

Plate 13.7 Maiden milker. Goatling with one-sided udder development.

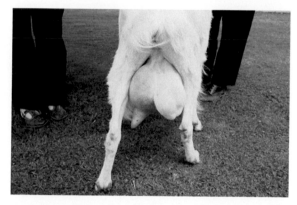

Plate 13.8 Gynaecomastia. Saanen buck showing left-sided mammary development and normal scrotum. Gynaecomastia does not generally affect fertility (Plate provided by Peter Jackson).

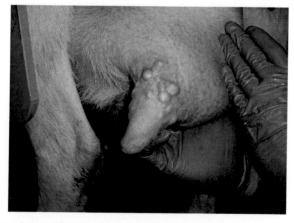

Plate 13.9 Cystic dilation of the teat sinuses (Plate provided by Katherine Anzuino).

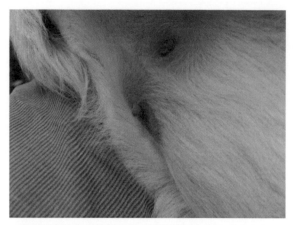

Plate 13.10 Double teats are a disqualifying fault in the show ring for dairy animals but acceptable in Boer goats.

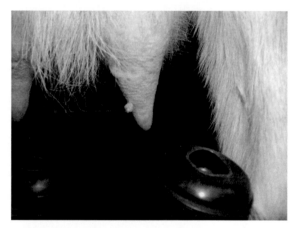

Plate 13.11 Tumours on the teat may be traumatized by milking (Plate provided by Katherine Anzuino).

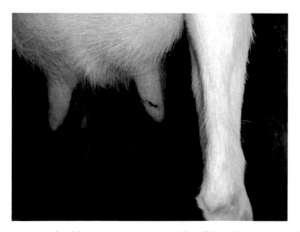

Plate 13.12 Healing teat injury – even superficial lesions can interfere with milking (Plate provided by Katherine Anzuino).

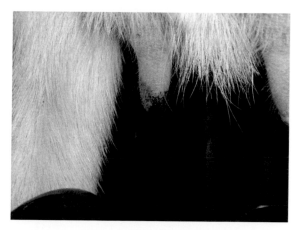

Plate 13.13 Bitten teat. Teat biting can present as a herd problem in commercial herds.

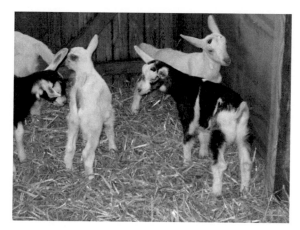

Plate 14.1 Provide clean, dry, well strawed pens for each batch of kids.

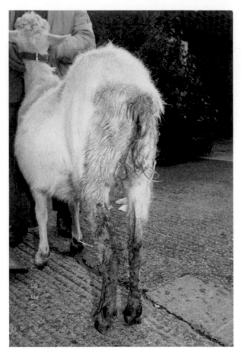

Plate 14.2 Acute enteritis – *Salmonella typhimurium* (Plate provided by Peter Jackson).

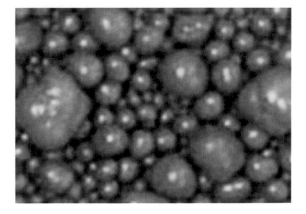

Plate 15.1 Carbonate stones.

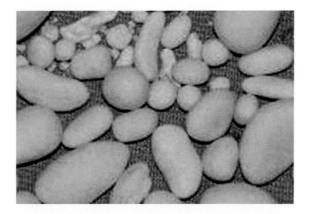

Plate 15.2 Phosphate stones.

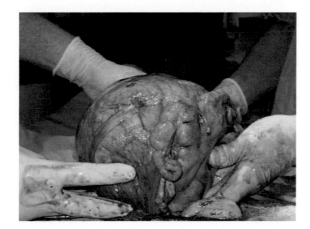

Plate 15.3 Leiomyoma.

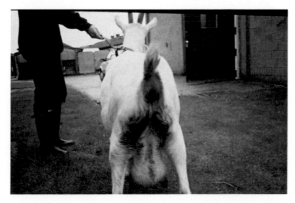

Plate 15.4 Chronic vaginal discharge caused by uterine leiomyoma (Plate provided by Peter Jackson).

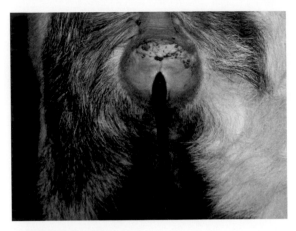

Plate 15.5 Bloody vaginal discharge in pygmy goat with a uterine tumour.

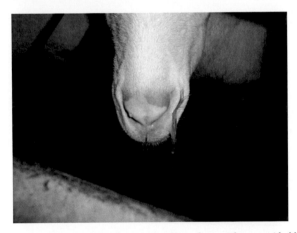

Plate 17.1 Mucoid nasal discharges are common in animals returning from shows (Plate provided by Katherine Anzuino).

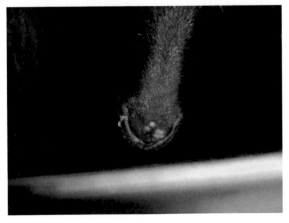

Plate 17.2 Mucopurulent nasal discharge (Plate provided by Katherine Anzuino).

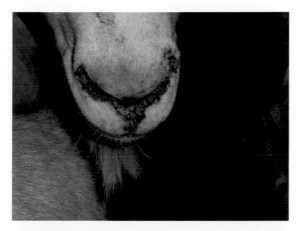

Plate 17.3 Bilateral nasal discharge with scabbing and adherent food material (Plate provided by Katherine Anzuino).

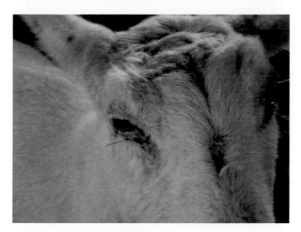

Plate 20.1 Allergic conjunctivitis.

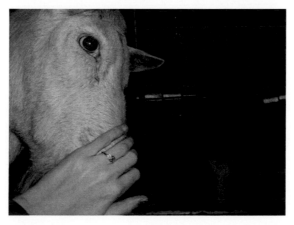

Plate 20.2 Mucopurulent ocular discharge.

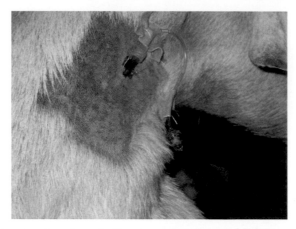

Plate 24.1 Jugular catheter; placing a jugular catheter facilitates anaesthetic induction, fluid therapy and administration of drugs.

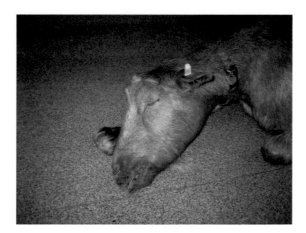

Plate 24.2 Diazepam provides about 30 minutes of sedation but no analgesia.

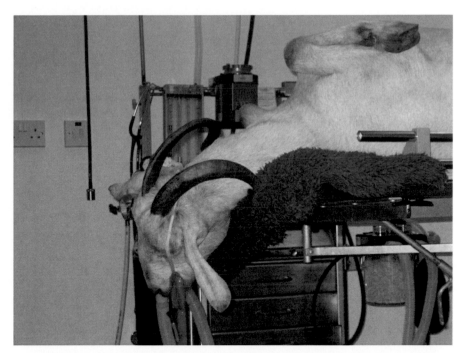

Plate 24.3 Gaseous anaesthesia; correct positioning of the goat on the table with the neck and thorax raised to lower the hindquarters, while the head is tilted downwards to allow free drainage of saliva.

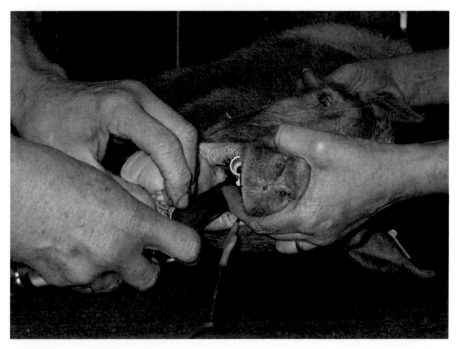

Plate 24.4 Intubation using a long-bladed laryngoscope.

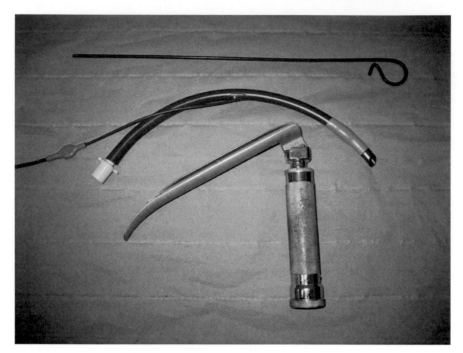

Plate 24.5 Equipment for successful inturbation.

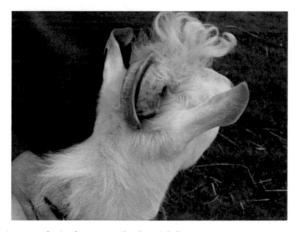

Plate 25.1 Poor disbudding technique results in the regrowth of unsightly scurs.

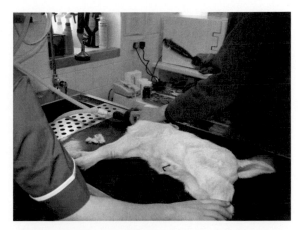

Plate 25.2 Kids should be disbudded between 2 and 7 days of age.

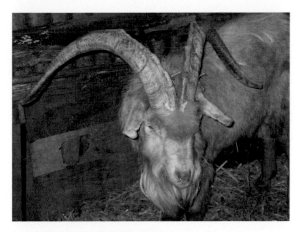

Plate 25.3 Removal of large horns from mature animals is contraindicated.

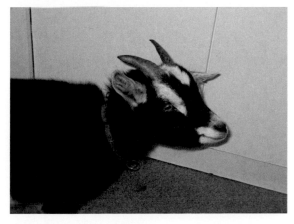

Plate 25.4 Dehorning; even relatively small horns have a large base.

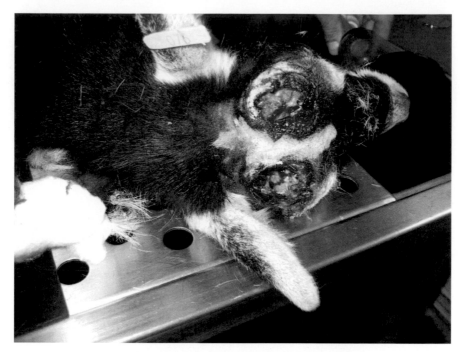

Plate 25.5 Dehorning exposes the frontal sinuses that extend into the hollow base of the horn.

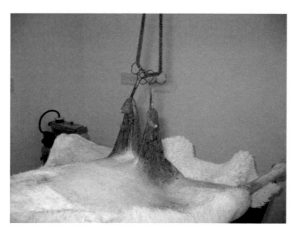

Plate 26.1 Mastectomy; suspending a pendulous udder above the operating table makes surgery much easier.

- Various sized actively swimming protozoa are present in normal fluid and can be examined by light microscopy using low (10×) magnification.

Clinical signs of colic

- Clinical signs may be continuous or spasmodic.
- Lethargic, depressed, reluctant to move or frequently gets up and down.
- Bleating.
- Pawing ground with front feet, shifting of weight between feet.
- Teeth grinding.
- Tachypnoea, shallow respirations.
- Tachycardia.
- Tenesmus.
- Arched back.
- Tucked up at abdomen, staring at abdomen, kicking at abdomen (uncommon).
- Goats rarely roll.

Colic in adult goats

Diarrhoea/enteritis
See Chapter 14.

Indigestion (ruminal atony)
Aetiology
- Minor degrees of dietary mismanagement, particularly inadequate protein and energy with a high fibre diet, mouldy or frosted feeds, a moderate overfeeding of concentrates or insufficient water, produce various degrees of ruminal impaction and atony.
- Oral dosing with antibiotics or sulphonamides (due to destruction of the normal ruminal flora).
- Lack of exercise.
- Oral dosing with linseed oil produces a foul-tasting cud which is often spat out and normal chewing of the cud ceases.

Clinical signs
- Reduced appetite or complete anorexia.
- Reduced milk yield.
- Constipation with small amounts of faeces or occasionally diarrhoea.

- Generally a firm, pliable rumen palpable on the left side, but occasionally moderate degrees of tympany as ruminal atony becomes established.
- No signs or only weak signs of rumination.
- Often few signs of abdominal pain, although occasionally typical spasmodic colic signs such as pawing the ground with the front feet, looking at the abdomen, frequent getting up and down and grinding of teeth.

Treatment
- Many mildly affected animals will recover spontaneously. In other cases, symptomatic treatment should be adopted.
- Use *200 g Epsom salts (magnesium sulphate)* in *300 ml water* as a drench on the first day, then 100, 75 and 50 g on successive days if necessary.
- Give *vegetable oil (30 ml)* in about *100 ml liquid paraffin* as a drench.
- Rehydration if necessary.
- Relief of pain where present.
- In animals with a recurrent problem, *bran mashes* two or three times weekly may help prevent impaction. Mix four handfuls of bran scalded with sufficient boiling water to make a crumbly mash and leave to stand for 10 minutes.
- Feed on browsings, leaves and branches, to encourage the resumption of cudding.
- Re-establish ruminal microflora with yoghurt, probiotics or by drenching fresh rumen contents or ground-up faeces. Cud can be obtained from the mouths of cudding goats (use a spoon!) and mixed with water to make a suitable solution for drenching, using a suitable plastic bottle.

Note: *abomasal impaction* may occur in animals with poor rumination. The abomasum is palpable in the low right abdomen. Treat as for ruminal atony.

Acute ruminal acidosis
Aetiology
- The rumen microbial system can only adapt to changes in diet slowly (3–10 days).
- Excess ingestion of high-energy feeds such as barley, wheat, dairy cake, etc., results in a rapid fermentation of the carbohydrate in the feed with the formation of large quantities of lactic acid, decreasing the rumen pH. As the pH falls, rumen motility decreases and the normal rumen microflora are destroyed and replaced

by lactobacilli and streptococci. The lactic acid produces a severe *rumentis* with necrosis of the mucous membrane, and lactic acid and the toxic products from the degeneration of the rumen bacteria are absorbed, causing a toxaemia. The ruminal contents are hypertonic to plasma, so fluids are lost into the alimentary tract resulting in sloppy rumen contents, diarrhoea and dehydration (PCV 30–40% = good prognosis for recovery, >45% poor prognosis).

- Certain feeds which are acidic in their own right, for example mangolds, apples, rhubarb, etc., may produce acidosis if they are suddenly fed in large quantities.
- Secondary infection by fungi or bacteria such as *Fusibacterium necrophorum* may lead to a more prolonged rumenitis after the animal has survived the acute disease.
- Reduced rumen function reduces thiamine (vitamin B1) synthesis by microbes and causes cerebrocorticonecrosis (CCN).

Clinical signs

There are different degrees of grain overload and hence varying degrees of ruminal acidosis. Animals with mild rumen acidosis, especially those that are more chronic (typically an overfed show animal) can have relatively normal rumen pH with little protozoal activity, whereas animals that are recumbent usually have metabolic acidosis as well as a rumen acidosis (diagnosed by low rumen pH on a sample of the fluid). The severity of clinical signs is similarly variable.

- Lethargy, sluggish palpebral reflex.
- Anorexia.
- Abdominal pain – grinding of teeth, kicking at abdomen.
- Subnormal temperature.
- Fast, weak pulse (<100 beats/minute has poor prognosis).
- Ruminal movements absent.
- Diarrhoea.
- Death.
- Laminitis (see Chapter 7) may develop in animals that have recovered due to changes in the corium of the feet.

Treatment

- Mild cases can be treated as for indigestion, particularly if treated early. *Epsom salts (magnesium sulphate)*

in *300 ml water* as a drench on the first day, then 100, 75 and 50 g on successive days if necessary, act as a laxative to move the grain through more rapidly and helps buffer the acid in the rumen.
- Drenching with 100 g *sodium bicarbonate* will help reduce the acidosis (but overdosing may lead to alkalosis); the bicarbonate can be mixed with a pinch of salt (to help replace the chloride lost with diarrhoea) and enough water to make a thick paste, which can be spooned into the back of the mouth.
- Alternatively, 15 ml *milk of magnesia* (suspension of hydrated magnesium carbonate in water) is a good antacid that will not convert to metabolic alkalosis if an excess is given. Repeat in 3 to 4 hours if necessary. Antacids containing *calcium carbonate* are also useful. Calcium and magnesium salts both increase gastrointestinal tract motility by stimulating smooth muscle contraction and help move the feed from the rumen.
- *Aluminium hydroxide gel*, 1–2 g, is an effective antacid by neutralising acid and absorbing hydrogen ions. It is also mildly astringent.
- Dehydration should be corrected with parenteral administration of *3 to 5 l of isotonic fluids* (Ringer's solution, *0.9% saline*).

Note: avoid lactic acid solutions, such as Hartmann's.

Oral fluids could be given via stomach tube or by dosing with a syringe; fluid will then be absorbed from the rumen.

- Metabolic acidosis can be corrected with intravenous *sodium bicarbonate*, given over 1 to 3 hours. Empirically give 500 ml of 4.2% sodium bicarbonate or estimate the base deficit (see Table 15.1) and the bicarbonate deficit (see Table 15.2) and treat accordingly. If the serum bicarbonate level is not known, the correction must be empirical. In severe acidosis, a base deficit of 10 nmol/litre can be safely assumed.
- *Thiamine, 10 mg/kg i.v. or i.m., 1 ml/10 kg* daily for 3 days may help prevent cerebrocortical necrosis.

Table 15.1 Estimation of base deficit.

Severity of clinical signs	% Dehydration	Base deficit (mmol/litre)
Mild	5	5
Moderate	8	10
Severe	10	15

Table 15.2 Estimation of bicarbonate deficit.

Body weight in kg $\times$ 0.3 $\times$ Base deficit = mmol bicarbonate required

where 0.3 is the extracellular fluid volume (ECFV) for **adult** animals

A 50 kg goat that is 10% dehydrated will have a base deficit of 15 mmol/litre and will need 50 $\times$ 0.3 $\times$ 15 = 225 mmol bicarbonate
1 ml of 1.26% sodium bicarbonate = 0.15 mmol bicarbonate
1 ml of 4.2% sodium bicarbonate = 0.50 mmol bicarbonate
1 ml of 8.4% sodium bicarbonate = 1.00 mmol bicarbonate

The goat will require 450 ml of 4.2% sodium bicarbonate

If sodium bicarbonate solutions are not available, sodium bicarbonate (baking soda) can be added to a litre of 0.9% saline:
13 g of baking soda in a liter water = 1.3% isotonic solution
1 g of sodium bicarbonate = 12 mmol bicarbonate
The 50 kg goat with 10% dehydration needs 18.75 g sodium bicarbonate = approximately 1.5 litres

---

Multivitamin preparations can be used if thiamine is not available, but must be given according to the thiamine content (usually 10 or 35 mg/ml).

- *Procaine benzylpenicillin, 10 mg/kg i.m.* every 12 hours for as long as 10 to 14 days will help eliminate or prevent anaerobic bacterial rumenitis.
- *Oral neomycin* may help stop fermentation.
- *Flunixin meglumine, 2.2 mg/kg i.v.*, can be given once the animal is rehydrated.
- *Rumenotomy* (see Chapter 23) should be performed in serious cases, the rumen completely emptied and washed out and the contents replaced by hay, water and preferably rumen contents from a normal goat.
- *Clostridium perfringens type D antitoxin* should be given if available.
- The re-establishment of the normal rumenal microflora should be assisted by dosing with yoghurt, probiotics, ground-up faecal pellets or transfaunation 12–24 hours after initial treatment.

Note: probiotic products containing *Lactobacillus* species are not suitable for ruminating animals. They readily ferment available carbohydrates to lactic acid, thus exacerbating the problem.

Subacute ruminal acidosis (SARA)
Incidence

The incidence of subacute ruminal acidosis is largely undocumented, but the incidence in commercial dairy herds appears much less than in dairy cattle. This may be because as browser feeders goats are more able to select food materials and maintain their fibre intake, even on total mixed rations and even if the overall ration is imbalanced. Similarly, the incidence in pet goats is unknown, despite the fact that they are often fed inappropriate and/or high grain diets. However, it is probable that the chronic laminitis, which is relatively common in pygmy and pet dairy goats is a direct result of ruminal acidosis.

Aetiology

The reticulorumen is a fermentation vat that for effective function requires a certain amount of fibre. It needs a mat of long fibre floating on top of the liquid to trap smaller particles – the thicker the mat of floating long fibre, the longer small particles are retained. The fibre mat stimulates receptors in the rumen wall stimulating rumination and long fibre stimulates eructation, cud chewing and salivation. Both the length and structure of the fibre in the feed is important – fine chopped straw is far less effective than unprocessed straw or hay with long fibres. As a rough rule of thumb, fibre particles longer than the animal's muzzle is wide will promote good levels of chewing and cudding, maximising saliva flow. The goat's dry matter intake (DMI) is usually about 2.5 to 3% of body weight, although lower during late pregnancy and after kidding, increasing over the first few weeks of lactation. DMI increases with age and with more digestible rations, depending on the palatability. Feeds that stimulate rumination are most useful for maintaining optimum conditions for fermentation within the rumen.

Saliva, which contains bicarbonate and phosphate ions, helps to buffer the rumen and maintain as near to the optimum pH of 7 as possible, although in practice the attainable pH is generally <6.5, because of the intake of cereal-based rations. Bacteria required for the fermentation of plant cell walls are sensitive to pH. The growth of rumen bacteria falls below pH 6 and below 6.2 fibre digestion is severely inhibited.

Low ruminal pH will:

- Depress voluntary feed intake.
- Increase the level of digestive disorders (acidosis, indigestion and bloat).
- Cause parakeratosis of the ruminal wall.
- Increase the incidence of laminitis/feet problems.
- Increase fat depots.
- Decrease milk fat concentration.
- Cause a relative decrease in milk production.

> Monitoring factors that influence rumen pH and function is an important component of a health programme.

Commercial goats may be susceptible to acidosis because of:

- High maize diets (maize silage) – maize silage contains significant amounts of starch (250 g/kg DM) so it is not all forage.
- High wheat diets.
- Low fibre intakes.
- Non-edible bedding, for example arabose, shavings, newspaper, rubber matting.
- Sudden changes in diet at kidding – freshly kidded animals need 2–4 weeks to adjust to an increased level of concentrates in their diet.

Pet goats may be susceptible to acidosis because of:

- Low fibre intakes.
- Inappropriate or poor quality forage.
- Overfeeding of goat mix.
- Inappropriate feeds – potatoes, bread waste, pub food, etc.
- Excessive supplements.
- Overfeeding.

Clinical signs
- Reduced feed intake.
- Reduced performance.
- Loose faeces or frank diarrhoea.
- Mild colic signs.

- Acute laminitis (chronic laminitis if acidosis persists for some time).

> Undegraded feed passing into the small intestine can cause an overgrowth of *Cl. perfringens*, epsilon toxin production and *enterotoxaemia*. Does shortly after kidding are particularly at risk.

Treatment
- Address dietary imbalances.
- Remove all sources of starch and put on good quality forage such as long-stemmed hay.
- Give sodium bicarbonate (20 g) or 15 ml milk of magnesia (suspension of hydrated magnesium carbonate in water) by mouth.

Prevention
- Add long fibre to the ration to stimulate chewing and saliva flow.
- Well-bedded straw yards provide an additional source of roughage and increase fibre intake.
- Long stemmy material will promote more rumination than a leafy precision-chopped silage, alleviate a subclinical acidosis and stimulate dry matter intake.
- Add sodium bicarbonate to the ration to increase the rumen buffering capacity.
- Feed whole uncrushed grains, rather than heavily rolled or crushed, so starch is released at a lower rate and the rumen pH is not so depressed.
- Feed starchy concentrates little and often. The amount of lactic acid produced is related to the amount of starch eaten at any one time, so lactic acid production is reduced by limiting the amount of concentrate eaten at any one time.
- Feed a complete diet (total mixed ration).

Ruminal tympany

Primary ruminal tympany (frothy bloat)
See Chapter 16.

Secondary ruminal tympany ('choke')
See Chapter 16.

Enterotoxaemia (*Clostridium perfringens* type D, pulpy kidney disease)

Clostridial bacteria and the goat

The most significant clostridial bacteria in goats are *C. perfringens* and *C. tetani*. Most disease in goats is associated with *C. perfringens* type D although *C. perfringens* types B and C may rarely cause acute haemorrhagic enteritis in young kids. Goats appear to be almost totally resistant to the clostridial gas gangrene conditions. The different types of *C. perfringens* are distinguished by their characteristic pattern of toxin production. The major toxin produced by types B and C is beta, whilst epsilon toxin is the most significant produced type D. Following the entry of spores via wounds, *C. tetani* produces tetanus toxin, which is a potent neurotoxin.

Aetiology

- *Clostridium perfringens* type D proliferates rapidly in response to dietary changes such as overgrowing lush pasture or overfeeding cereals. Epsilon toxin is produced as an inactive protoxin, which is activated by the proreolytic action of trypsin in the small intestine. The toxin increases intestinal permeability and is absorbed into the bloodstream causing vascular damage and oedema in organs such as the brain, lungs, kidneys and heart.

Transmission

- *Clostridium perfringens* is present in the intestine of normal sheep and goats and has also been isolated from soil.

Clinical signs

- Peracute – sudden death or terminal shocked condition with convulsions.
- Acute:
  o Diarrhoea, initially yellow-green and soft, later watery with mucus, blood and shreds of intestinal mucosa.
  o Sternal and later lateral recumbency.
  o Severe abdominal pain: pitiful intermittent cry of pain.
  o Shock: cold extremities.
  o Paddling movements and throwing back of head prior to death.

- A chronic form has been described in adult goats showing periodic bouts of severe diarrhea, reduced milk yield and wasting, which responds to vaccination.

Post-mortem findings

- Confirmation of the disease even at post-mortem is generally difficult and only possible in a freshly dead animal. 'Pulpy kidney', as seen in sheep, is rare in goats.
- Collect 20 to 30 ml of intestine contents to which 2 to 3 drops of chloroform have been added in a universal container and submit to the laboratory.
- Pericardial fluid that clots on exposure to air.
- Petechial or ecchymotic haemorrhages on the epicardium, endocardium, diaphragm, small intestine serosa and abdominal muscles.
- Mucosa of small intestine inflamed.
- Symmetrical areas of haemorrhage, oedema and liquefaction in the brain, particularly the basal ganglia; focal symmetrical encephalomalacia (see Chapter 12). Lesions produced by epsilon toxin in the brains of goats are pathognomonic for type D enterotoxemia.

Laboratory investigation

- All diagnostic tests for diagnosing *C. perfringens* infections have limitations.
- *Clostridium perfringens* type D is a normal inhabitant of the gut and may be found, with its toxin, in healthy animals. The presence of strains capable of producing a certain toxin does not necessarily mean that these toxins are either produced or produced in sufficient quantitiy to induce disease.
- Gram-stained impression smears from the small intestine show Gram-positive rods.
- Epsilon toxin can be demonstrated using mice protection tests with specific antisera or by an ELISA test.
- Urine collected from the bladder may contain glucose.

> **Glucosuria** is a consistent finding in enterotoxaemia.

Treatment

- *Clostridium perfringens* type D antitoxin, adults at least 12.5 ml, kids 5 ml, s.c. or i.m. (no longer available in the United Kingdom).

- Pain relief with:

  Flunixin meglumine, 2 mg/kg, 2 ml/45 kg i.v.
  Carprofen, 1.4 mg/kg, 1 ml/35 kg i.v.

- Supportive therapy – *intravenous balanced electrolyte solutions, 120 ml/kg* over 4 to 5 hours (not glucose saline as hyperglycaemia occurs terminally), warmth and company.

Prevention

- Avoid digestive disturbances – overeating of concentrates, high concentrate diet with insufficient fibre, excessive grazing of lush grass, etc. – and make any feed changes gradually.
- Diets should have a high fibre content with adequate fibre length (see subacute ruminal acidosis). Soluble carbohydrates passing too quickly through the rumen and abomasum are thought to encourage clostridial overgrowth in the small intestine.
- *Vaccination* with a multivalent clostridial vaccine will give some protection against enterotoxaemia, *Cl. perfringens* types B and C and tetanus. However, protective thresholds have not been established for goats and the antibody response to vaccination is often unclear. The immunity produced in goats appears less satisfactory than that produced in sheep – the levels of antibody capable of neutralising clostridial toxins seen in goats is usually less than in sheep given the same vaccines. It has been postulated that vaccination may give adequate protection against absorbed epsilon toxin but not against clostridial-induced damage to the intestinal mucosa. However, it has been shown experimentally that vaccination with epsilon toxoid can definitely protect against enterotoxaemia, so the reason for reported failures of routine vaccination is still unclear. There may be a fundamental difference between sheep and goats in their humoral or antibody mediated immunity, possibly in their B cell range of specificity, or perhaps the vaccine adjuvant, which is included to stimulate an immune response, has less effect in goats.
- There is some evidence from the field that 4 in 1 vaccines give better protection than 7 or 8 in 1 vaccines. However, any vaccine used should contain toxoids of *Cl. perfringens* types B, C and D and *Cl. tetani*. A 2 in 1 vaccine giving protection against enterotoxaemia and tetanus could be used if available. Other clostridial

Table 15.3 Vaccination regime for clostridial disease.

Primary course:	2 doses, 4 to 6 weeks apart
	The interval of 4 to 6 weeks is important and should not be reduced
Booster:	Every 6 months, with one dose
	4 to 6 weeks before kidding to ensure maximum transfer of immunity to kids
Kids:	Start primary course at 3 to 4 weeks of age (dam unvaccinated)
	8 weeks of age (dam vaccinated)
Dose :	2 ml

diseases are extremely rare in goats in the United Kingdom, so vaccines with more components should only be used if *Cl. novyi* or *chauvoei* infections have been confirmed in a herd (see Chapter 18).

- The use of combined clostridial and pasteurella vaccines is not recommended.
- The persistence of the response to vaccination is shorter in duration in goats than sheep, so it is necessary to shorten the interval between the booster vaccinations and vaccinations every 6 months; even more frequent vaccinations in problem herds are recommended (Table 15.3).

Vaccination for clostridial disease

Select the simplest vaccine available that contains the components most relevant to the herd in question.

Review and shorten the interval of booster doses, without automatically following the guidelines for sheep.

The animal will respond to maximal effect to a 2 ml dose. Doubling the dose to 4 ml is a waste and is likely to cause a larger local reaction at the site of injection.

- The length of persistence of maternally derived antibodies and their effect on vaccination is not clear. The age of immunological maturity in kids is likewise not well documented.
- The recommended site for injection is the lateral side of the neck or lateral thorax at the level of the elbow.
- Sterile swellings commonly occur as a reaction to vaccination and may range in size from small nodules to several centimetres in diameter.

Note: although generally considered a major disease of goats in the United Kingdom, difficulties in confirming the diagnosis mean that the true incidence in unknown.

Any 'sudden death' is usually attributed by goalkeepers to enterotoxaemia, so that other causes of sudden death, for example bacterial septicaemia or mesenteric torsion, are underdiagnosed. Even the finding of epsilon toxin in intestinal contents does not prove conclusively that death was caused by *Cl. perfringens* type D and histological examination of the brain is essential for diagnosis.

Abomasal ulceration
Aetiology
- Abomasal ulceration is poorly documented, but is probably due to a high concentrate/low roughage diet, particularly in early lactation!
- Ulceration may be a sequel to chronic acidosis and rumen stasis.

Clinical signs
- Many goats with superficial abomasal ulceration show no apparent illness, or only occasionally become inappetent. However, deeper ulceration will lead to more severe clinical signs.
- Changes in the abomasal tone and motility will in turn affect the motility of the rumen and reticulum.
- Perforation with omental adhesion that seals the perforation produces low-grade intermittent pain, with grinding of teeth, intermittent pyrexia, reduced ruminoreticular movement, weight loss, reduced milk yield, marked inappetence and intermittent diarrhoea.
- Perforation without the defect being sealed may result in an acute diffuse peritonitis and death.
- Severe haemorrhage may occur and produce displacement (see below) with adhesions to the left side of the abdomen.

Treatment
- Symptomatic; correct the diet.
- Metaclopramide, 0.5–1.0 mg/kg, 5–10 ml/50 kg i.v. initially, then i.m. twice daily (maximum two doses by i.m. injection) to restore abomasal tone and encourage gastric emptying.
- Broad-spectrum antibiotics.

Left-sided displacement of the abomasum
See Chapter 16.

Urolithiasis

> Any straining male goat should be assumed to have a blocked urethra until proved otherwise. Urolithiasis is common, constipation rare.

Urolithiasis is a metabolic disease of male goats, particularly castrates of any age and male kids, but occasionally males of any age, characterised by the formation of calculi within the urinary tract and urethral blockage. Urolithiasis is virtually always associated with concentrate feeding.

Aetiology: Anatomy
- Male animals are affected; females can pass calculi easily through their shorter, wider urethra.
- Castration arrests penile development, so the urethra remains narrow.
- Mature animals have a larger urethra than immature animals. *Young castrated animals are at greatest risk.*
- The most common sites of obstruction are the distal sigmoid flexure and the urethral process, although obstruction may occur anywhere from the renal pelvis to the distal urethra.

The development of uroliths
Uroliths are mineral concretions formed by the precipitation or crystalisation of mineral salts on an organic matrix. Their formation is, therefore, dependent on a number of factors, both dietary and environmental. Urolith development depends on the dietary mineral content, the dietary content of organic calculi-forming factors, the pH of the urine and urinary volume.

Phosphatic and calcium carbonate calculi are commonly found in intensively kept males.

Phosphatic calculi
These include magnesium ammonium phosphate (struvite) and calcium phosphate (Plate 15.1). They occur in alkaline urine and are associated with feeding of cereals and pelleted rations. High phosphorus levels are present in cereals, particularly wheat, maize, sorghum, oats and milo. Phosphorus should not exceed 0.6% of the total ration.
- High levels of urinary phosphorus increase the likelihood of the formation of insoluble phosphates and urinary calculi.

- Factors which increase urinary phosphorus excretion predispose to calculi formation.
- Urinary phosphorus excretion is normally very low in ruminants as any excess phosphorus absorbed is secreted back into the digestive system via saliva and excreted in the faeces. High fodder intake increases saliva production and phosphorus excretion. Conversely, saliva production is decreased if pelleted rations are fed rather than mixes.

A number of factors may lead to increased urinary phosphorus:

  ○ *High levels of dietary phosphorus*: at a certain level the salivary phosphorus recycling system becomes saturated and urinary phosphorus excretion occurs.

  ○ *Low levels of dietary calcium (low calcium:phosphorus ratio)*: because calcium opposes phosphorus absorption in the intestine, phosphate absorption, and therefore the urinary phosphate load, are increased if the dietary calcium: phosphate ratio is low (<1.5:1 calcium:phosphorus).

  ○ Conversely, a high calcium:phosphorus ratio in the diet reduces the incidence of calculi formation by decreasing the absorption of phosphorus from the gut, thus reducing urinary phosphate levels.

  ○ *Low fibre diet*: goats on high grain/low fibre diets secrete much lower amounts of saliva than animals on high roughage diets, thus decreasing the amount of phosphorus excreted in the faeces.

  ○ *Low urine output*: any reduction in voluntary water intake will lead to decreased urine volume and increased likelihood of calculi formation. Feeding concentrates instead of roughages significantly reduces the urine volume.

  ○ *Dietary magnesium levels*: some research has suggested that high magnesium levels *per se* do not cause urolithiasis and may in fact reduce the incidence of calculi formation by reducing urinary phosphorus excretion, but conversely levels of magnesium > 0.6% in the feedlot rations in the United States have been implicated in promoting struvite formation, even when the Ca:P ratio was 2–2.5:1, and it is recommended that magnesium does not exceed 0.6% of the total ration.

  ○ *Genetic predisposition*: in sheep, individual differences in phosphorus metabolism have been shown to have a genetic basis. Phosphorus is excreted mainly in the faeces by some sheep and in the urine by others. It is probable there is a similar situation in

goats – a FAMILIAL tendency to calculi formation has been shown in Saanen males. There are definite breed differences in sheep – it is not known if the same applies to goats. Genetics may also determine urethral size.

  ○ Mucopolysaccharides in urine can act as a matrix and cementing substance thus promoting calculi formation. They are associated with rapid body growth and feeding certain foods (cottonseed and milo) and pelleted feeds.

Calcium carbonate calculi

Calcium carbonate calculi (Plate 15.2) occur in alkaline urine.

- Plants high in calcium predispose and the calculi are typically associated with grazing clover-rich pastures or the feeding of lucerne (alfalfa) and other legume hays or chopped lucerne products, which contain more calcium than mature males require for maintenance.
- Increased urinary calcium excretion results in the precipitation of calcium carbonate crystals; 'green-gold ball bearings' of various sizes.
- In one retrospective study, goats with calcium carbonate uroliths were typically neutered males of African descent, > 1 year of age. Nigerian dwarf goats had a higher incidence of uroliths than did pygmy goats. Cross-bred, Anglo-Nubian and Toggenburg goats had the lowest incidence. It is not clear whether this reflects genuine genetic differences, differences in feeding regimes or other variables.

Calcium oxalate calculi

Urolithiasis can occur in goats grazing clover-rich pastures or where there is an abundance of oxalate-containing plants:

- Oxalate is the normal end-product of glycine and ascorbic acid metabolism and is a constituent of normal urine. Calcium oxalate is often present as crystals in the sediment of concentrated ruminant urine as it has a very low solubility.
- Calcium oxalate crystals may form in animals fed on oxalate-containing plants such as sugar beet tops, rhubarb leaves, docks (*Rumex* spp) and wood sorrel (*Oxalis acetosella*) (see Chapter 21). The amount of oxalate required to cause toxicity is variable, but because oxalate-degrading ruminal microflora develop in mature animals gradually introduced to oxalate (oxalate is metabolised to bicarbonate), the

incidence of poisoning by feeding oxalate-containing plants is uncommon.

> There is a widespread misconception among goatkeepers that sugar beet *pulp* should not be fed to male goats – there is no scientific evidence to support this theory.

Note: grazing lush clover pastures that are high in calcium and low in phosphorus but with a high oxalate content may lead to the formation of calcium *carbonate* calculi. Oxalate is degraded in the rumen, leaving excess calcium to be excreted in the urine and promoting the formation of calcium carbonate calculi in alkaline urine.

Silica calculi

Calculi of pure silica or mixed with calcium oxalate, calcium carbonate or organic materials are associated with the grazing of certain native grasses in parts of Australia and western North America (particularly during periods of water deprivation) and the eating of oat stubble, hay and grain.

Clinical signs

- Anorexia, lethargy.
- Signs of abdominal pain – grinding of teeth, looking at abdomen, kicking at abdomen.
- Reluctant to walk; stands with legs stretched out.
- Strains to urinate; may dribble urine before complete blockage occurs; small calculi may collect on preputial hairs.
- Palpation of the abdomen is resented.
- The distended bladder may be palpable in smaller animals and kids.
- Rupture of the urethra results in infiltration of urine into the perineal subcutaneous tissues; bladder rupture results in urine accumulation in the scrotum or intra-abdominally. Abdominal distension due to uroperitoneum must be distinguished from ruminal tympany, peritoneal tumours and gastrointestinal tract obstructions. Abdominal fluid can be identified by ballottement and the animal appears symmetrically enlarged and pear-shaped when viewed from behind.
- After rupture of the bladder or urethra, clinical signs will improve temporarily as pain is relieved, and the bladder is no longer palpable.

> Clinical signs may be mild. Careful examination of the goat on a hard concrete surface over a period of 1 or 2 hours may be required to establish if the goat is able to urinate.

Diagnosis

- Clinical signs.
- Examination of the preputial hairs may show gritty crystal deposits.
- In smaller animals, it may be possible to exteriorise the end of the penis, allowing examination of the urethral process and palpation of the urethra by sitting the animal on its rump or lying it on its back with front and hind legs tied together. However, in large animals this is generally impossible without sedation and even then is problematic.
- *Biochemistry* – a provisional diagnosis of urolithiasis is supported by greatly *increased levels of blood urea nitrogen (BUN) and creatinine* concentrations (up to a 10-fold increase or more). The normal level of BUN in the goat is 3.6 to 7.5 mmol/litre and creatinine 53 to 124 umol/1itre. In cases of urolithiasis, BUN concentrations may be greater than 40 mmol/1itre.

  In pre-renal azotaemia (e.g. dehydration, poor renal perfusion) urea may be moderately elevated but creatinine is normal or near-normal. If bladder rupture is suspected, the creatinine level of the fluid obtained by abdominocentesis can be compared with serum creatinine. If it is higher in the fluid than serum, uroabdomen is confirmed.
- *Radiography* – plain and contrast radiography will help determine the extent of urethral obstruction, the location of calculi, the numbers of calculi present or if there is urethral rupture. Calcium carbonate and calcium oxalate calculi can be seen in the bladder and urethra; struvite calculi cannot usually be identified.
- *Ultrasonography* – a distended bladder is identifiable by ultrasonography in the standing goat, using a 5 MHz sector or linear probe head in contact with the inguinal region. The bladder appears as an anechoic (black) area bordered by a hyperechoic (bright white) line.

  Ultrasonography can also readily identify the presence of free urine in the abdomen, following bladder rupture. Urine may leak through the distended bladder wall, without rupture of the bladder, so that free urine in the abdomen may be present even in the presence of a distended bladder.

Calculi can be identified in the dependent portion of the bladder. However, a variety of artifacts can generate acoustic shadows similar to those seen with calculi, particularly gas-filled intestine adjacent to the bladder – shadows from calculi tend to be rather anechoic, while those from gas are more hyperechoic.

Advanced hydronephrosis subsequent to prolonged urethral obstruction increases the size of the renal pelvis, which can be identified as the anechoic (fluid-filled) centre of the kidney.

- *Abdominocentesis* – in cases of bladder rupture, urine can be collected by abdominocentesis. Urine can be identified by its smell and urine dipsticks can be used for further analysis. The creatine level can be compared to that of serum (see above).

Treatment

Treatment is directed towards establishing a patent route of urine excretion, providing analgesia, correcting fluid deficits and correcting electrolyte imbalances, especially hyperkalaemia or hyperammonaemia.

- The urethral process should be examined in all cases of suspected urolithiasis as this is the commonest site of blockage. Gritty or sandy material can occasionally be milked out without resorting to surgery, particularly in kids and if the animal is sedated.
- Administration of a spasmolytic and analgesic agent (metamizole, hyoscine butylscopolamine, 0.5–5 ml i.v.; Buscopan Compositum, Boehringer Ingelheim) will relieve pain and aid passage of calculi. Alternatively, flunixin meglumine, 2 mg/kg, 2 ml/45 kg i.v. will provide analgesia and reduce inflammation.
- Sedation will aid the *exteriorisation of the penis* and may provide sufficient muscle relaxation to allow a stone to be passed. Diazepam (0.25–0.5 mg/kg slowly i.v.) is the sedative of choice, although it does not provide analgesia.

Note: the diuretic effect of xylazine may worsen bladder distension if the urethral obstruction is complete.Caudal epidural anaesthesia can be used instead of sedation and will also relieve the discomfort.

- If it is not possible to exteriorise the penis, it is possible to gain access to the penis by making a longitudinal incision through the prepuce, after anaesthetizing the skin with a small amount of local anaesthetic.

The urethral process can be exposed or, alternatively, if a blockage has been detected by palpation or ultrasound in the shaft of the penis, the obstructed area can be elevated and an incision made over the stones, allowing them to be removed. Small incisions can be closed with surgical glue, larger incisions may need closure of the mucosa with fine monofilament absorbable sutures.

- Pre-pubertal animals, and occasionally older animals castrated at a young age, may have a persistent frenulum, preventing exteriorising of the penis until this is broken down under anaesthesia. The frenulum is the anatomical attachment between the penis and preputial mucosa that typically breaks down between 4 and 6 months of age.

> In large animals, the exteriorisation of the penis may still be impossible even with sedation and can only be accomplished under general anaesthesia or lumbosacral epidural anaesthesia. It may be necessary to exteriorise the penis through a midline incision in the prepuce.

- The urethral process should *always* be removed with scissors. Amputation of the process may alleviate the blockage but even if the blockage is easily cleared, the process remains a prime site for blockage again in the future. Removal of the urethral process does not affect fertility of stud males.
- If urine does not flow immediately, catheterising the urethra and flushing with saline containing a few drops of lignocaine may allow sludge to be blown clear and urine to flow. The urine can now be acidified by instilling dilute vinegar through the catheter. Most commercial vinegar products contain 4 to 8% acetic acid, so diluting it 1 part in 5 (20% solution of vinegar) gives a suitable 1% acetic acid solution. This solution can also be used to flush the bladder, via the Foley catheter, after a tube cystotomy. In this case keeping the catheter plugged for 30–60 minutes will give time to dissolve crystals or stone still in the bladder and some will pass into the urethra to help dissolve any crystals there.

> Complete catheterisation to the bladder is anatomically impossible.

- Complete catheterisation to the bladder is anatomically impossible as catheters will not pass the ischial arch as they enter a diverticulum of the urethra, the urethral recess. Retrograde catheterisation from the bladder to the penis is possible after surgery.
- Even if urethral patency is restored, recurrent urethral blockage may subsequently occur as additional calculi enter the urethra from the bladder; 80% of animals initially relieved by amputation of the urethral process will re-obstruct as further stones pass from the bladder.
- Where further stones are present or the blockage is not at the urethral process, surgery will be necessary to locate and remove the obstruction. The surgical treatment of obstructive urolithiasis is discussed fully in Chapter 26. Financial constraints and the type of goat involved will impact on whether surgical treatment is justified or possible.
- Fluid therapy with 0.9% NaCl is indicated in any animals that are severely uraemic or depressed, initially using volumes sufficient to correct dehydration, and subsequently to encourage diuresis, reduce azotaemia and flush the urinary tract. Further correction of electrolyte and acid–base abnormalities may be necessary.
- Broad-spectrum antibiotic therapy should be given. Beta-lactams (penicillins and cephalosporins) have a good spectrum of activity and are excreted in urine.
- NSAIDs should be given, once adequate renal perfusion is attained, to decrease inflammation and help prevent urethral stricture formation.

General management for all male goats
- Ensure adequate water intake:
  - Clean water should always be available; change twice daily.
  - Give warm water in cold weather; use tank heaters where necessary in winter.
  - Check the height and suitability of any automatic drinkers and check that the goats know how to use them.
- The general nutritional approach to prevent urinary calculi is to decrease the intake of components that predispose to calculi formation by increasing the forage intake and decreasing concentrate/grain intake. Increased forage intake will additionally encourage water intake.
- Feed palatable fodder – good *grass* hay, pea straw, etc., if concentrates are being fed, while 50% grass/50%

lucerne (alfalfa) hay is suitable if no concentrates are fed. Grass hay has a calcium:phosphate ratio of 1:1; lucerne (alfalfa) hay 5.68:1; 50% grass/50% lucerne hay gives a ratio of approximately 2.3:1.
- Phosphorus levels in the total diet should be between 0.15 and 0.30% on a dry matter basis.
- Magnesium levels in the total diet should be between 0.12 and 0.18% on a dry matter basis.
- Feed dried grass products instead of concentrates, but *not* dried lucerne (alfalfa).
- Do not feed buffers, for example $NaHCO_3$.
- Feed a well-balanced diet with a 2:1 Ca:P ratio. Add calcium as calcium chloride to adjust the ration where necessary.
- Do not add P to concentrate diets.
- Feeding *ad libitum* rather than intermittently reduces the movement of water into the rumen in response to volatile acid production, which can lead to reduced urine output.

Additional control measures in problem herds/flocks
Control in the United Kingdom is generally directed towards prevention of phosphatic (struvite) calculi forming, but calcium carbonate calculi are common in animals fed high levels of dried lucerne (alfalfa). It is sensible to have the calculi analysed after each episode and to measure the urine pH before beginning control measures. Calculi can be analysed free of charge at the Minnesota Urolith Center (supported by Hill's Pet Nutrition): http://www.cvm.umn.edu/depts/minnesotaurolithcenter/. Stones that dissolve in a tube of 1% acetic acid are most likely to be struvite. If the stones dissolve, there is a better prognosis for the resolution of the urethral obstruction.

Measures are directed at changing the pH of the urine to increase the solubility of minerals that potentially form uroliths. Struvite crystals readily dissolve in acidic urine. Calcium carbonate stones will not dissolve in acid urine, but acidifying urine does prevent the formation of both phosphatic and carbonate stones. Anionic salts containing chlorides are used extensively. *The aim is to stabilise urine pH at around 5.5 to 6.5.*

- *Urine acidifiers* such as NH_4Cl (2% of concentrate ration, 0.5–1% dry matter intake), fishmeal, citrus pulp or maize gluten can be given as part of the concentrate ration, but the addition of salts as a simple percentage of the ration fails to consider the overall composition of the total ration. Some commercial diets may be naturally high in cations, which nullify the effect of adding anionic salts and can lead to inconsistent and unsuccessful maintenance of a low urinary pH. This is likely to occur with feedstuffs such as lucerne (alfalfa) and molassed feed. *NH₄Cl is not a universal panacea.* Ideally, complete rations with a balanced dietary cation–anion difference (DCAD) should be fed. The European Food Safety Authority (EFSA) has determined that a feed concentration of 1% ammonium chloride is considered safe for ruminants for approximately 3 months, but that for an unlimited period of administration, 0.5% ammonium chloride should not be exceeded. Unless a balanced ration is fed, these levels may not be enough to decrease the urine pH sufficiently. Some experimental work suggests that levels as high as 2.25% of the dry matter intake might be required. High doses of ammonium chloride could lead to metabolic acidosis.

- If complete rations are not formulated, *40 mg/kg of ammonium chloride* or a 100 g of commercial *anion dietary supplements* such as the acid-treated proteins Biochlor and Soychlor can be mixed with feed daily.

  Ammonium chloride is not very palatable and needs disguising with a palatable food such as granulated sugar (molassed feed should be avoided as its high potassium content may reduce the acidifying effect of ammonium chloride). Some goats will take these products mixed with mineral salts for free uptake – add 50 g of ammonium chloride to 1 kg of trace mineral mix. Soychlor (hydrochloric acid treated soybean meal) is more palatable.

- *Increasing the salt (NaCl) content* of the ration will increase the water intake – an increase to 4% of daily dry matter intake will be required to alter water intake, that is 80 g NaCl daily for an animal weighing 100 kg and ingesting 2% of its body weight in dry matter per day. Up to 9% NaCl can be fed before decreasing palatability. A saturated salt solution can be sprayed on the hay to increase salt intake.

- Individually animals can be given *ammonium chloride orally* daily or twice daily.

  The dose should be titrated for each individual goat, with urinary pH being determined using a pH meter or urine strips. *pH monitoring is the only way to gauge the efficiency of dosing, 10 g* being a reasonable starting point for a daily dose, but substantially higher levels may be necessary in large animals to ensure that the urine pH remains <6.0 for 24 hours. The salt can be dissolved in 40 ml of water for drenching and sweetened with sugar if necessary. Most goats readily take the necessary dose in orange juice.

- Continuous use of ammonium chloride can result in re-alkalisation of the urine so that clinical effectiveness is lost. This can occur in as little as 4 days. A *pulse dosing regime,* using a 3 day treatment period followed by 4 days without medication has been recommended.

- Lower calcium diets should be used if calcium carbonate or calcium oxalate uroliths are a problem.

Liver disease

A general increase in the size of the liver or specific parenchymal changes may result in abdominal pain, either a localised pain detectable by palpation or more generalised pain with changes in posture and unwillingness to move. Other clinical signs of liver disease include oedema, ascites, hepatic encephalopathy (Chapter 12), photosensitivity (Chapter 11), anorexia, constipation, diarrhoea (Chapter 14), jaundice (see below) or weight loss (Chapter 9).

Goats may become exposed to a variety of hepatotoxins, including toxic plants (see Chapter 21), mycotoxins and chemicals.

Diagnosis

- *Ultrasonography* – use a 5 MHz sector transducer; the liver can be viewed on the right side via the 8th to 10th intercostal spaces, with the probe head at a right angle to the thoracic wall.

- *Liver biopsy* – use a transthoracic approach via the right 9th intercostal space slightly above an imaginary line from the tuber coxae to the point of the elbow (with the animal standing) or the right 11th intercostal space (with the goat in left lateral recumbency). Blood vessels run along the caudal borders of the ribs and should be avoided. The goat is not starved, so the full rumen keeps the liver adjacent to the right body wall. The procedure can be carried out in the conscious animal, using light sedation where necessary.

  The site is surgically prepared and 2 to 3 ml of local anaesthetic infused subcutaneously and into the intercostal muscle. A stab incision is made through the skin and a 14 g, 11.5 cm liver biopsy instrument inserted through the incision and the intercostal muscles, with the biopsy instrument directed towards the opposite elbow, and then into the liver. The needle should be slowly advanced so that each tissue layer can be appreciated as it is reached – intercostal muscle, pleura, diaphragm and liver capsule. As the pleura is penetrated, there is slight resistance followed by a 'pop'; there is a slight 'pop' as the diaphragm is crossed and the needle moves strongly with each breath; a slight increase in resistance is felt on entering the liver and the needle activated to take the sample. The needle should be inserted about 2 cm into the liver. Real-time ultrasonography can help determine the direction and depth required and reduce the risk of penetrating a large vessel.

Samples can be taken for histopathology (in 10% formalin), culture (in a sterile, plain tube) and mineral analysis (in a plastic tube). Samples for mineral analysis should be washed thoroughly with deionised water before placing in the tube.

Biopsy may be useful in:

o Primary hepatocellular disease: necrosis of hepatocytes, cirrhosis, fatty changes, biliary hyperplasia, neoplasia.

o Bile duct obstruction: plugs of bile in canaliculi, biliary cirrhosis, etc.

The main risk factors include penetration of the gall bladder and haemorrhage from penetrating a large hepatic vessel. Peritonitis is rare. Animals occasionally exhibit diarrhoea after the procedure due to a pneumothorax, but does not cause a problem because of the complete mediastinum and resolves within 20 minutes.

■ *Biochemistry* – the biochemical profile shows whether there is significant liver disease and gives some indication of the type of liver pathology present: aspartate transaminase (AST), gamma glutamyl-transferase (GGT), glutamate dehydrogenase (GLDH), sorbitol dehydrogenase (SDH), albumin, globulin; serum protein electrophoresis.

o *Primary hepatocellular disease* – damage to hepatocytes gives an increase in serum of specific hepatocyte enzymes. In goats these are GLDH and SDH. In the absence of damage to the bile duct system, GGT remains low.

   ◆ Severe anaemia: haemorrhage, haemolytic disease, haemonchosis.
   ◆ Copper poisoning.
   ◆ Shock.
   ◆ Congestive cardiac failure.

   ◆ Bacteraemia: liver abscess, salmonellosis.

o *Cholangiohepatitis* – damage to the biliary system and the hepatocytes results in elevated serum GLDH and GGT.

   ◆ Fascioliasis.
   ◆ Bacterial cholangitis.
   ◆ Pyrrolizidine alkaloid poisoning.
   ◆ Primary neoplasia.
   ◆ Metastatic neoplasia.
   ◆ Aflatoxicosis.

o *Hepatic cirrhosis* – persistent liver damage and fibrosis from whatever cause results in a decrease in the functional liver mass. Early or moderate fibrosis is difficult to detect biochemically but when severe will result in decreased serum albumin and increased globulin; GGT and GLDH may be moderately elevated.

Jaundice is an uncommon sign in the goat even with severe hepatocellular damage, but may occur:

■ In *haemolytic disease* where there is excess production of bilirubin, for example copper toxicity, leptospirosis, eperylhrozoonosis and poisoning by brassicas or onions.

■ Following *bile duct obstruction*, for example Fascioliasis.

With haemolytic disease, most of the bilirubin is indirect as it has not been conjugated by the hepatocytes; in cholestatic disease more of the bilirubin will be direct. Urine bilirubin may not be elevated in haemolytic disease, because unconjugated bilirubin is bound to serum protein and will not be filtered by the kidney. Conjugated bilirubin in obstructive cholestasis is water soluble and may be detected in urine. Urine urobilinogen may be increased in haemolytic jaundice because of increased production, but is absent in obstructive cholestasis because no bilirubin is converted into urobilinogen in the intestine.

Toxic minerals

Copper poisoning

Goats are relatively more resistant to copper poisoning than sheep, but poisoning may occur from high copper mineral licks, eating pig rations containing high levels of copper, drinking footbaths, or dosing with copper sulphate. Calf milk replacers containing high copper levels have also been implicated. *Trifolium subterraneum* (clover) ingestion causes copper retention by the liver. The parenteral injection of copper compounds has been associated with collapse and sudden death.

Low dietary levels of zinc and molybdenum, which are copper antagonists, may increase copper intake, even when dietary copper levels are not obviously high. Copper accumulates in the liver until maximum hepatic levels are reached, when copper is released into the bloodstream, acting as an oxidant and causing an acute intravascular haemolysis, associated with the formation of Heinz bodies.

Clinical signs

The clinical onset of chronic copper poisoning may appear to be acute, although it is a chronic condition, which can take months or years to reach the hemolytic crisis stage.

- Often sudden death.
- Sudden depression and lethargy, pyrexia.
- Severe abdominal pain.
- Mucoid diarrhoea.
- Haemoglobinuria/anaemia if the goat survives long enough.
- Jaundice.
- Death within 24–48 hours after signs appear.

Laboratory findings

- Heinz body anaemia.
- Elevated serum liver enzymes (AST, GGT, GLDH) occur during the later stages of copper accumulation in the liver before clinical signs are apparent. Raised levels should prompt further investigation of the liver copper status by biopsy or post-mortem liver sampling of representative cull animals.
- Marked bilirubinaemia.
- Serum copper levels are often only marginally increased until the hepatic storage capacity is exceeded and of little diagnostic value, but are elevated during the haemolytic crisis.

Post-mortem findings

- Liver enlarged, friable, icteric (pale tan to bronze coloured).
- Entire carcase may be jaundiced.
- Kidneys dark green/black.
- Urine is dark-red coloured.

Diagnosis

- Liver, kidney and faecal copper levels markedly elevated – kidney levels > 314 µmol/kg DM; liver levels >6400–16 000 µmol/kg DM.

- Kidney iron concentrations increase markedly if there has been severe haemolysis >1600–18 000 µmol/kg DM.

Treatment

- Avoid stress.
- Interfere with copper absorption from the intestine (treat *all* exposed animals):
  o *Ammonium tetrathiomolybdate*, either *1.7 mg/kg i.v.* or *3.4 mg/kg s.c.* in three doses on alternate days. Ammonium tetrathiomolybdate is not licensed for use in food-producing animals and a meat withdrawal period of >6 months has been recommended. Tetrathiomolybdate can redistribute copper, bound to metallothionein, to extrahepatic sites and also blocks the transfer of copper to cuproenzymes by copper chaperones.
  o *Anhydrous sodium sulphate* (1 g) orally every 24 hours.
- Chelate copper in the blood:
  o *D-penicillamine*, 52 mg/kg orally every 24 hours for 1 week.
- Blood transfusion.

Lead poisoning

See Chapter 12.

Fertiliser ingestion

See Chapter 14.

Post-kidding problems

Metritis

See Chapter 4.

Retained kid

See Chapter 4.

Peritonitis

Peritonitis from whatever cause produces abdominal pain, ileus, pyrexia and possibly abdominal distension. Most infections occur post-kidding, following a uterine tear, as a sequel to metritis or following caesarian section, but peritonitis may also occur as a sequel to rumenitis, after trocharisation of the rumen or other abdominal catastrophe.

Cystitis

Cystitis occurs sporadically, particularly in does. Some does will merely show frequent urination with small amounts of urine being passed, but acute cases will show moderate abdominal pain and occasionally systemic illness.

Cystitis rarely occurs as a sequel to kidding, even when there is infection of the posterior reproductive tract, but stricture of the cervix and vagina, caused by fibrosis following trauma at kidding, has been associated with blockage of the urethra and ureter, obstructing urine flow and leading to cystitis and pyelonephritis.

Pyelonephritis occurs infrequently in goats, much less frequently than in cattle, possibly because there is a lower incidence of uterine infections post-partum. Most urinary tract infections involve *Corynebacterium renale*, which is susceptible to procaine penicillin. This is the drug of choice in treating cystitis and pyelonephritis as it is cheap and secreted unchanged by the kidney: *administer procaine penicillin, 10 mg/kg i.m.* daily.

Transabdominal ultrasonography of the standing goat with a 5 MHz sector scanner will identify the bladder and allow an assessment of bladder distension and the thickness of the bladder wall.

Note: (1) Many does will urinate frequently when nervous.

(2) It is sometimes difficult to distinguish between the end result of hydrometra (see Chapter 1), that is 'cloudburst', and cystitis. In most cloudbursts, the fluid is rapidly released with a sudden decrease in abdominal size and wetting of the flanks and perineum, but occasionally the fluid is released slowly over a few days with intermittent straining and passing of small amounts of fluid.

Uterine tumours

Although tumours of the urinary systems are uncommon, tumours of the uterus are reasonably common in old goats and *adenocarcinomas* and *leiomyomas* have been reported as a cause of abdominal straining and urinary

tenesmus. Leiomyomas are benign smooth-muscle tumours, which arise from the cervix, uterus or vagina (see Plates 15.3, 15.4 and 15.5).

Often the main presenting sign is *bleeding from the vulva*. The bleeding may occur spasmodically over quite long periods of time and by the time veterinary advice is sought the tumours are often quite large, so that a mass may be detectable by abdominal palpation. Large tumours may produce sufficient mass in the pelvic inlet to activate the pelvic reflex, as occurs during second-stage labour, or may obstruct the urethra, resulting in a distended bladder.

> In old female goats, persistent bleeding from the vulva, in the absence of obvious injury, is virtually diagnostic for a uterine tumour.

Intravaginal tumours can be detected by digital or speculum examination of the vagina. Intra-abdominal tumours can be detected by ultrasonography, using a 5 MHz sector scanner, as irregular hyperechoic structures distinct from the bladder.

Uterine torsion

Uterine torsion occurs rarely in heavily pregnant goats and can produce abdominal pain.

Plant poisoning

See Chapter 20.

Many plants can cause colic in goats, with the *Ericaceae* (rhododendrons, laurels, azaleas, Japanese pieris, lily of the valley) being prominent.

Colic in kids

> Any colic signs in kids should be treated as a potential emergency and the owner encouraged to seek veterinary help if the signs persist. Kids regularly die after quite short periods of abdominal pain.

Table 15.4 Causes of colic in kids.

Abomasal bloat	Diarrhoea	Urolithiasis
Mesenteric torsion Caecal torsion	*Clostridium perfringens* type D Enterotoxaemia	Visceral cysticercosis
Intussusception		
Ruminal bloat	Coccidiosis	Plant poisoning

Possible causes of colic in kids are listed in Table 15.4. Colic in kids is generally a sequel to feeding milk replacers by bottle or in *ad libitum* systems, as a result of nutritional mismanagement (incorrect concentration, incorrect temperature, overfeeding, etc.) (see Chapter 6). Abomasal bloat occurs in pre-ruminant and ruminant kids; ruminal bloat can occur if the oesophageal groove reflex does not function when the kid is stressed or its routine is altered and milk enters the developing rumen rather than the abomasum. Kids are more susceptible than adults to a number of abdominal catastrophes, including *mesenteric torsion*, *intussusception* and *caecal torsion*, all of which produce signs of severe colic.

Abomasal bloat

See Chapter 16.
Abomasal bloat is common in artificially reared kids and is a significant cause of death between 4 and 12 weeks of age.

Ruminal bloat

See Chapter 16.

Mesenteric torsion

Mesenteric torsion leads to infarction of the abomasum, intestine or caecum. Torsion should be considered in cases of bloat that do not respond to treatment.

Aetiology
- The aetiology of the condition is poorly understood, but it occurs most commonly in artificially reared kids, probably after an excessive feed of milk in a short time. Torsions occasionally occur in older animals,

but the predisposing factors in these cases are not known.

Clinical signs
- As for bloat, with severe abdominal pain, distended abdomen and intermittent piercing screams; the kid may throw itself about.
- Kids are often found dead.

Post-mortem findings
- The affected portion of the alimentary tract is enlarged, dark red and filled with gas or blood-stained fluid.
- Careful examination reveals a twist in the mesentery.

Treatment
- Surgical intervention to correct the torsion may be effective if the condition is diagnosed early. Supportive therapy with intravenous fluids is essential to combat shock, together with analgesics such as flunixin meglumine.

Coccidiosis

See Chapter 14.
In heavy coccidial infections, intense colic and shock can be produced by the damage to the intestinal cells during release of meronts and merozoites, so that kids may be found collapsed or dead.

Diarrhoea

See Chapter 14.

Clostridium perfringens type D (enterotoxaemia)

Enterotoxaemia is a potential problem in all ages of goat as the causative agent is present in most herds (see earlier in this chapter).

Urolithiasis

Urolithiasis (see earlier in this chapter) should be considered as a cause of colic in older male kids.

Visceral cysticercosis

Infection with large numbers of *Cysticercus tenuicollis*, the metacestode of the canine tapeworm *Taenia hydatigena*, occasionally causes acute disease in kids under 6 months because of damage to the liver parenchyma. Clinical signs include depression, anorexia, pyrexia, weight loss, abdominal discomfort and occasionally death due to acute haemorrhage.

Plant poisoning

See Chapter 21 and above.

Further reading

Clinical procedures and ultrasonography

Braun, U. (2011) Ultrasonographic characterization of the liver, caudal vena cava, portal vein and gallbladder in goats. *Amer. J. Vet. Res.*, **72**, 219–225.

Braun, U. *et al.* (2011) Ultrasonographic examination of the small intestine, large intestine and greater omentum in 30 Saanen goats. *Vet. J.*, **189** (3), 330–335.

Herdt, T.H. and Huff, B. (2011) The use of blood analysis to evaluate trace mineral status in ruminant livestock. *Vet. Clin. North Amer.: Food Anim. Pract.*, **27** (2), 255–283.

Mueller, K. (2010) Clinical procedures in goats. *Goat Vet. Soc. J.*, **26**, 15–18.

Scott, P. (2012) Abdominal ultrasonography as an adjunct to clinical examination. 1. Small ruminants. *In Pract.*, **34** (1), 12–21.

Copper poisoning

Cornish, J. (2007) Copper toxicosis in a dairy goat herd. *J. Am. Vet. Med. Assoc.*, **231**, 586–589.

Enterotoxaemia

Baxendell, S.A. (1984) Enterotoxaemia of goats. *Proc. Univ. Sydney Post. Grad. Comm. Vet. Sci.*, **73**, 557–560.

Blackwell, T.F. and Butler, D.G. (1992) Clinical signs, treatment, and postmortem lesions in dairy goats with enterotoxaemia; 13 cases (1979–1982). *J. Am. Vet. Med. Assoc.*, **200** (2), 214–217.

Deprez, P. (2015) Clostridium perfringens infections – a diagnostic challenge. *Vet. Rec.*, **177** (15), 388–389.

Dray, T. (2004) *Clostridium perfringens* type A and type A and β2 toxin associated with enterotoxemia in a 5-week-old goat. *Can. Vet. J.*, **45** (3), 251–253.

Green, D.S. *et al.* (1987) Injection site reactions and antibody responses in sheep and goats after the use of multivalent clostridial vaccines. *Vet. Rec.*, **120** (18), 435–439.

Houghton, S. (2006) Vaccination of goats against Clostridial disease. *Goat Vet. Soc. J.*, **22**, 17–20.

Uzal, F.A. and Kelly, W.R. (1998) Protection of goats against experimental enterotoxaemia by vaccination with *Clostridial perfringens* type D epsilon toxoid. *Vet. Rec.*, **142**, 722–725.

Uzal, F.A. and Songer, J.G. (2008) Diagnosis of *Clostridium perfringens* intestinal infections in sheep and goats. *J. Vet. Diagn. Invest.*, **20**, 253–265.

Leiomyoma

Cockcroft, P.D, and McInnes, E.F. (1998) Abdominal straining in a goat with a leiomyoma of the cervix. *Vet. Rec.*, **142**, 171.

Scott, P. (1998) Ultrasonography of the ovine urinary tract. *UK Vet.*, **3** (6), 67–73.

Liver disease

Ellinson, R.S. (1985) Some aspects of clinical pathology in goats. *Proceedings of the Course in Goat Husbandry and Medicine*, Massey University, 1985, pp. 105–122.

Pearson, E.G. (1981) Differential diagnosis of icterus in large animals. *Calif. Vet.* **2**, 25–31.

Pearson, E.G. and Craig, A.M. (1980) The diagnosis of liver disease in equine and food animals. *Mod. Vet. Pract.*, **61** (3), 233–237.

Ruminal acidosis

Andrews, A.H. (2003) Goat nutrition – notes on a few basic principles. *Goat Vet. Soc. J.*, **19**, 23–25.

Braun, U., Rihs, T. and Schefer, U. (1992) Ruminal lactic acidosis in sheep and goats. *Vet. Rec.*, **130**, 343–349.

Chamberlain, A.T. (2006) Acidosis in goats – Is it a problem and how will we know? *Goat Vet. Soc. J.*, **22**, 12–16.

Michell, R. (1990) Ruminant acidosis. *In Pract.*, **12**, 245–249.

Underwood, W.J. (1992) Rumen lactic acidosis. Part I. Epidemiology and pathophysiology. *Comp. Cont. Ed. Pract. Vet.*, **14** (8), 1127–1133.

Underwood, W.J. (1992) Rumen lactic acidosis. Part II. Clinical signs, diagnosis, treatment and prevention. *Comp. Cont. Ed. Pract. Vet.*, **14** (9), 1265–1270.

Urolithiasis

Baxendell, S.A. (1984) Urethral calculi in goats. *Proc. Univ. Sydney Post. Grad. Comm. Vet. Sci.*, **73**, 495–497.

Cuddeford, D. (1988) Ruminant urolithiasis: cause and prevention. *Goat Vet. Soc. J.*, **10** (1), 10–14.

EFSA Panel on Additives and Products or substances used in Animal Feed (FEEDAP) (2012) Scientific opinion on the safety and efficacy of ammonium chloride for bovines, sheep, dogs and cats. *EFSA J.*, **10** (6), 2738.

Franz, S. *et al.* (2008) Laparoscopic-assisted implantation of a urinary catheter in male sheep. *J. Amer. Vet. Med. Assoc.*, **232** (12), 1857–1862.

Gascoigne, E. (2015) Urinary tract disease in goats. *Goat Vet. Soc. J.*, **31**, 72–80.

George, J.W., Hird, D.W. and George, L.W. (2007) Serum biochemical abnormalities in goats with uroliths: 107 cases (1992–2003). *J. Amer. Vet. Med. Assoc.*, **230**, 101–106.

Janke, J.J. *et al.* (2009) Use of Walpole's solution for the treatment of goats with urolithiasis: 25 cases (2001–2006). *J. Amer. Vet. Med. Assoc.*, **234** (2), 249–252.

Jones, M.L., Streeter, R.N., Goad, C.L. (2009) Use of dietary cation anion difference for control of urolithiasis risk factors in goats. *Am. J. Vet. Res.*, **70**, 149–155.

Kannan, K.V. and Lawrence, K.E.(2010) Obstructive urolithiasis in a Saanen goat in New Zealand, resulting in a ruptured bladder. *N.Z. Vet. J.*, **58** (5), 269–271.

Kinsley, M.A. *et al.* (2013) Use of plain radiography in the diagnosis, surgical management and postoperative treatment of obstructive urolithiasis in 25 goats and 2 sheep. *Vet. Surg.*, **42** (6), 663–668.

Mavangira, V., Cornish, J.M. and Angelos, J.A. (2010) Effect of ammonium chloride supplementation on urine pH and urinary excretion of electrolytes in goats. *J. Amer. Vet. Med. Assoc.*, **237** (11), 1299–1304.

Miesner, M. (2009) Urolithiasis in small ruminants (Proceedings) CVC in Kansas City Proceedings. Available at: http://veterinarycalendar.dvm360.com/urolithiasis-small-ruminants-proceedings-1?rel=canonical.

Mueller, K. (2015) Soft tissue surgery, urethrotomy, tube cystotomy, dehorning and caesarian section. *Goat Vet. Soc. J.*, **31**, 67–71.

Nwaokorie, E.E. (2015) Risk factors for calcium carbonate urolithiasis in goats. *J. Amer. Vet. Med. Assoc.*, **247** (3), 293–299.

Oehme, F.W. and Tillman, H. (1965) Diagnosis and treatment of ruminant urolithiasis. *J. Am. Vet. Med. Assoc.*, **147**, 1331–1339.

Sprake, P. *et al.* (2012) The effect of ammonium chloride treatment as a long term preventative approach for urolithiasis in goats and a comparison of continuous and pulse dosing regimes. *J. Vet. Int. Med.*, **26** (3), 760.

CHAPTER 16

Abdominal distension

Abnormal distension must be distinguished from normal anatomical changes. Goats carry their fat deposits intra-abdominally rather than subcutaneously, so overweight goats may appear to have abdominal distension. Pygmy goats are achondroplastic dwarfs with relatively large abdomens, when compared to other breeds. In older goats of some breeds, particularly British Toggenburgs, the abdominal muscles may drop ventrolaterally in late pregnancy so that subsequently the abdomen remains permanently lower than normal. Many causes of abdominal distension will produce some degree of abdominal pain (see Chapter 15). Tables 16.1 and 16.2 list the causes of abdominal distension in adults and kids, respectively.

Initial assessment

- Age and sex, pregnant or non-pregnant.
- Sudden or slow onset of abdominal distension.
- Feeding history – type of feed, change in diet, age at weaning, kid feeding regime.
- Routine medication, including worming.
- General physical examination – most cases of abdominal distension will involve the alimentary tract or pregnant goats.
- Specific examination of the digestive system:
  o Visual inspection: abdominal contour from behind, position of distension.
  o Palpation of left abdominal wall and rumen: filling of rumen.
  o Percussion: tympanitic sounds, pain.
  o Auscultation: rumen mobility.

Table 16.1 Abdominal distension in adult goats.

	Distension
Normal goats	
▪ Abdominal fat	Bilateral
▪ Dropped stomach	Bilateral
▪ Pygmy goats	Bilateral
Ruminal distension	
▪ Primary ruminal tympany (frothy bloat)	Left paralumbar fossa initially, then entire left side, then also right ventral abdomen
▪ Secondary ruminal tympany (choke)	As primary tympany
▪ Impacted rumen	Low left
Abomasal distension	
▪ Abomasal impaction	Right ventral
▪ Left-sided displacement	
Reproductive	
▪ Pregnancy	Bilateral, particularly low
▪ False pregnancy (hydrometra)	Bilateral
▪ Hydrops uteri (hydroallantois, hydramnios)	Bilateral
▪ Ovarian tumour	Bilateral
Ventral hernia	Low right
Ascites	
▪ Chronic liver congestion	Bilateral
▪ Fascioliasis	Bilateral
▪ Cardiac failure	Bilateral
Abdominal tumour	Bilateral
Ruptured bladder (urolithiasis)	Bilateral ventral

Table 16.2 Abdominal distension in kids.

	Onset of distension
Birth to 1 week	
▪ Prematurity	Present at birth
▪ Congenital abnormalities	
○ Alimentary tract defect	Generally slow
○ Kidney defect	Slow
○ Heart defect	Slow
▪ High alimentary tract obstruction	
○ Pyloric obstruction	Sudden
○ Abomasal obstruction	Sudden
Older kids	
▪ Abomasal bloat	Sudden
▪ Ruminal bloat	Sudden
▪ Mesenteric torsion (intestinal bloat)	Sudden
▪ 'Pot belly'	
○ Inadequate nutrition	Slow
○ Gastrointestinal parasitism	Slow

Further investigations

- Abdominocentesis, trocharisation, passage of stomach tube (see Chapter 15).
- Ultrasonography in the standing goat, using a 5 MHz sector transducer, to determine the presence or absence of live fetuses.

Adult goats

Ruminal distension

Primary ruminal tympany (frothy bloat)
Aetiology
- Grazing lush pastures, particularly clover or lucerne in the spring; sudden introduction of grass clippings or excessive vegetable waste, etc., produces a rumen filled with gas or frothy material.

Clinical signs
- Depression.
- Abdominal pain – teeth grinding, shifting of weight of the feet, kicking at the abdomen.
- Abdominal distension – more obvious in left flank, but the whole of the abdomen is enlarged.

- Dyspnoea – mouth breathing, extension of the head, protrusion of the tongue.

Treatment
- First-aid treatment by owner:
  - Drench with
    - 100 to 200 ml of any non-toxic vegetable or mineral oil.
    - A proprietary non-ionic surfactant polymer (poloxalene) bloat drench (Bloat Guard, Agrimin).
    - 8 to 10 ml medical turpentine in 100 ml liquid paraffin.
    - 100–250 ml linseed oil with 15–20 ml turpentine oil.
    - In an emergency, 10 ml washing-up liquid will suffice.
    Massage the abdomen to spread the oil.
  - Stand the goat with the front feet raised, tie a 30 cm stick through the mouth like a bridle and smear honey or treacle on the back of the tongue to promote continual chewing. Gentle exercise may encourage eructation.
  - Trocharise the rumen on the left side with a 14 or 16 g 38 or 50 mm needle.
- Veterinary treatment continues the treatment started by the owner with release of gas by means of a stomach tube or trocharisation with a needle or sheep trocar and cannula. The oil or bloat remedy can be introduced directly into the rumen through a cannula.
- Increase the fibre in the diet by feeding hay before a return to feeding legumes or grazing.

Prevention
- Monitor animals carefully for the first 12 hours after access to the pasture.
- Allow only limited access to grazing:
  - Move animals on to the pasture in the afternoon, not in the morning, so the animals have already eaten.
  - Feed hay, silage or non-legume pasture in the morning before moving.
- Once moved, leave the animals on the pasture; the highest risk of bloat occurs in the first few hours after movement to the high-legume pasture.
- Frost increases the risk of bloat, so remove the animals before any frosts occur.
- The bloat risk is low in fields containing less than 50% legume.

- Some legumes, particularly those with a high tannin content like sanfoin, birdsfoot trefoil (*Lotus pedunculatus*) and *Sericea lespedeza* do not cause bloat.
- Wilting the forage significantly reduces the risk of bloat, so "cutting and carting" or allowing the animals to eat wilted forage off the ground is beneficial.
- Avoid any sudden introduction of fermentable material to the diet and provide sufficient fibre in the diet in the form of hay.
- Smearing vegetable oil on the coat before grazing will promote a regular intake of oil by licking so preventing gas buildup.
- A poloxalene pre-mix (Bloat Guard Premix, Agrimin/Phibro) is licensed for use in cattle (but not goats) at 22 mg of poloxalene/kg bodyweight daily sprinkled on the ration, starting 2–3 days before the period of risk.

Secondary ruminal tympany ('choke')
Aetiology
- A physical obstruction to eructation causes a buildup of gas in the rumen, for example oesophageal obstruction caused by a *foreign body,* such as a piece of apple or rootcrop, or a tumour at the region of the thoracic inlet, for example *thymoma* (see Chapter 10).
- Spasm of the reticuloruminal musculature in *tetanus* and interference with oesophageal groove functions in cases of *diaphragmatic hernia* may also lead to chronic ruminal tympany.
- A degree of ruminal tympany may be observed in diseases such as *listeriosis* because of phayngeal can produce large amounts paralysis.

Treatment
- First-aid treatment by the owner as for primary tympany. Small amounts of oil may help lubricate an obstruction.
- Veterinary treatment – trocharisation to relieve the buildup of gas.
- Administration of an antispasmolytic drug will aid relaxation of oesophageal musculature around a foreign body.

   Metamizole, Hyoscine butylbromide, 5 ml i.v.

- Consider oesophagostomy where the foreign body is palpable in the neck if conservative methods are unsuccessful.

Rumen impaction
Rumen impaction is uncommon in the United Kingdom unless goats are fed fibrous, low-energy diets. The distension is in the lower left ventral abdomen, where the rumen is palpably hard. Affected animals are lethargic and inappetent, with decreased milk yield. Some animals have mild bloat. Daily dosing with 100 to 200 ml of non-toxic mineral or vegetable oil may soften the impaction, but many goats will require a rumenotomy.

Abomasal distension

Abomasal impaction
Abomasal impaction is uncommon in the United Kingdom as diets do not generally predispose to the condition, which is the result of high-fibre, low-digestible feeds, particularly during pregnancy. There is progressive right ventral abdominal distension and the abomasum may be palpably hard and doughy. Affected animals lose weight and pass soft, fibrous, smelly faeces. Treatment with 100 to 200 ml of non-toxic mineral or vegetable oil daily, coupled with an improved, less fibrous diet, will resolve early cases. Severe impactions have a more problematical outcome.

Left-sided displacement of the abomasum
Aetiology
- Left-sided displacement of the abomasum is poorly documented in the goat, but is probably related to high levels of concentrate feeding in late pregnancy. During pregnancy the abomasum is pushed under the rumen by the expanding uterus. After parturition the rumen resumes its normal position, trapping the abomasum.

Clinical signs
- Selective anorexia – refuses concentrates but eats hay.
- Reduced ruminal contractions; rarely cuds.
- Initial constipation, then diarrhoea.
- Secondary ketosis – smell of ketones on breath, positive Rothera's reaction to milk.
- Auscultation of the left flank reveals abnormal sounds – high-pitched metallic tinkling and ringing sounds, which may be spontaneous or can be elicited.

Treatment

- A spontaneous cure may occur with exercise and access to browsings.
- Conservative treatment with starvation and rolling.
- Surgical replacement and anchorage.
- After spontaneous cure or surgery, concentrate feeding should be reintroduced very gradually over a period of 2 or 3 weeks.

Abomasal emptying defect (abomasal outflow defect)

Abomasal emptying defect (AED) is a sporadic cause of dysfunction of the alimentary tract of sheep, which has been reported in a limited number of goats.

Aetiology

- Unknown, but possibly deficiencies in the autonomic innervation of the abomasum.
- Progressive abomasal impaction leads to abdominal distension and passive hepatic congestion.

Clinical signs

- Abdominal distension.
- Decreased appetite.
- Cachexia.
- Weight loss.
- In sheep, firm pelleted faeces, frequently coated with thick mucus, but intermittent diarrhoea is reported in goats.
- Afebrile.
- Rumen motility may be increased.

Laboratory findings

- Liver enzymes (GGT and GLDH) may be elevated if hepatic congestion occurs.
- Rumen chloride concentrations are elevated in sheep because of the reflux of chloride-rich secretions from the abomasum into the rumen.

Post-mortem findings

- Abomasal enlargement and impaction.
- Abomasal contents firm, dry and fibrous, resembling rumen ingesta.
- Ascites.

Treatment

- None.

Note: animals with scrapie may present with marked abomasal impaction.

Other causes of abomasal distension

In sheep, *inadequate rumination* as a result of teeth problems, vagus indigestion and adenomata of the abomasal mucosa is reported to cause abomasal enlargement. Similar conditions could be expected to cause abomasal distension in the goat, although rarely reported.

Distension related to pregnancy and the reproductive tract

Normal pregnancy, *false pregnancy* (hydrometra) and *hydrops uteri* (hydrallantois and hydramnios) all cause abdominal distension (see Chapter 1). *Ovarian tumours* can produce large amounts of intra-abdominal fluid.

Ventral hernia

Rupture of the ventral abdominal muscles occasionally occurs following trauma or abdominal distension, resulting in abdominal swelling and dropping of the udder. Most cases occur in late pregnancy when increasing intra-abdominal pressure weakens the muscles and tendinous support of the abdominal wall, particularly the external and internal abdominal oblique muscles. Manual or surgical intervention at parturition is usually necessary. The hernia can be corrected surgically after kidding.

Ascites

Ascites is uncommon in goats, but may arise:

- In *fascioliasis* (see Chapter 9), as a result of blood loss and decreased hepatic synthesis of albumin.
- In *gastrointestinal helminthiasis*, secondary to hypoproteinaemia and anaemia.
- From *chronic liver congestion*.
- From *right-sided cardiac failure*.

Congestive cardiac failure

Congestive cardiac failure can arise in goats from a number of causes including *cardiotoxic plants* (see Chapter 21) and *thymoma* (see Chapter 10).

Clinical signs of congestive cardiac failure include exercise intolerance, ascites, tachycardia, increased jugular pulse, jugular distension, submandibular oedema, moist cough and chronic weight loss.

The heart can be auscultated over the ventral third of left thoracic wall between the 2nd and 4th or 5th ribs and is heard most clearly at the 4th intercostal space.

Heart rate: Kid: 120–140 beats/minute (adult rates attained by 3 months of age)

Adult: 70–95 beats/minute.

Normal heart rhythm: regular (a normal respiratory sinus arrhythmia is common).

Post-mortem findings include heart enlargement, hydrothorax, hydropericardium, hydroperitoneum and pulmonary oedema.

Treatment for heart failure is rarely attempted. Furosemide is licensed for use in cattle in the United Kingdom. Other drugs used in dogs, particularly diuretics, vasodilators and digoxin could be used, but are not licensed for use in food-producing animals.

Abdominal tumours

Both intestinal and ovarian adenocarcinomas have been associated with the accumulation of large amounts of intra-abdominal fluid.

Ruptured bladder (urolithiasis)

A blocked urethra as a result of urolithiasis in male goats will lead to the rupture of the urinary bladder and collection of urine in the abdomen (see Chapter 15). Abdominal fluid can be identified by ballottement and the animal appears symmetrically enlarged and pear-shaped when viewed from behind. The creatinine level of the fluid obtained by abdominocentesis can be compared with serum creatinine. If it is higher in the fluid than serum, uroabdomen is confirmed.

Kids from birth to 1 week old

Prematurity

Many premature kids have a flaccid, slightly distended abdomen. There may be additional evidence of abortions or stillbirths within the herd.

Congenital abnormalities

Alimentary tract defects – *atresia ani, atresia coli* and *atresia recti* occur occasionally in kids, leading to increasing abdominal distension with no production of faeces, decreasing appetite and lethargy. *Pyloric stenosis* produces a more rapid abdominal distension than alimentary tract blockages.

A *kidney defect* or *heart defect* (see Chapter 5) could produce ascites, with slowly increasing abdominal distension.

High alimentary tract obstruction

Rarely, *pyloric obstructions*, or example with milk curd, or *abomasal torsion* occur in very young kids.

Older kids

Abomasal bloat

Abomasal bloat is common in artificially reared kids and is a significant cause of death in kids between 4 and 12 weeks of age. It should be distinguished from other causes of abdominal distension (see Table 16.2).

Aetiology

- It is poorly understood, but probably related to the rapid ingestion of large quantities of milk, leading to excessive fermentation and rapid distension of the abdomen with gas and fluid. Proliferation of microorganisms that release an excessive quantity of gas has also been postulated.

Clinical signs

- Abdominal distension with drum-like tension on left and right sides.
- Colicky pain – grinding of teeth, yawning, constant stretching of the back.
- Diarrhoea.

- Shock.
- Death.

The condition may present as a 'sudden death' (Chapter 19) with the kid being found dead in the morning.

> All cases of bloat, even if mild, should be treated seriously and the kid checked at regular intervals.

Treatment

- Mild cases may respond to administration of a drench of a tablespoonful of vegetable oil or a proprietary bloat drench. Linseed oil is recommended in many older goat books but is not suitable as a drench as it may cause cessation of rumination since the regurgitation of stomach contents containing the oil is offensive in the mouth.
- More severe cases will require veterinary attention.
- Release pressure by trocharising the abdomen on the left side with a 16 or 18 g needle.
- Relieve spasm and pain:

  Metamisole, Hyoscine, 0.5–2 ml i.v. or i.m.

- Help restore abomasal tone and promote emptying:

  Metaclopramide, 0.5–1.0 mg/kg, 0.5–1 ml/5 kg i.v.

- Administer broad-spectrum antibiotics intramuscularly or intravenously.
- Fluid therapy for shocked kid.

Prevention

- Regular feeding with milk at the correct temperature and concentration.
- Consider feeding whole goats' milk in problem herds, but there is a danger of CAE spread.
- Kids fed from bowls rather than bottles are possibly more prone to bloat (due to more rapid intake of milk ?). Consider bottle feeding or a multisuckling system in these herds, but this is more time consuming.
- Early wean any kid that has repeat episodes of bloat.

Ruminal bloat

Ruminal bloat may occur in kids during weaning.

Aetiology

- Sudden dilation of the abomasum by rapid intake of milk causes inhibition of forestomach motility.
- Failure of the oesophageal groove closure reflex allows milk to leak into rumen, leading to excessive fermentation.
- Secondary to ruminal stasis and/or diarrhoea.
- Secondary to oesophageal obstruction (choke).

Clinical signs and treatment

- As for abomasal bloat.

Prevention

- Correct feeding technique – establish a routine to ensure oesophageal groove closure at feeding; smaller feeds more frequently.
- If the bloat is repetitive, wean the kid completely as early as possible.

Constipation

Constipation seems to be quite common in artificially reared kids in certain herds, presumably as a result of management practices.

Aetiology

- Excess of concentrates with insufficient water intake (?), as a sequel to abomasal Impaction (?).

Clinical signs

- Depressed.
- Frequent unsuccessful attempts to defaecate.
- Low-grade abdominal pain – stretching, yawning.
- Unwilling to feed or take milk.

Treatment

- Drench with a tablespoonful (15 ml) of liquid paraffin with about 2 teaspoonfuls (10 ml) of vegetable oil or proprietary colic drench containing turpentine oil and polymethylisoloxone.

Mesenteric torsion

See Chapter 15.

'Pot belly'

Poorly thriving kids will assume a 'pot bellied' appearance, coupled with a poor growth rate. This is generally due to too early inadequate nutrition or gastrointestinal parasitism.

Further reading

Displaced abomasum

Edwards, G.T. and Nevel, A. (2008) Abomasal emptying defect in two British Toggenburg goats. *Vet. Rec.*, **162**, 418–419.

Gerald, A.W., Thurston, D. and Ronald, F.M. (1983) Left displacement of the abomasum in a goat. *Vet. Med. Small Anim. Clin.*, **78**, 1919–1921.

Meimandi Parizi, A., Bigham, A. and Rowshan Ghasrodashti, A. (2008) Displacement of the abomasum to the left side and pyloric obstruction in a goat. *Iranian J. Vet. Res.*, **9** (1), Ser. No. 22, 81–83.

CHAPTER 17

Respiratory disease

Respiratory disease in goats is generally poorly researched worldwide. There is a paucity of information on the aetiology and frequency of respiratory disease in the United Kingdom, but it would appear to be relatively common, ranging from sudden death from peracute pneumonia to slight but persistent coughs and nasal discharges. Tables 17.1, 17.2 and 17.3 give differential diagnoses for nasal discharge, coughing and dyspnoea respectively.

Initial assessment

The preliminary history should consider:
- Individual or herd/flock problem.
- Possible exposure to infected animals – shows, brought-in stock, etc.
- Feeding, for example dusty hay, root crops, etc.
- Housing – ventilation, building design.
- Vaccination.
- Overall level of coughing/sneezing in the building.

Clinical examination

> Clinical signs of respiratory distress may arise from many conditions not directly related to the respiratory tract.

- A thorough clinical examination should be made – temperature, pulse, respiratory rate, auscultation of the lungs - to localise lesions to the upper and lower respiratory tract.

- Respiratory rates will be increased by stress, high environmental temperature, pain or metabolic acidosis.
- Many clinical conditions not directly involving the respiratory tract can result in hyperpnoea and tachypnoea, for example bloat, anaemia, pain, hyperthermia and acidosis. Hypocalcaemia may present as an apparently excited, pyrexic and pneumonic goat.

> Normal respiratory rate: adult 15 to 30 breaths/minute
> kid 20 to 40 breaths/minute

Auscultation

The cranioventral lung border is at the 6th rib, the middle of the thorax is the 7th rib and the caudal lung border is the 11th rib. This means that the lung field extends well forward under the elbow and it is important not to overlook this area during auscultation.

Normal breath sounds are loudest over the trachea and base of the lungs and loudest on inspiration, although in goats, as in sheep, the duration of expiration is also audible.

Harsh inspiratory sounds may be heard over the entire lung field in thin goats and increased sounds are heard in normal animals with increased rate and depth of respiration caused by stress, excitement, high environmental temperature, etc.

Thoracocentesis

The area is clipped and surgically prepared and an 18 g needle is inserted into the *7th intercostal space* at the costochondral junction level or slightly higher, just off the cranial border of the rib to avoid the intercostal vessels and nerves.

Diseases of the Goat, Fourth Edition. John Matthews.
© 2016 John Wiley & Sons, Ltd. Published 2016 by John Wiley & Sons, Ltd.

Table 17.1 Differential diagnosis for nasal discharge.

Bilateral	Unilateral
Rhinitis	Sinusitis
▪ Viral	▪ Infection post-dehorning
▪ Bacterial	▪ Tooth problem
▪ Mycoplasmal	▪ Horn injury
▪ Fungal (unlikely UK)	▪ Facial fracture
	▪ *Oestrus ovis* (rarely reported)
Pneumonia (see cough)	
Dusty conditions	Nasal tumour, e.g. nasal
Enzootic nasal tumour	adenocarcinoma
	Enzootic nasal tumour
	Foreign body

Table 17.2 Differential diagnosis for cough.

Pneumonia	Allergic bronchitis
▪ Bacterial	Congestive cardiac failure
▪ Inhalation	Oesophageal obstruction
○ Drench	Lymph node enlargement
○ Force feeding	
○ Dip	▪ Lymphosarcoma
○ Rhododendron poisoning	▪ Caseous lymphadenitis
▪ Parasitic	
▪ Fungal (unlikely UK)	Tuberculosis

Table 17.3 Differential diagnosis for dyspnoea.

Primary respiratory disease	Secondary respiratory disease	
Bacterial pneumonia	Heat stroke	Poisoning
Inhalation pneumonia	Anaemia	
	Cardiac disease	▪ Cyanide (*Prunus* family)
Chronic interstitial pneumonia (CAE)	▪ Congenital	▪ Nitrite/nitrate
	▪ Acquired	▪ Urea
Mycoplasma	Bloat	▪ Salt
Pulmonary adenomatosis	Selenium/vitamin E deficiency	▪ Organophosphorus
Lung tumours	Hypoglycaemia	
Nasal tumours	Trauma	Terminal stages of many disease conditions
Tracheal collapse	▪ Thoracic injuries	
	▪ Diaphragmatic hernia	

Radiographic examination of the thorax

Radiography is generally used for confirmation of extensive changes in the lung fields, for example pneumonia or multiple abscesses, or the presence of a thoracic mass, for example thymoma. It may also be useful for diagnosing infections or tumours of the sinuses.

Radiographic equipment and techniques used for dogs are suitable for goats. Sedation with diazepam or xylazine will be required if the goat is to be restrained in lateral recumbency.

The fore limbs need to be pulled forward to expose the cranioventral lung lobes.

Ultrasonographic examination of the thorax

Goats are better subjects than sheep for ultrasonographic examination of the thorax because they typically have less body fat. Ultrasonography, using a 5.0 MHz sector scanner, provides useful information about the condition of the pleural space and the peripheral pulmonary parenchyma because it allows the pleura and superficial lung surfaces to be visualised. A 5.0 MHz linear transducer allows examination of the pleura and superficial lung.

Ultrasonic examination is useful for identifying:

▪ Presence and extent of *pleural effusion*:

○ Ultrasonography is more sensitive than radiography in detecting small amounts of pleural fluid.

○ Pleural fluid appears as an anechoic area; as the cellular and protein content of the fluid increases, so does its echogenicity.

○ Gas-filled pockets within pleural fluid appear as bright hyperechoic spots within the anechoic area.

○ Ultrasonography allows the degree of effusion to be monitored during therapy.

▪ *Pleural fibrin deposits* and *adhesions*:

○ Pleura and lung lobes are separated by a hypoechoic area and the visceral pleura appears as a broad white line.

○ Fibrinous adhesions have a hyperechoic lattice-like appearance containing hyperechoic areas.

▪ *Consolidation of lung parenchyma*:

○ Consolidated lung parenchyma is a good acoustic medium and appears more hypoechoic than surrounding lung tissue.

■ *Abscesses*:
  o Fluid within an abscess appears more hypoechoic than surrounding lung tissue.
  o Abscesses may be obscured if they are deep to aerated lung.

It can also be used as a guide in determining the most useful site for *thoracocentesis* and *lung biopsy*.

Hair is clipped from both sides of the thorax, skin wet with tap water and ultrasound gel applied to ensure good contact. The thorax is examined in longitudinal and transverse planes by applying the transducer head to the skin over the intercostal muscles.

The *6th or 7th intercostal spaces* act as the reference site to start scanning, moving cranially to each intercostal space in turn for the cranial thorax and caudally to the *9th or 10th intercostal spaces* for the caudal thorax. Scanning starts dorsally in an attempt to identify normal lung tissue.

Endoscopy

Endoscopy is a useful tool to supplement clinical examination, ultrasonography and radiology, because it enables direct observation of the mucosal surfaces and anatominal structures of the pharynx, oesophagus and upper respiratory tract. Table 17.4 gives possible indications for endoscopy.

Endoscopes appropriate for dogs are suitable for goats, but goats have extremely sharp teeth, so that the use of a gag or speculum is required if the endoscope is passed

Table 17.4 Indications for endoscopy.

Endoscopy of the respiratory tract	Oesophagoscopy
Nasal discharge	Dysphagia
Chronic sneezing or coughing	Regurgitation
Epistaxis	Suspected foreign body
Stridor	Neoplasia
Suspected foreign bodies	Excess salivation
Deformation of nasal or frontal bones	Megaoesophagus
Tachypnoea	Pharyngeal abscesses
Dyspnoea	Biopsy
Bronchoalveolar lavage	
Biopsy	

through the mouth – polystyrene piping or wood with a hole drilled in it can be utilised as makeshift gags if necessary.

Passage through the nasal passages is preferable if a small enough diameter endoscope is available – a flexible endoscope with a diameter of 4 mm is suitable for yearling and adult goats. Good restraint of the head and neck is necessary and backward movement should be prevented. Sedation may be necessary if animals struggle. The endoscope is inserted quickly but carefully into the ventral nasal meatus – overaggressive insertion will result in haemorrhage. Coughing generally occurs when the endoscope is advanced into the trachea and it is easier to wait until coughing has stopped before advancing the endoscope distally. Oesophagastomy is tolerated well by most animals – swallowing is triggered by touching the arytenoid cartilage with the tip of the endoscope so that it enters the oesophagus through the lateral laryngeal recess.

Bronchial alveolar lavage

Bronchial alveolar lavage(BAL) produces cells from the lower airways and can be a useful diagnostic technique in acute outbreaks of respiratory disease in older animals. There is less likelihood of contaminants or commensals from the nasopharynx confusing the diagnostic picture compared with sampling with a nasopharyngeal swab.

Apparently healthy in-contacts are ideal candidates for BAL without the risk of causing them respiratory distress. The technique is obviously unsuitable for dyspnoeic animals.

Technique

With the head of the animal fixed with the neck in extension, a Portex tube (8 mm bore, 1.75 mm wall thickness) is inserted through the nasal passage to the larynx. As the animal inhales, the larynx opens and the tube can be advanced, triggering a cough reflex.

A smaller tube (4.5 mm bore, 0.9 mm wall thickness) is passed through the outer tube to the level of a bronchus, when resistance is felt. Obstetric lubricant aids the passage of the inner tube through the outer tube. Then 50 ml of sterile phosphate buffered saline is flushed through the inner tube. After about 20 seconds fluid is aspirated and transferred to a sterile container. Up to 30 ml of fluid is normally recovered.

Tracheal wash

A tracheal wash is easier to achieve than a true bronchial alveolar lavage and can provide useful information.

Technique

An area over the mid-trachea is clipped, surgically prepared and 1–2 ml of local anaesthetic injected. A 16 gauge needle is inserted between two tracheal rings and fifteen to 20 ml of phosphate buffered saline (or isotonic saline if not available) is injected into the traches. Suction is applied immediately to harvest as much fluid as possible. The fluid is placed in a sterile container.

A tomcat catheter can be inserted through a 14–16 gauge needle and advanced towards the distal trachea, allowing a flush closer to the bronchial bifurcation. The needle is withdrawn with the catheter in situ to avoid the sharp needle bevel slicing off the end of the catheter.

The procedure can be carried out in a standing animal with the head lowered but is easier with the animal in lateral recumbency.

Nasal discharge

Possible causes of nasal discharge are listed in Table 17.1. Healthy goats do not normally have a nasal discharge. Clinically normal goats have a wide variety of aerobic bacteria in their nasal passages, including potential pathogens such as *Mannheima haemolytica* and *Pasteurella multocida*.

Any cause of rhinitis will lead to a nasal discharge – bacteria, mycoplasma, fungi and dusty conditions. *Oestrus ovis* (see Chapter 12) and enzootic nasal tumours (see Plate 17.1) both occur in sheep in the United Kingdom and could potentially infect goats. Nasal tumours and foreign bodies are rare. Nasal and cutaneous aspergillosis has been described in Brazil in an adult goat that presented with clinical signs of severe respiratory distress due to partial nasal obstruction, bilateral mucopurulent nasal discharge, skin nodules on the ears and dorsal nasal region and focal depigmentation of the ventral commissure of the right nostril.

Animals returning from shows commonly develop a clear nasal discharge (Plate 17.1), generally without other clinical signs, although there may be an accompanying loss of appetite and decreased milk yield, together with a mild keratoconjunctivitis. The condition is usually self-limiting. Antibiotic therapy does not appear to alter the course of the disease in most animals and is unnecessary if the goat is otherwise well. It is tempting to suggest a viral aetiology for these conditions (see later this chapter), but the role of viruses is uncertain. Mycoplasma are known to cause mild respiratory signs in goats in the United Kingdom (see Chapter 13) and are probably at least partly responsible for these cases.

Animals with a bilateral purulent nasal discharge (Plate 17.2) are often clinically ill; unilateral purulent discharges can be due to a foreign body, trauma, *Oestrus ovis* or enzootic nasal tumour. Unilateral infections can also occur as a result of a horn injury or post-dehorning infection.

The nostrils of goats with a chronic discharge can be become sore, with scab formation and adherent food material (Plate 17.3), which may obstruct the nares. Animals fed chopped, preserved material, such as dried lucerne (alfalfa), may get food material stuck around the lips and nostrils and this may need distinguishing from an infectious cause.

Cough

Possible causes of coughing are given in Table 17.2.

Goats do not normally cough. Any cough in a goat should be considered abnormal and is the result of infection, allergy or environmental irritation (dust, dry feed, fumes), or in individual animals from an oesophageal obstruction, lymph node enlargement or from inhaling foreign material. Upper respiratory tract infections generally produce a dry, hacking cough. In goats with bronchopneumonia, the cough is generally moist and less vigorous.

Sinusitis

Aetiology

- Sinusitis involving the frontal sinuses can be a sequel to dehorning.
- Maxillary sinusitis is generally secondary to tooth problems.
- Inflammation of both sinuses can as a result of:
  o Neoplasia, for example nasal adenocarcinoma.
  o Facial fractures.
  o Horn injuries.

o Nasal myiasis caused by *Oestrus ovis* larvae (see Chapter 12).

Clinical signs

- Nasal discharge.
- Head shaking or pressing.
- Rubbing head.
- Abnormal smell.
- Pus may be visible in the sinus.
- Pyrexia, lethargy, anorexia if systemic infection.

Treatment

- Topical antibiotics – oxytetracycline spray; intramammary infusions.
- Systemic antibiotics if animal is depressed.
- NSAIDs.
- Open sinuses can be rinsed with a 0.1% chlorhexidine solution.
- Closed sinuses may need flushing through holes drilled in the frontal sinus.

Infectious respiratory disease

> Respiratory disease may have a multifactorial aetiology.

Aetiology

Although several organisms known to produce severe respiratory disease in goats are absent from the United Kingdom, including the mycoplasma responsible for contagious caprine pleuropneumonia (CCPP) and peste des petits ruminants virus (PPRV), a number of infectious agents have been isolated from clinical cases or experimentally shown to produce disease in goats in the United Kingdom.

Bacteria

Pasteurella

Mannheimia haemolytica (formerly *Pasteurella haemolytica*) and *P. multocida* have been isolated from pneumonic lungs of goats. *Mannheimia haemolytica* serotypes Al, A2 and A6 are the most common isolates in the United Kingdom. The disease may be precipitated by stress, for example weather, transport, etc., and may be secondary to a primary Mycoplasma infection.

Bibersteinia (formerly *Pasteurella*) *trehalosi* appears to have no role in caprine respiratory disease.

Clinical signs

- The disease syndrome of '*pasteurellosis*' may involve other aetiological agents such as viruses or other bacteria and a wide variety of clinical signs ranging from occasional coughing to sudden death, but often an acute pneumonia, particularly in kids.
- Lethargy, anorexia, pyrexia.
- Tachypnoea, hyperpnoea, dyspnoea.
- Abnormal lung sounds – rales, rhonchi, noisy expiration.

Pasteurella multocida rarely causes disease in the United Kingdom, but has been shown to produce an atrophic rhinitis with nose bleeding, sneezing and nasal turbinate atrophy.

Post-mortem findings

- Exudative bronchopneumonia.
- Extensive consolidation of the lung.
- Fibrinous pleurisy.

Diagnosis

> Identification of *M. haemolytica* from a swab does not prove the goat has pasteurellosis.

- There is no confirmatory laboratory test in the living goat, so preliminary diagnosis depends on the clinical signs.
- *Mannheimia haemolytica* may be isolated from a nasal or nasopharyngeal swab as an incidental finding and does *not* indicate that the goat has pasteurellosis.
- Post-mortem confirmation depends on bacteriology and histology of lung lesions.

Treatment

See treatment of infectious respiratory disease later in this chapter.

Antibiotics suitable for treating pasteurellosis in goats include *tulathromycin*, 2.5 mg/kg; *oxytetracycline*, 3–10 mg/kg i.v.; *florfenicol*, 40 mg/kg s.c. and *cetiofur*, 1 mg/kg s.c.

Enrofloxacin (Baytril, Bayer) is licensed for goats in the United Kingdom for the treatment of infections of the respiratory tract caused by enrofloxacin susceptible strains of *Pasteurella multocida* and *Mannheimia haemolytica*: 5 mg of enrofloxacin/kg bw, corresponding to 1 ml/20 kg bw, once daily by subcutaneous injection for 3 days.

Not more than 6 ml should be administered at one subcutaneous injection site.

> Do not use *tilmicosin* (Micotil, Elanco) as this drug is associated with a high death rate in goats.

Control

See control of infectious respiratory disease later in this chapter.

Vaccination

- Ideally vaccines should contain *M. haemolytica* serotypes Al, A2 and A6 and all serotypes of *P. multocida*, but no vaccine available in the United Kingdom meets these requirements.
- The cattle vaccine Pastobov (Merial) has been used in goats. Pastobov contains serotype Al, but some cross-immunity to other types, including A6, can be expected, but not to *P. multocida*. The vaccine also stimulates development of antileuco-toxin antibodies.
- The sheep vaccine Ovipast plus (MSD) contains *M. haemolytica* serotypes A1, A2 A6, A7 and A9:

    Primary course, 2 ml, two injections at 3 to 4 week intervals
    Booster dose, 2 ml annually

The vaccination can be given at the same time as clostridial vaccination, but at a separate site.

> It is not recommended to use combined clostridial and pasteurella vaccines.

Mycoplasma

> Mycoplasma are increasingly reported from cases of respiratory disease in the United Kingdom.

Depending on the species of mycoplasma, mycoplasma infections produce various clinical conditions in goats – respiratory disease, keratoconjunctivitis (Chapter 20), arthritis (Chapter 8), mastitis (Chapter 13), abortion (Chapter 2) and septicaemia (Table 17.5). Infection can range from a severe disease resulting in death to a subclinical disease with few clinical signs. Both host immunity and the virulence of the mycoplasma strain influence the progression of the disease. Disease is introduced into a herd by carrier animals or animals with subclinical infections or by the mixing of animals at shows. Transmission may be via respiratory secretions or vertically in kids from colostrum or milk.

- *Mycoplasma ovipneumoniae* and *M. arginini* are widely distributed in goats in the UK, causing mild respiratory signs, such as nasal discharge and coughing, particularly in kids and occasionally in adults. They are implicated in the mild respiratory disease often acquired by goats attending shows. *Mycoplasma arginini* appears to be of limited pathogenicity, but is often isolated with *M. ovipneumoniae* in cases of atypical pneumonia. They may act synergistically with *Mannheimia haemolytica*.
- *Mycoplasma capricolum*, *M. conjunctivae* and *Acholeplasma oculi* have been isolated from animals in the United Kingdom. Their role in respiratory disease is uncertain.
- Out-with the United Kingdom, severe respiratory disease is produced by a number of mycoplasma, for example *M. capricolum* subspecies *capripneumoniae*, *M. mycoides* subspecies *capri* (which now includes mycoplasma, formerly designated *M. mycoides* subspecies *mycoides* – alarge colony type). Clinical signs of pneumonia vary in severity and include pyrexia, cough and dyspnoea, often progressing to chronic interstitial pneumonia and resulting in an unthrifty, emaciated animal. The pneumonia may be severe enough for cor pulmonale and congestive cardiac failure to occur. Respiratory signs may be accompanied

Table 17.5 *Mycoplasma* spp. involved in caprine disease.

Species	Disease	Geographic distribution
M.ovipneumoniae	Mild respiratory disease, initiator of pneumonia, keratoconjunctivitis?	UK, worldwide
M. arginini	Mild respiratory disease, initiator of pneumonia, keratoconjunctivitis?, vulvovaginitis, arthritis?	UK, worldwide
M. conjunctivae	Keratoconjunctivitis, pneumonia, arthritis	UK, worldwide
M. capricolum subsp. capricolum	Polyarthritis, mastitis, pneumonia, neonatal death, keratoconjunctivitis	UK, Europe, Australia, India, USA, Egypt
Acholeplasma oculi	Keratoconjunctivitis?	UK, worldwide
Ureaplasmas	Keratoconjunctivitis?, vulvovaginitis?	UK, worldwide
M. mycoides subsp. *capri* (*M. mycoides* subsp. *mycoides* (large- colony type))	Pleuropneumonia, mastitis, arthritis, keratoconjunctivitis, neonatal death/abortion	Europe, Africa, Asia, Australia, North America
M. putrefaciens	Mastitis, arthritis	USA, France, Australia
M. agalactiae	Contagious agalactia (CA), arthritis, pneumonia, keratoconjunctivitis, vulvovaginitis	Europe, United States, former USSR, Asia, North Africa
M.capricolum subsp. *capripneumoniae*	Contagious caprine pleuropneumonia (**CCPP**)	Africa, Middle East, India, Pakistan

by a chronic indurative mastitis and chronic bony joint enlargement.

- *M. mycoides* subspecies *capri* is prevalent throughout the United States, often causing a multisystemic disease. Clinical signs in kids include septicaemia, pneumonia, meningitis and arthritis, with adults showing pyrexia, pleuropneumonia, mastitis and polyarthritis. The organism is transmitted to kids in milk or colostrum from carrier does and between does at milking. Ear mites (*Psoroptes* species) are thought to act as vectors for *Mycoplasma* organisms.

Asymptomatic carriers act as a reservoir of an infection within the herd. Prevention is by maintaining a closed herd, hygiene at milking and by separating kids at birth and feeding heat-treated colostrum and pasteurised milk or milk-replacer (see Chapter 23).

Diagnosis

Definitive diagnosis requires isolation or identification of the organism or serological test results:

- Culture of mycoplasmas is relatively easy in acute cases, producing colonies with a characteristic 'fried egg' appearance, but becomes more difficult in chronically affected animals. Mycoplasma have special growth requirements and will not grow in standard bacteriological media.
- Polymerase chain R\reaction testing can be used for the detection and differentiation of mycoplasma species, but some closely related species may be misdiagnosed. PCR/denaturing gradient gel electrophoresis (PCR/DGGE) detects and identifies nearly all *Mycoplasma* species including mixed infections.
- Fluid can be examined under a dark field microscope or stained with 5% nigrosine solution to identify the pleomorphic, coccoid, ring and filamentous organisms.
- Novel or unusual species can be identified by DNA sequencing.

Treatment

- When clinical signs are mild, no treatment is necessary.
- Mycoplasmas are sensitive to tulathromycin, fluoroquinolones and tylosin and they have been used when disease outbreaks are more severe. They are potentially less sensitive to tetracyclines. Because mycoplasmas lack a cell wall, drugs that act on the cell wall are not effective.
- Treatment may not eliminate the carrier state.
- Ear mites and other ectoparasites should be controlled using an ectoparaciticide such as ivermectin.

Contagious caprine pleuropneumonia

M. capricolum subspecies *capripneumoniae* causes *contagious caprine pleuropneumonia* (*CCPP*), a highly contagious condition of goats with morbidity approaching 100% and mortality from 60 to 100%. It is prevalent in most of Africa, the Middle East, India and Pakistan.

Suspect CCPP when goats have pyrexia, respiratory distress, coughing, nasal discharge and a high mortality rate.

Most likely to be introduced to a previously free country by the introduction of infected goats. It is spread by close contact between goats and by the respiratory route.

Clinical signs

Peracute and acute forms of the disease occur when it is introduced into fully susceptible flocks. Incubation is between 2 and 28 days.

Peracute form: minimal respiratory disease with death in 1 to 3 days.

Acute form:

- Pyrexia.
- Mucopurulent nasal discharge.
- Excess salivation.
- Coughing and painful dyspnoea.
- Diarrhoea.
- Anorexia.
- Rapid loss of condition.
- Mortality rate up to 90%.

Chronic cases occur in endemically affected areas:

- Chronic cough and nasal discharge.
- Debility.

Post-mortem findings

- Severe fibrinous pleuropneumonia:
  o Unilateral or bilateral pneumonia with varying degrees of lung consolidation.
  o Cut surface of lung has a granular appearance with copious straw-coloured exudate.
  o Serofibrinous pleuritic.
- Bronchial lymph nodes enlarged.
- In chronic cases lungs will be in various stages of resolution with encapsulation of acute lesions and numerous fibrous adhesions.

Differential diagnosis

- Bacterial pneumonia (for example pasteurellosis).
- Other mycoplasma pneumonia.
- Caseous lymphadenitis.

Specimens required for diagnosis

- At post-mortem, pleuritic fluid and exudate fluid from lung lesions should be collected, together with fresh active lung lesions and duplicate lung samples in neutral buffered formalin for histopathology.
- Blood samples should be collected from several animals in the affected flock for serology.

Control

- Slaughter of all infected and in-contact goats with quarantine and movement controls.
- Tylosin, terramycin or streptomycin can be used to treat clinical cases where the disease is endemic.
- No vaccine is available for general field use.

Tuberculosis (TB)

TB is a chronic, primarily respiratory infectious disease of mammals caused by the *Mycobacterium tuberculosis* (MTB) complex, a group of closely related bacteria that includes *M. bovis* responsible for TB in cattle and other mammals, including occasionally people. Cattle are the natural host of *M. bovis*, but nearly all warm-blooded animals, including goats, deer, pigs, camelids and badgers are susceptible to the infection. This broad range of animal hosts complicates the eradication of bovine TB. Goats are also susceptible to *M. tuberculosis*, the primary cause of TB in people, *M. avium* and *M. Kansasii*, but these rarely cause caprine TB. A goat-adapted strain of the *M. tuberculosis* complex, known as *M. Caprae*, occurs in central and southern Europe. Bovine TB in goats, caused by *M. bovis*, is a notifiable disease in the United Kingdom.

Epidemiology

TB can spread either directly (animal to animal), particularly by aerosol or indirectly (via infective material, for example manure, urine, bedding, contaminated feed and water). The organisms can survive for long periods in moist conditions or organic matter. Spread from dam to kid through the feeding of milk from animals with TB of the udder is also possible.

- In the United Kingdom, goats appear to be 'spill-over hosts', that is TB occurs in goats only so long as there is input from an external source (maintenance host), for example infected badgers or cattle, when the challenge level is relatively high and they cannot sustain the infection within their own populations in the absence of infected cattle or a wildlife reservoir.

- Goats also act as 'amplifier hosts', that is they have the ability to spread the disease to other goats as well as other species (including humans) cohabiting with them. Once infection is established within a herd, it appears to spread rapidly within the herd.
- In other European countries, including France, Spain and Italy, goats are classified as 'maintenance hosts', where TB infection persists within the species without the need for input from other species.

Clinical signs

Clinical signs are non-specific, making a diagnosis of TB difficult.

TB should be considered in cases of chronic loss of condition and appetite, reduced milk yield and debilitating disease, with or without respiratory signs. A chronic cough can be a sign of TB in goats and should in particular be considered when a goat has failed to respond to antibiotic treatment for a respiratory infection.

- Goats may have extensive lesions without obvious clinical signs.
- Occurs as a disseminated disease involving the thorax (mediastinal lymph nodes, lungs, pleura) and abdomen (peritoneum, liver, spleen, mesenteric lymph nodes); occasionally superficial lymph nodes are enlarged and palpable.
- Chronic weight loss ± diarrhoea.
- Chronic cough due to bronchopneumonia.
- Skin lesions occasionally present – fistulae, ulcers and nodules.

Post-mortem findings

- Tuberculosis granulomas in one or more lymph nodes.
- Caseous tubercles in the lung, liver or spleen.
- The lungs and associated lymph nodes were the sites most frequently affected in recent cases in the United Kingdom. Although tubercle production is classically described in goats as in cattle, these cases often did not develop tubercle lesions in the lungs, producing instead large abscesses with liquid white or cream pus, which often quickly eroded into the airways, resulting in a greater propensity for disease spread by aerosol. Lung lesions were white or cream, multifocal and often occurred in areas of purple consolidation. Bronchial and mediastinal lymph nodes contained lesions varying from pinpoint foci to large caseous lesions with mineralisation. Lesions were also present in the mesenteric and retropharyngeal lymph nodes.

Diagnosis

- *Tests for cell mediated immune response*:
  - *Single intradermal comparative cervical tuberculin (SICCT) test* (specificity 99.5%, sensitivity >80%) compares the skin reaction to *M. bovis* antigen and *M. avium* antigen. Some countries, including the United States, use a single intradermal test using the tail fold. Intercurrent paratuberculosis can reduce the sensitivity of the test and false positives can occur in herds infected with, or vaccinating against, paratuberculosis.
  - *Gamma-Interferon (IFN)* tests are being evaluated for use in goats. The test is based on measuring the response to specific tuberculosis antigens by T cells, which release interferon gamma (IFN-γ). The test is considered to have a better sensitivity (>80% in goats) than the SICCT, presumably because it is able to detect infection earlier, but has poorer specificity. False positives can occur when animals are infected with other pathogenic mycobacteria and does not distinguish between infected and vaccinated animals.
  - The greatest sensitivity is obtained when the SICCT and IFN-γ are used together, although this results in a lower specificity than using the SICCT alone.
- *Serology tests*. It is now recognised that antibodies are produced soon after infection, so that serological tests are useful if they are sensitive enough. Three serological tests that identify the presence of antibodies to *Mycobacterium bovis* are available (two in the UK) – Idexx, StatPak and Enferplex.
  - *Enferplex ELISA* (SureFarm) is being evaluated for specificity and sensitivity in goats. It appears to offer greater reliability in identifying early cases of TB in goats when compared to the skin test. It gives a quantitative result using chemiluminescence and has better sensitivity than the other serological tests because it uses a greater number of separate antibodies (7).
- *Post-mortem examination* – histology (with acid fast stains; tubercle bacilli are Gram-positive, acid-fast and aerobic) and culture.

Public health considerations

The transmission of TB from goats to people can occur:
- From the consumption of raw (unpasteurised) milk or dairy products made with unpasteurised milk from goats infected with bovine TB (effective pasteurisation removes the risk of transmission of TB to humans).

- By inhaling the bacteria shed by infectious animals in respiratory and other Secretions.
- Through contamination of unprotected cuts or abrasions in the skin while handling infected animals or their carcases.

Other bacteria

Trueperella pyogenes (*Corynebacterium pyogenes*), *Staphylococcal* spp., *Streptococcal* spp., *Haemophilius* spp. and *Klebsiella pneumoniae* among others have been isolated from infected goats.

Respiratory caseous lymphadentis (CLA) caused by *Corynebacterium pseudotuberculosis* is rare in the United Kingdom, but infected animals may present with pulmonary abscesses.

Viruses

> The role of viruses in the aetiology of respiratory disease in goats is poorly documented, but they do not appear to play a significant role in the development of disease in the United Kingdom.

Several viruses have been isolated from or shown serologically to be present in association with clinical disease, but there is only limited evidence of natural infection occurring in the UK:

Infectious bovine rhinotracheitis (IBR, BHV-1) virus has been isolated from goats with respiratory and ocular disease, although the goat may not be a natural host for the virus.

Parainfluenza (PI3). A role for parainfluenza virus in respiratory disease in goats has been suggested, possibly as a predisposing agent for pasteurellosis.

Respiratory syncytial virus (RSV). Although respiratory syncytial virus has been isolated from goats in the United Kingdom, its role in respiratory disease is unclear. In the United States, RSV has been associated with nasolacrimal discharge, pyrexia and coughing, particularly in goats attending shows or 4-H events. Bovine RSV vaccines have been used empirically to protect goats travelling to shows with young stock vaccinated 60 and 30 days prior to the start of show season and booster vaccinations for pregnant females

with one dose 30 days prior to parturition and one dose to adults 30 days prior to show season.

Multivalent cattle vaccines containing modified attenuated strains of live virus should not be used, because their virulence has not been tested in goats.

Other viruses are occasionally implicated in respiratory disease in goats:

Bluetongue (BTV). See Chapter 10. Although not primarily a disease of goats, serous or mucopurulent nasal discharges are occasionally reported in infected animals.

Caprine arthritis encephalitis. See Chapter 7. Kids infected with CAE may have a subclinical interstitial pneumonia and some adult goats develop a slowly progressive interstial pneumonia, with similar signs to ovine maedi-visna, characterised by a chronic cough and weight loss. Pneumonia may occasionally be the major presenting sign.

Pulmonary adenomatosis (jaagsiekte, pulmonary carcinoma) is a contagious tumour of the lungs of sheep, which has been transmitted experimentally to goats. There is a chronic progressive pneumonia with adenomatosis lesions of the lung alveoli, resulting in chronic weight loss.

Caprine herpesvirus 1 (CpHV-1/BHV-6), which causes vulvovaginitis and infertility in New Zealand and Australia (see Chapter 1) does not appear to be a significant cause of respiratory disease, although the virus proliferates in the upper respiratory tract and experimental challenge can produce rhinitis.

Strains of caprine herpes virus in the United States have caused severe systemic illness including dyspnoea in 1 to 2 week old kids.

Peste de petit-ruminants (PPR)

> Suspect PPR when there is apparent sudden death of several animals with others showing variable clinical signs including pyrexia, oculonasal discharge, oral erosions, enteritis and bronchopneumonia. Animals may have foul-smelling oral pathology and foetid diarrhoea.

The clinical signs are similar to rinderpest, which has now been eradicated, but PPR is the more severe disease in goats. There is high morbidity (up to 90%) and mortality (50 to 80%) in susceptible populations.

Sheep, goats, wild ungulates and experimental American white tailed deer are susceptible.

The disease would only be introduced by the movement of live animals, as virus transmission is essentially through direct contact with infected animals or through contact with fresh secretions or faeces from infected animals. The virus does not survive for long in normal environments, being susceptible to heat, UV light, dehydration and high and low pH.

Present distribution

- Sub-Saharan Africa, North Africa, the Middle East and South-Western and Central Asia. In recent years an increasing number of outbreaks have been reported in Turkey. The disease has spread over the past 10 years and is considered by the World Organisation for Animal health (OIE) as a top priority disease and a possible candidate for eradication, following the successful eradication of rinderpest.

Aetiology

- Paramyxovirus (genus *Morbillivirus)* that replicates in lymphoid and epithelial cells, especially those in the alimentary tract.

Clinical signs

The clinical signs of PPR and rinderpest are very similar. Peste des petits ruminants is the more important disease in goats. Goats were often only mildly affected by rinderpest and frequently experience only subclinical infections, but were then a source of infection for cattle.

The severity of clinical signs depends on the immune status of the animal, so in endemic areas young, old and newly introduced animals are most severely affected.

- Pyrexia.
- Depression.
- Anoxia.
- Hyperpnoea/tachypnea.
- Reddening of mucous membranes.
- Mucopurulent lacrimation.
- Excessive salivation.
- Necrosis/ulceration and erosion of oral mucosa; foul smell.
- Profuse malodorous haemorrhagic diarrhoea with necrotic debris and mucus.
- Severe tenesmus.
- High mortality – death in 8 to 12 days.

The clinical signs are very similar to contagious pleuropneumonia and pneumonic pasteurellosis except for the lack of oral lesions and diarrhoea (which may be absent in mild PPR).

Laboratory diagnosis

- Virus detection by antigen capture ELISA, RT-PCR or cell culture techniques.
- Serological methods, competition ELISA and virus neutralization are also available.

Treatment

- There is no specific treatment.
- Infected animals would be compulsorily slaughtered if the disease was introduced.
- Homologous live attenuated virus vaccines are used in endemic areas.
- Development of a genetically modified (recombinant) vaccine would enable. Differentiation of vaccinated and infected animals.

Laboratory investigation of infectious respiratory disease

- Bacteriology. Isolation of bacteria from nasal swabs does not confirm an organism as being responsible for disease, merely that it is present in the nasal passages; nasopharyngeal and oropharyngeal swabs are more useful.
- Virology. Nasopharyngeal swabs can be used for virological examination.
- Biochemical and haematological changes may indicate an inflammatory response but are not specific for respiratory disease.
- Paired serum samples 10 to 14 days apart may be of value.
- Post-mortem examination – histopathology, bacteriology/virology, etc.
- Laboratory confirmation of Mycoplasma infection is by PCR/denaturing gradient gel electrophoresis (PCR/DGGE).

Treatment of infectious respiratory diseases

- Isolate affected animal(s) and carefully observe other animals for early signs of disease.
- Provide a *warm, draught-free environment.*

- Use *antibiotics* to control bacterial pneumonias or prevent secondary bacterial infection.
- Long acting oxytetracycline (20 mg/kg) and danofloxacin are usually effective in early cases of *Mannheimia* (*Pasteurella*) infection.
- Penicillin-based microbials are effective against some, but not all, *Mannheimia* (*Pasteurella*) strains.
- Enrofloxacin (Baytril, Bayer) is licensed for goats in the United Kingdom for the treatment of infections of the respiratory tract caused by enrofloxacin susceptible strains of *Pasteurella multocida* and *Mannheimia haemolytica*: 5 mg of enrofloxacin/kg bw, corresponding to 1 ml/20 kg bw, once daily by subcutaneous injection for 3 days.
- Do *not* use tilmicosin (Micotil, Elanco) as this drug is associated with a high death rate in goats.
- Mycoplasmas are sensitive to tulathromycin, fluoroquinolones and tylosin, but are potentially less sensitive to tetracyclines.
- Use *non-steroidal anti-inflammatory drugs* to reduce pulmonary congestion and pyrexia: Flunixin meglumine, 2 mg/kg, i.v. or i.m., Carprofen, 1.4 mg/kg, i.v. or s.c., Ketoprofen, 3 mg/kg, i.v. or i.m., Meloxicam, 2 mg/kg i.v. or s.c.

Control of infectious respiratory diseases

The prevention and control of respiratory disease is based on the elimination, or at least the minimisation, of factors predisposing towards disease, combined with strategic prophylactic treatments to reduce the impact of respiratory pathogens. Trigger factors for respiratory disease are shown in Table 17.6.

- *Strong, well-nourished kids* will be less susceptible to respiratory infection.
- *Avoid mixing different age groups* in one air space.
- Operate an *'all-in-all-out' policy* for batches of kids, with a minimum of 2 weeks rest period between batches.
- *Isolate* purchased animals for at least 2 weeks in a separate air-space.
- *Minimise handling stress.*
- *Manage concurrent disease* such as parasitic gastroenteritis.
- Ensure a *well ventilated draught-free environment.* (Table 17.7). Expert advice should be taken when

Table 17.6 Factors associated with respiratory disease.

Management factors	Natural factors
Overcrowding	Age (kids more susceptible)
Poor ventilation	Extremes of weather conditions, particularly temperature and humidity
Excessive buildup of bedding in deep litter systems leading to high humidity and ammonia levels	
Mixing different age groups	Breed/genetics
Failure to isolate purchased animals	
Failure to operate an 'all-in-all-out' policy for kids	
Malnourished kids	
Transportation	
Handling	

designing new buildings and particular care is needed when adapting buildings designed for other animal species to ensure that suitable environmental conditions can be met.

o *Temperature.* Goats are homeothermic animals needing to maintain a constant body temperature of between 38.7 and 40.7 °C. Correct building design enables the animals to operate most efficiently.

The ability to tolerate extremes of temperature varies with breed and their natural habitat and is also influenced by the amount of body fat, thickness of coat and diet. Goats are able to withstand quite cold temperatures, provided water troughs are not frozen and they are well fed, but do not like sudden variations in temperature. Sudden decrease in temperature alters the moisture content of the air and produces condensation on metal structures. Most breeds of goats found in a temperate country like the United Kingdom have a lower critical temperature of 0 °C, below which they feel cold and need to convert feed into heat.

o *Moisture.* Adult goats evaporate 1.2 to 1.5 litres of water/day. Additional moisture is added to the atmosphere by the evaporation of urine from deep litter systems and any leakage from troughs, etc. Optimal relative humidity is 60–80%.

Increased humidity influences the goat's thermal neutral zone, in winter by making the coat wet

Table 17.7 Suitable environmental conditions for goats.

Temperature	Optimum 10 –12 °C	Minimum 0 °C[a]	Maximum 27 °C[a]
Relative humidity	Optimum 60–80%		
Ventilation	Winter 30 m³/hour/goat	Summer 120–150 m³/hour/goat	Maximum air speed 0.5 m/s adults 0.2 m/s kids
	Air intake >2× surface area of air exit Air flow < 0.5 m/s at the level of the animals Volume of air, optimum 8–10m³/goat (minimum 5–6 m³/goat)		
Lighting	Window area equal to 1/20 of ground surface area		
Space allowance	**Adult**		**Kid**
	Yard 2.0–2.5 m² doe 2.5–3.0 m² buck	Pen 4.0 m²	Pen 1.0 m² (Maximum 25 kids/pen)
Trough space	0.4 m/goat		
Air space	5–6 m³ per goat		

[a]The temperature of a range that goats find comfortable varies with their breed and natural habitat.

reducing the insulating properties and in summer by reducing evaporation and limiting heat loss.

o *Ammonia*. Deep litter systems release significant quantities of ammonia, hydrogen sulphide, etc., which if not controlled, can irritate the eyes and respiratory tract.

Clearing deep litter systems every 6 weeks limits the release of ammonia and reduces fly nuisance. Reducing the height of the bedding also increases the volume air available per goat, helping to reduce temperature and humidity. Bedding should be 130–150 cm thick on concrete and provide for good drainage of urine and faeces. Dirt floors will require 70–100 cm.

o *Ventilation*. Bad ventilation is a major cause of pneumonia, especially for young stock. There should be adequate air flow in the building – 30 m³/h/animal in the winter; 120–150 m³ in the summer. Draughts should be avoided. Air flow should be less than 0.5 m/s at the level of the animals (0.2 m/s for kids).

Ventilation may be static - adjustable shutters, 'Yorkshire' boarding, plastic netting, perforated sheets, etc., with ridge tiles, or dynamic with electric extractors. Placement and size of air inlets, extractors and fans are very important.

Good ventilation:

◆ Maintains a supply of fresh air.

◆ Removes water vapour from the goats.

◆ Helps evaporation from bedding, faeces and water spillage.

◆ Removes odours and gases from animal waste.

◆ Reduces dust levels.

◆ Reduces the build-up of micro-organisms.

◆ Reduces the risk of pneumonia.

◆ Minimises condensation.

◆ Provides a satisfactory minimal temperature in winter and maintains a summer temperature inside the building approximately the same as outside.

o *Insulation*. In temperate areas, additional insulation is generally not justified, but in areas with colder winters may be necessary, particular in kid housing, and will help prevent temperature fluctuations. The addition of insulation will also prevent warm air in the building condensing on cold walls.

o *Animal density*. The minimum space requirement is 2.0–2.5 m² per adult and 1.0 m² per unweaned kid.

> It is not possible to appreciate the air-speed and air-flow in a building without special apparatus. First impressions can be misleading.

■ *Vaccination* may be useful to control *Mannheimia* (*Pasteurella*) infection (see page?), but at present there is no convincing evidence that vaccination against respiratory viruses, such as RSV or P13, is useful in controlling respiratory disease in goats, although they have been used empirically to protect goats regularly attending shows.

Parasites

Dictyocaulus filaria

The lungworm *Dictyocaulus filaria*, found in the trachea and bronchi, infects both sheep and goats. The life cycle is direct with larvae being passed in faeces. It is not often a major pathogen; respiratory signs being most likely in the south of England during late summer/autumn following larval buildup on pasture during the summer.

Epidemiology

- Larvae overwinter on pasture.
- Carrier animals perpetuate the infection.

Clinical signs

- Coughing, tachypnoea, naso-ocular discharge.
- Inappetence, weight loss.
- Secondary infection may result in pyrexia and dyspnoea but severe clinical parasitic bronchitis is rare.

Diagnosis

- Larvae in faeces after a Baerman or $ZnSO_4$ flotation.

Treatment

- Levamisole 12.5 mg/kg, orally (limited efficacy against larval stages of worms; may need to repeat after two weeks).
- Mebendazole, 22.5 mg/kg; Febental, Fenbendazole, Oxfendazole, 7.5 mg/kg, orally.
- Ivermectin, 10 mg/50 kg, 12.5 ml/50 kg orally.
- Abamectin, Doramectin, Ivermectin, Moxidectin, 10 mg/50 kg, 1 ml/50 kg s.c. (potential persistent activity against *D. filaria* worms for four weeks or more).

> Do not use injectable levamisole in goats with possible lung worm infection.

Muellerius capillaris

The lungworm *Muellerius capillaris*, found in the alveolar ducts, small bronchioles, subpleural connective tissue and lung parenchyma, infects both sheep and goats; goats are more susceptible to disease. The life cycle is indirect, with slugs and snails ingesting the larvae and acting as intermediate hosts.

Epidemiology

- Goats are infected during their first summer on pasture by eating intermediate hosts on herbage. The level of infection increases with age so that clinical disease is generally seen in adult goats over 3 years old.

Clinical signs

- Variable, ranging from mild cough to severe chronic cough and dyspnoea.

Diagnosis

- Larvae in faeces after Baerman or $ZnSO_4$ flotation.

Treatment

- Fenbendazole, 30 mg/kg in single dose or 15 mg/kg daily for 3 to 5 days orally.
- Abamectin, doramectin, ivermectin, moxidectin, 10 mg/50 kg, 1 ml/50 kg s.c.
- Immature worms may not be eliminated by treatment, which should therefore be repeated after about 3 weeks.
- Levamisole, particularly in injectable form, may produce a hypersensitivity reaction in the lungs due to the death of large numbers of *M. capillaris* and should not be used in any animals suspected of having a heavy worm burden.

Protostrongylus rufescens

The lungworm *Protostrongylus rufescens*, found in the bronchioles, has not been reported as pathogenic in goats in the United Kingdom but large numbers can cause respiratory distress and weight loss in sheep and it has been reported as leading to secondary pneumonia and pleuritis in the United States. Like *Muellerius capillaris*, it has a mollusc intermediate host that requires wet ground for survival.

Hydatid cysts

Hydatid cysts are the metacestode stage of the carnivore tapeworm *Echinoccus granulosus*. A proportion of hydatid cysts reach the lungs and may produce respiratory signs, particularly if a secondary pasteurellosis occurs.

Fungi

Cryptococcosis

Cryptococcus neoformans are saprophytic and opportunistic fungal pathogens that have on rare occasions been reported to cause pneumonia, mastitis or meningitis.

Airway obstruction

Foreign bodies in the trachea or oesophagus (see 'Secondary ruminal tympany ('choke')', Chapter 16) can result in coughing and signs of respiratory distress.

Lymph node enlargement in the neck can impede air flow (may be caused by caseous lymphadenitis).

Tracheal collapse has been recorded in kids, resulting in exercise intolerance, stertorous breathing and coughing.

Tumour – thymomas or thymic involvement in **multicentric lymphosarcoma** may affect the respiratory or cardiovascular systems. Thymomas are relatively common in goats. They may extend into the chest cavity (or be entirely contained within it), producing respiratory or cardiac dysfunction.

Inhalation pneumonia

Inhalation pneumonia may follow drenching, stomach tubing, etc., or *rhododendron poisoning* (Chapter 21), where vomiting results in inhalation of rumen contents.

Trauma

Injury to the throat from drenching guns or barbed plant material (Chapter 21) can result in cellulitis, pharyngitis and respiratory signs. Penetrating thoracic wounds, fractured ribs, etc., will result in respiratory signs and *diaphragmatic hernia* occasionally occurs after parturition or major trauma, with the reticulum herniating through the diaphragm.

Heat stress

Goats being transported, confined in buildings or attending agricultural shows in hot weather will often show heat stress – excessive panting, increased heart rate, excessive thirst, etc. Severe cases progress to respiratory and circulatory collapse, convulsions, coma and death.

Allergic alveolitis

Exposure to dusty conditions or mouldy feed may result in an allergic alveolitis with a chronic non-productive ('winter') cough in older goats that have been sensitised.

Treatment
- Remove from the cause and feed damp hay.
- Clenbuterol, 0.8 mcg/kg, 1.25 ml/50 kg, slow i.v. or i.m., 2.5 g/50 kg orally in feed twice daily. (The use of Clenbuterol is illegal in the United States.)

Neoplasia

- *Primary and secondary lung tumours* are very rare.
- *Enzootic nasal tumours,* caused by the enzootic nasal tumour virus (ENTV), have been described in goats in many countries worldwide and sporadically in sheep in the United Kingdom. Tumours may be unilateral or bilateral. The first clinical sign is a small amount of seromucous fluid from the nostrils, resulting in hair loss around the nostrils. Affected animals snore, cough, sneeze and head shake. Later, animals present with a continuous serosanguinous nasal discharge, stertorous breathing and dyspnoea. Mouth breathing develops because the tumour fills up the nasal passages and sinuses. As much as 300 ml of fluid can be produced daily. Cranial bones may soften from the pressure, leading to fistula formation, and exophthalmos develops if the neoplasm presses on retrobulbar structures. Animals remain alert and are afebrile but lose weight. There is no treatment and death occurs in 3 to 5 months.

Other conditions producing respiratory signs as part of a clinical syndrome

Hypocalcaemia (Chapter 12) may present as an apparently excited, pyrexic and pneumonic goat. When in doubt give calcium and magnesium.

Poisoning:

o Nitrites/nitrates (see Chapter 21).

o Urea (see Chapter 12).

o Organophosphorus (see Chapters 12 and 19).

Bloat

See Chapter 16.

Anaemia

See Chapter 18.

Cardiac disease

Congenital or acquired (see Chapter 5).

Selenium/vitamin E deficiency

See Chapter 8.–

Kids with white muscle disease may show dyspnoea, coughing and abnormal respiratory sounds.

Further reading

General

Chakraborty, S., Kumar, A., Tiwari,R. *et al.* (2014) Advances in diagnosis of respiratory diseases of small ruminants. *Vet. Med. Inter.*, **2014**, Article ID 508304, 16 pages, 2014. DOI: 10.1155/2014/508304.

Harwood, D.G. (1989) Goat respiratory disease. *Goat Vet. Soc. J.*, **10** (2), 94–98.

Martin, W.B. (1983) Respiratory diseases induced in small ruminants by viruses and mycoplasma. *Rev. Sci. Tech. Off. Int. Epizool.*, **2** (2), 311–334.

McSporran, K.D. (1985) Pneumonia. *Proceedings of the Course in Goat Husbandry and Medicine*, Massey University, November 1985, pp. 123–125.

Robinson, R.A. (1983) Respiratory disease of sheep and goats. *Vet. Clin. North Amer.: Large Anim. Pract.*, **5** (3), 539–556.

Aspergillosis

do Carmo, P.M. *et al.* (2014) Nasal and cutaneous aspergillosis in a goat. *J. Comp. Pathol.*, **150** (1), 4–7.

Cryptococcus

Chapman, H.M., Robinson, W.F., Bolton, J.R. and Robertson, J.P. (1990) *Cryptococcus neoformans infection in goats. Aust. Vet. J.*, **67**, 263–265.

Stiwell, G. and Pissarra, H. (2014) Cryptococcal meningitis in a goat – a case report. *BMC Vet. Res.*, **10**, 84.

Endoscopy

Stierschneider, M. *et al.* (2007) Endoscopic examination of the upper respiratory tract and oesophagus in small ruminants: technique and normal appearance. *Vet. J.*, **173** (1), 101–108.

Enzootic nasal tumours

De las Heras, M. *et al.* (2003) Enzootic nasal adenocarcinomas of sheep and goats. *Current Topics Micro. Immunol.*, **275**, 201–223.

Housing and ventilation

Collins, E.R. (1990) Ventilation of sheep and goat barns. *Vet. Clin. N. Amer.: Food Anim. Pract.*, **6** (3), 635–654.

Pocknee, B.R. (2013) Housing and ventilation of goat buildings. *Goat Vet. Soc. J.*, **29**, 23–26.

Lungworms

Hoste,H., Sotiraki S. and de Jesús Torres-Acosta, J.F. (2011) Control of endoparasitic nematode infections in goats. *Vet. Clin. North Amer.: Food Anim. Pract.*, **27** (1), 163–173.

Mycoplasma

Gonçalves, R., Mariano, I., Núñez, A., Branco, S., Fairfoul, G. and Nicholas, R. (2010) Atypical non-progressive pneumonia in goats. *Vet J.*, **183** (2), 219–221.

Jones, G.E. (1983) Mycoplasmas of sheep and goats. *Vet. Rec.*, **113**, 619–620.

Nicholas, R., Ayling, R. and McAuliffe, L (2008) *Mycoplasma Diseases of Ruminants*. CABI, Wallingford, Oxfordshire, UK.

Rifatbegović, M., Maksimović, Z. and Hulaj, B. (2011) Mycoplasma ovipneumoniae associated with severe respiratory disease in goats. *Vet. Rec.*, **168**, 565–566.

Peste de petit-ruminants (PPR)

Baron, M.D., Parida, S. and Oura, C.A.L. (2011) Peste des petits ruminants: a suitable candidate for eradication. *Vet. Rec.*, **169** (1), 16–21.

Tracheal wash

Mueller, K. (2010) Clinical procedures in goats. *Goat Vet. Soc. J.*, **26**, 15–18.

Tuberculosis

Crawshaw, T. *et al.* (2008) TB in goats caused by *Mycobacterium bovis. Vet. Rec.*, **163**, 163–164.

Crawshaw, T., de la Rua-Domenech, R. and Brown, E. (2013) Recognising the gross pathology of tuberculosis in South American camelids, deer, goats, pigs and sheep. *In Pract.*, **35**, 490–502.

Daniel, R. *et al.* (2009) Outbreak of tuberculosis caused by *Mycobacterium bovis* in Golden Guernsey goats in Great Britain. *Vet. Rec.*, **165**, 335–342.

George, A. (2015) Tuberculosis in goats. *Goat Vet. Soc. J.*, **31**, 32–37.

Gordejo, F.J. *et al.* (2008) Interference of paratuberculosis with the diagnosis of tuberculosis in a goat flock with a natural mixed infection. *Vet. Microbiol.*, **128**, 72–80.

Hayton, A. (2014) The diagnosis of tuberculosis. *Goat Vet. Soc. J.*, **30**, 26–32.

Ultrasonography

Scott, P.R. (2007) Ultrasonographic examination of the thorax. In: *Sheep Medicine*, pp. 139–140. Manson Publishing Ltd, London.

Scott, P.R. (2015) Diagnostic imaging in small ruminants. *Goat Vet. Soc. J.*, **31**, 19–31.

Scott, P.R. and Gessert, M.E. (1998) Ultrasonic examination of the ovine thorax. *Vet. J.*, **155** (3), 305–310.

Streeter, R.N. and Step, D.L. (2007) Diagnostic ultrasonography in ruminants. *Vet. Clin. North Amer.: Food Anim. Pract.*, **23** (3), 541–574.

CHAPTER 18

Anaemia

Initial assessment

The preliminary history should consider:
- Individual or flock/herd problem.
- Grazing – haemonchosis and Fascioliasis common in certain areas; access to poisonous plants.
- Feeding – brassicas, onions, cow colostrum to kids.
- Trauma – accidents, fights or dog attacks, obstetric trauma.
- Anthelmintic treatment.

Clinical examination

Individual animals should be examined for signs of:
- Trauma/lacerations – may be internal haemorrhage without obvious external signs.
- External parasite infestations, for example sucking lice.
- Diarrhoea.
- Haemoglobinuria.
- Oedema – bottle jaw, ascites, ventral abdominal oedema.
- Many anaemic animals are also hypoproteinaemic.
- The mucous membranes should be carefully examined – pale or cyanotic or jaundiced.
- Cardiac rhythm may be altered with severe anaemia.
- Jaundice (but see below).

Both intravascular and extravascular hemolysis produce pale mucous membranes and lethargy and possibly jaundice and bilirubinuria. Intravascular hemolysis will also be accompanied by haemoglobinemia and haemoglobinuria. Since haemoglobin is a pyrogen, pyrexia is common with intravascular hemolysis, whatever the cause. Haemoglobin is also renotoxic, and secondary acute renal failure can occur with severe intravascular hemolysis.

Note: red urine indicates pigmenturia, that is haematuria, haemoglobinuria or myoglobinuria, all of which will be positive on a urine dipstick. With haematuria, centrifugation will produce a pellet of red cells (the supernatant may still be red).

Jaundice

> Jaundice is uncommon in goats and always has a poor prognosis.

Jaundice is an uncommon sign in the goat even with severe hepatocellular damage. However, it may occur:
- In haemolytic diseases, for example *copper toxicity, leptospirosis, eperythrozoonosis* and *poisoning by brassicas or onions*, where indirect (unconjugated) bilirubin levels are elevated.
- Following *bile duct obstruction* in fascioliasis or *tumours* where direct (conjugated) bilirubin levels are raised.
- In some cases of liver dysfunction, for example hepatitis or photosensitisation, both direct and indirect bilirubin levels may be elevated.
- Rift Valley fever.

Laboratory investigation

Blood samples
For normal haematological values, see Table 18.1.
- EDTA, serum, fixed smears.
- Examination of smears may show parasitised red blood cells (eperythrozoonosis) or abnormal shaped cells (poikilocytosis) associated with formation of a different type of haemoglobin (HbC).

Diseases of the Goat, Fourth Edition. John Matthews.
© 2016 John Wiley & Sons, Ltd. Published 2016 by John Wiley & Sons, Ltd.

Table 18.1 Red blood cell parameters.

Test	Range	Units
RBCC	10–18	x 10^{12} /litre
Hb	8–15	g/dl
PCV	0.24–0.39	l/litre
MCH	7–9	pg
MCHC	31–42	g/dl
MCV	16–34	fl
Platelets	3–6	10^5/litre

Table 18.2 Type of anaemia and possible aetiology.

Normcytic anaemia	Macrocytic anaemia	Microcytic anaemia
Infection	Haemonchosis	Copper deficiency
Carcinomas	Recovery from trauma	Chronic blood loss
Protein deficiency	Eperythrozoonosis,	
Cobalt deficiency	Subacute/chronic	
Plant poisoning	fascioliasis	
Acute fascioliasis		

Table 18.2 shows types of anaemia and possible aetiologies. Table 18.3 shows laboratory findings with different causes of anaemia and suggests possible aetiologies.

Faecal sample

- Egg counts for haemonchosis and trichostrongylosis (see Chapters 14 and 18).
- Egg counts for Fasciola if in 'fluke' area.
  Use the sedimentation technique.

Treatment

> Avoid stress by handling the patient as little as possible.

A healthy goat can cope with an acute loss of up to 25% of its red cell mass and up to 50% over 24 hours. With chronic blood loss, a PCV as low as 9% can be tolerated without overt signs of clinical disease, provided the goat is not stressed, or exerted, or is not suffering from another concurrent disease.

- Specific therapy for particular diseases.
- Supportive therapy to correct anaemia and hypoproteinaemia.
  o Avoid stress: it is better to leave untreated than severely stress the patient.
  o Fluid replacement:

  Lactated Ringer's (Hartmann's) solution, 20–80 ml/kg slowly i.v.,depending on the severity of the blood loss.

  o Multivitamin/mineral preparations, i.m. or slow i.v. every 48 hours.
  o Parenteral iron is indicated in cases of severe anaemia due to chronic parasitism, using ferrous sulphate or ferrous gluconate orally.
  o High protein diet.
  o *Blood transfusion* is probably only indicated in shocked animals following severe acute blood loss, that is PCV <20% (Table 18.4) or in chronic conditions when the PCV is 10 or less. Aim to increase the PCV to 25% if possible.

  Red cells transferred into a goat survive about 4 days, that is long enough to treat an acute crisis but not long enough to help a chronically anaemic animal. Avoid repeat transfusions; use adrenaline if transfusion reaction (rare) occurs. An immediate improvement should be evident following intravenous transfusion and within 12 to 14 hours of peritoneal administration.

  If a commercially prepared collection bag is not available, a suitable bag can be produced by draining a litre bag of saline using an IV administration set, leaving 25–50 ml in the bag. Then 5000 units of heparin or 100 ml ACD per litre of blood are added and mixed thoroughly.

  Note: a goat has 55–80 ml of blood per kg of bodyweight. An upper limit of 15% of blood volume is recommended for repeated blood donations at, for instance, fortnightly intervals.

- *Hydroxyethyl starches* (Pentastarch and Hetastarch) are colloids that can be used in animals with hypoalbuminaemia at a rate of 10–20 ml/kg of a 6% solution.

Table 18.3 Cause of anaemia and possible aetiology (after Bennett, 1983).

Cause of anaemia	PCV	Haemoglobin	Hypoproteinaemia	Bilirubin	Possible aetiology
Blood loss	Low	Low	Yes	Normal	Haemonchosis Trichostrongylosis Rumen fluke Coccidiosis Lice Trauma
Haemolytic anaemia	Low	Low	No	High	Rape, kale or onion poisoning Copper poisoning Leptospirosis Eperythrozoonosis
Hepatic disease	Low or normal	Low or normal	Yes	High	Pyrrolizidine alkaloid poisoning
Hepatic disease + blood loss	Low	Low	Yes	High	Fascioliasis
Aplastic anaemia	Low	Low	No	High	Chronic inflammatory disease Protein deficiency Copper deficiency Cobalt deficiency
Protein loss	High or normal	High or normal	Yes	Normal	Coccidiosis Johne's disease Salmonellosis, Trichostrongylosis

Table 18.4 Blood transfusion.

Donor (CAE seronegative):
10 ml/kg from the jugular vein into a blood bag with 50–100 ml of 4% sodium citrate per 400 ml of blood, using a 14 or 16 g needle. Blood is collected by gravity flow.
A healthy adult goat of 50 kg can donate 450–500 ml blood (up to 20% of blood volume; blood volume is 8% of body weight).
The amount of blood taken can be replaced by lactated Ringer's solution.
Recipient:
The amount of blood in litres needed by the recipient can be calculated by:

$$\frac{(\text{Desired PCV} - \text{Actual PCV})}{(\text{Donor PCV})} \times 0.08 \times \text{body weight (kg)}$$

10-20 ml/kg i.v. into jugular or cephalic vein at **10 ml/kg/hour** through a blood filter set or more rapidly in kids intraperitoneally.
10 ml/kg will increase PCV by 3%.

- *Oxyglobin®* is a colloid used in small animals as an initial resuscitation fluid when reduced oxygen-carrying capacity is causing clinical signs. It could be used in valuable animals or neonates, but is too expensive for general use.
- *Hypertonic saline* is a crystalloid solution that has properties that mean that it acts like a colloid and has been used to resuscitate animals in haemorrhagic/hypervolaemic shock, by rapid plasma volume expansion and associated increase in systemic arterial pressure and cardiac output.

> *Hypertonic saline* (7.2%, 2400 mOsm/litre), 5 ml/kg rapidly i.v. (in <7 minutes)

Immediately after infusion animals will often drink large amounts of warm water to which oral electrolytes can be added if appropriate. Treatment with hypertonic saline should be followed by full replacement of fluid deficits using isotonic solutions.

Helminthiasis

Haemonchosis

> Haemonchosis may present as sudden death.

Haemonchus contortus thrive in warm/wet climates, needing warm (15.5 °C), moist conditions to complete its life cycle. In many parts of the world Haemonchosis is the most important nematode infection. In cooler regions, such as the United Kingdom, a sudden hot spell can produce rapid development of larvae on pasture and the sudden development of disease in kids or even adults in the spring or summer. It is a blood-sucking roundworm that pierces the mucosa of the abomasum, causing blood and protein loss to the host. Each day 10% of total blood volume may be consumed by parasites. Severe anaemia and hypoproteinaemia may be produced very rapidly, before loss of condition is observed and a kid may be found dead.

Chronic haemonchosis occurs in cooler years, with ingestion of low to moderate numbers of larvae, leading to prolonged chronic blood loss and anaemia.

Epidemiology
- Long transmission season and short direct life cycle (<3 weeks under optimum conditions and as short as 7 days).
- Very fecund, producing 5000+ eggs/day (300 worms = 1.5 million eggs/day/animal; 30 goats = 1 billion eggs over 3 weeks).
- 20% of the herd responsible for 80% of egg output.
- Very adaptable:
  o Can go into a hypobiotic (arrested) state in the animal to survive poor environmental conditions.
  o Can survive on pasture for a long time.
  o Larvae survive over winter.
- It is estimated that 80% of the worm larvae is found in the first two inches of grazing vegetation.

Clinical signs
Young animals and highly stressed adults are most vulnerable to its effects. Kids have relatively small blood volume, poor immunity and poor resilience and anaemia can progress rapidly from moderate to severe.
- Death.
- Loss of body condition.
- Ill thrift.
- Anemia.
- Oedema – 'bottle jaw' accumulation of fluid under jaw.

Diagnosis
- Anaemia/hypoproteinaemia.
- Abomasal contents reddish/black with 'barber pole' in large numbers.
- Faecal egg counts.

Treatment and control
The treatment and control of gastrointestinal parasites, including the use of anthelmintics and vaccination against *Haemonchus contortus*, are discussed fully in Chapter 14. Vaccination is likely to play an important role in the control of *Haemonchus* throughout the world as vaccine becomes available.

The control of *Haemonchus contortus* in areas where it is the predominant parasite raises additional problems and alternative solutions in the face of increasing resistance to anthelmintics. In particular, selecting individual animals for treatment rather than treating all animals at fixed intervals, or the whole group when some animals show signs of clinical disease, reduces drug costs and delays the development of anthelmintic resistance by reducing the number of anthelmintic treatments administered. Importantly, it also maintains a population of anthelmintic susceptible larvae *in refugia* on pasture to dilute out resistance genes carried by worms that survive treatment.

It has been estimated that 20–30% of the herd or flock carry most of the worms and are responsible for 80% of the egg output. A large proportion of the other goats can live with their small worm burden and need worming infrequently.

Determining the need for treatment can be based on combinations of body condition scores, weight change and *faecal egg counts*.
- Monitoring worm egg counts can be used together with larval differentiation to monitor for the presence of *Haemonchus*, but the samples must not be

refrigerated as this may adversely affect the hatching of these eggs.

- *Haemonchus contortus* eggs can also be identified by fluorescent assay. Peanut agglutinin binds to *Haemonchus* eggs but not those of other trichostrongyle species. A fluorescent isothiocyanate marker can then be attached to peanut agglutinin.

FAMACHA®[1] is a novel system for monitoring *Haemonchus* infection in small ruminants. It was developed in South Africa due to the widespread emergence of drug resistant worms in sheep, but has been validated for sheep and goats in the United States.

- The system is only available through veterinary surgeons, who can then train goat keepers to receive certification to use the system. The system must be used as part of an overall strategy for integrated parasite control developed for each individual farm. It can only help the control of *Haemonchus* and other worms, such as *Teladorsagia* and *Trichostrongylus,* will need to be included in management programmes on individual farms.
- The colour of the ocular mucous membranes is used to estimate the degree of anaemia of each animal by comparison to a laminated colour chart of sheep conjunctivae, where colours range from red or healthy to almost white or anaemic. The lighter the colour the more anaemic the goat is. Animals with red colour are left untreated, whereas paler scores indicate that an animal should be treated.
- FAMACHA examination of the whole herd should occur regularly (every 2–3 weeks) and most frequently on weaned kids and late pregnant/early lactation does.
- *Herd* faecal egg counts should be monitored every 4–6 weeks
- Culling the most chronically heavily parasitised goats will remove susceptible animals and improve the genetics for resistance over time, because host resistance to infection with *H. contortus* is a moderately heritable trait and the same animals tend routinely to have the highest faecal egg count and PCV.
- Failure to identify correctly animals requiring treatment could result in the death of these animals.
- Other causes of anaemia must be identified and the overall health and nutritional status of the herd monitored.

It is extremely important that the efficacy of anthelmintics is known, because animals are not treated until they become anaemic.

Trichostrongylosis

See 'Gastrointestinal parasitism', Chapter 14.

In trichostrongylosis, anaemia is generally present as part of a clinical syndrome involving diarrhoea, weight loss, unthriftiness and hypoproteinaemia.

Diagnosis

- Anaemia/hypoproteinaemia.
- Egg counts.

Fascioliasis

See Chapter 9.

Generally, fascioliasis is a chronic condition in goats, resulting in hypoproteinaemia and anaemia.

Diagnosis

- Anaemia/hypoproteinaemia.
- Faecal egg counts.
- Post-mortem findings.

Rumen fluke

See Chapter 14.

Severe infections with *Paramphistomum cervi* and *Calicophoron duabneyi* cause profuse, projectile, watery diarrhoea with mucus and traces of blood and a characteristic foetid smell, with weight loss, dehydration, mild to moderate anaemia and submandibular oedema and death in 5 to 10 days. Young goats are more frequently and seriously affected than older goats.

Protozoal causes

Coccidiosis

See Chapter 14.

Haemorrhage in the intestine caused by coccidiosis may result in anaemia and hypoproteinaemia.

Diagnosis

- History.
- Clinical signs.
- Faecal occyst counts.
- Post-mortem findings.

Babasiosis

Babasiosis, a tick-borne protozoan parasite, infects goats out-with the United Kingdom. Like *Mycoplasma ovis*, it produces extravascular hemolysis by parasitising red blood cells, leading to their destruction by the reticuloendothelial system.

Sarcococystosis

See Chapter 2.

Bacterial causes

Eperythrozoonosis

Infection with *Mycoplasma ovis* (formerly *Eperythrozoon ovis*) have been reported worldwide. As the organism occurs in the United Kingdom and may infect goats, it should be considered as a remote possible cause of anaemia. It is a small bacteria lacking cell walls, previously classified as a rickettsial bacteria, but now classified as a *Mycoplasma*.

The organism is transmitted mechanically by arthropods – lice, fleas and mosquitos have been implicated in transmission to goats. Transmission may also occur via surgical procedures through blood contamination of instruments and needle contamination during vaccination.

Eperythrozoonosis in goats is generally regarded as an innocuous disease and usually causes only mild anemia. In naïve or debilitated animals, clinical disease with inappetence, wasting, anaemia, malaise and depression may become apparent. Body temperature may be elevated but is often normal. Young goats are most severely affected and the effects are most severe if there are concomitant infections such as gastrointestinal parasites or malnutrition, when eperythrozoonosis can be a component of an ill thrift problem (see Chapter 6). Older animals develop immunity following exposure, but the organism remains in the bloodstream and if the animal is stressed can result in clinical disease.

Extravascular haemolysis occurs because the organism parasitises red blood cells, leading to their destruction by the reticuloendothelial system. Haematology shows a macrocytic haemolytic anemia, with anisocytosis, poikilocytosis and a marked left shift in erythrocyte maturation. The leukocyte count is normal or slightly elevated.

Diagnosis can be made with the detection of organisms on blood smears stained with Giemsa, Romanowsky or acridine orange, but in chronic infections parasitaemia can be cyclic and organisms can disappear from circulation in as little as 2 hours so the failure to detect the organism does not preclude the diagnosis. Sensitive PCR tests have been developed that are more sensitive than the detection organisms in blood smears and are capable of discriminating between various *Mycoplasma* species.

Oxytetracyclines, 20 mg/kg i.v. once daily for 5 days, have been used for treatment, but reinfection may occur if the development of immunity is compromised.

Anaplasmosis

Anaplasma phagocytophilum (formerly *Ehrlichia phagocytophila*), an intracellular parasite of the Rickettsia family, transmitted by the tick vector *Ixodes ricinus*, causes tick-borne fever and abortion (see Chapter 2) in sheep and goats in the United Kingdom. Feral goats in Scotland and Northern Ireland have tested positive for the parasite and may be a significant wildlife reservoir of the disease in some areas.

Anaplasma ovis infects animals out-with the United Kingdom and produces similar clinical signs to those for eperythrozoonosis. *A. marginale* can cause latent infections in small ruminants. Goats are more resistant than sheep to the development of clinical disease. Known arthropod vectors include ticks and horse-flies. Treatment is with tetracyclines.

A. ovis is present in the wild Bighorn sheep population in the United States.

Leptospirosis

Goats do not appear to act as primary reservoirs of leptospiras, infection occurring spasmodically from contact with the organism in their environment or from carrier animals of other species.

Infection is generally poorly documented worldwide, with the serovar *pomona* the most common reported. Serological surveys in New Zealand have shown the serovars *Bratislava*, *Ballum* and *Copenhagi* to predominate, followed by *Pomona*, *Hardjo*, *Tarassovi* and *Australis*, but, despite serological evidence of widespread exposure to leptospira species, there has been little evidence of active infection. In Poland, goats had antibodies to 11 different serovars, with *Zanoni*, *Autumnalis*, *Bratislava*, *Australis* and *Javanica* being the most common, but no abortions or other clinical manifestations of leptospirosis were observed. No serological surveys of goats in the United Kingdom have been carried out.

Most animals exposed to *Leptospira* do not develop the clinical disease, but, out-with the United Kingdom, sporadic reports of acute disease have been recorded. Severely affected animals are pyrexic and dyspnoeic, with anaemia, haemoglobinuria and occasionally jaundice as a result of intravascular haemolysis. In goats, abortion is reported to occur only following septicaemia in acute infections, although, in sheep, the serovars *Hardjo*, *Pomona*, *Ballum* and *Bratislava* have been implicated in late-term abortions, stillbirths and the birth of weak lambs in the United Kingdom, without other clinical signs of disease. *Hardjo* infection in sheep has been shown to produce an agalactia similar to that seen in cows, with soft udders, return to milk in 3 to 4 days and starvation of lambs if not hand reared. *Hardjo* has also been recovered from the brains of young lambs showing meningitis.

Diagnosis

- Serology: microscopic agglutination test (MAT); ELISA.
- Isolation and identification of *Leptospira* spp. in the doe's urine, placenta or fetal fluids and kidney tissues.

Treatment and prevention

- Vaccines labelled for cattle could be used if considered necessary.
- Treatment has a limited effect on the course of the disease, unless antibiotics are given early, when oxytetracyclines, ampicillin, amoxicillin, tylosin and intravenous penicillin G may be successful.
- Management methods to reduce transmission, include controlling rodents, keeping the herd away from potentially contaminated streams and ponds and keeping goats away from wildlife.

Plant poisoning

The production of anaemia by plant poisoning is discussed more fully in Chapter 21.

Bracken (*Pteridium aquilinum*)

Goats seem less susceptible to bracken poisoning than sheep, but prolonged grazing of the plant may result in an acute haemorrhagic syndrome or blood loss due to tumours in the bladder or intestine.

Pyrrolizidine alkaloids

Pyrrolizidine alkaloids, for example found in ragwort, result in haemorrhages following liver damage.

Brassicas

Prolonged feeding of kale and other brassicas such as rape, cabbage, Brussels sprouts and swede tops in large quantities results in haemolytic anaemia as a result of the conversion of *S*-methyl cysteine sulphoxide (SMCO) to dimethyl disulphide, which destroys red blood cells.

Onions

Onions can be fed over long periods without signs of poisoning, but in large amounts produce haemolytic anaemia.

Mouldy sweet clover (*Melilotus* spp.)

Melilots can be safely grazed as they are not poisonous and only become dangerous when the coumarins in the plant become changed into dicoumarol by the action of moulds in hay or silage. Dicoumarol interferes with the metabolism of vitamin K, impairing blood clotting and leading to internal and external haemorrhages.

External parasites

Sucking lice

See Chapter 11.

Lice infestations are common in goats, especially in the wintertime. The blood-sucking louse *Linognathus stenopsis* affects goats in the United Kingdom, producing pruritus and hair loss, particularly on the head, neck and back, as well as anaemia. Sucking lice can be treated with injectable ivermectin or dormectin, or topical treatments. However, topical treatments may be preferable, because mixed infections of biting and sucking are common and only topical treatments are effective for biting lice. Treatments (both topical and injectable) should be repeated in 10 to 14 days to kill any lice that have emerged from eggs or that were in the environment. All animals of the same species in contact with the infested animal should also be treated.

Keds

Keds can also affect goats and produce anaemia.

Trauma

Chronic blood loss from internal or external wounds, for example dog bites or excessive bleeding following castration, will result in anaemia.

Cow colostrum

Feeding bovine colostrum to kids may produce an immune-mediated extravascular hemolysis and a haemolytic syndrome similar to that seen in lambs. Affected kids have severe anaemia and sometimes jaundice. The PCV declines to below normal by 7 days after birth and below 10% within 2 weeks, when clinical signs will be noticed. Initial signs are lethargy and failure to feed, progressing to collapse and death. In practice, this is probably a problem related to feeding colostrum from individual cows, so that pooled colostrum is unlikely to cause a problem.

Laboratory findings
- Direct Coombs test demonstrates bovine IgG on erythrocytes.

Post-mortem findings
- Extreme pallor, very watery blood; creamy appearance to bone marrow.

Treatment
- Blood transfusion, corticosteroids, antibiotics and supportive therapy. Treat any other kids that have received the same batch of colostrum.

Mineral deficiencies

Copper deficiency
See Chapter 5.

Copper deficiency may occur alone, or in combination with cobalt deficiency. Anaemia occurs as a result of poor iron absorption, with a resultant deficiency in haemoglobin synthesis and microcytic, hypochromic non-regenerative anaemia.

Cobalt deficiency
See Chapter 9.

Cobalt deficiency results initially in normocytic, normochromic anaemia, often with haemoglobin and erythrocyte levels within the normal range because of haemoconcentration. Later there may be marked poikilocytosis and macrocytic anaemia with polychromasia.

Mineral poisoning

Copper poisoning
See Chapter 15.

Goats are not as sensitive to copper toxicosis as sheep, but excess intake of copper can cause intravascular hemolysis, resulting in an acute haemolytic crisis with sudden release of copper into the bloodstream when maximum hepatic levels are exceeded.

Protein deficiency

Primary protein deficiency due to *malnutrition* and secondary protein deficiency due to disease, for example *Johne's disease*, may both result in anaemia.

Chronic disease

Chronic disease states (such as Johne's disease or alimentary tumours) may result in non-regenerative anaemias through chronic blood loss or secondary protein deficiencies.

Rapid changes in plasma osmolality

Rapid changes in plasma osmolality due to rapid intravenous injection of hypotonic fluids or ingestion of large quantities of water, following water deprivation or dehydration, can also cause intravascular haemolysis.

Congenital disease

Myelofibrosis is an inherited lethal disease of pygmy goats in California. Kids are normal at birth but become weak and inactive as early as 2 weeks of age as a progressive profound anaemia, neutropaenia and thrombocytopaenia become established because of a primary bone marrow dysfunction. There is no treatment and kids are usually euthanised.

Further reading

General

Bennett, D.G. (1983) Anaemia and hypoproteinaemia. *Vet. Clin. North Amer.: Large Anim. Pract.*, **5** (3), 511–524.

Cornell University College of Veterinary Medicine online textbook on Veterinary Clinical Pathology, eClinPath. Available at : http://www.eclinpath.com/.

Ermilio, E. and Smith, M.C. (2011) Treatment of emergency conditions in sheep and goats. *Vet. Clin. North Amer.: Food Anim. Pract.*, **27** (1), 33–45.

Jones, M.L. and Allison, R.W. (2007) Evaluation of the ruminant complete blood cell count. *Vet. Clin. North Amer.: Food Anim. Pract.*, **23** (3), 377–402.

Mews, A. and Mowlem, A. (1981) Normal haematological and biochemical values in the goat. *Goat Vet. Soc. J.*, **2** (1), 30–31.

Anaplasma

Stuen, S. and Longbottom, D. (2011) Treatment and control of Chlamydial and Rickettsial infections in sheep and goats. *Vet. Clin. North Amer.: Food Anim. Pract.*, **27** (1), 193–202.

Fluid therapy

Jones, M. and Navarre, C. (2014) Fluid therapy in small ruminants and camelids. *Vet. Clin. North Amer.: Food Anim Pract.*, **30** (2), 441–453.

Haemonchosis

See Helminthiasis, Chapter 14.

Leptospirosis

Czopowicz, M. *et al.* (2011) Leptospiral antibodies in the breeding goat population of Poland. *Vet. Rec.*, **169** (9), 230.

CHAPTER 19

Sudden death, post-mortem examination and euthanasia

> Genuine sudden death is rare in animals inspected regularly.

Investigations into a sudden death in a goat or group of goats can be divided into four stages:

- Identification of the animal(s) and history taking.
- External assessment.
- Initial dissection and display of the body cavities.
- Detailed examination and sampling.

Initial assessment

The preliminary history may play a major role in deciding the cause of death. The cause of death may be evident from the history. Consider:

- Individual or group of animals involved.
- Location – housed, yarded, access to pasture.
- Recent introduction or movement of animal(s) involved.
- The interval between the last inspection and the animal(s) being found dead.
- Time period over which deaths have occurred.
- Age of animal, breed, sex.
- Pregnant/non-pregnant (expected kidding date if relevant), stage of lactation.
- Body condition compared to others in the group.

- Feeding – recent changes, access to feed, etc.; weaned or unweaned, artificial rearing of kids, milk or milk replacer.
- Grazing – possible access to poisonous plants.
- Vaccination.
- Known disease status.
- Signs of ill health.
- Weather.
- Season of year.
- Recent management tasks – transport, weaning, mixing of groups.

Examination of the carcase

- Position of body – possibility of trauma or electrocution.
- Signs of struggling? Terminal convulsions.
- An animal in ventral recumbency will have died quietly from conditions such as starvation, dehydration, exposure or hypocalcaemia.
- Condition of body:
  - Emaciated/good condition.
  - Bloat.
  - Discharges from orifices.
- Signs of predation whilst alive or after death.
- Extent of post-mortem decomposition.
- Take a digital photograph of the undisturbed carcase, including a close-up of the ear tags, leg bands, tattoos or other means of identification.
- Take photographs of any lesions and abnormalities.

Diseases of the Goat, Fourth Edition. John Matthews.
© 2016 John Wiley & Sons, Ltd. Published 2016 by John Wiley & Sons, Ltd.

Post-mortem examination

> Post-mortem examination is only of use if carried out very shortly after death.

A thorough, prompt post-mortem examination should be carried out, although some causes of death, including many poisons and hypomagnesaemia, produce no obvious post-mortem changes. Post-mortem autolysis and decomposition may already be present depending on the time interval from death to examination and will be greater in higher environmental temperatures, in fat animals or animals with a dense coat or pyrexia and where bacterial pathogens, such as clostridia, were the cause of death. Table 19.1 shows some common autolytic/agonal changes. Delay will result in further decomposition and reduce the chances of a successful outcome. Tissues with naturally high levels of bacteria, such as the intestine, or in contact with proteolytic enzymes, such as the intestine, gall bladder and pancreas undergo decomposition more rapidly than other body tissues. Rigor mortis can be quite variable in onset, duration and severity and may be easily missed.

Suitable health and safety precautions must always be taken to minimise the risk to human health during the post-mortem examination, including the use of waterproof, protective clothing, cut-resistant and waterproof gloves and Wellington boots.

Post-mortem examinations should be carried out in a consistent and systematic manner. Detailed descriptions of how to carry out a post-mortem examination are available on the Internet:

http://www.veterinaryhandbook.com.au/Content-Section.aspx?id=10 and http://www.esgpip.org/pdf/Technical%20bulletin%20No.33.pdf

Table 19.2 gives an outline of a post-mortem examination for goats which have died suddenly.

A standard procedure should be adopted for examining each particular organ:

- Assess position, colour, shape, size, contents (volume, colour, turbidity), smell, consistency.

Table 19.1 Some common autolytic/agonal changes.

Distension of the abdomen	Animals bloat quickly after death and develop signs resembling true bloat Rapid distension of the rumen is common after death and is not diagnostic of frothy bloat unless also full of frothy foam
Viscera darker red than normal	Blood from the limbs is forced centrally into the viscera, especially the lungs and liver
Bloody froth/discharge at nose	Nasal congestion with rupture of vessels occurs normally during autolysis
Corneal opacity	Occurs as the external surface of the cornea dries and aqueous humour is absorbed
Hypostasis	After death, blood is forced into the lower parts of the body by gravity The skin on the ventral part of the carcase becomes coloured red to purple. The lower parts of the lungs, liver and kidney are darker and heavier than the upper parts
Pulmonary congestion	Reddening of the lungs on the dependent side from hypostatic congestion is a common post-mortem change and should not be mistaken for pneumonia
Sloughing of the rumen mucosa	Normally occurs within an hour of death
Abomasal rupture	May occur due to post-mortem digestion by stomach acids
Bile leakage	Bile may stain surfaces of organs in contact with the gall bladder and leak into the duodenum, which becomes thin walled, dilates and develops a dark green colour
Predation	Damage to the body after death by predators is very common

- Note size, location, appearance and number of any lesions.
- Photograph organs and lesions as necessary.
- Make multiple cuts in the parenchyma of solid organs (liver, spleen, lung).

Table 19.2 Post-mortem examination of goats found dead.

External examination	General	Record ear tag or tattoo
		Body condition
		Trauma or predation – take photographs if legal proceedings are likely
		Record external lesions – ante-mortem trauma will be associated with haemorrhage, erythema and swelling
		Diarrhoea or faecal staining
		Discharges from any orifices
		Loss of hair or evidence of external parasitism
	Head	Eyes (conjunctiva), nose – check for discharges; collect aqueous/vitreous humour
		Ears (including ear canal)
		Mouth (including lips, gums and tongue) – check for haemorrhage, erosions, ulcers, blisters or discoloration and damage from predation
		Mucous membranes – anaemia, jaundice, haemorrhage, ulceration, vesicles
		Estimate age from eruption and wear of incisor teeth
	Skin and hair	Part hair at several sites – check for external parasites
	Neck and superficial lymph nodes	Lymph nodes, including supramammary nodes, should be evaluated for size
	Body	General body condition – fat and muscle cover
		Check the umbilicus in kids
	Udder or testicles	Mastitis; check for predation
	Prepuce, anus, vulva, tail	Check for crystals on preputial hairs (urolithiasis), damage from predation
	Feet	Including interdigital spaces, coronets, joints for swellings, erosions, ulceration
	Subcutaneous tissues	Check for anaemia, jaundice, haemorrhage (petechial, ecchymotic)
		Check for evidence of predation, including bite wounds, claw marks, bruising, haemorrhage
		Check and assess superficial lymph nodes – enlargement, abscess, haemorrhage
	Upper alimentary tract	**Pharynx:** check for inflammation, haemorrhage, necrosis; possible dosing gun injuries
		Oesophagus: check for ulceration or obstruction
	Abdomen	**Abdominal fluid:** identify excessive fluid (serous, ascetic) – consistency, appearance, fibrin, pus
		Examine organs in situ before opening into the alimentary tract
		Rumen: fill, content (plant material, excess grain, foreign material, foam, gas); check for mucosal inflammation/ulceration; check pH if indicated
		Abomasum: check for abomasitis, ulceration, presence or absence of milk in kids. *Haemonchus contortus* are grossly visible. Collect contents for worm egg counts
		Intestines: check for thickening, pigmentation; torsion, neoplasia, intussusception. Collect contents for worm counts, ileal contents for clostridial toxin testing, sample ileocaecocolic lymph nodes
		Liver: determine size, colour, texture, shape of liver lobes, degree of hepatic lipidosis, check for fluke. Collect liver samples for trace element and heavy metal analysis

(continued overleaf)

Table 19.2 (*continued*)

Urinary tract	**Bladder:** check for calculi (collect for analysis); collect urine from bladder and check colour **Urethra** and **urethral process:** check for calculi (collect for analysis) **Kidneys:** strip capsule; check for nephrosis, hydronephrosis, colour. Collect kidney samples for copper and lead analysis
Respiratory tract	**Larynx:** check for obstruction **Trachea** and **bronchi:** check for froth, parasites, foreign body **Pleura:** check for pleural effusion, pleurisy, adhesions **Lungs:** check for consolidation, neoplasia, abscesses (swab for culture). Post-mortem and agonal changes will alter the colour of lung tissue **Lymph nodes:** check and access size, haemorrhage, abscessation
Circulatory system	**Heart:** check muscle thickness, colour, kids for congenital abnormalities, pericarditis, endocarditis **Pericardial fluid:** check for excess fluid, fibrin
Reproductive tract	Check for pregnancy (stage), evidence of abortion, metritis
Musculoskeletal system	**Joints:** incise, examine and collect joint fluid, swab for bacteriology **Muscles:** check for areas of discoloration
Central nervous system	**Brain:** remove if necessary (e.g. if CCN, clostridial enterotoxaemia, listeriosis suspected)

Sample collection

> Aqueous humour is a useful sampling fluid in dead animals as concentrations of minerals and metabolites are stable for up to 48 hours.

Samples that may be of value from freshly dead animals include serum, vitreous and aqueous humour and a faecal sample. In addition, any ectoparasites, for example sucking lice, can be collected and swabs taken of any discharges.

Analysis of blood is only possible if it is collected very soon after death and before coagulation, whereas aqueous humour (AH) and vitreous humour (VH) can be used for up to 48 hours for the post-mortem determination of chemicals such as calcium, magnesium, beta-hydroxybutyrate, urea, creatinine and nitrates that are not protein bound. They are thus useful for the diagnosis of conditions such as renal disease, nitrate poisoning, hypomagnesaemia and for determining calcium status (Table 19.3).

- Aqueous humour is collected by inserting a 21 gauge, 25 mm needle horizontally into the anterior chamber with the bevel towards the cornea to avoid damage to and contamination from the iris.
- Vitreous humour is collected with a 14 or 16 gauge, 25 mm needle inserted vertically through the sclera behind the iris.
- Where possible the gel-like samples should be centrifuged before analysis.

When collecting tissue samples:
- Use clean instruments.
- Use sterile swabs or vacutainers to collect fluids.
- Take representative samples of the pathology present.
- Solid tissue sections should include a margin of normal tissue.
- Label all samples with the tissue or site of origin.
- Use clean leakproof containers.

Sudden death in kids

Non-infectious causes
Trauma and abdominal catastrophe are the most common causes of sudden death in kids.

Kids regularly die after short periods of abdominal pain or as a result of trauma, for example strangulation in hay nets. In some areas, predation can be responsible for high kid mortality.

Other causes of sudden death in kids are listed below:
- Hypothermia/hypoglycaemia –see Chapter 5.
- Abomasal bloat – see Chapter 16.
- Ruminal bloat - see Chapter 16.
- Mesenteric torsion - see Chapter 15.
- Disbudding meningoencephalitis – see Chapter 12.
- Trauma.
- Anaphylactic shock. It is commonly believed that goats are more likely than other species to suffer anaphylactic shock following repeated injections, particularly of procaine penicillin but also local anaesthetics and occasionally clostridial vaccines, although there is no convincing evidence to support this supposition.
- Plant poisoning – see Chapter 21. Plant poisons may produce no obvious pathological changes, so that evidence of consumption, or leaves in the mouth or forestomachs may provide vital information.
- Chemical poisoning – uncommon:
  o Copper poisoning – see Chapter 15).
  o Arsenic, lead (see Chapter 12) and other metal poisonings produce acute or chronic illness, but occasionally present as sudden death.
  o Organophosphorus insecticides produce no obvious gross lesions at post-mortem.
- White muscle disease – see Chapter 8.
- Acute selenosis – see Chapter 8.
- Predators.
- Snakebites. Kids are more likely to be bitten by snakes than adults, because of lack of caution and greater curiosity. Many of them are bitten on the nose or head as they attempt to investigate the snake. Snakebites can be recognised by fang marks in a localised oedematous area, but may be difficult to identify without careful examination and they may be obscured by decomposition.

Infectious causes
- Septicaemia, for example Pasteurella, Streptococci.
- Coccidiosis – see Chapter 14.
- Enterotoxaemia (*Clostridium perfringens* type D) – see Chapter 15.
- Listeriosis – see Chapter 12.
- Pasteurellosis – see Chapter 17.

Table 19.3 Chemical levels in aqueous and vitreous humour.

Chemical	Levels in recently dead animal[a]	Comments
Urea	**Renal disease** AH > 30 mmol/litre (180 mg/dl)	VH urea levels are more stable than AH levels and are about 0.84 times the serum levels for up to 36 hour after death Stable for longer if refrigerated
Calcium	**Hypocalcaemia** AH < 1 mmol/litre (4 mg/dl) Recently dead	Fresh AH more useful than VH as a rapid fall in calcium equilibrates quicker with AH than VH in equilibrium with plasma ionised calcium as protein-bound calcium excluded
Magnesium	**Hypomagnesaemia** AH <0.33 mmol/litre (0.80 mg/dl) Recently dead VH <0.65 mmol/litre (1.58 mg/dl) up to 48 h post-mortem	VH more stable than AH Magnesium leaks from the iris into AH and VH after death, increasing the ocular levels
β-hydroxybutyrate	**Pregnancy toxaemia** AH >2.5 mmol/litre (26 mg/dl)	
Sodium and chloride	**Salt poisoning** AR and VH elevated	
Nitrate	**Nitrate poisoning** AH levels < 35% serum levels	Useful for 60 hours after death if very high

[a]Sheep levels (Edwards *et al.*, 2009).

- Haemonchosis – see Chapters 14 and 18.
- Salmonellosis – see Chapter 14.
- Foot and mouth disease. Peracute death from myocarditis may occur in kids less than 2 weeks of age, even though older animals may show no clinical signs (see Chapter 7).
- Bluetongue – see Chapter 10.

Predators

In many parts of the world, more goats are injured or killed by domestic and feral dogs than by any other predator. In the United Kingdom, the dog is the only significant predator, although foxes will occasionally take neonatal kids. In the United States, coyotes can cause significant losses. Other predators, such as big cats, feral pigs, bears and eagles can be of economic importance in certain areas. Many animals, including rats, foxes and dogs, and birds, such as crows, are opportunist scavengers and will feed off body parts removing teats, noses and vulvas or pecking out eyes from weak or dead animals.

Management problems resulting in the death of kids can be blamed erroneously on predation. Predators frequently taken carrion, so it is important to ascertain if kids have died from predation, or were stillborn, mis-mothered or died of disease before being eaten. The general condition of the kid should be evaluated for evidence of dehydration, such as sunken eyes, the presence or absence of milk in the abomasum and the condition of the hooves. A neonatal kid that has not walked will have smooth, soft hooves. Even if bite marks are present, the absence of external or subcutaneous haemorrhage suggests that the animal was dead before being bitten.

Which predator?

Predators frequently feed on carrion and the kills of other predators and several species may feed on the same carcase, so it not always obvious which predator, if any, is responsible for the death of a particular animal without careful investigation. The carcase should be as fresh as possible as decomposition will make identification of a predator more difficult. Some stages of decomposition can resemble extensive bruising. Table 19.4 gives information on the most common predators of goats.

When investigating a possible death by predation, it is important to consider:

- Mode of attack. Although most predators follow a general pattern of attack, individuals vary in food preferences, method of attack and feeding behaviours and these can overlap extensively between individuals of different species. Most predators attack the head and neck. Kids may be killed by a single bite on the head, neck, shoulders or back. Larger goats may be bitten repeatedly as they attempt to escape, with smaller or inexperienced predators, such as foxes, coyotes and dogs, tending to inflict multiple injuries. Foxes rarely crush the skull or spine of kids, but coyotes, bobcats and larger carnivores commonly inflict such injuries.
- Type and extent of damage:
  o Examine carcases for wounds, haemorrhage, bruises, broken bones and evidence of feeding, remembering that injuries can arise from a multitude of causes other than predation, such as nails, barbed wire and vehicles.
  o Check for the presence or absence of subcutaneous haemorrhage. Haemorrhage is only present if skin and tissue damage occurred while the animal was alive.
  o Note the sites of damage, particularly the throat, back of head, neck and back. Foxes rarely crush the skull or spine of kids, but such injuries are commonly inflicted by coyotes, bobcats and larger carnivores. Injuries to the hind quarters are common with dog attacks.
  o Note the number of bites. The skin should be removed when necessary, particularly around the neck, throat and head, and the area checked for tooth marks, subcutaneous haemorrhage and tissue damage. Experienced predators may kill by suffocating the animal with a single bite to the throat, leaving only limited external evidence. Larger predators, like bears and cougars, may leave little external damage if blows from the fore legs break the victim's neck or back, but extensive bruising may be obvious when the animal is skinned. Dense hair may hide claw marks caused by bobcats or mountain lions.
  o Note the size and location of tooth/talon marks. The size and spacing between the canine teeth are characteristic for each species and may indicate a particular predator, but there are close similarities in species of similar size.
  o Note the location of the carcase. Animals that are killed are usually lying in an unnatural position. Predators such as cougars, bobcats and black bears move their kills to feed in secluded areas. Foxes,

bobcats and coyotes frequently carry small animals away, but scavengers may also disturb or move the carcase while feeding. Big cats feed in a limited area and usually cover the carcase with dirt or vegetable debris. Coyotes tend to scatter body parts, wool and hair over a large area during feeding.

Sudden death in adult goats

Non-infectious causes

- Ruminal bloat – see Chapter 16.
- Acidosis (ruminal impaction) – see Chapter 16.
- Trauma.
- Cold stress – Angoras and Cashmere goats shorn in inclement weather without adequate shelter or nutrition.
- Anaphylactic shock – see 'Sudden death in kids'; earlier in this chapter.
- Plant poisoning – see 'Sudden death in kids'.
- Chemical poisoning – see 'Sudden death in kids'.
- Hypomagnesaemia - see Chapter 12 (Plate 12.3).
- Hypocalcaemia – See Chapter 4.
- Transit tetany - see Chapter 12.
- Predators – see 'Sudden death in kids'.
- Lightning/electrocution.

Infectious causes

Where bacterial pathogens, such as Clostridia, were the cause of death, the rate of autolysis after death is likely to be accelerated.

- Gangrenous mastitis – see Chapter 13.
- Enterotoxaemia (*Clostridium perfringens* type D) – see Chapter 15.
- Listeriosis – see Chapter 12.
- Pasteurellosis – see Chapter 17.
- Haemonchosis – see Chapters 14 and 18.
- Acute fascioliasis – see Chapter 9.
- Anthrax.
- Black leg.
- Malignant oedema.
- Black disease.
- Botulism.

Anthrax

Anthrax is rare. The peracute form may produce death in 1 to 2 hours. Acute cases may show pyrexia, tremor, dyspnoea and mucosal congestion. After death,

Table 19.4 Predators.

Predator	Animals at risk	Mode of attack
Dog (domestic and feral) Dingo	All ages of goats are at risk. Dogs often attack the goats from behind injuring the hindquarters, flanks and head. Horned animals may be attacked from the side, to avoid the horns, and males may be bitten on the testicles. They rarely kill as effectively as coyotes.	Inexperienced animals, or those that kill for fun, often severely mutilate the goat, causing significant damage to the hind legs, neck and shoulders with multiple bites and flaps of skin pulled away from the animal. The ears are often badly torn.	The flight behaviour of small ruminants encourages attacks on several animals at once by both single dogs and packs of dogs and only a small proportion of the injured or killed goats are eaten.
Fox (red fox)	Only kids at risk because of the small size of the fox. Unlike wild dogs, foxes rarely challenge older kids and mature goats, unless their food is very limited.	Multiple bites on the back and neck or may attack the throat.	Small kids may be taken away from the kill location, often to a den.
Coyote	All ages are at risk. Normally kill goats by biting the throat, penetrating and collapsing the trachea. A young, inexperienced coyote may bite wherever it can catch the animal, attacking the side, hindquarters and udder. The upper canine teeth may penetrate the top of the neck or the skull of small kids	Death occurs by suffocation, sometimes after a rather prolonged struggle, leaving considerable haemorrhage beneath the skin.	Commonest and most serious predator of livestock in the United States. Carcases are frequently completely dismembered and eaten. The rumen and intestines may be removed and dragged away from the carcase.
Bobcat	All small ruminants at risk as will take prey up to 8 times its weight. Kids often killed by a bite through the back of the neck at the base of the skull or on the side of the head. Also bite the back of the jaw and lower part of the skull, leaving claw marks on the goat's side, back, flank and shoulders. Canine teeth marks 1.9 to 2.5 cm.	Death is usually caused by crushing the spine and/or skull. Jugular vein may be punctured, but the victims usually die of suffocation and shock.	Carcase may be eaten immediately or it may be taken away to be eaten later and partially covered with debris. Bobcats reach 30 to 35 cm when scratching litter, compared to the 90 cm reach of a mountain lion. Rumen is usually untouched. Will scavenge the remains of animals killed by other predators.
Mountain lion (Cougar)	Often kill large numbers of animals in one night, typically 5 to 10 animals. Bites are inflicted from above, frequently biting the top of the neck or head and may bite through the skull or the throat. Canine teeth marks 3.8 cm.	Vertebral column severed and neck broken. This differs from the typical coyote bite in the throat and the general mutilation caused by dogs.	Usually feed on the front quarters and neck region first. The rumen is generally untouched. Large leg bones and ribs may be crushed and broken. Like bobcats they drag and then hide the carcase, covering it with litter and sometimes urinating and defecating on top of it. Often return to feed on a kill for three or four nights.

(continued overleaf)

Table 19.4 (*continued*)

Predator	Animals at risk	Mode of attack	
Feral pigs	Kids are particularly vulnerable and predation usually occurs in kidding areas. The presence of afterbirths may attract the pigs. Pigs can have a devastating effect on kid populations and occasionally adult animals giving birth are attacked and killed.		Typically almost the entire carcass is consumed or carried off, so often no evidence of predation is found. Kids may be missing or the does may have distended udders. May find skin with hooves or skull attached or just blood and tracks where feeding occurred.
Bear (Black and Grizzly)	Predation is most common in the spring and summer during times of poor feed availability. Bears usually kill by biting the neck or with blows from the forelegs.	Goats may be consumed almost entirely, leaving only the rumen, skin and large bones . Torn, mauled, and mutilated carcases are characteristic of bear attacks, with extensive shoulder and back injuries and substantial bruising. The udders of does may be eaten, possibly to obtain milk.	Body is often moved to a more secluded spot. The carcase is usually opened ventrally, the heart and liver eaten and the intestines spread out around the kill site. The goat may be partially skinned during eating.
Eagle (Bald, Golden and Wedge-tailed)	Although capable of killing adults, almost all predation on goats is directed at kids in the first few months of life. Over a certain size, they are too heavy to carry to the nest. Golden eagles are more likely to prey on goats than bald eagles.	The bird lands on the goat's back or neck, gripping tightly with its talons and riding its prey until it collapses, either as result of exhaustion, shock or internal injury. Talons cause triangular wounds up to 5 cm in the shoulders, ribs, back, brisket and abdomen of kids. Internal bleeding is common when talons enter the abdominal or thoracic cavities. Compression skull fractures are seen in kids.	Eagles eat carrion and carcases left by foxes and coyotes. It is probable that more kids are taken as carrion than being taken alive. They have been known to drive goats and sheep off hillsides and cliffs.

dark unclotted blood discharges from the nostrils, mouth, anus and vulva. The carcase undergoes rapid decomposition and there is absence of rigor mortis.

If anthrax is suspected, the carcase should not be opened until the disease has been proved absent. If a post-mortem has been carried out inadvertently, there will be evidence of widespread haemorrhage and a grossly enlarged spleen.

Diagnosis

- Blood smears from an ear vein should be air dried, fixed with heat and stained with polychrome methylene blue to show *Bacillus anthracis* rods with purple staining reaction of the capsule.

Black leg

Black leg is also rare. Goats appear less susceptible than sheep.

Aetiology

- Acute infection by *Clostridium chauvoei* spores, which enter by skin wounds, or via the vulva and vagina at kidding, or occasionally via the intestines, and settle in muscle masses of the hindquarters, shoulder or lumbar areas. Bruising in these areas provides the anaerobic environment suitable for germination of spores.

Clinical signs

- Generally the goat is found dead, often in a characteristic position with the affected limb stuck out stiffly and gas and oedema at the affected site.
- Decomposition and bloating occur rapidly and there may be blood from the nostrils and anus.

Malignant oedema

Malignant oedema is characterised by acute anaerobic wound infection caused by *Clostridium septicum* or other Clostridial organisms. Goats appear less susceptible than sheep, but the disease may occur following fighting and head butting in males ('swelled head' or 'big head').

Clinical signs

- Death occurs within 12 to 24 hours of first appearance of clinical signs; affected areas are swollen with emphysema, erythema and extensive frothy exudate from the wound.

Note: multivalent Clostridial vaccines should be used as a herd preventative whenever black leg or malignant oedema have been diagnosed in a herd.

Black disease (infectious necrotic hepatitis)

Black disease is rare. It causes acute toxaemia by combined infection with the liver fluke, *Fasciola hepatica* and *Clostridium novyi* (*Cl. oedematiens*). Animals are generally found dead with blood-stained froth from the nostrils. Decomposition occurs rapidly. Post-mortem shows dark subcutaneous tissue, blood-stained fluid in body cavities and a dark liver with scattered necrotic areas. In fluke areas, routine Clostridial vaccination should include *Clostridium novyi*.

Botulism

See Chapter 12.

Ingestion of botulism toxin, produced by *Clostridium botulinum* in food, has occasionally been reported to cause an acute onset of paralysis or sudden death.

Euthanasia

Handling of animals prior to euthanasia should be as stress free as possible.

A variety of methods are available for the emergency killing of animals. These include:

- Lethal injection.
- Captive-bolt stunning, followed by bleeding or pithing.
- Free-bullet firearms.
- External trauma, followed by bleeding.

The choice of method depends on the size of the animal, the availability of equipment and drugs, the location of the animal and, in the case of pet animals, the preference of the owner.

Death must always be confirmed before leaving the owner's premises or disposing of the animal's remains.

Lethal injection

An intravenous injection of a lethal dose of a barbiturate drug is a convenient method of euthanising pet goats.

- In the United Kingdom, secobarbital sodium (quinalbarbitone sodium) 400 mg with cinchocaine Hydrochloride, 25 mg, 1.0 ml/10 kg (Somulose, Dechra Veterinary Products Ltd), is licensed for euthanasia in cattle. The full dose should be administered over 10 to 15 seconds in order to minimise premature cardiac arrest. If the injection rate is too slow, the period until death may be prolonged.

- Pentobarbital sodium 20% w/v is licensed for euthanasia in smaller farm animals (Lethobarb, Pentobarbital for Euthanasia, Ayrton Saunders Ltd) of 140 mg/kg bodyweight; 0.7 ml/kg bodyweight by rapid i.v. injection.

The jugular vein is generally the most accessible vein capable of taking a large volume of fluid rapidly. In recumbent animals, particularly when the neck is twisted, the use of a rope or baler twine tourniquet around the neck makes raising the vein easier. An 18 gauge needle is suitable for most juvenile and adult goats, or an indwelling jugular catheter can be placed if desired. Where necessary, another suitable superficial vein, such as the cephalic, can be used.

In fractious animals, pre-medication with an appropriate sedative (Chapter 24) may be appropriate. After a barbiturate injection, the carcase cannot be used for human or animal consumption and the body should be kept away from wild scavengers such as foxes.

Potassium chloride and magnesium sulphate are effective methods of euthanising animals that have previously been anaesthetised, with death generally more rapid after potassium chloride injection. Using an 18 gauge needle, 60 to 100 ml of either solution is administerd into a suitable vein.

Note: although α_2 agonists, such as xylazine, produce a state resembling general anaesthesia, they should not be used alone before the administration of i.v. potassium chloride or magnesium sulphate.

Captive bolt stunning

The humane killing of goats using captive-bolt equipment is a two-stage procedure. The captive bolt administers a severe percussive blow to the skull of the animal rendering it insensible and it must then be bled or pithed immediately to ensure rapid death. It is the bleeding or pithing that actually kills the animal.

To ensure that the percussive blow is not deflected by the thick mass of bone on the top of the skull, all goats should be treated as though they have horns. Therefore, the muzzle of the stunner should be placed behind the bony mass on the mid-line and aimed towards the base of the tongue (Figure 19.1). The muzzle of the captive-bolt stunner must always be held

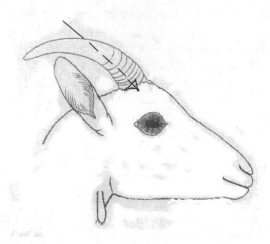

Figure 19.1 Captive-bolt stunning.

firmly against the head. It is essential that equipment is well maintained and that stunning is carried out accurately, using the appropriate cartridge strength for the animal, to ensure that animals are effectively and irreversibly stunned.

Following an effective stun, the goat collapses and exhibits exaggerated tonic activity for 10 to 20 seconds, becoming rigid with its head extended and its hind legs flexed towards the abdomen. This is followed by gradual relaxation and involuntary kicking movements.

Pithing

Pithing involves inserting a flexible wire or polypropylene rod through the entry site produced in the skull by a penetrative captive-bolt. The rod is then slid backwards and forwards ('fiddling') to destroy brainstem (and spinal cord tissue if the rod is long enough). Violent muscle activity occurs during the pithing process, but reflex muscle movement then becomes inhibited.

Note: in the United Kingdom, animals that have been pithed cannot be used for human consumption in case the carcase has been contaminated with brain tissue.

Bleeding

Animals must be bled as soon as possible after stunning, ideally within 15 seconds, whilst still in the tonic (rigid) phase. Bleeding involves severing the carotid arteries and jugular veins, or the blood vessels from which they arise. All the major blood vessels must be severed to ensure a rapid death and this can be achieved by making a deep transverse cut across the animal's throat at the angle of the jaw, until the blade of the knife touches the spine, transecting skin, muscle, trachea, oesophagus, carotid arteries and jugular veins. This requires a very sharp knife with a rigid blade at least 12 cm long.

Note: in the EU, the trachea and oesophagus of animals intended for human consumption must remain intact during bleeding, except in the case of slaughter according to a religious custom.

Free-bullet firearms

Firearms should only be used by a trained, competent operator, using the correct ammunition, in accordance with the relevant regional and national legislation controlling firearm use. In the United Kingdom, this means that in most situations only a humane killer, shotgun or .22 long rifle is likely to be available. In other parts of the world, handguns of a suitable high calibre can be used. The use of firearms in enclosed spaces, or when animals are on hard surfaces, should be avoided whenever possible, because of the risk of ricochet if the bullet exits the animal's body. Shooting from behind the poll is recommended for all goats (see captive-bolt stunning above). On hard ground, where there is an increased danger of ricochet, using a shotgun is safer than a firearm with a free bullet.

Except for humane killers, firearms should never be placed closer to the head than 15 to 30 centimetres to avoid self-inflicted injury.

The animal should collapse immediately when shot and may bleed from the bullet entry point, its nose and its mouth. There is no need to bleed or pith an animal following shooting.

About a minute after shooting, involuntary movement of the limbs may occur and does not necessarily indicate consciousness. Although one correctly placed bullet usually results in immediate loss of consciousness, the animal should be monitored until death is confirmed in case an additional shot is necessary.

A *humane killer* is a single-shot, free-bullet pistol with a vented barrel. The muzzle of the gun is placed against the forehead of the animal and a bullet fired into the brain.

Shotguns are the best firearm for on-farm destruction of goats. Because the shot disperses within the head, the accuracy of the shot is not as critical as with other firearms and there is not the same danger of ricochet.

.22 Rifles can be used to kill goats, but it needs an accurate shot.

Handguns. Although hollow-point bullets increase brain destruction and reduce the chance of ricochet, solid point bullets have better penetration and are more suitable for larger animals.

Euthanasia of kids

In pet animals, a lethal injection of barbiturate into the jugular or cephalic vein is a suitable method of euthanising kids. If no other method is immediately available, neonatal kids can be humanely killed by delivering a heavy blow to the head. This should only be done by someone who has received adequate instruction in suitable techniques. The Humane Slaughter Association has descriptions of the techniques available: http://www.hsa.org.uk/publications/publications.

Further reading
General

Ensley, S. and Rumbeiha, W. (2012) Ruminant toxicology diagnostics. *Vet. Clin. North Amer.: Food Anim. Pract.*, **28** (3), 557–564.

Herdt, T.H. and Hoff, B. (2011) The use of blood analysis to evaluate trace mineral status in ruminant livestock. *Vet. Clin. North Amer.: Food Anim. Pract.*, **27** (2), 255–283.

King, J.M. (1983) Sudden death in sheep and goats. *Vet. Clin. North Amer.: Large Anim. Pract.*, **5** (3), 701–710.

Lovatt, F., Stevenson, H. and Davies, I. (2014) Sudden death in sheep. *In Pract.*, **36**, 409–417.

Nietfeld, J.C. (2012) Neuropathology and diagnostics in food animals. *Vet. Clin. North Amer.: Food Anim. Pract.*, **28** (3), 515–534.

Osweiler, G.D. (2011) Diagnostic guidelines for ruminant toxicoses. *Vet. Clin. North Amer.: Food Anim. Pract.*, **27** (2), 247–254.

Stegelmeier, B.L. (2011) Identifying plant poisoning in livestock: diagnostic approaches and laboratory tests. *Vet. Clin. North Amer.: Food Anim. Pract.*, **27** (2), 407–417.

Valentine, B.A., Cebra, C.K. and Taylor, G.H. (2007) Fatal gastrointestinal parasitism in goats: 31 cases (2001–2006). *J. Amer. Vet. Med. Assoc.*, **231** (7), 1098–1103.

Euthanasia

American Veterinary Medical Association Guidelines for the Euthanasia of Animals. Available at: https://www.avma.org/KB/Policies/Documents/euthanasia.pdf.

Callan, R. *et al.* (2012) *Veterinary Euthanasia Techniques: A Practical Guide.* Wiley-Blackwell, Oxford.

Humane Slaughter Association. Available at: http://www.hsa.org.uk/publications/publications.

Shearer, J.K. and Ramirez, A. *Procedures for Humane Euthanasia*. Iowa State University College of Veterinary Medicine. Available at: http://vetmed.iastate.edu/vdpam/extension/dairy/programs/humane-euthanasia.

Post-mortem examinations

Australian Livestock Export Corporation Limited (2015) *Veterinary Handbook for Cattle, Sheep and Goats*. Available at: http://www.veterinaryhandbook.com.au/ContentSection.aspx?id=10.

Debien, E. *et al.* (2013) Proportional mortality: a study of 152 goats submitted for necropsy from 13 goat herds in Quebec, with a special focus on caseous lymphadenitis. *Canadian Vet. J.*, **54**, 581–587.

Edwards, G. *et al.* (2009) Use of ocular fluids to aid post-mortem diagnosis in cattle and sheep. *In Pract.*, **31**, 22–25.

Ethiopia Sheep and Goat Productivity Improvement Program (2010) Technical Bulletin No. 33, Postmortem techniques for sheep and goats. Available at: http://www.esgpip.org/pdf/Technical%20bulletin%20No.33.pdf.

Fodstad, F.H. and Gunnarsson, E. (1979) Post-mortem examination in the diagnosis of Johne's disease in goats. *Acta Veterinaia Scandinavica*, **20** (2), 157–167.

Harwood, D. (2016) Approach to post mortem in the goat and some common pathological presentations. *Goat Vet. Soc. J.*, **32** (in print).

Mearns, R. (2009) Ovine necropsy and fetal examination. *Livestock*, **14** (2), 46.

Otter, A. and Davies, I. (2015) Disease features and diagnostic sampling of cattle and sheep post-mortem examinations. *In Pract.*, **37** (6), 293–305.

Predators

Cearley, K. (2000) Predator Management. Available at: http://www2.luresext.edu/goats/training/predator.html.

Vantassel, S.M. (2012) *The Wildlife Damage Inspection Handbook*, 3rd edition, Lincoln, NE.

Transport of casualty animals

Defra (2000) Guidance on the Transport of Casualty Farm Animals (PB1381). Available at: www.nifcc.co.uk/publications/44.

Defra (2011) Goats: Welfare of Animals During Transport. Advice for Transporters of Goats (PB12544b). Available at: http://adlib.everysite.co.uk/adlib/defra/content.aspx?id=2RRVTHNXTS.98BB68ONT9KZ0.

Live Transport: Welfare Regulations – Detailed Guidance. Available at: https://www.gov.uk/farm-animal-welfare-during-transportation.

CHAPTER 20

Eye disease

Non-infectious conjunctivitis

Conjunctivitis in individual animals can occur as a result of irritation by dusty hay (particularly if fed from overhead racks), dust, wind, bright sunlight or localized trauma or foreign objects in the conjunctivae, or as a result of allergy (Plates 20.1 and 20.2).

Infectious keratoconjunctivitis

Infectious keratoconjunctivitis ('pink eye' or contagious ophthalmia) is an acute contagious disease characterised by inflammation of the conjunctiva and cornea in one or both eyes.

Aetiology
- The causal agents of the disease are still unclear; it is probable that several agents are involved.
- Predisposing factors include dusty hay, wind, bright sunlight and dust; overcrowding; long grass; flies.

Mycoplasma
There is strong evidence that *Mycoplasma conjunctivae* is a major causal agent of keratoconjunctivitis in the United Kingdom. *Ureaplasma*, *M. ovipneumoniae*, *M. arginini* and *Acholeplasma oculi* have also been isolated from keratoconjunctivitis in sheep and goats, but their role in natural disease remains debatable. Predisposing factors such as wind or dust probably play an important part.

Chlamydia
Clamydophila pecorum (formerly *Clamydia psittaci*) produces keratoconjunctivitis in both sheep and goats. There may be abortions (see Chapter 2) occurring in

the same herd/ flock and polyarthritis in kids (see Chapter 8).

Colesiota
Colesiota conjunctivae, previously classified as a rickettsia-like organism, is a member of the Chlamydiaceae, similar to *C. psittaci*. It is reportedly a common cause of keratoconjunctivitis in sheep and possibly goats out-with the United Kingdom, although in goats only a mild conjunctivitis is produced. It is probable that many cases attributed to this organism were in fact produced by *Mycoplasma* spp.

Bacteria
Bacteria probably act as secondary invaders where the primary damage is produced by smaller organisms, increasing the severity of the condition. *Staphylococcus aureus*, *Escerichia coli* and *Branhamella ovis* are commonly isolated from sheep with affected eyes. *Moraxella* spp. may also be involved.

Listeria monocytogenes (Chapter 12) may also cause keratoconjunctivitis (silage eye) as part of a syndrome involving neurological signs and/or abortion. Individual goats occasionally only show the ocular lesions – conjunctivitis, nystagmus, hypopyon and endophthalmitis.

Yersinia pseudotuberculosis is a significant cause of disease in goats, causing enterocolitis, mesenteric lymphadenitis, septicaemia, placentitis/abortion and mastitis and it is a zoonotic infection. It can also cause ocular disease – mucopurulent ocular discharge, blepharospasm, chemosis, conjunctival hyperemia, corneal opacity and neovascularisation.

Viruses
Infectious bovine rhinotracheitis (IBR) can cause a mucopurulent conjunctivitis in goats.

Diseases of the Goat, Fourth Edition. John Matthews.
© 2016 John Wiley & Sons, Ltd. Published 2016 by John Wiley & Sons, Ltd.

Transmission of infectious keratoconjunctivitis

- Flies and lice are possible vectors for the disease.
- Carrier goats exist for *Mycoplasma* spp. and *C. pecorum* and can thus introduce the disease into a new herd; carriers continue the disease within a herd and, as immunity is poor, individual goats may suffer repeated infection.
- Contact at shows will facilitate spread between herds.
- Close contact at feeding or even at grass will spread the disease within a herd.
- Cross-infection occurs between sheep and goats.

Clinical signs

- This is a herd/flock problem as it is very infectious. Angoras may be more severely affected than dairy breeds; older goats may be more severely affected, following previous exposure.
- Conjunctivitis with marked hyperaemia, excessive lacrimation and blepharospasm, so animals stand with affected eyes closed.
- Later corneal opacity and vascularisation; corneal ulceration in severe cases with a purulent ocular discharge and possible rupture of the anterior chamber of the eye.
- Vision is affected in severe cases so animals may have difficulty feeding and lose condition.
- Cloudiness of the cornea may persist for several weeks.

Note: *Cobalt deficiency* ('pine') (see Chapter 9) and *iodine toxicity* (see Chapter 5) can produce excessive lacrimation, which might be confused with keratoconjunctivitis.

Diagnosis

- Clinical signs as herd/flock.
- Swab early cases – vigorously swab conjunctivae and cornea:
  o Submit dry or in Stuart's medium for bacteriology.
  o Place in mycoplasma transport medium.
  o Place in Chlamydia transport medium.
- Scrapings of everted conjunctivae can be placed on a slide, fixed in methanol and stained with Giemsa or examined using fluorescent antibody techniques for *Mycoplasma* or *Chlamydophila.*.
- Blood samples for *Chlamydophila* serology.

Treatment

Treatment will not eliminate the organism in all cases, so carrier animals will remain to perpetuate the infection.

- Topical tetracycline ointments daily for 5 to 6 days, together with long-acting tetracycline injections intramuscularly, are generally effective if started early in the course of the disease.
- Long-acting tetracycline injections can be used prophylactically in the rest of the herd.
- Subconjunctival injections with oxytetracycline can be used additionally to achieve a high concentration of antibiotic.

    The conjunctivae can be anaesthetised with 0.5% proparacaine; a maximum of 0.5 ml is administered in the dorsal conjunctival fornix with a 25 gauge needle. Sedation and/or an auriculopalpebral nerve block can be used in fractious animals.

- Subconjunctival injections of a combination of oxytetracycline and dexamethasone have been used to treat Listerial infections.
- Fluoroquinolones drugs, including danofloxacin and florfenicol administered parenterally have been used empirically because of the effectiveness of these drugs in treating respiratory disease caused by *Mycoplasma* spp.
- Tilmicosin has been used effectively in sheep, but should not be used because it is associated with a high death rate in goats.
- Severely affected animals should be penned separately in dark surroundings with easy access to food and water.
- With severe corneal ulceration, third eyelid flaps can be used to protect the cornea.

Foreign bodies

Foreign bodies, such as seeds, shavings, etc., will result in severe conjunctivitis and possible corneal ulceration if untreated. Foreign bodies may lodge behind the third eyelid and will need careful removal, with the goat securely held. Sedation and/or the use of a topical anaesthetic, such as 0.5% proparacaine, is advisable. After removal of the foreign body, treatment is as for infectious keratoconjunctivitis.

Corneal trauma

The cornea of goats is commonly traumatised, often by stalks of hay or straw; overlarge tags on the ears of Angora kids may irritate the eye and the eye will also be damaged when entropion is present. Treatment involves correcting or removing the cause of the trauma and then treating the resultant conjunctivitis or corneal damage.

Treatment

- Simple corneal ulcers and non-penetrating lacerations can be treated with topical antibiotic ointments and 1% atropine drops; atropine should be used to effect a moderately dilated pupil and stopped as soon as this is achieved and the animal is more comfortable.
- Third eyelid flaps can be used to assist healing; an alternative 'eye-patch' can be made by gluing a piece of water resistant cloth to the hair around the orbit, using livestock adhesive. The eye should be cleaned thoroughly and checked for foreign bodies before the cornea is covered. A subconjunctival injection of penicillin helps prevent bacterial infection.
- Alternatively, blood can be drawn from the affected animal, allowed to clot and the serum decanted. Then 0.5 to 1 ml of serum can be injected subconjunctivally into each eye using a 23 gauge needle. The serum leaks out through the injection hole over the next few days, promoting healing. Whilst healing of the ulcer takes place, the eye can be protected by suturing the eyelids together.

Entropion

Entropion has been reported as an occasional congenital condition in all breeds of dairy goats and Angoras, but is uncommon in the United Kingdom. Because it is an inheritable defect, possible carriers, especially male goats, should be identified wherever possible. Acquired entropion can arise following trauma and scar formation.

Clinical signs

- Inversion of the lower eyelid, which rolls inwards so the lid and eyelashes rub the surface of the cornea.
- Epiphora, blepharospasm and photophobia.

- Keratitis.
- Temporary blindness in advanced cases if bilateral.

Treatment

Most cases of entropion can be treated with simple, non-surgical techniques:

- 0.5 ml of liquid paraffin or long-acting penicillin is injected subcutaneously into the eyelid in a linear fashion parallel to the affected eyelid margin, using a 21 gauge needle. The initial bleb produces immediate reversal the eyelid, followed by a degree of fibrosis, which often prevents recurrence.
- The lower eyelid can also be everted with staples, Michel clips or skin sutures. Two vertical (inverting) mattress sutures are placed in the eyelid, using 3 metric non-absorbable material and a small cutting needle. The size of the bite depends on the degree of eversion required and the exact degree of eversion is controlled by drawing together the ends of the suture in the knot. The suture ends are cut short.

  Michel clips are thin metal strips, which are placed in the skin at right angles to the palpebral fissure and closed using special forceps, pulling the lower eyelid down and away from the corneal surface. The clips will fall off naturally in time and do not need removal.

- Superglue can be used to evert the eyelid – glue is applied down one side of a toothpick, then rolled down the lower lid on the hair away from the eye. The glue sticks to the hair better than to the toothpick and the eyelid is rolled into the proper position before the toothpick sticks to the hair.
- Surgical correction of the defect can be carried out simply using similar techniques to those used in the dog, removing a strip of skin from the lower eyelid as necessary.

Secondary bacterial infection may occur where chronic irritation of the cornea has been present for some time and should be treated with topical ophthalmic antibiotic ointments.

Additional pain relief with injectable NSAIDs may be required because of the concomitant keratitis.

Tumours of the eyelids

Reported tumours of the eyelids include *squamous cell carcinoma, fibroma, fibrosarcoma, melanoma and lymphoma.*

Tumours of the third eyelid are occasionally observed and include squamous cell carcinoma, adenocarcinoma and lymphoma. Excision is generally curative.

Exophthalmos

Protrusion of the eyeball may be due to a *retrobulbar abscess* or a *tumour*, such as lymphosarcoma or enzootic nasal tumour (see Chapter 17).

Ultrasonography can be used to examine the retrobulbar area and the contents of the orbit.

Photosensitisation

Photosensitisation (Chapter 11) from whatever cause will affect the head, resulting in swelling of unpigmented skin of the muzzle, drooping ears, swollen eyelids and ocular lesions, that is conjunctivitis, keratitis, excessive lacrimation, corneal oedema, blepharospasm and photophobia.

Affected animals should be removed from exposure to sunlight and any possible photosensitising substance.

Blindness

Blindness is an uncommon presenting sign in goats, usually in conjunction with other neurological signs (see Chapter 12) or severe keratoconjunctivitis. The following conditions should be considered in apparently blind goats:

- Keratoconjunctivitis.
- Cerebrocortical necrosis. Blindness is always present in advanced cases of polioencephalomalacia, so thiamine administration is indicated for every goat where there is blindness without any external visible defect in the visual system (amaurosis).
- Pregnancy toxaemia.
- Pituitary abscess syndrome.
- Cerebral abscess.
- Coenuris cerebralis (gid).
- Caprine arthritis encephalitis virus.
- Listeriosis.
- Poisoning:

  ○ Lead (not a prominent sign in goats).
  ○ Plant, for example rape, *Stypandra* spp. (Australia), *Astragulus* spp., *Helichrysum* spp. (South Africa).
  ○ Rafoxanide.
  ○ Closantel.
- Focal symmetrical encephalomalacia.
- Scrapie.
- Louping ill.

Cyclopia

In the western United States, the cyclops condition, that is birth with a single eye, is associated with the consumption of a toxin contained in *Veraturum californicum* (skunk cabbage) on day 14 of gestation. One day later, the eye fields have already divided to make two eyes and a cyclops can no longer be created. The condition may be associated with other deformities such as anophthalmia, hydrocephalus, shortening and absence of the maxillary and nasal bones and cebocephalus (monkey face).

Ultrasonography

Ultrasound is used primarily to assess internal structures of the globe, including assessment of intraoccular masses, particularly when direct visualisation is obscured by haemorrhage or infection, due to swollen eyelids or the prominence of the third eyelid, or corneal oedema. It can also be used to investigate extraocular neoplasms, such as squamous cell carcinomas and the causes of exophthalmos, such as abscess or tumour.

The internal structures of the eye and retrobulbar space can be evaluated by ultrasonography, either through the upper eyelid or directly through the cornea using a 7.5 to 13 MHz linear transducer. A transcorneal approach provides better images with fewer artifacts, but is less well tolerated by the animal. The transpalpebral approach is better tolerated, but is associated with more artifacts. If the ocular condition being investigated is unilateral, the normal eye can be examined for comparison. An examination glove filled with water can be used as a stand-off pad between the transducer and the eye.

Normal chamber fluid is hypoechoic and the posterior lens capsule and retina hyperechoic.

Table 20.1 Normal ophthalmic diagnostic test values.

Schirmer tear test	15.8 (10–30) mm/min	Adult Pygmy goat[a]
	13.8 (4–35) mm/min	Adult Saanen goat[b]
	18.0 (11–30) mm/min	Adult Angora goat[c]
Intraocular pressure	11.8 (9–14) mmHg (Tonovet d mode)	Adult Pygmy goat[a]
	7.9 (6–12) mmHg (Tonovet p mode)	Adult Saanen goat[b]
	10.8 (8–14) mmHg (Tonopen XL)	Adult Angora goat[c]
	9.79 (4–21) mmHg	
	13.9 (8–20) mmHg (Tonopen)	

Intraocular pressure and tear secretion values are lower in kids and increase until about 6 months of age in parallel with increases in the anterior chamber, lens, vitreous chamber and axial globe length.
[a]Broadwater, J. *et al.* (2007),
[b]Ribeiro, A. *et al.* (2008),
[c]Whelan, N. and Thompson, D. (2008).

Normal ophthalmic diagnostic test values

Normal ophthalmic diagnostic test values are shown in Table 20.1.

Further reading

Drugs

Whelan, N.C., Castillo-Alcala, F., Lizarraga, I. (2011) Efficacy of tropicamide, homatropine, cyclopentolate,atropine and hyoscine as mydriatics in Angora goats. *N. Z. Vet. J.*, **59** (6), 328–331.

General

Baxendell, S.A. (1984) Caprine ophthalmology. *Proc. Univ. Sydney Post Grad. Comm. Vet. Sci.*, **73**, 235–237.

Moore, C.P. and Whitley, R.D. (1984) Ophthalmic diseases of small domestic ruminants. *Vet. Clin. North Amer.: Large Anim. Pract.*, **6** (3), 641–665.

Wyman, M. (1983) Eye disease of sheep and goats. *Vet. Clin. North Amer.: Large Anim. Pract.*, **5** (3), 657–676.

Exophthalmos

Valentine, B.A. *et al.* (2011) Exophthalmos due to multicentric B-cell lymphoma in a goat. *Canadian Vet. J.*, **52**, 1350–1352.

Keratoconjunctivitis

Erdogan, H. M. (2010) Listerial Keratoconjunctivitis and Uveitis (Silage Eye). *Vet. Clin. North Amer.: Food Anim. Pract.*, **26** (3), 505–510.

Greig, A. (1990) Keratoconjunctivitis. *Goat Vet. Soc. J.*, **11** (1), 7–8.

Hosie, B.O. (1989) Infectious keratoconjunctivitis in sheep and goats. *Vet. Annual*, **29**, 93–7.

Wessles, M. E. *et al* (2010) *Yersinia pseudotuberculosis* as a cause of ocular disease in goats. *Vet. Rec.*, **166**, 699–700.

Mycoplasma

Jones, G.E. (1983) Mycoplasma of sheep and goats. *Vet. Rec.*, **113**, 619–20.

MacOwan, K.J. (1984) Mycoplasmoses of sheep and goats. *Goat Vet. Soc. J.*, **5** (2), 21–4.

Ophthalmic examination and diagnostic test values

Broadwater, J. J. Schorling, J.J., Herring, I. P., Pickett, J.P. (2007) Ophthalmic examination findings in adult pygmy goats. *(Capra hicus) Vet. Ophthalmol.*, **10** (5), 269–73.

Isler, C.T., Altug, M.E. and Kilic, S. (2013) Evaluation of tear fluid secretion and intraocular pressure in normal Merino sheep and Saanen goats. *Revue Med. Vet.*, **164** (5), 278–282.

Piso, D.Y.T., Padua, I.R.M. *et al* (2010) Intraocular pressure and tear secretion in Saanen goats with different ages. *Pesq. Vet. Bras.*, **30** (9), 798–802.

Ribeiro, A.P. *et al*, 2008 Ocular biometry in a colony of Saanen goats with different ages (Abstract) Annual Meeting of the American College of Veterinarian Ophthalmologists, Boston, DC, USA. *Vet. Ophthalmol.*, **11** (6), 419.

Townsend, W/M. (2010) Examination Techniques and Therapeutic Regimens for the Ruminant and Camelid Eye. *Vet. Clin. North Amer.: Food Anim. Pract.*, **26** (3), 437- 458.

Whelan, N. C., & Thompson, D. (2008) Normal ophthalmic diagnostic test values in Angora goats (Abstract) Annual Meeting of the American College of Veterinarian Ophthalmologists, Boston, DC, USA. *Vet. Ophthalmol.*, **11** (6), 419.

Reflexes

Raoofi, A., Mirfakhraie, P & Yourdkhani, S. (2011) The development of the pupillary light reflex and menace response in neonatal lambs and kids. *Vet. J.*, **187**, 411–412.

Surgery

Dun, K. (2009) Practice Tip: Treatment of entropion in newborn lambs. *Livestock*, **14** (1), 4142.

Donnelly, K.S., Pearce, J.W., Guiliano, E.A *et al* (2014) Surgical correction of congenital entropion in related Boer kids using a combination Hotz-Celsus and lateral eyelid wedge resection procedure. *Vet. Ophthalmol.*, **17** (6), 443–7.

Shaw-Edwards, R. (2010) Surgical Treatment of the Eye in Farm Animals. *Vet. Clin. North Amer.: Food Anim. Pract.*, **26** (3), 459–476.

Tumours

Ahmed, A.F. and Hassanein, K.M.A. (2012) Ovine and caprine cutaneous and ocular neoplasms. *Small Ruminant Research*, **106** (2), 189–200.

Ultrasonography

Hallowell, G. and Potter, T. (2010) Practical guide to ocular ultrasonography in horses and farm animals. *In Pract.*, **32**, 90–96.

Riberiro, A.P., Silva, M.L., Rosa, J.P. *et al.* (2009) Ultrasonographic and echobiometric findings in the eyes of Saanen goats of different ages. *Vet. Ophthalmol.*, **12** (5), 313–317.

CHAPTER 21

Plant poisoning

> Goats frequently consume small amounts of potentially harmful plants with no apparent ill effect.
> *'The dose makes the poison' – Paracelsus*

Many plants worldwide are potentially toxic to animals. Australia alone has about 1000 species of poisonous plants and approximately 10% of these produce cyanide. Goats, being of an inquisitive nature and of browsing habit, coupled with a tolerance of bitter or high tannin material, commonly consume small quantities of poisonous plants without ill effect, particularly when the rumen is full of other foodstuffs, and there are very few well documented cases of plant poisoning occurring in Britain, where most goats are kept in well defined and limited areas.

Poisonous plants may be pasture species, native or naturalised species or garden plants. In Britain, most cases of poisoning are caused by garden shrubs, in particular rhododendrons, azaleas and laurels. *It seems safest to assume that all evergreen shrubs are poisonous and to keep goats and such plants well separated with adequate fencing.*

Many plants are listed in goat publications as being poisonous, but there are equally as many reports of goats eating 'poisonous' plants without harm. *The goat is poisoned only when it consumes too much of the plant, too quickly and when conditions are right for the plant to be poisonous.* Some of the plants listed, for instance walnut, are generally safe when eaten in small amounts, but large quantities should not be given to stall-fed goats. Ivy is regularly fed to sick goats in winter when no other fresh green fodder is available and, because of their binding properties, oak leaves are used by goatkeepers as a treatment for diarrhoea.

Several ornamental plants grown outdoors or indoors are highly toxic. For example, goats should not have access to, or be fed, oleander (*Nerium oleander*), lily-of-the-valley (*Convallaria majalis*), larkspur (*Delphinium* spp.), or bulbs and their leaves, such as daffodil, tulip, aconite and anemone. Oleander and larkspur are established as range plants in parts of North America.

Many woodland and hedgerow plants, including buttercup (*Ranunculus* spp.), lesser celandine (*Ranunculus ficaria*), deadly nightshade (*Atropa belladonna*), bryony (*Bryonia* spp.), woody nightshade or bittersweet (*Solanum dulcamara*), old man's beard or traveller's joy (*Clematis vitalba*), wild mustard or charlock (*Sinapis arvensis*), fool's parsley (*Aethusa cynapium*) and spindle berry (*Euonymus europaeus*) are potentially toxic, at least under certain circumstances. Honeysuckle (*Lonicera* spp.) is readily eaten by goats, but the berries are poisonous.

There may be a difference in toxicity levels between different varieties of plants growing in different climates or soils. *Sambucus nigra*, the European variety of elderberry, is less toxic than the American variety *Sambucus canadensis* and *Sambucus racemosa* (red elderberry). *Sambucus nigra* has been used for centuries in a wide range of medicinal and culinary products.

Garden by-products, which are potentially poisonous when fed to excess, are commonly fed to goats. These include forage brassicas – turnip, swede, Brussel sprouts, cauliflower and cabbage – which have been variously implicated in nitrate poisoning, goitre, anaemia, photosensitisation and ruminal stasis, at least in cattle and sheep, if seldom in goats.

Goats are regularly utilised as effective environmentally friendly *biocontrol agents* to reduce weed populations to economically acceptable levels in pas-

Diseases of the Goat, Fourth Edition. John Matthews.
© 2016 John Wiley & Sons, Ltd. Published 2016 by John Wiley & Sons, Ltd.

tures, abandoned farmland and rangeland, removing brush and undergrowth of invasive species, weeds and dead plant material, so allowing the natural grasses and woodlands to recover. Goats typically consume a diet of 65–70% browse, 20–25% grasses and 5% other herbaceous flowering plants. Because goats consume a large number of different plant species within the day, they have fewer problems than sheep or cattle with plant toxicity. Goats can improve rangeland and reduce the risk of cattle being poisoned by grazing toxic plants. Shrubs controlled by goats include gorse (*Ulex eurpeaus*) and broom (*Cystisus scoparius*) and they will feed on some herbaceous weeds avoided by other livestock, such as the various varieties of thistle – Scottish (*Cirsium vulgare*), Californian (*Cirsum arvense*) and variegated (*Silybum marianum*) – and docks (*Rumex* spp.) Many of the weeds targeted and eaten, like bracken (*Pteridium aquilinum*), poison oak (*Toxicodendron* spp.) and variegated thistle, are listed as poisonous.

Potentially poisonous plants can be found in most areas likely to be grazed by goats. *Where goats are extensively grazed, the veterinary surgeon and the goat-keeper should become acquainted with the poisonous plants local to that area*, learning to identify these plants at all stages of growth, *and the conditions in which grazing is safe or potentially dangerous*. The same plant may provide useful forage or be toxic under different conditions of management or season. Usually only a small number of species of poisonous plants will be responsible for losses in a particular geographical area and losses will only occur under specific grazing conditions. *Herd health plans should include recommendations to perform routine examinations of pastures for potentially toxic plant species, as well as suitable control measures*. Most poisonous weeds and cultivated plants can be controlled. Grazing programmes should be planned, so areas where poisonous plants exist can be used when the plants are least toxic. Fencing can be used to prevent access to particularly hazardous areas. Overgrazing should be avoided.

Toxic plants can also be conserved in hay and it is important that both the producers and purchasers of hay are able to recognise potentially poisonous plants. Careful inspection of hay is important and contaminated hay should be discarded. In Britain, ragwort (*Senecio jacobea*), which contains pyrrolizidine alkaloids, can be a particular problem and in parts of North America plants that are nitrate accumulators or contain pyrrolizidine alkaloids or cardiac glycosides like oleander (*Nerium oleander*) can be found in alfalfa hay. Although there is some degradation in silage, the pyrrolizidine alkaloid level in hay remains constant for months.

> The major reason for plant poisoning in free-range goats is starvation.

Is it plant poisoning?

Plant identification is essential to confirm poisoning. However, although the presence of a plant in the environment, together with evidence that it has been eaten, might suggest poisoning, the presence of a plant alone is not diagnostic and other possible risk factors such as lack of other feed, together with relevant clinical signs, should be considered.

The rumen provides a significant protection from plant poisons for the goat compared to monogastric animals. Moderate levels of oxalates, as found in sugarbeet tops or rhubarb, can be metabolised in the rumen, and glycosidic steroidal alkaloids, as found in solanaceous plants such as green potatoes and tomatoes, can be safely hydrolysed. Mature goats are less susceptible than sheep and cattle to the effects of some toxins, including hypericum in St John's wort and tannins in acorns, and are also more discriminatory in selecting feed. Further, the browsing habit of the goat means that some pastures are safer for goats than for sheep or cattle.

To prevent poisoning, it is important to understand the factors that convert valuable forage into a poisonous plant. Many factors influence whether eating a potentially poisonous plant is dangerous:

- Goats grazing a particular area for extended periods may become accustomed to eating small amounts of toxic plant material. Goats often adjust to specific plant communities, minimising plant poisoning. New animals introduced to the area may be poisoned, because of lack of acclimatisation and curiosity as they browse the new area. Curiosity may kill the goat as well as the cat.
- Most poisonous plants are unpalatable and animals will not consume them if adequate alternative forage is available. Hungry or thirsty animals should never

be grazed on areas heavily infested with poisonous plants. A well fed animal with a full rumen is less likely to be poisoned than a hungry animal. Goats are very discriminatory and will generally reject unpalatable plants, but hungry animals may eat plants that are not very palatable. Animals are often poisoned because hunger or other conditions cause them to graze abnormally. Overgrazing should always be avoided.

- Palatability may be increased by herbicide treatment or forage conservation.
- The various parts of a plant vary in their toxicity. Only certain parts of a plant, such as the root or the leaves, may be toxic. Farm operations, such as ditching, may expose the dangerous part.
- Previously safe pasture or rangeland can become dangerous when toxins accumulate in certain plants or plants become more palatable. The relative toxicity of plants may vary because of:
  o The season and the stage of plant growth. Early spring can be dangerous as a particular poisonous plant may represent a disproportionately high percentage of the pasture and, during dry summer months, lack of alternative grazing may lead animals to eat plants usually avoided. The amount of toxin may also vary with stages of growth.
  o Growth in particular soil types.
  o Stressful growth conditions, such as drought, insect attack or the effects of frost.
  o Wilting in dry conditions, or conversely rapid growth after rain.
  o Concentration of toxins, such as nitrates, during drought conditions.
  o Rapid growth after fertiliser treatment. Fertiliser treatment can also promote the accumulation of nitrates.
- Some plants are equally toxic when fresh or when fed dry in hay, for example ragwort.
- Some plants are harmless when fresh, but poisonous when dry and wilted, for example leaves of the *Prunus* family.
- The age of the animal may also (but not always) be important, with young animals often more susceptible than older ones.
- Many plants cause an *immediate poisoning*, e.g. yew (*Taxus baccata*), *Rhododendron* species, but some plants cause *delayed poisoning* as well as immediate, for example ragwort (*Senecio jacobaea*) and St John's wort (*Hypericum perforatum*).

If plant poisoning is suspected

To diagnose any plant poisoning, a detailed history of all events leading up to the time when the animals were found affected and a careful description of the clinical signs noticed are essential.

Obtain a detailed grazing history

This should be obtained for the goat(s) immediately before the incident, or, where applicable in extensively grazed animals, in the weeks before the incident, including any feed or pasture changes.

- Carefully observe where the goats have been grazing and attempt to identify any unusual or toxic plants. *Identification of the plant* is important, whatever its stage of growth. Sometimes plant material can be removed from the goat's mouth or it can be found in the rumen contents of a dead animal.
- If the suspect plant cannot be identified, collect as much of the whole plant as possible, including leaves, flowers, stem, roots and fruit. Parts of the plant can be preserved by drying and pressing in a rolled-up newspaper or magazine.
- Try to identify the plant by using the links below or by contacting a local reference centre.
- Consider the weather conditions leading up to the incident (drought, rainfall, snow, season) and the effect on forage growth and forage availability.
- *Obtain a description of the course and progression of the clinical disease so far*, including unusual behaviour, lesions, morbidity and mortality and carefully examine any remaining animals.

Eliminate other possibilities

- Consider breed, sex, ages and number of animals involved, body condition, vaccination status, known trace mineral deficiencies in the area and trace mineral supplementation, other routine treatments such as deworming. Mineral deficiencies may cause animals to develop cravings and eat plants they would normally refuse.
- Look for other potential sources of poisoning, such as old batteries, lead paint and contaminated feed or water.

Further investigation

- *Metabolic profiles* are useful for some toxicities, but blood tests are usually of little value in identifying specific plant toxins and chemical analysis of rumen contents to identify toxins is generally not practical or cost-effective.

- Any dead animal should be submitted to a veterinary diagnostic laboratory for *post-mortem examination* or a post-mortem examination carried out in the field, noting the condition of the animal and any obvious lesions, examining the mouth, rumen and gastrointestinal tract and their contents.
- Suitable samples for histologic examination (brain, lung, heart, liver, spleen, digestive tract, kidney, skeletal muscle and any gross lesions) should be fixed in 10% neutral buffered formalin.
- Tissues for chemical or microscopic studies should be stored in plastic bags and frozen (rumen and gastrointestinal contents, whole eye, liver, kidney, body fat, serum, whole blood, bone, urine, and milk if lactating).
- Where appropriate, feed and water samples should be collected and sent to the laboratory as soon as possible, freezing the sample if it has a long distance to travel.

A tentative diagnosis may be possible if the following information is available:

- The goat's grazing history is compatible with ingestion of a poisonous plant.
- The clinical signs seen match those for a known poisonous plant in the grazing area.
- A change of management may have caused an animal to change its diet or grazing habits.
- A change in environmental conditions (drought, rainfall, season) may have increased the toxicity of the plant, or increased the likelihood of the goats eating the plant, such as lack of alternative forage.
- Local soil conditions, including mineral deficiencies or excess, may have altered plant toxicities.

Finding information on poisonous plants

Many potentially poisonous plants occur worldwide; other plants are restricted to specific countries or localities within these countries. Plants may be garden or household plants in one country, but a widespread range plant in another. The following links provide information on plants that cause poisoning in farm and pet animals, including native, introduced and cultivated outdoor plants as well as indoor plants. Most of them have searchable databases and are well illustrated to help with the identification of plant species.

Australia
Rural Industries Research and Development Corporation The palatability, and potential toxicity, of Australian weeds to goats https://rirdc.infoservices.com.au/items/00-139

Canada
Canadian Poisonous Plants Information System http://www.cbif.gc.ca/eng/species-bank/canadian-poisonous-plants-information-system/?id=1370403265036

New Zealand
New Zealand Plant Conservation Network http://www.nzpcn.org.nz/page.aspx?flora_vascular_poisonous_plants

South Africa
University of Pretoria Poisonous Plants of South Africa http://www.ais.up.ac.za/vet/poison/bnames.htm

United Kingdom
Royal Horticultural Society Potentially harmful garden plants https://www.rhs.org.uk/advice/profile?pid=524

The Smallholder Series

Plant Poisons on the Farm http://www.smallholderseries.co.uk/index.php?option=com_content&view=article&id=181:poisonous-plants17&catid=89:gardening&Itemid=193

Royal Botanic Gardens Kew http://www.kew.org/science/ecbot/poisonous-plants.html

Telephone 44 (0)20 8332 5000 (weekday office hours)

Natural History Museum http://nhm.ac.uk/nature-online/british-natural-history/uk-biodiversity-portal/identification-information/index.html

United States
Cornell University http://www.ansci.cornell.edu/plants/index.html

FDA Poisonous Plant Database http://www.accessdata.fda.gov/scripts/plantox/Provides access to references in the scientific literature (primarily print literature through about 2007), describing studies and reports of the toxic properties and effects of plants and plant parts.

University of Illinois, Plants Poisonous to Animals http://www.library.illinois.edu/vex/toxic/

University of Pennsylvania School of Veterinary Medicine Poisonous Plants Directory http://research.vet .upenn.edu/Home/tabid/5034/Default.aspx

General

Pyrrolizidine Alkaloid - Containing Toxic Plants (Senecio, Crotalaria, Cynoglossum, Amsinckia, Heliotropium and Echium spp.) digitalcommons.unl.edu/ cgi/viewcontent.cgi?article=1882&context

Clinical signs of plant poisoning

Table 21.1 lists clinical signs that have been attributed to plant poisoning.

Plants affecting milk

A variety of ingested plant compounds and their metabolites, once absorbed into the blood, are secreted by the mammary gland into the milk (Table 21.2). There are toxins that cause changes in milk flavour (Table 21.3) and may pose a hazard to animals and people drinking the milk. Milk taints are discussed in Chapter 13. The excretion in milk of toxins from poisonous plants is unlikely in the United Kingdom, at least at high enough levels to provide a human health hazard. The quantities of toxins are generally very low because most of the toxins are more readily excreted through the liver and kidneys. However, the possibility of toxins in milk affecting humans should always be considered, particularly as milk from an individual goat may be consumed by a limited number of people over a long period.

Certain plant toxins, for example bracken toxins, are carcinogens and *pyrrolizidine alkaloids*, known to be excreted in goats' milk, may be carcinogenic and cause chronic liver disease. *Quinolizidine* and *piperidine alkaloids* are capable of causing congenital defects in the fetus. Thyroid gland enlargement (goitre) may occur in young animals and human babies drinking the milk of animals that have eaten plants containing *glucosinolates*, which are hydrolysed to compounds that have an antithyroid hormone effect. Mycotoxins, such as aflatoxin M1, have been demonstrated experimentally to be excreted in milk. Tremetol is excreted in milk

and causes a syndrome called milk sickness in humans drinking the milk.

Table 21.4 lists plants that may produce a reduction in milk yield. Many of these plants may also have far more serious affects, particularly if consumed over a long period of time.

Treatment of plant poisoning

Advice to owners

- Separate the goat from the plant. It may be possible to actually remove the plant material from the goat's mouth.
- Keep the goat walking slowly, so that it does not settle and start cudding.
- Give large quantities of strong tea (do not attempt to dose a vomiting animal).

  The tannic acid in the tea will precipitate many alkaloids and salts of heavy metals and will also have a useful stimulant effect. Strong coffee will also have a stimulant effect.

Note: poisoning by acorns is due to their high tannic acid content. Tea should not be given in cases of acorn poisoning.

- Large doses (500 ml) of liquid paraffin are also commonly used as a first-aid remedy.
- Treat shock.
- Give demulcents, for example a mixture of eggs, sugar and milk, to soothe and relieve irritation of the stomach linings.
- Charcoal, 2–9 g/kg orally in a water slurry, may be beneficial with some poisonings, such as rhododendron and oxalate.
- If possible, identify the source of poisoning. Where animals are grazed extensively, either remove all the animals from danger or fence off the suspect area.
- Improve the nutritional status of the remaining animals where necessary by providing good quality roughage.

Veterinary treatment

- In most cases there is no specific antidote to the toxic principle involved in the poisoning, and first aid should be continued together with symptomatic, supportive treatment, for example spasmolytics, intravenous fluids, oral laxatives, B vitamins and antibiotics if there is a danger of inhaling vomit.

Table 21.1 Clinical signs of plant poisoning.

Anaemia	Rape (*Brassica napus*), turnip rape (*Brassica campestris*), kale (*Brassica oleracea*), cabbage, Brussels sprouts (*Brassica oleracea*), swede tops (*Brassica napus*)
Cardiotoxicity	**Cardiac glycosides containing plants**: foxglove (*Digitalis purpurea*), lily-of-the-valley (*Convallaria majalis*), oleander (*Nerium oleander*), *Helleborus* spp., spindle (*Euonymus europaeus*), Indian hemp or dogbane (*Apocynum* spp.) and milkweed and red cotton (*Asclepias* spp.) Crassulaceae (such as the genera Tylecodon, Cotyledon and Adromischus) and some *Kalanchoe* spp., chinkerinchee (*Ornithogalum toxicarium*), pig's ear or round-leafed navel-wort (*Cotyledon orbiculata*)
	Yew (*Taxus baccata, Taxus cuspidata*), Jimsonweed or thornapple (*Datura stramonium*), false hellebore (*Veratum* spp.), avocado (*Persea americana*), gifblaar or poison leaf (*Dichapetalum cymosum*)
	Grayanotoxin containing plants: rhododendron and azaleas (*Rhododendron* spp.), pieris (*Pieris* spp.), and laurels (*Kalmia* spp.).
Constipation	Oak (acorns and old leaves) (*Quercus* spp.), ragwort (*Senecio jacobaea*), linseed (*Linum usitatissimum*), lantana (*Lantana camara*)
Diarrhoea	Hemlock (*Conium maculatum*), oak (*young* leaves) (*Quercus* spp.), cuckoo pint or wild arum (*Arum maculatum*), castor seed (in foodstuffs), foxglove (*Digitalis purpurea*), water dropwort (*Oenanthe crocata*), box (*Buxus sempervirens*), potato (green) (*Solanum tuberosum*), rhododendron spp, linseed (*Linum usitatissimum*), oleander (*Nerium oleander*), lantana (*Lantana camara*), blue-green algae, freshly harvested mangel and beet roots (*Beta vulgaris*), corn cockle (*Agrostemma githago*), soapwort (*Saponaria officinalis*), cow cockle (*Saponaria vaccaria*), broomweed (*Gutierrezia sarothrae*) charlock (*Sinapsis arvensis*) and wild radish (*Raphanus raphanistrum*)
Discoloured Urine	**Haematuria:** bracken (*Pteridium aquilinum*), oak
	Haemaglobinuria: rape (*Brassica napus*), kale, cabbage, Brussels sprouts (*Brassica oleracea*)
Frothy bloat	Legumes, e.g. rapidly growing lucerne
Goitre and stillbirth	Brassica spp., linseed *(Linum usitatissimum),* some clovers
Haemorrhage	Bracken (*Pteridium aquilinum*)
Hepatotoxicity	**Pyrrolizidine alkaloid poisoning:** *Compositae* family – ragwort (*Senecio jacobaea*), common groundsel (*S. vulgaris*), Riddell's groundsel *(S. riddelli)* and threadleaf groundsel (*S. fiaccidus*)
	Boraginaceae family - hound's tongue (*Cynoglossum officinale, Cynoglossum cinale*), European heliotrope (*Heliotropium europaeum*), Paterson's Curse or salvation Jane (*Echium lycopis; Echium plantagineum*), rattleweed (*Crotalaria retusa*), comfrey (*Symphytum* spp.)
	Photosensitisation: see below
	Other: Sacahuista or beargrass (Nolina texana), kraalbos (*Galenia africana*), lechuguilla (*Agave lecheguilla*), mycotoxins (aflatoxin, B, rubratoxin B, ochratoxin A), some fungi (*Amanita* spp. and *Galerina* spp.)
Nephrotoxicity	**Oxalate-containing plants**: sugar beet tops and mangold tops (*Beta vulgaris*), rhubarb leaves (*Rheum rhabarbarum*), docks (*Rumex* spp.), wood sorrel and soursob (*Oxalis* spp.), halogeton (*Halogeton glomeratus*), greasewood (*Sarcobatus vermiculatus*), elephant grass (*Panicum* spp.), lambsquarter, goosefoot and fat hen (*Chenopodium* spp.), Russian thistle **(***Salsola tragus),* common purslane or pigweed (*Portulaca oleracea*), bassia (*Bassia hyssopifolia*), Palmer amaranth or Palmer's pigweed (*Amaranthus palmeri*) and pigweed amaranth or common tumbleweed (*Amaranthus retroflexus*), acorns + oak *(Quercus spp)*, sacahuista or beargrass (Nolina texana), some fungi (*Drechslera campanulata; Aspergillus flavus*)
	Calcinogenic plants: Solanaceae family, including *Solanum malacoxylon, Solanum torvum* and *Cestrum diurnum*; yellow/golden oat grass (*Trisetum flavescens*)
Nervous signs	Ragwort (*Senecio jacobaea*), horsetails (*Equisetum* spp.), hemlock (*Conium maculatum*), water dropwort (*Oenanthe crocata*), potato (*Solanum tuberosum*), black nightshade (*Solanum nigrum*), male fern (Dryopteris spp.), rhododendron spp., laburnum (*Laburnum anagyroides*), rape (*Brassica napus*), rhubarb (*Rheum rhaponticum*), common sorrel (*Rumex acetosa*), sugar beet tops (*Beta vulgaris*), *Prunus* family, blue-green algae, fool's parsley (*Aethusa cynapium*), milkweeds (*Asclepia* spp.), cycad poisoning (*Cycas* spp., *Bowenia* spp., *Macrozamia* spp., *Zamia* spp.), caltrop (*Tribulus terrestris*), locoweeds, Oxytropis spp., Astragalus spp., Swainsona spp., *Ipomoea* spp., *Turbina* spp. and *Sida* spp., rayless goldenrod or jimmyweed (*Isocoma pluriflora*), white snakeroot (*Ageratina altissima*)

Table 21.1 (*continued*)

Oestrus	Some clovers (*Trifolium* spp.)
Photosensitisation	**Primary**: St John's wort (*Hypericum perforatum*), Buckwheat (*Fagopyrum esculentum*), Giant hogweed (*Heracleum mantegazzianum*), rape (*Brassica napus*), clovers (*Trifolium* spp.), St Anne's lace (*Ammi majus*), Dutchman's breeches (*Thamnosma texana*), spring parsley (*Cymopterus* spp.) **Secondary (hepatogenous)**: Bog asphodel (*Narthecium ossifragum*), pyrrolizidine alkaloid toxicosis? (from *Senecio* spp., *Crotolaria* spp. and *Heliotropium* spp.), mycotoxins, white and Alsike clover (*Trifolium* spp.), bitter (bitterkarroo) bush *Chrysocoma ciliata* (*C. tenuifolia*), kleingrass (*Panicum* spp.), caltrop (puncture vine, yellow vine or goathead) (*Tribulus terrestris*), lechuguilla (*Agave lecheguilla*), *Lantana* spp., sacahuista or beargrass (*Nolina texana*), boobialla tree, Ellangowan poison bush, ngaio (*Mycoporum* spp.), blue-green algae
Respiratory signs (acute)	**Cyanogenic plants**: *Prunus* family - cherry trees, cherry laurel (*Prunus laurocerasus*) peach (*Prunus persica*), plum (*Prunus domestica*), black cherry (*Prunus serotina*), choke cherry (*Prunus virginiana*), crab apple (*Malus sylvestris*), marsh arrow grasses (*Triglochin maritima* and *T. palustris*), gum trees (*Eucalyptus* spp.), bracken fern (*Pteridium aquillinum*), linseeds and flaxes (*Linum* spp.), corn (*Zea mays*), hydrangias (*Hydrangia* spp.), California holly (*Heteromeles arbutifolia*), poison suckleya (*Suckley suckleyana*), oleander (*Nerium oleander)*, cassava (*Mannihot esculentum*), Sudan grass; Johnson grass, sorghum or durra (*Sorghum* spp.) **Plants containing excess nitrites/nitrates**: mangels, fodder beet, sugar beet (*Beta vulgaris*), turnips (*Brassica campestris*), swedes (*Brassica napus* var. *naprobrassica*), kale (*Brassica oleracea*) and rape (*Brassica napus, Brassica campestris*), corn and oat silages, sorghums (Sudan grass, Johnson grass), oats (*Avena sativa*), silage, rye (*Secale cereale*), wheat (*Triticum vulgare*), alfalfa/lucerne (*Medicago sativa*), maize/corn (*Zea mays*) and white clover (*Trifolium refens*), pigweed (*Amaranthus palmeri*), variegated thistle (*Silybum marianum*), *Chenopodium* spp. (lambsquarters, goosefoot), oatgrass (*Arrhenatherum* spp.), Canada thistle (*Cirsium arvense*), jimsonweed (*Datura stramonium*), cockspur, barnyard grass (*Echinochloa crusgalli*), silverleaf povertyweed (*Ambrosia tomentosa*), ragweed, bursage (*Ambrosia* spp.), wild sunflower (*Helianthus* spp.), fireweed (USA), rosebay willowherb (UK), great willowherb (Canada) (*Chamerion angustifolium*), sweet clover (*Melilotus* spp.), smartweed (*Persicaria* spp.), Russian thistle (*Salsola tragus*) **Cardiotoxic plants**: see above Mouldy sweet potatoes (Ipomoea batatus), purple or perilla mint (Perilla frutescens, P. maculatta), blue-green algae, fool's parsley (*Aethusa cynapium*)
Stomatitis	Giant hogweed (*Heracleum mantegazzianum*), cuckoo pint or wild arum (*Arum maculatum*)
Sudden death	Yew (*Taxus baccata*), laurels (*Kalmia* spp.), linseed (*Linum usitatissimum*), foxglove (*Digitalis purpurea*), oleander (*Nerium oleander*), water dropwort (*Oenanthe crocata*), blue-green algae
Vomiting	Rhododendron (*Rhododendron species*), azalea, pieris (*Pieris japonica*), black nightshade (*Solanum nigrum*), gladiolus spp. corms

- Administration of activated charcoal, 2–9 g/kg in a water slurry given orally (1 g charcoal/5 ml), will help adsorb toxins by surface binding, protecting the ruminoreticular mucosa from further injury, but is less effective than in monogastric animals.
- Rumenotomy should be considered to remove plant material, particularly if this can be done before clinical signs of poisoning have developed.
- Specific antidotes, such as methylene blue, are available to treat some poisonings (see under individual plants), but these may not be authorised for use in food-producing animals.

- Treatment of nervous disease depends on clinical signs:
  - If cholinergic signs predominate, that is salivation, diarrhoea: Atropine sulphate 80–160 micrograms/kg s.c.
  - If anticholinergic signs predominate, that is dilated pupils, gastrointestinal tract stasis: Physostigmine 10–30 mg s.c., 0.01–0.02 mg/kg
  - Convulsions can be controlled with diazepam. The dose depends on the degree of CNS depression required and each animal should be treated according to response.

Table 21.2 Plant toxins excreted through milk.

Pyrrolizidine alkaloids		Glucosinolates	
Senecio spp.	Ragwort, groundsel	Amoacia	Horseradish
Crotalaria	Rattleweed	Brassica	Cabbage, broccoli, etc.
Heliotropium	European helioptrope	Nasturtium	Watercress
Echium	Salvation Jane Paterson's curse	Raphanus	Radish
Symphytum Cynoglossum	Comfrey	Limnanthes	Meadowfoam
Amsinckia	Hound's tongue	Thlaspi	Stinkweed
Festuca	Fiddlenecks		
	Tall fescue		
Piperidine alkaloids		**Mycotoxins**	
Conium	Hemlock	Legumes	Slaframine
Nicotiana spp.	Tobacco		
Unknown toxin		**Quinolizidine alkaloids**	
Chrysocoma ciliate	Bitter bush	Lupinus	Lupins
Tremetol		**Colchicine/colchiceine alkaloids**	
Ageratina altissima	White snakeroot Rayless	Colchicum autumnale	Autumn crocus
Haplopappus spp.	goldenrod		
		Selenium	
		Astragalus, Oonopsis, Stanleya, Xylorrhiza, Aster, Atriplex, Sideranthus, Machaeranthera	

Table 21.3 Plants that can taint milk.

Achillea millefolium	Yarrow	Matricaria recutita	Scented mayweed
Aethusa cynapium	Fool's parsley	Melilotus spp.	Sweet clover
Arctium minus	Common burdock	Mentha spp.	Mint, penny royal
Allium spp.	Onion and garlic	Narthecium ossifragum	Bog asphodel
Ambrosia spp.	Ragweed	Nasturtium officinale	Watercress
Anthemis cotula	Stinking chamomile	Oxalis spp.	Wood sorrel
Arctotheca calendula	Capeweed	Pinguicula vulgaris	Butterwort
Beta vulgaris	Beet	Pissum spp.	Pea
Brassica campestris	Turnip	Polygonum aviculare	Knotgrass, wireweed
Brassica oleracea	Kale	Pteridium aquilinum	Bracken
Caltha palustris	Kingcup, marsh marigold	Quercus spp.	Oak
Capsella bursa-pastoris	Shepherd's purse	Ranunculus spp.	Buttercup, marsh marigold, etc.
Compositae spp.	Various	Raphanus raphanistrum	Radish
Conium maculatum	Hemlock	Rhamnus spp.	Buckthorn
Coronopus	Cress	Rumex spp.	Docks
Daucus carota	Queen Anne's lace, wild carrot	Senecio madagascariensis	Fireweed
Equisetum spp.	Horsetail	Sium latifolium	Water parsnip
Foeniculum vulgare	Fennel	Silaum silaus	Pepper saxifrage
Hedera helix	Ivy	Solanum tuberosum	Potato (green)
Helenium spp)	Bitterweed, sneezeweed	Sisymbrium officinale	Hedge mustard
Hyoscyamus niger	Henbane	Tanacetum vulgare	Tansy
Lactuca virosa	Wild lettuce	Taxus baccata	Yew
Lepidium hyssopifolium	Pepperwort	Thlaspi arvense	Penny cress
Lotus corniculatus	Birdsfoot trefoil	Xanthium strumarium	Cocklebur
Laburnum anagyroides	Laburnum		
Leucanthemum vulgare	Ox-eye daisy		

Table 21.4 Plants affecting milk causing a reduction in milk yield.

Aconitum napellus	Monkshood	Hypericum perforatum	St John's wort
Allium spp.	Onion and garlic	Laburnum anagyroides	Laburnum
Beta vulgaris	Beet	Mercularis spp.	Mercury
Bryonia dioica	White bryony	Papaver spp.	mycotoxins
Chenopodium album	Fat hen	Pteridium aquilinum	Poppy
Cicuta virosa	Cowbane	Quercus spp.	Bracken
Claviceps purpurea	Ergot	Ranunculus spp	Oak
Colchium autumnale	Meadow saffron	Raphanus raphanistrum	Buttercup
Conium maculatum	Hemlock	Rhododendron ponticum	Radish
Crataegus monogyna	Hawthorn	Rhamnus spp.	Rhododendron
Cupressus spp.	Cypress	Ricinus communis	Buckthorn
Cynoglossum officinale	Hound's tongue	Rumex spp.	Castor oil plant
Endymion non scriptus	Bluebell	Scrophularia aquatic	Sorrel
Equisetum spp.	Horsetail	Solanum tuberosum	Water Betony
Frangula alnus	Alder	Taxus baccata	Potato (green)
Fraxinus excelsior	Ash	Trifolium spp.	Yew
Hedera helix	Ivy		Clover
Hyoscyamus niger	Henbane		

Specific plant poisoning

Cardiotoxic plants

> Gastrointestinal helminthiasis and liver fluke disease may also present with signs suggesting congestive cardiac failure.

Plants containing cardiac glycosides

Plants containing cardiac glycosides include foxglove (*Digitalis purpurea*), lily-of-the-valley (*Convallaria majalis*), oleander (*Nerium oleander*), *Helleborus* spp., Spindle (*Euonymus europaeus*), Indian hemp or dogbane (*Apocynum* spp.) and milkweed and red cotton (*Asclepias* spp.). They grow all over the world and can be found as ornamental plants, woodland plants, or in scrubland and hedges. The widest variety grows in southern Africa, where poisoning with cardiac glycoside-containing plants is collectively the most important plant-associated poisoning of livestock.

Asclepias spp. are established in the natural grasslands of North America and have become naturalised in parts of Australia. Those species with narrow, grass-like leaves

are the most poisonous. Oleanders are cultivated widely in the southern United States.

The many cardiotoxic plants of South Africa include Crassulaceae (such as the genera Tylecodon, Cotyledon and Adromischus) and some *Kalanchoe* species, which contain bufadienolide cardiac glycosides. This is a particular problem in the native range of many *Kalanchoe* species in the Karoo region of South Africa, where the resulting animal disease is known as krimpsiekte (shrinking disease) or as cotyledonosis. Chinkerinchee (*Ornithogalum toxicarium*) has also been implicated in this disease.

Similar poisonings have occurred in Australia and pig's ear or round-leafed navel-wort (*Cotyledon orbiculata*) is now naturalised in New Zealand.

The plants are generally unpalatable and goats appear to be relatively resistant to poisoning compared with other ruminants.

Aetilogy

- Toxic principles are cardiac glycosides, such as oleandrin and digitoxin. The concentrations of glycosides within the plants vary with the stage of growth and season. The toxins inhibit the cellular membrane sodium/potassium ATPase pump, thereby causing electrolyte disturbances that affect electrical conductivity of the heart.

- The toxins are widely distributed throughout the body, including the fetus and milk.
- All parts of the plants, whether fresh or dry, should be considered poisonous and poisoning is often associated with dried leaves after trimming. Plants are most toxic during rapid growth.
- Glycosides and resinoids in these plants are also gastrointestinal irritants and have direct effects on the respiratory and nervous systems.

Clinical signs

As well as their cardiotoxic effect, cardiac glycosides also affect the gastrointestinal, respiratory and nervous systems, although death is usually a result of the cardiotoxic effect. Clinical signs usually develop 4 to 12 hours after ingestion of the plants and may present as sudden death.

- Lethargy, weakness and anorexia.
- Increased salivation.
- Rumen stasis and distension.
- Colic – vocalization, teeth grinding.
- Tachypnoea, dyspnea, periods of apnoea.
- Bradycardia, then cardiac arrhythmias associated with second degree heart block.
- Polyuria.
- Mucoid or haemorrhagic diarrhoea.
- Neurotoxins in plants such as thin-leafed *Asclepias* spp. can cause muscle tremors, seizures and head pressing.
- Death in 12 to 36 hours.
- If sublethal quantities are eaten, the clinical signs may persist for 2 to 3 days.
- Relapse may occur from the continued release of the glycoside from the rumen.

Treatment

- Removal of the plant from the rumen by rumenotomy, then transfaunation to help reestablish rumen function.
- Symptomatic and supportive treatment such as fluid therapy.
- Large doses of activated charcoal (2–9 g/kg) orally in a water slurry.
- Atropine sulphate for heart block, 0.04 mg/kg i.m. (preferably) or 0.02 mg/kg i.v. to effect.
- Other animals in the affected group should also be given activated charcoal after removal from the source of the poisoning.

Plants that accumulate selenium

Selenium toxicity is discussed in Chapter 8. Recognition of seleniferous plants, proper land management and grazing control are all necessary to completely prevent selenosis.

When growing on seleniferous soils, several plant species accumulate selenium in sufficient amounts to be toxic, including locoweeds and milk vetches (*Astragalus* spp.), goldenweed (*Onopsis*), woody asters (*Zylorhiza*) and prince's plume (*Stanleya*).

Indicator plants require selenium for growth and can accumulate very high levels of selenium (1000 to 10 000 parts per million). They are generally unpalatable, with a bitter taste and strong odour, and not readily eaten, but will be consumed when other forage is sparse.

Facultative or *secondary selenium absorbers* do not need selenium for growth and accumulate lower amounts. They belong to a number of genera and include aster (*Aster*), saltbush (*Atriplex*), paint-brush (*Castilleja*), gum-plant (*Grindelia*) and matchweed (*Gutierrezia*).

A third group includes crop plants and grasses such as barley, wheat and lucerne (alfalfa) that normally do not accumulate selenium to levels above 50 parts per billion (ppb), even when grown in selenium-laden soils. Plants containing more than 5 ppm are potentially toxic to livestock and it is these more palatable plants growing on selenium-rich soil that pose the greatest hazard.

Other cardiotoxic plants

Yew (*Taxus baccata, Taxus cuspidate*)

All *Taxus* spp. and all parts of the plant, fresh and dried, should be considered poisonous. Most poisonings are caused by yew clippings.

Aetiology

Yews contain 10 or more toxic alkaloids, the most toxic of which are taxine A and B. Taxine alkaloids cause depression of cardiac depolarisation and conduction, by inhibiting normal sodium and calcium exchange across the myocardial cells.

Clinical findings

Sudden death, tremor, dyspnoea, excitation, abdominal pain, death in one to three days.

Post-mortem findings
Plant in the rumen.

Treatment
Supportive and symptomatic.

Jimsonweed or thornapple (*Datura stramonium*)

Jimsonweed prefers rich soils, growing in cultivated fields and being a major weed in soybeans worldwide. It is common on overgrazed pastures and waste land and is found in hedgerows, on embankments and road-sides throughout the United States, in most southern Canadian Provinces and in limited areas of the south of England. It was introduced into Australia in the 1800s and is common in many parts of New Zealand. All parts of the Jimsonweed are poisonous. It is generally unpalatable with a strong odour and unpleasant taste, so poisoning is unlikely unless hungry animals are grazed in areas with no alternative food.

Aetiology
All parts of the green or dried plant contain toxic tropane alkaloids, L-hyoscyamine (atropine) and scopolamine (L-hyoscine), which act as competitive antagonists of acetylcholine.

Clinical signs
Clinical signs, involving the neuromuscular, ophthalmic and gastrointestinal systems, are attributable to the effects of the toxins on the parasympathetic nervous system.
- Lethargy, weakness, drowsiness, recumbency and altered locomotion.
- Tremors.
- Mydriasis; photophobia.
- Anorexia with decreased activity of the gastrointestinal tract, ruminal atony, constipation.
- Decreased salivation, dry mucous membranes.
- Increased vagal tone; sinus tachycardia.
- Tachypnoea.

False Hellebore (*Veratum* spp.)
Aetiology
Plants of *Veratum* spp., such as *Veratrum californicum*, contain over 50 complex alkaloids. Goats readily eat the leaves and plant tops, but although the plants are toxic from the start of their growth period until they are killed by freezing, with toxicity decreasing as the plants mature, severe toxicity in grazing goats is rare and is usually not lethal. The roots are more poisonous than the leaves or stems.

Clinical signs
Salivation, vomiting and abdominal pain; cardiac irregularities (bradycardia, conduction abnormalities), hypotension; convulsions, coma and death.

Treatment
Activated charcoal followed by supportive care, including fluid replacement, antiemetics for persistent nausea and vomiting, atropine for treatment of bradycardia, and vasopressors for the treatment of hypotension.

Rhododendron and azaleas (*Rhododendron* spp.), pieris (*Pieris* spp.) and laurels (*Kalmia* spp.)

Contain grayanotoxins, which have cardiotoxic effects.

Spindle tree (*Euonymus europaeus*)

The spindle tree is found throughout Britain, often as part of ancient woodlands or hedgerows. It has long been recognised as poisonous to goats – John Gerard, in his *Herbal or General History of Plants* (1597), describes goats as 'especially at risk'. Parts of the plant have been used medicinally. However, all parts of the plant – twigs, leaves and fruit – are poisonous, with gastrointestinal and cardiac effects. The toxic principles include cardiac glycosides and alkaloids.

Avocado (*Persea americana*)

The avocado is native to Mexico and Central America but is cultivated in tropical and Mediterranean climates throughout the world. The leaves are the most toxic part, but fruit, stems and seeds are also poisonous. The Guatemalan varieties of avocado have been most commonly associated with toxicosis.

Aetiology
The toxic compound is persin.
- Avocado causes necrosis and hemorrhage of the mammary gland epithelium of lactating mammals. Goats are highly susceptible to the mammary effects of avocado poisoning with levels above 20 g/kg producing a severe non-infectious mastitis within 24 hours of exposure to avocado and a marked decrease in milk

yield or agalactia. Lactation may provide a degree of protection against myocardial injury when avocado is ingested at lower doses.

- In non-lactating mammals, or at higher doses, myocardial insufficiency may develop within 24–48 h of ingestion In goats 30 g/kg body weight of fresh leaves can produce cardiac effects.

Clinical signs

- Intake of high doses of toxin may result in apparent sudden death.
- Affected mammary glands are firm, swollen and produce watery, curdled milk of a cheesy consistency, with markedly elevated somatic cell counts. The toxin causes destruction of the lacteal cells and milk production does not recover after removal from the plant.
- In animals with cardiac insufficiency, signs of severe cardiomyopathy are seen – lethargy, exercise intolerance, tachycardia, tachypnoea, muffled heart sounds, cough, cyanosis, subcutaneous oedema and death.

Post-mortem findings

- Congestion of lungs and liver, pulmonary edema.
- Ascites, pleural and pericardial effusion.
- Flabby heart with pale streaks.
- Histopathological lesions in the mammary gland include degeneration and necrosis of secretory epithelium, with interstitial edema and hemorrhage.
- Myocardial lesions include widespread degeneration and necrosis of myocardial fibres.

Diagnosis

History of exposure and clinical signs. There are no readily available specific tests that will confirm diagnosis.

Treatment

NSAIDs and analgesics may benefit animals with mastitis. Diuretics and antiarrhythmic drugs could be used for congestive heart failure in pet goats.

Gifblaar or poison leaf (*Dichapetalum cymosum*) is a South African plant containing *monofluoroacetateic acid*. Ingestion causes dyspnoea, cardiac arrhythmias and neurological signs, such as trembling, twitching and convulsions, with death in 4 to 24 hours from cardiac failure.

Gousiekte (quick sickness) is a syndrome, seen in South Africa, caused by plants in the family Rubiaceae

(*Pachystigma* spp., *Fadogia homblei* and *Pavetta* spp.) with affected animals dropping dead after exercise or when stressed because of congestive cardiac failure.

Plants containing grayanotoxins

> Vomiting in goats is almost always due to plant poisoning.

Rhododendron and Azaleas (*Rhododendron* spp.), Pieris (*Pieris* spp.), and Laurels (*Kalmia* spp.) are members of the *Ericaceae*. All contain grayanotoxins and are highly toxic either growing or dry.

Aetiology

- Rhododendron is the most common plant poison of goats in Britain, from browsing on the living shrubs or eating discarded prunings.
- Ingestion of 0.1% of the animal's body weight of fresh foliage is considered toxic.
- Toxic principles are the polycyclic diterpines grayanotoxins I (rhodotoxin or andromedotoxin, II and III). These act on the autonomic nervous system stimulating the vomiting centre via the vagus nerve.

Clinical signs

Clinical signs appear about 6 hours after ingestion of leaves, with the initial clinical signs being related to the gastrointestinal tract.

- Lethargy, anorexia.
- Excessive salivation, repeated swallowing.
- Abdominal pain, vocalisation.
- *Vomiting* (considered pathognomonic for plant poisoning in the UK).
- Ruminal bloat and atony.
- Cardiovascular signs include irregular heart rate, initially bradycardia then tachycardia.
- Recumbency and death.
- *Inhalation pneumonia* may occur secondarily to the vomiting.

Post-mortem findings

- No characteristic lesions.
- Evidence of leaves in rumen.

Treatment

- Symptomatic and supportive therapy.

- Spasmolytics, B vitamins, analgesics (NSAIDs; pethidine, 3 mg/kg every 12 hours).
- Antibiotics to treat aspiration pneumonia.
- Charcoal 2–9 g/kg orally in a water slurry.
- Atropine sulphate, 80–160 micrograms/kg s.c.
- Rumenotomy to remove eaten leaves.

In Britain, vomiting is virtually pathognomonic for poisoning by members of the *Ericaceae*, but isolated incidents of vomiting in goats have been reported following ingestion of radish (*Raphanus sativus*), black nightshade (*Solanum nigrum*) and gladiolus corms.

Plants causing nephrotoxicity

Plants with a high oxalate content

Oxalate poisoning results from the ingestion of plants containing oxalic acid or its salts. These include rhubarb leaves (*Rheum rhabarbarum*), docks, common sorrel, sheep's sorrel (*Rumex* spp.), wood sorrel, yellow sorrel, soursob (*Oxalis* spp.), greasewood (*Sarcobatus vermiculatus*), lambsquarter, goosefoot and fat hen (*Chenopodium* spp.), Russian thistle (*Salsola tragus*), bassia (*Bassia hyssopifolia*), Palmer amaranth or Palmer's pigweed (*Amaranthus palmeri*) and pigweed amaranth or common tumbleweed (*Amaranthus retroflexus*) and various grasses such as elephant grass (*Panicum* spp.), setaria grass (*Setaria sphacelata*), Kikuyu grass (*Pennisetum clandestinum*) and buffel grass (*Cenchrus ciliaris*).

Leaves and roots of sugar beets, fodder beets, mangolds (*Beta vulgaris*) and turnips (*Brassica campestris*) can contain up to 12% of soluble and insoluble oxalates. The oxalate content of mangels, sugar beet leaves and roots decreases as the plants mature.

The most common cause of oxalate poisoning in goats in Australia is *pigweed* or common purslane (*Portulaca oleracea*), often from ingesting the rapidly growing leaves with high oxalate (and nitrate) content after rain following a dry period. Soursob (*Oxalis pes-caprae*) is a common oxalate-rich plant in the medium rainfall districts of Australia. In North America, halogeton (*Halogeton glomeratus*) is a range plant introduced from Asia. Sodium oxalate may comprise 30-40% of the dry matter content of the plant. Poisoning generally occurs in naïve or hungry animals, whereas it can be used as a winter forage in animals that have been slowly adapted to the plant.

Aetiology

- The amount of oxalate required to cause toxicity is variable because of the proliferation of oxalate-degrading ruminal microflora that develop in mature animals gradually introduced to oxalate. Over a period of 4 days, the ability of the rumen to detoxify oxalates can increase by up to 30%.
- Goats can detoxify large amounts of ingested oxalates, so poisoning is only likely to arise if large amounts are eaten over a short period. Plants like sugar beet and mangolds are generally a safe livestock feed, which will only give rise to poisoning under special circumstances.
- The concentration of oxalate in the plant varies with stage of plant growth, weather, soil and geographical area.
- Soluble oxalates are readily absorbed from the rumen and bind with serum calcium and magnesium. The production of insoluble calcium oxalate lowers the serum calcium levels, resulting in severe *hypocalcaemia,* resulting in the typical clinical signs. Oxalates also interfere with cellular energy metabolism, contributing to the acute death of the affected animals. In animals that survive, death can occur from oxalate nephrosis.

Clinical signs

- Depression, inappetence.
- Muscular tremors, ataxia, staggering.
- Dyspnoea.
- Paralysis, recumbency and death.
- May present as sudden death.

Post-mortem findings

- Calcium oxalate crystals in kidneys and urinary tract.
- Hyperaemia of the lungs; scattered haemorrhages.
- Rumenitis.

Confirmation of diagnosis

- Oxalate can be detected in kidneys and rumen contents.

Treatment

- Calcium borogluconate 20%, 80–100 ml, slowly i.v. or s.c., or half by each route.
- Oral calcium chloride or dicalcium phosphate can precipitate oxalate within the rumen and prevent further absorption.

- Provided treatment is early and kidney damage has not occurred there is rapid response to treatment.

> The feeding of dried sugar beet to male goats does *not* lead to urolithiasis.

Note: (1) In castrated male goats, the urethra may become blocked by calcium oxalate crystals. This association of *sugar beet tops* with urolithiasis has led to the common misconception among goalkeepers that sugar beet pulp should not be fed to male goats.

(2) *Ethylene glycol* (antifreeze) poisoning occasionally occurs in goats because they like the sweet taste and will preferentially drink it to water. Metabolites of ethylene glycol, for example glycolic acid formed by the liver, are responsible for metabolic acidosis and hyperosmolality. Glycolic acid is excreted or further converted to oxalic acid with formation of oxalate crystals and signs of oxalate poisoning. Because of the ability of rumen microorganisms to degrade oxalate, adult ruminants are more resistant than monogastric animals to poisoning. Poisoning results in increased salivation, ataxia, staggering, seizures, recumbency and death. Ethylene glycol can be detected in rumen contents and glycolic acid in urine, serum or ocular fluid.

Acorns and oak (*Quercus* spp.)
Aetiology
The toxic principles are simple phenols and tannins (e.g. gallic acid and pyrogallol), which produce severe intestinal irritation and nephrosis. Higher numbers of cases usually occur in years with a bumper crop of acorns or on drought stricken pastures. The level of tannins in the acorns fluctuates from year to year, so toxicity may occur in animals that have grazed the same pasture for years without previous cases of toxicity. Deer produce proline-rich salivary proteins (PRPs), which render the tannins inactive. Goats produce more PRPs than cattle and sheep, making them much less susceptible to toxicity.

Clinical signs
- Lethargy.
- Alimentary signs of colic, anorexia, ascites.

- Weight loss and oedema.
- Constipation, followed by black tarry mucoid faeces.
- Haematuria.

Laboratory findings
- Blood urea and creatinine levels elevated; elevated liver enzymes.

Post-mortem findings
- Gastrointestinal ulceration and haemorrhage.
- Nephritis – kidneys pale and enlarged.
- Liver degeneration.

Treatment
- Remove the goat from the source of the oak; oral purgatives such as mineral oil and/ or magnesium sulphate; intravenous fluid therapy to correct dehydration and acidosis.

Calcinogenic plants

Most calcinogenic plants are from the Solanaceae family, including *Solanum malacoxylon*, *Solanum torvum* and *Cestrum diurnum*. They contain an active metabolite of vitamin D_3, which directly interferes with calcium metabolism.

Yellow/golden oat grass (*Trisetum flavescens*) has been reported as causing calcinosis in goats, but, despite it being a common grass in England and Wales, calcinosis has not been reported there. Young growing plants are generally more calcinogenic than mature plants. Flowering plants and hay are not calcinogenic.

Enzootic calcinosis is characterised by widespread calcification of soft tissues, osteopetrosis, hypercalcemia and hyperphosphatemia and mineralisation of the arteries, cardiac valves, lungs and kidneys. Destruction of connective tissues precedes tissue mineralisation in which calcium, phosphorus and magnesium are involved.

Calcinosis results in loss of condition and weight loss, progressing to emaciation, with a stiff and painful gait and dyspnoea even at rest. In advanced cases, joints cannot be extended completely and animals tend to walk with an arched back. Animals recover rapidly if they are removed in the early stages from dangerous pasture, but mortality is high after prolonged exposure.

Cyanogenic plants

A wide variety of plants contain cyanogenic glycosides. Most cases of cyanide poisoning are caused by consumption of plants in the families *Rosaceae*, *Leguminosae* and *Gramineae*.

The leaves of the *Prunus* family, for example cherry trees, cherry laurel (*Prunus laurocerasus*) peach (*Prunus persica*) and plum (*Prunus domestica*) contain a cyanogenic glycoside amygdalin. Commercial orchard species are often bred for low cyanide content, but ornamental bushes and trees can be very poisonous. In Britain, cherry laurel is associated with most poisonings, although, for goats browsing woodland, wild cherry can be a problem. In North America, various cherry trees, including black cherry (*Prunus serotina*) and choke cherry (*Prunus virginiana*) can present a serious risk. Poisoning has also occurred in goats in Britain after eating crab apple (*Malus sylvestris*) leaves and fruit. Amygdalin is converted into hydrogen cyanide and sugar by enzymes in crushed and wilted plants, or plants damaged by drought, frost or insects. This means that fresh leaves are not toxic, but after wilting they become toxic and also more attractive to goats than fresh leaves. As goats browse, smaller branches can break and leaves become damaged by chewing, causing leaves to wilt, which can lead to poisoning. Fallen branches or tree prunings should not be fed and fallen branches should be removed after storms. Care should be taken during droughts and after frosts.

Amongst many others, the following plants also contain cyanogenic glycosides and have the potential to cause poisoning, but there are few reports of poisoning in goats: marsh arrow grasses (*Triglochin maritima* and *T palustris*), gum trees (*Eucalyptus* spp.), bracken fern (*Pteridium aquillinum*), linseeds and flaxes (*Linum* spp.), maize or corn (*Zea mays*), hydrangias (*Hydrangia* spp.), California holly (*Heteromeles arbutifolia*), poison suckleya (*Suckley suckleyana*), oleander (*Nerium oleander)*, cassava (*Mannihot esculentum*), sudan grass, Johnson grass, sorghum or durra (*Sorghum* spp.).

The stage of growth, mineral and moisture content of the soil, time of year and even time of day can affect the amount of cyanogenic glycosides in plants. Sudan grass, sorghum, sorghum/Sudan hybrids and their aftermaths are particularly dangerous if they sprout after an early frost and should not be grazed once frozen. Normal ensilage fermentation renders the grasses non-toxic after about 2 weeks. Some pasture species, including *Trifolium* spp. (clovers), *Vicia* spp. (vetches) and *Lotus* spp. (bird's-foot trefoils) have been bred for low cyanogenesis.

As plants are chewed, the cyanogenic glycosides are catabolised by plant enzymes producing hydrogen cyanide. A neutral ruminal pH favours plant enzyme action and ruminal bacterial enzymes also hydrolyse the cyanogenic glycosides. Animals fed mainly a grass or lucerne (alfalfa) hay diet tend to release the poison faster, because the rumen is more alkaline than in goats fed a grain ration, which have an acidic rumen. As with the majority of plant toxins, the actual amount of the toxin, in this case hydrogen cyanide, absorbed over a short period, determines whether poisoning occurs or not. Once absorbed, hydrogen cyanide reacts with the trivalent iron of cytochrome oxidase in mitochondria inhibiting cellular respiration and depriving the cells of oxygen. Poisoning occurs when the absorption of hydrogen cyanide is faster than it can be detoxified. Although cyanide poisoning is usually rapidly fatal, an animal may tolerate a higher dose of cyanide if the stomach is full of plant matter and carbohydrates. Fatalities can also occur if small amounts of cyanide are eaten consistently over a long period of time.

Clinical signs

- Sudden death – death can occur within 15 to 60 minutes of exposure.
- Dyspnoea, cardiac arrhythmias.
- Muscular tremors, frothing at the mouth, dilated pupils, ataxia, convulsions.
- Mucous membranes bright red.

Post-mortem findings

- Blood bright red.
- Bitter almond smell of rumen contents.

Confirmation of diagnosis

- Cyanide estimation on rumen contents, liver, muscle or blood (preserve with 1% sodium fluoride). Tissue samples and rumen contents must be collected within a few hours of death and frozen immediately in airtight containers before sending to an appropriate laboratory.

Treatment

- Rumenotomy.

- *1% sodium nitrite, 25 mg/kg* i.v. – induces formation of methaemoglobin to which hydrocyanic acid is preferentially bound; followed by *25% sodium thiosulphate, 600 mg/kg* i.v. combines with hydrocyanic acid to form non-toxic thiocyanate; then sodium thiosulphate, 30 g orally every hour to fix free hydrocyanic acid in the rumen and prevent further absorption of cyanide.

Plants containing excess nitrites/nitrates

Nitrates occur in many plants, including barley, wheat, rye, maize (corn) and sorghum and Sudan grasses and many common annual weeds, but, under normal circumstances, the concentration of nitrate in plants is not high enough to poison livestock. Under certain conditions, however, plants have the ability to accumulate large quantities of nitrates, which are potentially toxic to goats. Use of large quantities of nitrogenous fertilisers can result in excess accumulation of nitrate, so that plants become toxic. Livestock may also be poisoned by water that has been contaminated by fertiliser. As sources of nitrate are cumulative, toxic levels can be reached by a combination of moderately increased nitrogen levels in both water and forage.

Poisoning is uncommon in Britain, but in the United States and Australia may be caused by consumption of common pasture grasses and weed species that accumulate nitrate, such as pigweed (*Amaranthus palmeri*), variegated thistle (*Silybum marianum*), *Chenopodium* spp. (lambsquarters, goosefoot), oatgrass (*Arrhenatherum* spp.), Canada thistle (*Cirsium arvense*), jimsonweed (*Datura stramonium*), cockspur, barnyard grass (*Echinochloa crusgalli*), silverleaf povertyweed (*Ambrosia tomentosa*), ragweed, bursage (*Ambrosia* spp.), wild sunflower (*Helianthus* spp.), fireweed (United States), rosebay willowherb (United Kingdom), great willowherb (Canada) (*Chamerion angustifolium*), sweet clover (*Melilotus* spp.), smartweed (*Persicaria* spp.), Russian thistle (*Salsola tragus*). Toxic levels of nitrate can be found during periods of rapid growth, particularly when warm rains follow a very dry summer, when plants have low levels of soluble sugars and rumen metabolism of nitrates/nitrites is reduced.

Poisoning in ruminants has also been associated with the feeding of sorghums (Sudan grass, Johnson grass), oats (*Avena sativa*), silage, rye (*Secale cereale*), wheat (*Triticum vulgare*), lucerne/alfalfa (*Medicago sativa*), maize/corn (*Zea mays*) and white clover (*Trifolium refens*). In North America and Australia forages, especially corn and oat silages, green chop or pasture and weeds, are most commonly implicated in nitrate poisoning.

In the United Kingdom, the plants most likely to accumulate nitrates are: mangels, fodder beet, sugar beet (*Beta vulgaris*), turnips (*Brassica campestris*), swedes (*Brassica napus* var. *naprobrassica*), kale (*Brassica oleracea*) and rape (*Brassica napus, Brassica campestris*). Nitrates are present in freshly harvested roots and sugar beet tops. Leafy tops of turnips can contain from 5 to 9% of nitrates as well as oxalates. Sheep in Britain have been poisoned by eating various species of mallow (*Maliva* spp.) and the marsh mallow (*Malva parviflora*) is recognized as poisonous in Australia, South Africa and the United States.

Aetiology

- In the rumen, nitrates are converted to much more toxic nitrites and then to ammonia. Excessive nitrite concentrations lead to nitrite being absorbed from the gastrointestinal tract into the blood, where they combine with haemoglobin to form methaemoglobin, preventing the uptake of oxygen and resulting in *hypoxia*. Methaemaglobin concentrations of 30 to 40% lead to clinical signs and death occurs with concentrations > 80%.
- Nitrate concentrations are highest in the stem and leaves, whereas flowers, seeds and fruit do not contain nitrate. High nitrate levels persist in hay, but the levels may be significantly reduced in well-made silage. Cereal grains do not contain high levels of nitrogen.
- Nitrates accumulate in plants grown in acidic soils and in soils deficient in sulphur, phosphorus and molybdenum.
- Herbicide use increases the nitrate level in plants and also increases the palatability.
- Weather conditions may affect nitrate concentrations within the plants. Nitrates can accumulate in plants when adverse growing conditions such as drought, hot weather, cool weather or frost slows the growth of the plants. Levels of nitrogen can also increase in rapidly growing plants when rain follows drought conditions.
- Parasitism or other conditions causing anaemia increase susceptibility to nitrate poisoning.

Clinical signs

- Depression.
- Abdominal pain, diarrhoea (due to high *nitrate* levels).
- Dyspnoea, convulsions, tachycardia, purple and dark cyanotic mucous membranes (due to *nitrite* absorption).
- Ataxia, incoordination, coma and death, usually within 12 to 24 hours after ingestion.
- Pregnant animals may abort because of lack of oxygen to the fetus, without other clinical signs of poisoning, 10 to 14 days after exposure.

Post-mortem findings

- Chocolate-coloured blood, petechiation of mucous membranes.

Confirmation of diagnosis

- Diphenylamine test on clear body fluids (urine, serum, CSF, aqueous humour).
- Nitrate levels in aqueous humour of 20–40 mg/litre (ppm) are suspect and levels >40 mg/litre are diagnostic. Increased nitrate concentrations can be detected for up to 24 hours at room temperature (very high concentrations may be diagnostic of nitrate poisoning up to 60 h following death).
- Nitrite estimation in blood or urine (but nitrite is rapidly converted to nitrate after death).
- Methaemoglobin estimation (stabilise sample in pH 6.6 phosphate buffer).

Treatment

- Adrenaline (Epinephrine), 20 µg/kg, i.v. or s.c.
- Methylthioninium chloride (methylene blue), about 10 ml of 2% aqueous solution i.v. (4 to 15 mg/kg). Repeat if necessary after 6 to 8 hours.
- Conversion of nitrate to nitrite in the rumen may be decreased by ruminal lavage with cold water or by administration of oral antibiotic.
- Diluted vinegar given orally by stomach tube will acidify the rumen and decrease nitrate conversion to nitrite by rumen bacteria. Alternatively, cold water with added broad-spectrum antibiotics can be used.

Reducing the risk of nitrate toxicity

- Avoid rapid diet changes that can trigger nitrate poisoning.
- Forages known to accumulate nitrates such as oat hay and Sudan grass should be tested before feeding – care should be taken when nitrate levels exceed 1%.
- Water sources should also be tested. Nitrate levels in water should be less than 45 ppm, although in some situations levels of up to 400 ppm can be tolerated.
- The total nitrogen intake can be reduced by feeding hay with no nitrates together with high nitrogen forage or low nitrate forages can be fed before turning animals out on to pastures with a high nitrogen content.
- Allow animals to adjust to low levels of nitrate before increasing the nitrate content of the ration. Nitrate is not normally accumulated in the animal because it is continually converted to other nitrogen compounds that are utilised or excreted in the urine and faeces, but the ability to utilise and effectively excrete the nitrogen compounds requires adaptation by the animal.
- As with most plant poisoning, starved animals are most at risk, because they are less selective grazers. Increasing the total energy of the diet with carbohydrate-rich cereals improves the tolerance for high nitrate levels. In well-fed animals, rumen organisms convert nitrates to microbial protein and nitrite to ammonia. Goats should be fed a balanced ration for the level of production expected.
- If zero-grazing, feed the ration in two or three meals per day rather than just one meal per day.
- Beet and mangel roots may contain high levels of nitrates when freshly harvested and should be 'ripened' by storage in clamps for 3 to 4 months before feeding. Sugar beet tops should be left to wilt for at least a week before feeding.

Plants causing anaemia

Members of the *Brassica* family, including common cultivated crops such as kale, broccoli, Brussels sprouts, cabbage and rape all contain a toxic constituent *S*-methyl cysteine sulphoxide (SMCO), a chemical that is converted by normal rumen fermentation to dimethyl disulphide, which can cause haemolytic anaemia in livestock by destroying red blood cells. The SMCO content increases as the plants mature and secondary growth and flowering occurs. In general, cases of livestock poisoning only occur when animals are fed large amounts of these crops, without other fodder being available, so poisoning can be avoided by restricting the amount of *Brassica* crops fed. Modern *Brassica* cultivars have lower quantities of SMCO, greatly diminishing or virtually eliminating the risk of poisoning.

Clinical signs

The clinical signs depend on the extent of the haemolysis and the ability of the animal to replace the red blood cells. *Anaemia* is generally detectable in blood samples 1 to 3 weeks after commencing feeding, with haemoglobin levels falling significantly over the next couple of weeks. If the anaemia is not too severe, haemoglobin levels return to normal in 3 to 4 weeks after stopping *Brassica* feeding.

- Lethargy, inappetence, depressed milk yield.
- Anaemia, haemoglobinuria (reddish-brown or black urine), jaundice.
- Pyrexia, tachypnea, tachycardia.
- Diarrhoea.
- Collapse and death from respiratory failure secondary to the anaemia.
- Sudden death, if earlier signs of anaemia are not noticed.

These plants also produce glucosinolates, bitter tasting compounds that can taint the milk of animals eating the plants. Hydrolysis of the glucosinates produces compounds, such as isothiocyanates, thiocyanates and goitrin, that have an *antithyroid* effect, preventing accumulation of iodine in the thyroid gland, resulting in thyroid enlargement and decreased growth rates (see 'Goitre', Chapter 10). The secondary iodine deficiency can lead to suboptimum fertility, embryonic mortality and the birth of death or very weak kids.

Brassica species have been associated with *primary and secondary* **(hepatogenous)** *photosensitisation* (see this chapter).

Laboratory investigations

- Heinz bodies and decreased haemoglobin levels on complete blood counts.

Treatment

- Remove Brassicas from the diet.
- Treat the anaemia, including blood transfusion in severely affected animals.
- Avoid stress and exertion during recovery.

Other plants implicated in causing anaemia include:

Bracken (*Pteridium aquilinum*). Goats seem less susceptible to bracken poisoning than sheep, but prolonged grazing of the plant may result in an acute haemorrhagic syndrome or blood loss due to tumours in the bladder or intestine.

Plants containing pyrrolizidine alkaloids (see this chapter). Pyrrolizidine alkaloids may result in haemorrhages following liver damage.

Onions (*Allium cepa*). Goats are relatively resistant to onion toxicity and onions can be fed over long periods without signs of poisoning, but in large amounts could produce haemolytic anaemia as in other ruminants. This is the result of the precipitation of haemoglobin and the formation of Heinz bodies in red blood cells, which leads to their destruction and removal from the circulation. Animals may have dark urine, drastic drop in milk yield and milk taint.

Mouldy sweet clover (*Melilotus* spp.). Although melilots are naturalised in Britain, they are unlikely to cause a problem as they are not grown as fodder crops. Melilots can be safely grazed as they are not poisonous and only become dangerous when the coumarins in the plant become changed into dicoumarol by the action of moulds in hay or silage. In areas where sweet clover plants are conserved, such as the north-western United States, ruminants are at risk, although sheep and goats have some resistance. Large weathered bales usually contain the highest levels of toxin. Cultivars of sweet clover have been developed that contain low levels of coumarin. Dicoumarol interferes with the metabolism of vitamin K, impairing blood clotting and leading to internal and external haemorrhages, with subcutaneous haematoma formation, epistaxis, blood in urine and faeces, pale mucous membranes, stiffness and lameness due to bleeding into joints and muscles. Death can occur rapidly. Animals should not receive sweet clover hay or silage for 3 to 4 weeks before elective surgery or parturition.

Affected animals can be treated with phytomenadione (vitamin K1), 1 to 3 mg/kg body-weight daily by i.m. injection (initially this can be given slowly i.v.). The dose should be divided between injection sites.

Plants causing bloody or dark urine (haematuria or haemoglobinuria)

- **Onions (*Allium cepa*).** See plants causing anaemia above.

- **Brassica spp.** See plants causing anaemia above.
- **Mouldy sweet clover (*Melilotus* spp.).** See plants causing anaemia above.

Hepatotoxic plants

Hepatotoxins are found in numerous plants. Often they are responsible for chronic poisoning, with the toxic agent being ingested over weeks or months, as in pyrrolizidine alkaloid toxicity. In all cases, prognosis is guarded and depends on the particular hepatotoxin. Affected animals and those in the same group should be denied access to the source of the poisoning if known as soon as possible. Hepatotoxicity can occur with or without photosensitisation (see below in this chapter). Many plant hepatotoxins, additionally, have toxic effects on multiple organs, particularly the kidneys, lungs and gastrointestinal tract.

Treatment for acute poisoning
- Administration of activated charcoal or mineral oil.
- Rumenotomy.
- Supportive therapy including fluid therapy to correct electrolyte, metabolic, and glucose imbalance and dietary management.

Treatment for chronic poisoning
- Supportive therapy as for acute poisoning.
- Control hepatic encephalopathy (see Chapter 12).
- Avoid sunlight if photosensitisation is present.
- Antibiotics to control/prevent secondary pyoderma.

Hepatoxic plants containing pyrrolizidine alkaloids

Plants containing hepatotoxic pyrrolizidine alkaloids are found worldwide. Goats demonstrate an apparent tolerance to pyrrolizidine alkaloids (PAs) in plants, but are susceptible if enough is consumed over a long period. However, the large amounts that need to be consumed, together with the low palatability of plants like ragwort, mean that poisoning is unlikely (a total plant intake of ragwort (*Senecio jacobaea*) in excess of 100% of body weight may be required for toxicity to occur). Goats are sometimes used to graze pastures that are recognised as dangerous to horses and cattle.

Three plant families, *Compositae*, *Leguminosae* and *Boraginaceae*, contain the majority of PA-containing plants. Members of the *Compositae* family are most likely to cause poisoning in Britain, where ragwort (*Senecio jacobaea*) is widespread, and the United States, where common groundsel (*S. vulgaris*), tansy ragwort (*S. jacobaea*), Riddell's groundsel (*S. riddelli*) and threadleaf groundsel (*S. fiaccidus*) are present. Hound's Tongue (*Cynoglossum officinale, Cynoglossum cinale*), a member of the *Boraginaceae* family, has poisoned cattle in both countries.

Comfrey (*Symphytum* spp.), a member of the *Boraginaceae* family, contains pyrrolizidine alkaloids and, although goats have some resistance to these toxins, long-term consumption could lead to poisoning. The feeding of comfrey and the use of dietary supplements containing comfrey should be discouraged. Comfrey preparations used externally are not a cause for concern.

Although the families *Amsinckia*, *Crotalaria*, *Heliotropium* and *Echium* also contain PSs they are rarely reported to cause poisoning. European Heliotrope (*Heliotropium europaeum*) and Paterson's Curse or Salvation Jane (*Echium lycopis; Echium plantagineum*) have produced toxic liver cirrhosis in sheep in Australia. Vipers bugloss (*Echium vulgare*) has poisoned sheep in Britain. Rattleweed (*Crotalaria retusa*) has been associated with a natural poisoning outbreak in goats in Brazil.

Aetiology
Pyrrolizidine alkaloids are hepatotoxic. Poisoning can occur from the fresh plant or hay or silage, although, because of the lack of palatability of most fresh plants, ingestion of the preserved plant is more likely to cause poisoning, unless there is heavy infestation of pasture and no other grazing is available.

PAs are absorbed from the gastrointestinal tract and undergo extensive metabolism in the liver, where some are detoxified to harmless metabolites and some are converted to highly toxic bound pyrroles.

Sheep and goats are relatively resistant to PAs, apparently as a combination of rumen metabolism breaking down the alkaloids to less toxic products and species-specific hepatic metabolism moderating their conversion to toxic pyrroles.

Clinical signs
- Clinical signs generally develop slowly, with hepatic and neurological signs superficially resembling other diseases. Goats are unlikely to eat sufficient toxic

material to produce acute onset signs of hepatoen-cephalopathy. Young animals are considered more susceptible to poisoning than adults. Nursing animals may develop hepatic disease despite their lactating mothers being unaffected.

- Depression, inappetence, emaciation.
- Incoordination.
- Jaundice, anaemia.
- Hepatic neurotoxicity (aimless walking, head pressing, ataxia, blindness), coma, death.

Post-mortem findings
- Enlarged cirrhotic liver.
- Petechial haemorrhages in the digestive tract.
- Spongy degeneration of brain and spinal cord due to ammonia accumulation because of liver damage.

Treatment
None.

Other hepatotoxic plants

Cocklebur (*Xanthium strumarium*) contains a potent glycoside hepatotoxin, carboxyactractyloside, which is present in high concentrations in the seeds and two cotyledon stages, but gradually declines and is absent in the mature plant. Seedlings are toxic even when dead and dry. Poisoning has been reported from North America, but not from Britain, where it is an introduced plant with local distribution. Clinical signs generally occur 12 to 48 hours after cocklebur seedlings are eaten, with lethargy, depression and weakness with subnormal temperature; unsteady gait; hyperpnoea and tachypnoea with a weak, rapid pulse; regurgitation, convulsions, opisthotonus and death.

Sacahuista or beargrass (*Nolina texana*) is a common range plant in the southwestern United States, which contains an unidentified hepatotoxin in the buds, flowers and fruit, but not the leaves, so that it is only toxic for a short time in the spring. Hepatic and renal toxicity leads to lethargy, anorexia, jaundice and photosensitisation, with dark urine and yellowish ocular and nasal discharges.

The South African plant **kraalbos** (*Galenia africana*) is not normally eaten, except during drought in heavily grazed areas when it leads to a condition known as *'water belly'*, characterised by the development of liver damage with ascites and heart lesions with decreased cardiac function. Other plants occasionally implicated in hepatotoxicity in goats in South Africa are *Cestrum* spp., which contain kaurene glycosides, the Springbokbush (*Hertia pallens*) and Scholtzbos/poor man's bush (*Pteronia pallens*).

Lantana (*Lantana camara*), a shrub found in tropical and subtropical regions, contains hepatotoxic lantadenes, which cause chronic toxicity with slow hepatic failure resulting in lethargy, jaundice, cholestasis, ruminal atopy and constipation with photosensitisation sometimes being reported. Jaundice and bloody diarrhoea occur after 2 to 4 days, with death occurring from hepatic and renal failure over a period of several weeks. Goats are susceptible to poisoning, but are rarely naturally poisoned. However, poisoning of goats has been reported from Australia, South Africa and the United States. Lantana is occasionally sold as a house plant in more temperate or colder regions.

Blue-green algae (cyanobacteria) can produce hepatotoxins, as well as neurotoxins and skin allergens (see this chapter). Poisoned animals develop muscle tremors and staggering within 30 minutes of drinking toxic water, followed by recumbency, coma and death, usually within 24 hours. Animals may be found dead. Animals that survive longer develop liver damage, jaundice, diarrhoea and photosensitisation, dying within 1 to 2 weeks.

Although **lupinosis**, resulting from the ingestion of a mycotoxin associated with *Diaporthe toxica* fungus growing on the stalks of lupine plants (*Lupinus* spp.), is important in other species in Australia and South Africa and has been reported from New Zealand and Europe, natural occurrence in goats appears rare, although it has been produced experimentally. It can be expressed as either a severe acute disease or as a chronic liver dysfunction syndrome. Lupinosis may also predispose sheep to a nutritional muscle disease, lupinosis-associated myopathy. Most stands of lupins in Western Australia will be infected and colonised to some degree by *Diaporthe toxica*. Resistant narrow-leafed lupin varieties have been developed and under most conditions have very low levels of toxicity, so the stubbles provide a valuable food source for sheep and goats.

Photosensitisation

Photosensitisation is caused by the accumulation of photodynamic chemicals in the skin, which become stimulated by sunlight on exposed, non-pigmented areas. It is less likely to occur in the United Kingdom, where sunlight is less intense, than in warmer climates.

Goats with black and/or brown coloration over the entire body have an advantage over white goats under range conditions in warm climates, because of decreased susceptibility to sunburn, photosensitisation and skin tumours, coupled with enhanced camouflage from predators.

Primary photosensitisation is due to ingestion of plants such as St John's wort (*Hypericum perforatum*), buckwheat (*Fagopyrum esculentum*), rape (*Brassica napus*), clovers (*Trifolium* spp.), giant hogweed (*Heracleum mantegazzianum*), and *Lantana* spp. Primary photosensitisation may also occur due to direct contact with plants such as giant hogweed.

Secondary photosensitisation in animals with hepatic dysfunction is due to accumulation of phylloerythrin, a breakdown derivative of chlorophyll. Normally the liver degrades phylloerythrin, keeping serum levels negligible. Any liver damage affecting bile excretion may be implicated – liver disease, hepatotoxic drugs, chemicals, mycotoxins or plant toxins. Although many plants in diverse parts of the world have the potential to cause liver damage and photosensitisation, there are a relatively few well documented reports of photosensitisation in goats (Table 21.1). *Pyrrolizidine alkaloid toxicosis* from *Senecio* spp., *Crotolaria* spp. and *Heliotropium* spp. is unlikely in goats, because substantially larger doses of toxin are required compared with horses and cattle.

Ingestion of *mycotoxins* has the potential to cause photosensitisation in goats. In South Africa, Boer goats were poisoned by a mycotoxin of the fungus *Drechslera campanulata* growing on green oats (*Avena sativa*).

Some species of *Trifolium*, particularly white and Alsike clover may cause primary photosensitisation and secondary photosensitisation as a result of liver damage.

In South Africa, *Kaalsiekte* is a problem in goat kids less than 3 weeks of age when the mothers graze on the usually unpalatable bitter (bitterkaroo) bush *Chrysocoma ciliata* (*C. tenuifolia*) pre-partum, ingesting large amounts and excreting a toxin in their milk. Kids are born with normal coats, but between 3 and 14 days of age exposure to sunlight leads to pruritus with the resultant pulling out of hair over the non-pigmented areas of the rump, shoulders and body, producing alopecia leading to sunburn during the day and hypothermia at night.

Kleingrass (*Panicum* spp.), an imported grass from South Africa, sporadically causes photosensitisation

in goats in the southwestern United States. New basal leaves can be very toxic when rains bring rapid growth after a period of drought. The toxic principle is sapogenin.

Caltrop (*Tribulus terrestris*), found worldwide, particularly in areas with a Mediterranean climate, has been associated with hepatogenous photosensitisation disease ('yellow big head', 'geeldikkop') in Australia, California and South Africa. It has also been associated with nitrate poisoning and nervous disorders – the ingestion of large amounts of caltrop over many months can result in a progressive and irreversible weakness in the hind legs. Photosensitisation due to the ingestion of caltrop only occurs spasmodically. The plant contains steroidal saponins, which accumulate when the plant wilts in hot dry weather after summer rains, and these are thought to be responsible for the hepatotoxicity and photosensitisation The toxic effects are believed to be enhanced by a mycotoxin of *Pithomyces chartarum*, a fungus that grows on caltrops under the same climatic condition.

In Texas, New Mexico and Mexico 'goat fever' or 'swell-head' is the result of *hepatogenous photosensitisation* from the ingestion of lechuguilla (*Agave lecheguilla*), during drought conditions, with swelling of the face and ears and coma.

Animals that recover from the acute phase of *blue-green algae poisoning* may develop photosensitisation secondary to liver disease (see above).

Clinical signs

- Pruritus, erythema, oedema and swelling of the skin, with blistering and scab formation, particularly of non-pigmented areas of the face, eyelids, muzzle, ear and tail.
- Head shaking and rubbing of the face and head.
- Affected areas may ooze serum with development of secondary bacterial infection.
- Necrosis of the ear tips.

Treatment

- Prevent access to any photosensitising plant.
- Protect from sunlight.
- Symptomatic and supportive therapy; corticosteroids during the early stages will help reduce oedema; antibiotics because of secondary bacterial infection.
- Treatment of primary disease if liver damage is present.

Plants causing diarrhoea

A variety of plants have been implicated as causing diarrhoea in goats, although other clinical signs may predominate. They include *plants containing cardiac glycosides, hepatotoxic plants* and *plants with excess nitrate*. Hemlock (*Conium maculatum*), oak (*young* leaves) (*Quercus* spp.), cuckoo pint or wild arum (*Arum maculatum*), castor seed (in foodstuffs), foxglove (*Digitalis purpurea*), water dropwort (*Oenanthe crocata*), box (*Buxus sempervirens*), potato (green) (*Solanum tuberosum*), rhododendron spp., linseed (*Linum usitatissimum*), oleander (*Nerium oleander*), lantana (*Lantana camara*), blue-green algae, freshly harvested mangel and beet roots (*Beta vulgaris*) and spurges (*Euphorbia* spp.) have been implicated amongst many others.

Plants containing *saponin glycosides* produce severe gastroenteritis with colic and diarrhoea, in addition to neurological signs. Pokeweed (*Phytolacca americana*) is native to North America and introduced into Britain as a garden plant. All parts are potentially poisonous, particularly the tap root and berries, but goats will generally avoid it because of its acrid taste. There are anecdotal reports of young shoots being eaten with no apparent ill-effect. Toxic constituents include saponins, the alkaloids phytolaccine and phytolaccotoxin, and a glycoprotein. Clinical signs become apparent after 2 or more hours: retching or vomiting, watery diarrhoea (often bloody) with spasms, dyspnoea, tremors, convulsions, collapse and death if a sufficient quantity is eaten. Several rangeland weeds in the United States including corn cockle (*Agrostemma githago*), soapwort (*Saponaria officinalis*), cow cockle (*Saponaria vaccaria*) and broomweed (*Gutierrezia sarothrae*) contain *saponins* and have caused serious toxicity problems in sheep and cattle. Although common British plants, including Christmas and Easter Rose (*Helleborus niger*) and horse chestnut trees (*Aesculus hippocastanum*) contain saponins, poisoning of livestock is rarely seen.

Members of the *Cruciferae* may contain mustard oil glycocides, including charlock (*Sinapsis arvensis*) and wild radish (*Raphanus raphanistrum*) and can cause severe colic and diarrhoea.

In Texas, abnormal leaf flower or spurge (*Phyllanthus abnormis*) causes poisoning if young green plants are eaten, although the toxin is degraded by drying. Affected animals are lethargic, unthrifty and anorexic and develop diarrhoea. The plant is also suspected of causing hepatogenous photosensitisation.

All parts of allamanda (*Allamanda cathartica, A. blanchetti*) are poisonous (particularly the sap and roots), acting as gastrointestinal tract irritants with resultant excessive salivation, ruminal atony, abdominal cramps, diarrhoea, dehydration and electrolyte imbalance on digestion. There are also minor cardiotoxic effects and the sap can cause skin and eye irritation. It is widely naturalised and cultivated as an ornamental in warm, tropical and subtropical climates around the world, including Australia.

Severe diarrhoea is produced in South African goats consuming large amounts of bitterbush (*Chrysocoma ciliate*).

Meadow saffron or autumn crocus (*Colchicum autumnale*) has poisoned goats. All parts of the plant are poisonous, especially the corms and seeds, which contain high levels of the alkaloids colchicine and colchiceine. These are absorbed slowly, so that clinical signs may be delayed several hours – severe diarrhoea, colic, salivation, depression, incoordination, collapse and death. Colchicine is excreted in milk, so kids may be poisoned.

Plants toxic to the nervous system

Many different plant species are associated with the development of nervous signs in livestock. They affect the nervous system in various ways, including stimulation, depression, tremors, convulsions, paresis, paralysis and abnormal behaviour. Although nervous disease associated with plant toxity is regularly reported in cattle and sheep, it is only sporadically reported in goats. Most reported incidents in the United Kingdom, as with the majority of plant poisonings, involve goats gaining access to garden plants. In North America and Australia, range animals are exposed to plants such as bitterweed (*Hymenoxys odorata*), pingue or Colorado rubberweed (*Hymenoxys richardsoni*), coyotillo (*Karwinskia humboldtiana*), *Astragulus* spp., guajillo (*Acacia berlanderi*), caltrop (*Kallstroemia hirsutissima*) and milkweeds (*Asclepias*), which are all capable of poisoning the nervous system. In Australia, sheep have shown neurological signs after grazing branched onion weed (*Trachyandra divaricata*), Jimson weed or thornapple (*Datura stramonium*), long-spined thornapple (*D. ferox*), native tobacco (*Nicotiana suavolens*) and tree tobacco (*N. glauca*), *Stypandra* spp. and *Ipomoea* spp. Blue-green algae can also produce neurotoxins.

In addition to toxins, which have direct pathogenic effects, some plants can induce specific diseases through metabolic or dietary mechanisms:

- Toxic plants that cause *hepatic neurotoxicity* (aimless walking, head pressing, ataxia, blindness, coma) include those containing pyrrolizidine alkaloids (see this chapter).
- Many plants containing *cyanogenic glycosides* (see this chapter) also cause neurotoxicity.
- *Hypocalcaemia* can be induced by exposure to plants high in oxalate (see this chapter).
- A number of ferns and related species contain thiaminase I: horsetail (*Equisetum* spp.), bracken (*Pteridium aquilinum*) and common bracken fern (*Pteridium esculentum*). Normally ruminants are fairly resistant to thiamin deficiency, because rumen microbes provide the animal with sufficient amounts of thiamin, so that *polioencephalomalacia* (see Chapter 12) is more likely in horses grazing plants containing thiaminase or from eating bedding or hay containing these plants.

Nardoo (*Marsilea drummondii*) is an Australian fern that can contain thiaminase activity up to one hundred times that of bracken fern and is responsible for the deaths of sheep in Australia and New Zealand. Rock fern (*Cheilanthes sieberi*) is another Australian fern with a high level of thiaminase activity. Ruminants grazing on summer cypress or fireweed (*Kochia scoparia*) in desert regions of the south-western United States have developed polioencephalomalacia, but it is unclear whether this effect is due to the presence of a thiaminase or a hepatotoxin, which interferes with thiamin utilisation as infected animals develop liver necrosis. Signs of polioencephalomalacia include disorientation and wandering, head-pressing, sudden onset blindness, opishotonus, nystagmus and convulsions.

Hemlock (poison hemlock) (*Conium maculatum*)

All parts of hemlock contain a number of poisonous alkaloids that act on the nervous system producing paralysis, convulsions and death from respiratory paralysis. Signs usually appear within an hour after an animal eats the plant. Animals die from respiratory paralysis in 2 to 3 hours.

Goats are more resistant than cattle to poisoning, but may develop a craving for the plant.

Clinical signs

- Initial stimulation, followed by depression.
- Salivation and regurgitation, ruminal atony, signs of abdominal pain.
- Diarrhoea.
- Tachypnea and rapid weak pulse, followed by respiratory paralysis.
- Muscle tremors, lack of coordination, difficulty in moving, convulsions.
  Convulsions are more common with hemlock water dropwort
- Death.
- Skeletal deformities or cleft palate occur in kids when goats eat hemlock between 30 and 60 days gestation. These are similar to the deformities induced by lupine poisoning.

Hemlock water dropwort (water hemlock, water dropwort) (*Oenanthe crocata*)

Hemlock water dropwort is the most toxic plant in Britain to both humans and animals and is a particular risk after ditching operations have exposed the poisonous roots (often referred to as 'dead man's fingers'). The toxic principle is oenathetoxin, a polyunsaturated higher alcohol, which is unaffected by drying or storage. Very small amounts cause death.

Clinical signs

- Salivation, dilated pupils.
- Respiratory distress.
- Spasmodic convulsions.
- Collapse and death.
- Animals that do not die may develop diarrhoea for two days, then slowly return to normal.

Cowbane or northern water hemlock (*Cicuta virosa*)

Cowbane contains a convulsant poison, cicutoxin, particularly in the roots, but also in the stems and leaves. Signs of poisoning include vomiting, salivation, abdominal pain, muscular spasms, violent convulsions and death from asphyxia. Animals eating a sublethal dose will recover if not stressed.

Fool's parsley (*Aethusa cynapium*)

Common in pastures in Britain, but generally unpalatable, although poisoning has been reported in goats in Holland with clinical signs of ataxia, hyperpnoea, panting and indigestion.

Locoweeds and poison peas

A small number of species of plants, mostly in the genera *Fabaceae*: Oxytropis and Astragalus in North America and Swainsona in Australia, produce swainsonine, a phytotoxin harmful to livestock. Other range plants producing swainsonine include *Ipomoea* spp., *Turbina* spp. and *Sida* spp. The North American species of *Oxytropis* and *Astragalus* are often called locoweed. They are rare in Britain and unlikely to cause poisoning in goats, but are recognised as some of the most poisonous plants in North America. *Ipomoea carnea* caused neurological disease in goats in Mozambique.

Chronic ingestion of large amounts of swainsonine produces a lysosomal storage disease, alpha-mannosidosis, known as *locoism* (swainsonine disease, loco disease) in North America and *pea struck* in Australia. Swainsonine inhibits a lysosomal enzyme alpha–mannosidase, particularly neurons and epithelial cells to this genus. Locoweeds are relatively palatable to goats once they have become habituated to them and some individual animals will seek them out. Goats will recover if prevented from further intake of the plants early in the disease as the vacuolation resolves, but some irreversible and permanent neurologic damage may occur with more chronic intake. Clinical signs appear 6 to 8 weeks after the onset of grazing – generalised depression, intention tremors, proprioceptive defects, hind limb weakness, ataxia and partial paresis – with death 4 to 6 weeks later if ingestion is prolonged.

Experimentally, *Astragalus* spp. have been shown to effect fetal and placental development in goats. The placenta is most susceptible during the first 90 days of pregnancy. Some species of *Astragalus*, including a few that produce swainsonine, act as selenium accumulators. This has led to confusion between swainsonine poisoning and selenium poisoning (see Chapter 8) due to this genus.

An acute neurologic condition caused by nitro-containing compounds in *Astagalus* spp. has been demonstrated experimentally in goats – depression, anorexia, recumbency, weakness and death in 1 to 2 days. Less severe cases developed a pronounced ataxia, particularly evident in the hind limbs and which persisted for up to a year after removal from the plant.

Black nightshade (*Solanum nigrum*)

Black nightshade has a worldwide distribution. All parts of the plant, particularly the green, unripe berries, contain the glycoalkaloid solanine. The toxic content of the leaves increases as the plant matures. It also contains nitrates and nitrates in varying amounts, which may contribute to its toxic effects. Animals show severe abdominal pain, vomiting, depression and staggering movements.

Laburnum (*Laburnum anagyroides*)

Although goats appear to be rarely affected, laburnum is a very toxic plant and goats are thus at risk, particularly if fed trimmings or grazing under trees in gardens. All parts of the tree, particularly the bark and seeds, contain a quinolizidine alkaloid, cystisine, a nicotinic receptor agonist, which effects the nervous system, causing incoordination, muscle tremors convulsive movements, coma and death if large amounts are eaten, together with signs relating to the gastrointestinal system, including abdominal pain, vomiting and diarrhoea.

Common sorrel (*Rumex acetosa*), sheep's sorrel or sourgrass (*Rumex acetosella*) and rhubarb (*Rheum rhaponticum*)

These contain varying amounts of oxalates. Acute poisoning causes hypocalcaemia with clinical signs of depression, inappetence, muscular tremors, ataxia, staggering, dyspnea, paralysis, recumbency and death (see this Chapter). Although goats often seem to eat small amounts of rhubarb with impunity, there are also reports of animals being poisoned after eating rhubarb leaves.

Potato (*Solanum tuberosum*)

Potatoes contain toxic glycoalkaloids, including solanine and chaconine. Solanine is also found in other plants in the family *Solanaceae*. Most poisoning of ruminants has involved green potatoes, as a result of eating sprouting tubers or tubers that have been exposed to light. Poisoned animals show nervous signs including restlessness, incoordination and convulsions or may be found dead.

Larkspur poisoning (*Delphinium* spp.)

Although toxicity and the concentration of toxins vary greatly among species, all larkspurs should be considered to be potentially toxic and all parts of the plant should be considered toxic. Larkspurs primarily affect the neuromuscular system. Signs of poisoning include salivation, arched back, stiff gait, tremors, collapse and death within 3 to 4 hours from either paralysis of the respiratory system or asphyxiation caused by bloating or vomiting. Toxic alkaloid concentrations are highest in the spring after flowering and gradually decrease as the plant matures.

Cycad poisoning (*Cycas* spp., *Bowenia* spp., *Macrozamia* spp., *Lepidozamia* spp., *Zamia* spp.)

Various tropical plants of the genera *Cycas*, *Bowenia*, *Macrozamia* and *Zamia* produce a toxic glycoside, cycasin, in the nuts, leaves and young shoots. Natural poisoning of goats has been reported from Australia and the disease has been produced experimentally. Chronic poisoning causes ataxia and incoordination, particularly of the hind limbs, with knuckling, abnormal placement of feet and stumbling due to demyelination and axonal degeneration in the spinal cord white matter. Hepatotoxicity has been demonstrated experimentally in goats.

Milkweeds (*Asclepia* spp.)

Milkweeds are generally only eaten if no other forage is available, but retain their toxicity in hay. They contain a number of toxins – resinoids, alkaloids and cardiac glycosides. The cause of neurotoxicity is unknown, but ingestion produces clinical signs within a few hours – depression, weakness, staggering gait, laboured respiration, tetanic convulsions, dilated pupils, coma and death.

Caltrop (*Tribulus terrestris*)

Caltrop causes hepatogenous photosensitisation disease ('yellow big head', 'geeldikkop') in Australia, California and South Africa (see this chapter) and nitrate poisoning. Chronic ingestion is associated with outbreaks of a nervous disorder – progressive and irreversible assymetrical hindquarter paresis, when the plant is eaten in the months following periods of drought. Ingestion of the related *Tribulus micrococcus* (yellow vine) has been associated with a transient ataxia of sheep.

Rayless goldenrod or jimmyweed (*Isocoma pluriflora*) is a native plant of Texas, Arizona and New Mexico containing tremetol toxins. White snakeroot (*Ageratina altissima*) also contains tremetone toxins, which have been shown experimentally to be potent myotoxins in goats. Poisoned animals are depressed, anorexic and reluctant to move and develop violent trembling when forced to move. The skeletal muscle and myocardial lesions are due to diffuse and severe muscle degeneration and necrosis with subsequent fibrosis and atrophy. Some animals become tachypnoeic and tachycardic with ascites and hydrothorax. Secondary poisoning of nursing neonates by the toxins or one of their metabolites excreted in milk has been reported, sometimes without apparent maternal toxicity and this represents a potential risk to humans drinking the milk.

Phalaris staggers is an incoordination syndrome associated with the ingestion of phalaris (*Phalaris aquatica*), which contains dimethyltryptamine alkaloids. Goats can be affected by phalaris toxicity, although they appear to be less vulnerable than sheep. There are also two potentially related forms of phalaris 'sudden death' syndrome, a cardiac form, possibly caused by acute hydrocyanic acid toxicity in combination with nitrate poisoning and other potentially toxic compounds and a neurological polioencephalomalacia-like syndrome. Sheep that survive exhibit blindness, wandering behaviour, head pressing, tremors, excess salivation and general depression.

Blue-green algae (cyanobacteria) can produce neurotoxins as well as hepatotoxins and skin allergens (see this chapter) Poisoned animals develop muscle tremors and staggering within 30 minutes of drinking toxic water, followed by recumbency, coma and death, usually within 24 hours. Animals may be found dead. Animals that survive longer develop liver damage, jaundice, diarrhoea and photosensitisation, dying within 1 to 2 weeks.

Plants that cause abortions and fetal defects

In Britain, goats are very unlikely to be exposed to plants with teratogenic properties. This compares to the rangelands of the United States, where it has been estimated that approximately 1% of livestock are born with birth defects from maternal ingestion of teratogenic plants. Where plants with known teratogenic effects are present in pastures, the access of pregnant animals should be restricted and only non-pregnant animals grazed. The fetus is generally most susceptible to teratogenic effects during the first third of pregnancy. Plant toxic components cross the placenta, resulting in physical deformities, fetal resorption, abortion and stillbirth. Many of these plants are also responsible for other acute or toxic poisoning. Plants from the following genera have been identified as having teratogenic effects: *Veratrum*, *Lupinus*, *Conium*, *Nicotiana*, *Astragalus* and *Solanum*.

At least one alkaloid (anagyrine) found in lupins (*Lupinus* spp.) is teratogenic. The proposed mechanism of action for *Lupinus*-induced skeletal defects has been attributed to reduction in fetal movement over a protracted time during specific stages of gestation, resulting in leg deformities and spinal curvatures, with abnormal tendon and ligament development. A cleft palate may sometimes develop as a result of mechanical interference by the tongue between the palatal shelves at the programmed time of closure. Anagrine is found in the milk of lactating animals. The mechanism of action of the teratogenic effects of hemlock (*Coninum maculatum*) and tobacco (*Nicotiana* spp.) is believed to be identical.

Plants of *Veratum* spp., such as false hellebore (*Veratrum californicum*) (see also page 300), produce a variety of teratogenic effects in kids born to dams that ingested the plant early in gestation, depending on the stage of embryonic development. Severely deformed kids may result in dystocia. Day 14: cyclopia and other eye deformities, including anophthalmia; congenital deformities of the head (monkey-faced kids) – with underdeveloped upper and protruding lower jaws, a proboscis-like nose, harelip and hydrocephaly; days 17–19: tracheal stenosis; days 28–31: shortened metatarsal and metacarpal bones. Several *Solanum* spp. contain similar steroidal alkaloids to *Veratrum* spp. and experimentally have produced similar defects.

When fed to excess over a long period, the goitrogenic properties of kale are reported to cause infertility in cattle and sheep by suppression of oestrus, reduced conception rate, embryonic mortality and stillbirth. In a herd of goats in France, kale was suspected of causing the birth of mummified or weak, non-viable kids 5–15 days after the expected parturition date.

Although cattle may abort after eating *Pinus* spp., such as ponderosa and juniper pines, goats and deer are apparently unaffected. Similarly, although poisoning of goats by milk vetch, locoweed (*Astragulus* spp.) occurs (see this chapter), abortion is not generally recognised.

Perennial broomweed (*Gutierrezia sarothrae*) is a toxic plant that occurs throughout much of western United States and northern Mexico. Goats have a relatively high resistance to poisoning but abortion, stillbirths, weak offspring and retained placentae can occur as the result of chronic poisoning.

Bitterbos (bitter bush) (*Chrysocoma ciliate*) produces alopecia with photosensitisation in kids whose dams have consumed the plant during pregnancy.

Plants causing mechanical injury

Plant structural features like awns, sharp barbs, spines, thorns, or trichomes – hairs on the leaf often with barbs spines and thorns, which are particularly prevalent in some members of the grass family (*Gramineae*) – reduce feeding by herbivores by restricting the herbivores' feeding rate or by wearing down the molars. These features can cause both internal and external physical or mechanical injury to animals, through ingestion and contact. Plant material can damage the mouth and gums, resulting in ulcers and infection, become lodged in an eye, causing conjunctivitis and corneal ulceration, act as foreign bodies in the nose or throat or form bezoars in the stomach and intestines. Mouth lesions lead to increased salivation, halitosis and dysphagia. Damage may also be caused to the skin or hair. Raphides, sharp needles of calcium oxalate or calcium carbonate in plant tissues, are an additional plant defence mechanism that makes ingestion painful, damages the mouth and oesophagus and permits entry of the plant's toxins. Raphides are found in many species in the families *Araceae* and *Commelinaceae*.

In Britain, only individual animals are likely to be affected, usually by trauma from grass awns or seeds, particularly to the eye, but in extensively grazed animals mechanical injury can be more problematic. In North America, a variety of plants have been implicated: cheatgrass, downy brome (*Bromus tectorum*), cocklebur (*Xanthium* spp.), crimson clover (*Trifolium incarnatum*), foxtail barley, squirreltail grass, wild barley (*Hordeum jubatum*), porcupine or needle grass (*Stipa* spp.), poverty (oat) grass, (*Danthonia spicata*), puncture vine (*Tribulus terrestris*), rip-gut grass (brome) (*Bromus rigidus*), wild oat (*Avena fatua*), sandbur (*Cenchrus* spp.) and creeping (Canada) thistle (*Cirsium arvense*).

> Fields being cut for hay should be checked for contamination by plants that can cause mechanical injury.

The sap from some plants, including the spurges (*Euphorbia* spp.) and buttercups (*Ranunculus* spp.), can irritate the skin, causing inflammation and blistering, and irritate the mouth and pharynx, producing swelling and ulceration. In Britain, a pygmy goat became depressed, inappetent, developed mouth ulcers and drooled excessively after access to giant hogweed (*Heracleum mantegazzianum*), a plant in the family Apiaceae, which contains toxic furanocoumarins in the leaves, roots, stems, flowers, and seeds of the plant. Cuckoo pint or wild arum (*Arum maculatum*) contains conicine-type alkaloids, including conicine, aroine and toxic saponins. Due to its bitter taste, direct ingestion of the plant is rare, but does occur during periods of food shortage or drought. Poisoning results from livestock feeding on the plant while grazing or consumption of contaminated fresh forage. Small amounts of sap from the plant are highly irritant to the skin, mouth and digestive mucosae and its berries are also toxic. Ingestion of plant material causes diarrhoea, sometimes haemorrhagic, trembling, moderate to severe colic, rectal spasm and neurological signs – ataxia, weak hindquarters, collapse, convulsions and opisthotonus. Treatment is symptomatic. There is generally a good prognosis for recovery after removal from the plant.

Mycotoxins

Filamentous fungi such as *Aspergillus*, *Penicillium* and *Fusarium* can contaminate crops in the field or grow on foods during storage if the temperature and humidity are favourable. Mycotoxins are secondary metabolites produced by these fungi. Some fungi produce more than one mycotoxin and some mycotoxins are produced by more than one fungal species. Affected foods often contain more than one mycotoxin. Multiple

toxins can have a synergistic effect. Although there are approximately 300 known harmful mycotoxins, seven are of major concern to livestock keepers – aflatoxin, deoxynivalenol (vomitoxin), ochratoxin, zearaleone, fumonisin, T-2 toxins and PR toxin, together with ergot alkaloids and the silage-associated Roquefortin C and Mycophenolic acid. Mycotoxins found in forages may differ from those found in grains and are of major importance in mycotoxicoses of ruminants.

To some extent, ruminants, including goats, are able to metabolise and detoxify mycotoxins (ochratoxin A, zearalenone, T-2 toxin and deoxynivalenol) in the rumen, conferring a degree of resistance over simple stomached animals. However, not all toxins are degraded or transformed. Only about 10% of aflatoxin is transformed, with 90% being undegraded. Metabolism of mycotoxins in the rumen can result in the production of new and more toxic metabolites – 90% of zearalenone may be converted to a-zearalenol, which is ten times more toxic. Toxin metabolism is generally more efficient in animals with a more neutral rumen pH in comparison to goats on a high grain/low fibre diet, where the rumen pH is more acidic.

Growth, production and fertility can all be affected when goats consume mycotoxin-contaminated feed for extended periods, but this is difficult to quantify in the absence of specific experimental and field data and because of the difficulties in gathering representative feed samples during sampling and in analysing feedstuffs for mycotoxins. Fungal growth is inconsistent and mycotoxins are not uniformly distributed within a feedstuff; large amounts of mycotoxins can be produced in small areas, 'hot-spots', making the mycotoxin concentrations highly variable within the food being sampled.

The response of individual animals to mycotoxins will vary depending on physiological, genetic and environmental factors, the amount ingested and length of exposure.

Clinical signs are often non-specific and will vary depending on the mycotoxin(s) involved and their interactions with other stress factors, but they are likely to be the result of:

■ *Reduced food intake or feed refusal.* As well as the direct effect on the animal, fungal contamination will also reduce the nutritional value of the affected feeds, causing additional economic loss. Goats, being fussy eaters, may refuse unpalatable feed completely.

However, some contaminated feed, particularly conserved fodder, may remain palatable.

- *Reduced nutrient absorption and impaired metabolism.*
- *Suppression of the immune system.*
- *Hormonal changes.*

These lead directly or indirectly to:

- *Reduced food consumption.*
- *Poor rumen function.* Rumen function is likely to be adversely affected by the presence of mycotoxins, with decreased rumen motility, starch digestion and microbial growth.
- *Reduced production* (milk, meat or fibre).
- *Infertility.* In sheep and cattle, zearalenone has been associated with infertility and lower conception rates. In goats, it has been suggested that one cause of swollen vulvas and vaginal or rectal prolapses (see Chapter) could be mycotoxicosis.
- *Intermittent diarrhoea*, possibly haemorrhagic. In dairy cattle, T2-toxin has been associated with gastrointestinal lesions, enteritis, intestinal haemorrhage and haemorrhagic diarrhoea and it has been suggested that herd outbreaks of diarrhoea or haemorrhagic diarrhoea in goats may similarly involve mycotoxins. Mycotoxins and Shiga toxin-producing *E. coli* (STEC) have been implicated in the disease complex *Haemorrhagic Enteritis* in dairy goats in Canada consuming mouldy corn (maize) silage.
- *Non-specific increased disease incidence.* Mycotoxins have a significant immunotoxic potential, depending on the type and degree of exposure, resulting in impaired immune responses and poor response to challenge by disease.
- *Muscle tremors.*

Goats are most likely to be affected by contaminated cereals in hard feed or conserved forages, such as maize (corn) silage. *Ensiled forages* are more likely to be contaminated by moulds and their associated mycotoxins than dry preserved forages such as hay, but poorly stored hay can be contaminated. Poorly made silages, where the fermentation and anaerobic conditions were not strictly controlled, are particularly risky and increasing the storage time gives greater opportunity for fungal growth. Plastic-wrapped bales still permit some oxygen ingression and any damage to the plastic increases the oxygen flow.

Moist or poorly-kept *by-products* such as brewers and distillers grains and fruit pulp have increased potential for fungal growth and *bedding*, such as poor quality straw, can also be contaminated with mycotoxins.

Various *mycotoxin binders* can be added to feed, reducing the exposure of any animals eating them to potentially harmful toxins, but no product currently meets all the characteristics of a desirable binder. Diets can be treated with other decontaminants and animals can be supplemented with *antioxidants, pre-* and *pro-biotics* and other beneficial substances, which may reduce the morbidity and production losses associated with mycotoxicosis.

Forage toxicosis of fungal origin can affect goats as well as sheep and cattle. Fresh grasses can be contaminated by several mycotoxins. These include *tall fescue toxicosis* caused by endophytic alkaloids, *ergotism* and *dicoumarol poisoning* from ingestion of fungal-infected sweet clover and sweet vernal grass (see this chapter). Syndromes of unthriftiness and impaired reproduction associated with *Fusarium*, perennial ryegrass staggers and slobbers syndrome occur in other species of ruminant and could potentially affect goats. Ryegrass staggers and sweet vernal poisoning have been recorded in Britain, but not in goats.

Fescue toxicosis (associated with tall fescue grass, *Festuca arundinacea*) and *ergotism* (generally associated with grasses, rye, triticale and other grains) are both caused by ergot alkaloids, and referred to as '*ergot alkaloid intoxication*'. The primary toxicological effect of ergot alkaloid involves vasoconstriction and/or hypoprolactinaemia. A range of effects are produced by ingestion of ergot alkaloid including poor weight gain, reduced fertility, hyperthermia, convulsions, gangrene of the extremities and death.

Fescue toxicosis of livestock is reported from Australia, New Zealand and the United States, where approximately 90% of tall fescue pastures are infected with a fungal endophyte, *Neotyphodium coenophialum*, that produces harmful toxins, including ergot. Goats rarely exhibit the clinical signs recorded in other species, possibly because of their selective feeding behaviour and ability to detoxify ergot alkaloids in the liver. Tall fescue is often unpalatable to goats, but they will eat it in the absence of other food, during early spring growth and after a hard frost. Few studies have assessed fescue toxicosis in goats, but, experimentally, reduced weight gain has been demonstrated. However, in other studies, weight gain and body condition score were not affected. Anecdotally, reproductive problems such as low conception rates, delayed parturition, leading to oversized kids, weak uterine contractions, failure of cervical dilation and poor offspring survival have been reported but these remain to be substantiated and goats often appear to successfully breed, give birth and lactate while consuming a diet high in fescue pastures and hay.

In Europe, intoxications of livestock with ergot toxins have largely been associated with cereals. Ergotism, caused by the fungus *Claviceps purpurea*, is visible and infects the outside of the plant seed.

In North America, consumption of clovers and other legumes parasitised by the fungus *Rhizoctonia leguminicola* can cause excessive salivation ('*slobbers disease*') in livestock. The fungus produces an alkaloidal mycotoxin, slaframine. Goats metabolise the toxin more effectively than cattle and thus have a shorter salivary response. Slaframine passes into milk and is thus a potential hazard for lactatating kids and humans drinking the milk or consuming milk products.

Ryegrass staggers, due to intoxication with an indole-diperpene, Lolitrem B, and metabolites from the fungal endophyte *Neotyphodium lolii*, is a nervous disorder of cattle, sheep, horses and deer eating perennial ryegrass (*Lolium perenne*), which has not been recorded in goats, although they may be susceptible to the disease. Goats may be protected by their grazing/browsing habits, which mean they are less likely to graze close to the ground so they are less exposed to the tremogenic fungal toxin, which occurs mainly in the leaf sheaths at ground level.

Mouldy sweet potato (*Ipomoea batatus*) toxicity

Mouldy sweet potatoes have killed cattle in the United States and the United Kingdom when infested with the fungus *Fusarium solani*, which produces the furanoterpenoid pneumotoxin 4-ipomeanol. Acute respiratory distress occurs within a day of ingesting the toxin, with death from anoxia in 2 to 5 days. Mild cases will recover without treatment.

The leaves and seeds of purple or perilla mint (*Perilla frutescens, P. maculatta*), found in the southern United States and New Zealand, contains a ketone pneumotoxin, which cause pulmonary oedema and pleural effusion, dyspnoea and acute death. Goats are susceptible, but rarely eat a toxic amount.

Lupinosis results from the ingestion of a mycotoxin associated with *Diaporthe toxica* fungus growing on lupine plants (*Lupinus* spp.) (see this chapter).

The three main grasses that cause a tremorgenic syndrome due to the presence of indole-diterpenoid alkaloids are *Paspalum* spp., *Cynodon dactylon* and *Lolium perenne*. Poisoning by consumption of Bermuda grass (*C. dactylon*) infected with *Claviceps cynodontis* has been reported in cattle in Uruguay, Argentina, the United States and South Africa and in horses in California and has been demonstrated experimentally in goats. Dallas grass, Bahia (*Paspalum* spp.), infested by *Claviceps paspali* also causes incoordination and tremors in sheep.

Blue-green algae (cyanobacteria)

Cyanobacteria are Gram-negative bacteria with a thick protective peptidoglycan layer. During warm weather, they grow rapidly in stagnant bodies of water containing a good supply of nutrients, resulting in blooms on the water surface. Growth may be particularly profuse in water enriched by fertiliser runoff from adjacent fields. During the winter, they persist in the sediment of lakes and reservoirs, providing the inoculum for the next year's bloom. Bloom-forming cyanobacteria synthesise a variety of cyanotoxins, including neurotoxins, hepatotoxins and skin allergens. These toxins are released into the water when cells die. In the United Kingdom, the most important species are *Microcystis aeruginosa*, *Anabaena* spp., *Aphanizomenon* and *Oscillatoria* spp.

Goats are susceptible to poisoning and can be poisoned by drinking water containing the algae, or where algal death has released toxins into the water, or by ingestion of algae found as dried mats on the shore. Animals may succumb to haemorrhagic shock and be found dead, close to the water. Poisoned animals develop muscle tremors and staggering within 30 minutes of drinking toxic water, followed by recumbency, coma and death, usually within 24 hours. Animals that survive longer and develop liver damage with intrahepatic haemorrhage and diffuse centrilobular hepatocellular degeneration, are weak, ataxic and anorexic with gastrointestinal signs – ruminal atony, abdominal pain, jaundice and haemorrhagic diarrhoea – and generally die within 1 to 2 weeks. Animals that recover may show hepatogenous photosensitisation.

Treatment is symptomatic and supportive, including intravenous fluids, corticosteroids and calcium.

M. aeruginosa can produce both neurotoxins (lipopolysaccharides) and hepatotoxins (microcystins). Microcystins, which are the most common cyanobacterial toxins found in water and the ones most likely to cause poisoning, are extremely stable in water, surviving in both warm and cold water and tolerating radical changes in water chemistry.

Anabaena spp. produce alkaloid neurotoxins (anatoxins and saxatoxins), which cause muscle weakness, loss of coordination, convulsions and paralysis similar to organophosphorus poisoning by acting as an agonist of acetylcholine on the nicotinic acetylcholine receptor. Death is caused by respiratory paralysis.

Further reading

General

Angus, K.W. (2007) In: *Plant Poisoning in Britain and Ireland. Diseases of Sheep* (ed. Aitken, I.), 4th Edition, pp. 405-423. Wiley-Blackwell, Oxford.

Bischoff, K. and Smith, M.C. (2011) Toxic plants of the Northeastern United States. *Vet. Clin. North Amer.: Food Anim. Pract.*, **27** (2), 459–480.

Botha, C.J. and Penrith, M.-L. (2008) Poisonous plants of veterinary and human importance in Southern Africa. *J. Ethnopharmacol.*, **119**, 549–558.

Burrows, G.E. and Tyrl, R.J. (2013) *Toxic Plants of North America*, 2nd Edition. Wiley-Blackwell, Iowa.

Clarke, E.G.C. (1975) *Poisoning in Veterinary Practice*. Association of the British Pharmaceutical Industry, London.

Cooper, M.R. and Johnson, A.W. (1984) *Poisonous Plants in Britain*. MAFF Book 161, HMSO, London.

Ensley, S. and Rumbeiha, W. (2012) Ruminant toxicology diagnostics. *Vet. Clin. North Amer.: Food Anim. Pract.*, **28** (3), 557–564.

FDA Poisonous Plant Database. Available at: http://www.accessdata.fda.gov/scripts/plantox/. Provides access to references in the scientific literature (primarily print literature through about 2007) describing studies and reports of the toxic properties and effects of plants and plant parts.

Knight, A.P. (2007) *A Guide to Poisonous House and Garden Plants*. Teton NewMedia, Jackson, WY.

Knight, A.P. and Walter, R.G. (2001) *A Guide to Plant Poisoning of Animals in North America*. Teton NewMedia, Jackson, WY.

McKenzie, R. (2012) *Australia's Poisonous Plants, Fungi and Cyanobacteria: A Guide to Species of Medical and Veterinary Importance*. CSIRO Publishing, Collingwood, Australia.

Payne, J. and Murphy, A. (2014) Plant poisoning in farm animals. *In Pract.*, **36**, 455–465.

Seawright, A.A. (1984) Goats and poisonous plants. *Proc. Univ. Sydney Post Grad. Comm. Vet. Sci.*, **73**, 544–547.

Spratling, R. (1980) Is it plant poisoning? *In Pract.*, **2**, 22–31.

Stegelmeier, B.L. (2011) Identifying plant poisoning in livestock: diagnostic approaches and laboratory tests. *Vet. Clin. North Amer.: Food Anim. Pract.*, **27** (2), 407–417.

Wagstaff, D.J. (2008) *International Poisonous Plants Checklist: An Evidence-Based Reference*, CRC Press.

Miscellaneous plant poisons

Andrews, A.H., Giles, C.J., Thomsett, L.R. (1985) Suspected poisoning of a goat by giant hogweed. *Vet Rec.*, **116** (8), 205–207.

Baker, I. (1993) Poison, laburnum. *In Pract.*, **15** (1), 20.

Barbosa, R.R. *et al.* (2008) Toxicity in goats caused by oleander (*Nerium oleander*). *Res. Vet. Sci.*, **85**, 279–281.

Boermans, H.J., Ruegg, P.L. and Leach, M. (1988) Ethylene glycol toxicosis in a Pygmy goat. *J. Am. Vet. Med. Assoc.*, **193** (6), 694–696.

Braun,U., Diener, M., Camenzind, D., Thoma, R. and Flückiger, M. (2000) Enzootic calcinosis in goats caused by golden oat grass (*Trisetum flavescens*). *Vet. Rec.*, **146** (6), 161–162.

Gunn, D. (1992) Poison, water dropwort. *In Pract.*, **14** (5), 203.

Gunn, D. (1992) Poison, cyanobacteria (blue-green algae). *In Pract.*, **14** (3), 132.

Jacob, R.H. and Peet, R.L. (1987) Poisoning of sheep and goats by *Tribulius terrestris* (caltrop). *Australian Vet. J.*, **64** (9), 288–289.

Maia, L.A., de Lucena, R.B., Nobre, V.M., Dantas, A.F., Colegate, S.M. and Riet-Correa, F.J. (2013) Natural and experimental poisoning of goats with the pyrrolizidine alkaloid-producing plant *Crotalaria retusa*. *Vet. Diagn. Invest.*, **25** (5), 592–595.

Mayor, S. (1990) Ragwort poison. *In Pract.*, **12**, 112.

Mayor, S. (1991) Poison, acorns. *In Pract.*, **13** (4), 167.

Mayer, S. (1991) Poison, rhododendron. *In Pract.*, **13** (6), 232.

Mayer, S. (l991) Poison, brassicas. *In Pract.*, **13** (5), 216–217.

Stegelmeier, B.L. (2011) Pyrrolizidine alkaloid-containing toxic plants (*Senecio, Crotalaria, Cynoglossum, Amsinckia, Heliotropium* and *Echium* spp.). *Vet. Clin. North Amer.: Food Anim. Pract.*, **27** (2), 419–428.

Fetal development

Panter, K.E., Welch, K.D., Gardner, D.R. and Green, B.T. (2013) Poisonous plants: effects on embryo and fetal development. *Birth Defects Research. Part C: Embryo Today: Reviews*, **99**, 223–234.

Riet-Correa, F. Medeiros, R.M.T. and Schild, A.L. (2012) A review of poisonous plants that cause reproductive failure and malformations in the ruminants of Brazil. *J. Appl. Toxicol.*, **32**, 245–254.

Milk

Painter, K.E. and James, L.F. (1990) Natural plant toxins in milk: a review. *J. Animal Sci.*, **68**, 892–904.

Mycotoxins

Baines, D.D.S. *et al.* (2011). Characterization of haemorrhagic enteritis in dairy goats and the effectiveness of probiotic and prebiotic applications in alleviating morbidity and production losses. *Fungal Genomics and Biology*, **1** (1), 1000102.

Canty, M.J., Fogarty, U., Sheridan, M.K., Ensley, S.M., Schrunk, D.E. and More, S.J. (2014) Ergot alkaloid intoxication in perennial ryegrass (*Lolium perenne*): an emerging animal health concern in Ireland? *Irish Vet. J.*, **67**, 21.

Iheshiulor, O.O.M., Esonu, B.O., Chuwuka, O.K., Omede, A.A., Okoli, I.C. and Ogbuewu, I.P. (2011) Effects of mycotoxins in animal nutrition: a review. *Asian J. Anim. Sci.*, **5**, 19–33.

Mostrom, M.S. and Jacobsen, B. J. (2011) Ruminant mycotoxicosis. *Vet. Clin. North Amer.: Food Anim. Pract.*, **27** (2), 315–344.

Riet-Correa, F., Rivero, R., Odriozola, E., de Lourdes Adrien, M., Medeiros, R. and Schild, A. (2013) Mycotoxicoses of ruminants and horses. *J. Vet. Diagn. Invest.*, **25** (6), 692–708.

Neurological disease

Finnie, J., Windsor, P. and Kessell, A. (2011) Neurological diseases of ruminant livestock in Australia. II: toxic disorders and nutritional deficiencies. *Australian Vet. J.*, **89**, 247–253.

Nitrate/nitrite poisoning

Jones, T.O. (1988) Nitrate/nitrite poisoning in cattle. *In Pract.*, **10**, 199–203.

Photosensitisation

Qui, J.C. *et al.* (2014) Secondary plant products causing photosensitization in grazing herbivores: their structure, activity and regulation. *Int. J. Molec. Sci.*, **15** (1), 1441–1465.

CHAPTER 22

The geriatric goat

Geriatrics are either animals retired from the milking herd or 'retired' pets, usually owned by hobbyists, often pygmy goats or castrated males. The life span of goats is very variable, but is comparable to that of dogs, with ages of 16 to 18 years being regularly attained by non-milking females and castrated males, although high-yielding dairy animals are considered geriatric by 10 or 11 years old, with 'veteran' classes in the show ring starting at 6 years old.

Geriatric goats present with many of the same age-related problems as other companion animals. Loss of, or excess, body condition, decreased activity, and stiffness or lameness due to arthritis or foot problems are common presenting signs, but, with a little common sense and small adjustments to meet changing needs, the ageing goat can be helped to a longer and more comfortable life.

In older animals, there is likely to be a generalised decrease in immune function and a decreased ability to absorb available nutrients from the gastrointestinal tract, together with an increased susceptibility to parasites, both external and internal. Thus, in addition to a thorough physical examination, it is important for the veterinary surgeon to review nutrition and ensure that preventative health programmes, in particular worming and vaccination, are adequate. In some cases, blood tests for haematology and biochemistry may be indicated to screen for ongoing disease or organ failure.

Although most geriatric goats are being kept purely as pets, there is no legal distinction between them and 'food-producing animals', even if it is the clear intention of the owner that they will never enter the food-chain, so that regulations covering drug supply are exactly the same as for other farm livestock. In the United Kingdom, the cascade should be followed and legally only drugs licensed for use in food-producing animals should be used. The same difficulties arise when treating geriatrics as other classes of goats, so, for instance, it is impossible to follow best anaesthetic practice and still meet legal requirements.

Does can continue to conceive for as long as physiologically possible, providing that they are in good body condition and free from debilitating conditions like arthritis. Productivity gradually diminishes with age, and older does produce fewer offspring, so that single kids are common in does reaching the end of their reproductive life. Older goats are likely to be more prone to pregnancy toxaemia and pregnant does should be monitored carefully to ensure adequate food intake and regular exercise.

Milk production gradually declines with age, after peaking at the 2nd or 3rd lactation. The age at which an individual goat becomes unproductive is highly variable. It is very dependent on the care the animal has received, the work (milk production and parturitions) it has undertaken and the individual's genetic makeup. Some lines of goats remain productive much longer than others. In general, high-yielding dairy goats have a much shorter life span than goats that have been kept as pets and not regularly bred.

Buck fertility also declines with age. Although the male retains normal breeding interest, falling sperm counts may render him infertile and arthritis may prevent him serving the doe. The testicles often show signs of atrophy.

Body condition scoring (see Chapter 9) can be used to assess an animal's condition initially and to monitor changes with time. Loss of weight and muscle mass is common in older animals, but some animals will be overweight because of reduced activity, due to lameness, for instance, without a corresponding decrease in food consumption. However, body scoring should be used sensibly. Because it was originally designed for use in animals in their production years and does not take into account changes in body shape caused by age, older animals may lose condition over their top-line, but still remain in an ideal weight range.

Housing

Changes in management may be required to assist older animals. Older goats may need to be housed separately from the rest of the herd or, at least, individually penned at certain times of the day to ensure that they are not competing with younger, stronger animals for food and shelter. Lameness or stiffness caused by arthritis can decrease both the ability and willingness of an animal to move to food and water.

Older animals are also likely be less tolerant of extremes of weather conditions, because of decreased metabolism, lower body weight and muscle mass, decreased activity, and sparser hair coats. In particular, they will need protection from very cold or wet weather by the provision of warm, dry, draught-free shelter, adequately bedded. In very cold weather or if animals are unwell, the use of blankets or rugs (which are usually well tolerated by goats) is beneficial. Heat lamps can provide additional warmth in cold weather, provided cables and bulbs are out of reach of enquiring mouths.

Nutrition

The nutritional management of older goats is an essential component of their overall care. Dental disease and resulting tooth loss may impair the animal's ability to prehend or masticate food. Animals with impaired movement may be unable or unwilling to reach hay racks and feeders and younger, more aggressive animals may actively stop them feeding. Individual penning or separate feed areas may need to be provided and food and water may need to be brought to the animal, especially if it is recumbent for any length of time.

Goats are fussy eaters at the best of times and generally become more so as they get older, so feeding will have to be tailored to meet the requirements of the individual animal.

A high-quality, easily digested diet, which maintains an adequate fibre intake for correct rumen function, is important, so roughage must still be provided, but

should be finer stemmed and easy to chew. Good quality hay should always be available. When goats can no longer manage long stemmed forage, the next step is to try an equine hay replacer product that combines short-chop high-temperature dried grasses and/or lucerne (alfalfa). Most goats prefer dried, chopped products to pellets.

Increasing calories in a ruminant is generally more challenging than with a monogastric animal. Many goats find dried sugar beet pulp palatable and this is a good source of energy, although low in protein. Others goats prefer soaked beet nuts. Equine products containing a mixture of lucerne (alfalfa) and beet pulp are also available. Soaking feed to a mash or gruel consistency can help make it easier to consume, but will not be eaten by every goat. If the goats are used to eating dairy nuts, fat can be increased in the diet by the addition of a rumen bypass fat.

Vitamin/mineral supplementation is best provided as part of the concentrate ration, but mineral licks should be available for all animals.

Water should be readily accessible, particularly for animals with impaired movement. Warm water during cold weather will encourage consumption.

Older males with a reduced fibre intake will be more susceptible to developing urolithiasis, especially if the cereal intake is increased to try to maintain body weight.

Teeth

Dental problems are common in the older goat. Geriatric goats' teeth should be checked on a regular basis and a thorough dental examination should be undertaken if loss of body condition is the presenting sign in the older animal. As well as difficulty in eating, dental disease can also result in a decrease in water intake as the teeth become sensitive to cold water.

Incisor teeth

Because goats are preferentially browsers and do not graze close to the ground, they do not generally have the same problems with the premature loss of incisor teeth as sheep. The incisors do not usually wear completely down, but, with normal dental work, undergo a change in shape from rectangular to round, develop an elongated appearance and slant further forward as the goat ages, to give the appearance of an undershot jaw. However, with time, and depending on the type of feed and management, the incisors become loose and are eventually lost. Most old goats cope well with loss of incisor teeth, without significant problems eating.

Cheek teeth

Molar teeth are present at birth, erupt continuously throughout life and are worn down during feeding. Uneven wear of the teeth can make chewing and rumination difficult. Any uneven wear of the molars becomes more evident with age. Sharp points or hooks on the teeth may lacerate the inside of the mouth or tongue, causing significant pain, and the goat may try to chew preferentially on one side of the mouth, holding the head to one side when eating. Cud may be found lodged between the teeth and cheek (quidding) or the goat may drop the cud because of pain when chewing. Such animals are often interested in food, but stop eating due to pain. The accumulation of cud in the mouth is often accompanied by a foul smell.

Tooth loss can result from fractures or periodontal disease. Loss of a molar tooth will allow the opposing molar to grow excessively and food may accumulate in the empty socket.

Oral tumours will cause mouth pain, loose incisors or molars and lost teeth – sarcomas, adenocarcinomas, osteomas, fibrosarcomas and fibromas have all been reported from older goats. In contrast, lymphosarcomas are commoner in young adult goats.

Tooth root abscesses may present as firm swellings along the jaw line with or without the presence of a superficial abscess. These abscesses may resolve with the administration of broad-spectrum long-term antibiotic therapy.

Dental treatment

Loosening and/or loss of incisor teeth is easily recognised and molar teeth can be palpated through the cheeks, but visual examination of the molar teeth is difficult because goats have a narrow mouth that does not open very wide, so that careful examination of the cheek teeth almost always requires sedation and some form of mouth gag (sheep gag; self-retaining thoracic retractors or similar) is needed. A small mouth speculum or larnygoscope and a good light source facilitate the examination.

Because the goat chews with a lateral grinding motion, normal molars have sharpened points on the lateral (buccal) aspect of the upper arcade and the medial (lingual) aspect of the lower arcade. These do not need routine removal if they are not causing damage to the oral mucosa or tongue, but larger spurs or points will need reducing. Any flat rasp (with protected corners), dental floats of suitable sizes, orthopaedic bone files or a high-speed dental hand piece with an appropriate burr can be used to file sharp points. Very long points can be cut with pliers, gigli wire or bone cutters, dramatically reducing filing time and thus minimising oral trauma. The goal of filing sharp points is to file only those that protrude above the surrounding teeth or appear to be causing sores inside the cheeks or on the tongue, not to smooth the entire dental arcade. Most loose teeth can be hand-pulled with fingers or pliers. Major extractions are rarely necessary and may be overly traumatic. Following extractions, the opposing teeth will grow long because of lack of wear.

Sedation for dental work

Suitable sedative regimes for goats are discussed in Chapter 24.

Butorphanol 0.07–0.1 mg/kg mixed with *xylazine 0.01–0.03 mg/kg i.v.* provides good sedation and analgesia without general anesthesia. The xylazine can be reversed with antipamezole (or yohimbine) if necessary. See Chapter 24 for other anaesthetic/sedative combinations.

Arthritis

Most old goats eventually develop some degree of arthritis, ranging from a little stiffness on rising to a severely debilitated animal with difficulty in moving. In the United Kingdom, where the *caprine arthritis encephalitis (CAE)* virus infection rate is extremely low, *osteoarthritis* is the most likely cause of lameness in old goats, but blood samples should be taken if CAE infection is suspected.

The hooves of all older goats should be trimmed regularly – any overgrowth will potentially increase the discomfort and lameness and reduction in movement will reduce the natural wear on the hooves. *Chronic laminitis* (see Chapter 7) is relatively common, particularly in old pygmy goats, so it is important to check the depth as well as the overall shape of the hooves, especially the front feet.

In animals suffering from osteoarthritis, *weight management* is a crucial part of the treatment plan. Carrying excess weight will exacerbate the lameness.

Lameness in goats is often very painful, so pain relief/anti-inflammatory treatment should be given as necessary. Non-steroidal anti-inflammatory drugs are effective for the provision of daily pain relief. Goats generally tolerate non-steroidal anti-inflammatory drugs (NSAIDs) well, with none of the gastrointestinal side-effects that can effect dogs, and the drugs are relatively easily to administer orally long-term in tablet or liquid form. Although no NSAIDs are licensed specifically for goats in the United Kingdom, several are licensed for cattle and so can be used under the cascade system, provided the statuatory withhold times are observed. For short-term use, injectable NSAIDs licensed for cattle are suitable (see Table 22.1). For long-term use, oral preparations – tablets, liquid or granules – have proved useful, although not specifically licensed for small ruminants (see Table 22.2). Start with higher doses initially, possibly twice daily with drugs like carprofen, and then continue with a daily maintenance dose. The dose should be reduced to the lowest effective dose. At lower doses, it may be possible to repeat the dose every 24 hours, but animals should be closely monitored.

Like people, arthritic goats feel better when the weather is warm and dry and worse when it is cold and damp, so some goats may need only intermittent or seasonal therapy. Once an animal can move about with a minimum of pain, it is important to provide exercise on a daily basis, especially with pregnant does.

Chondroprotective agents, such as *chondroitin sulphate* and *glucosamine*, are not licensed for use in farm animals, but could theoretically prove useful at doses similar to those used in horses.

The following have all been used empirically in non-lactating pet goats, where permitted, with dose rates extrapolated from those for other species as there are no published results of clinical trials in goats:

- *Polysulphated glycosaminoglycan* (Adequan, Novartis Animal Health) is licensed for use in horses in the United Kingdom and has been used empirically in adult dairy goats (50–80 kg) at a dose rate of *125 mg (1.25 ml) i.m.* weekly, with a single injection every 4–6 months as needed. Large animals may require a bigger amount.

Table 22.1 Injectable NSAIDs.

Drug	Dose	Route
Carprofen	**1.4mg/kg** repeat once after 48–72 hours	s.c. or i.v.
Flunixin meglumine	**2.2 mg/kg** sid for 3–5 days	i.v.
Ketoprofen	**3 mg/kg** sid for 3 5 days	i.m. or i.v.
Meloxicam	**0.2 mg/kg** initially then **0.5 mg/kg** every 36–48 hours	s.c. or i.v.
Tolfenamic acid	**2–4 mg/kg** repeat once after 48 hours	s.c. or i.v.
Phenylbutazone[a]	**4 mg/kg**	i.v.

[a]Phenylbutazone is banned from use in food-producing animals in the EU.

Table 22.2 Oral NSAIDs.

Drug	Dose	Route
Carprofen	**1–2 mg/kg** once daily	Oral
Meloxicam	**0.4 mg/kg** once daily	Oral
Aspirin[a]	**50–100 mg/kg** every 12 hours	Oral
Phenylbutazone[b]	*10 mg/kg* for 2 days, then once daily for 3 days, then every other day or as needed	*Oral*

[a]Aspirin is poorly absorbed from the rumen so relatively high doses are needed. Aspirin is not licensed for use in food-producing animals in the UK.
[b]Phenylbutazone is banned from use in food-producing animals in the EU.

- *Pentosan polysulphate sodium* (Cartrophen, Arthropharm) is also licensed for use in horses and has been used at the dog dose of *3 mg/kg s.c.* weekly for 4 weeks, and then a single injection every 4 to 6 months as necessary. It should not be given concurrently with steroids or non-steroidal anti-inflammatory drugs, including aspirin and phenylbutazone.

- *Sodium hyaluronate*, 20 mg, 2 ml i.v. (Hyonate, Bayer).

Further reading

Wolff, P.L. (2007) The geriatric small ruminant – dental care, body condition scoring and nutrition, *North American Veterinary Conference*, January 13, 2007.

CHAPTER 23

Herd health and biosecurity

Herd health plans

A herd health plan should be produced for each farm, taking into consideration the diseases of greatest concern and their modes of transmission, identifying possible areas of risk and implementing management systems to reduce these risks. The establishment of the plan demonstrates a commitment to the health and welfare of the herd and to the health and safety of the personnel involved with the caring and treatment of the goats. *Biosecurity* underpins the maintenance of a healthy herd.

The plan should aim to:

- Prevent exposure to disease:
  o Keep out any diseases not already present.
- Identify the diseases already on the farm:
  o Treat/control/eradicate diseases already present.
  o Cull affected animals where necessary.
- Protect animals on the farm:
  o By vaccination.
    The plan should include details of vaccines required, the target animals and a protocol for vaccine administration.
  o By drug use.
    Records should be kept of all medicines used, including those administered by a veterinary surgeon.
    Drugs should be correctly labelled and securely stored.
    There must be an effective procedure for identifying treated animals that is known to all farm staff, so that the correct withdrawal times for milk and meat can be observed.

The plan should include:

- A parasite control plan that specifies strategies and worming programs, including target animals and the medicines to be used.

- Protocols for routine foot care.
- In dairy herds, a mastitis action plan to prevent and control mastitis in the herd, including methods for detection and treatment protocols for clinical procedures and procedures for drying off.
- Procedures for the management of casualty animals, including responsibilities and methods of humane slaughter.
- Protocols for kid rearing: nsure kids receive colostrum as soon as possible after birth.

Record keeping should be designed so that the process is easy, whether handwritten or computer-based, and the results purposeful and useful for making strategic management decisions. Records should be maintained of:

- Chronic infectious disease
- Mastitis
- Fertility, reproductive disorders, problems at kidding, including kids born dead
- Foot problems
- Metabolic disorders
- Kid diseases

The plan should be written down and reviewed annually, with veterinary guidance, or more often if problems arise, with changes adopted in response to the monitoring of the health and welfare of the animals in the herd.

Written health plans are a specific requirement of many welfare codes and farm assurance schemes and are often required by the purchaser of the end product (milk, cheese, yoghurt, meat, etc.) and/ or the retailer, particularly the large supermarkets. They act as a reminder for all those concerned of the various procedures to be adopted and are always there as a reference for future consultation.

To be of any lasting use to the farmer, the plan needs to demonstrate and indicate thought in relation to

Diseases of the Goat, Fourth Edition. John Matthews.
© 2016 John Wiley & Sons, Ltd. Published 2016 by John Wiley & Sons, Ltd.

disease, welfare and management and should not just be a 'tick-box exercise' to satisfy the demands of a farm assurance scheme, so it is important to establish from the outset what problems the farmer and the farm staff consider significant. The health plan must be clear and concise and establish objectives and targets, which should be SMART:

- **S**pecific
  Objectives and targets should relate to specific diseases and issues on the particular farm.
- **M**easurable
  Targets should be capable of being measured, so that improvement or deterioration can be easily assessed and obvious.
- **A**chievable
  Targets should be realistic. Gradual sustained improvement is often the most effective way forward.
- **R**elevant
  The most relevant objectives are those that will bring the most benefit.
- **T**ime-based
  The time for objectives and targets to be met should be clearly defined and realistic.
  Progress should be monitored regularly.

Preventing exposure to disease

Starting out

- Buy healthy goats from established goatkeepers where the animals:
  o Have a known health history.
  o Established genetics.
- Ideally the goatkeeper and veterinary surgeon should visit the vendor before the purchase to:
  o Discuss any health problems in the herd, including abortion, neurological disease, chronic wasting, mastitis, diarrhoea and lameness.
  o Examine individual animals; animals with defects or obvious health problems should be rejected.
- Animals from herds belonging to official 'health schemes' which are tested and monitored for specific diseases such as CAE and scrapie have a higher health status than other animals.

Before purchase

- *Check the preventative measures on the vendor's farm,*
  o Vaccination.
  o Deworming (including liver fluke).
- *Consider blood tests for specific diseases.*
  o CAE.
  o Enzootic (*Chlamydophila*) abortion.
  o Screening for Johne's disease is probably not worthwhile because of the number of false negatives during the subclinical and early stages of the clinical disease, although positive serological tests are likely to be significant.
- *Reject* goats vaccinated against orf, Johnes disease and enzootic abortion as vaccination does not guarantee freedom from disease.

Transport

- Animals should only be moved in properly cleaned and disinfected vehicles.
- Avoid sharing transport and mixing animals from different sources.
- Farmers should preferably use their own transport to move the animals.

On arrival

- *Quarantine the new goats.*
  o Preferably for 6 weeks (minimum 28 days).
  o At a distance 2 m away from any building housing goats or sheep.
  o Double fence paddocks with 3 m separation.
  o Handle/feed after caring for existing stock, with dedicated clothing and footwear.
  o Use disinfectant footbaths.
  o Manure from the quarantine area should be composted for 12 months before being spread on fields.
- *Observe quarantined animals regularly.*
  Diseases to watch for:
- Johne's disease
- Caseous lymphadenitis (CLA)
- Caprine arthritis encephalitis virus (CAEV)
- Scrapie
- Mycoplasma (out-with the UK)
- Chlamydophila
- Toxoplasmosis
- Respiratory disease, including tuberculosis
- Orf
- Gastrointestinal parasites
- Ectoparasites – lice, mange
- Footrot

Maintaining a herd free from CAE, Johne's and CLA provides an excellent basis for future sales of goats locally and abroad. All three diseases are debilitating, chronic and result in marked loss of income through decreased production and culling of goats.

- *If the goats have been grazed*:
  o Treat with an *effective* anthelmintic on arrival. The aim is to *deworm* the goats not just give an anthelmintic! Check egg counts on faecal samples.
  o The best current advice is to treat introduced goats with the correct dose per weight of a *combination of drugs from all three anthelmintic groups, for example Albendazole 20 mg/kg, Levamisole 12 mg/kg and Ivermectin 400 ug/kg* or a *combination of moxidectin and levamisole* (given as <u>separate drenches</u> *straight after each other*; do not mix drugs together). Moxidectin should not be used for goats producing milk for human consumption and prolonged withholding times are required for other macrocyclic lactones.

    Monepantel (Zolvix, Elanco AH) can be used as a quarantine dose at *5 mg/kg, 2 ml/10 kg (2 times the sheep dose rate)*.
  o Yard or house animals on concrete for 48 hours after treatment to ensure that any viable nematode parasite eggs have been expelled before the animals go on to pasture.
  o Goats that are to be kept extensively should then be placed in a field that has recently been grazed by the farm's original goats, so that nematode eggs are likely to be present. Any resistant nematode eggs passed by the newcomers will be diluted out by eggs already on the pasture.
- *Ectoparasites*
  o Treatment with an avermectin will also help control sucking lice and partially control biting lice, but only topical treatments are totally effective against biting lice. Animals should be checked carefully for lice and treated with a pyrethroid pour-on preparation or eprinectin (see Chapter 10) where necessary.
  o Fibre goats should be shorn on arrival, dipped and isolated. If shearing and dipping are not possible, a pyrethroid pour-on preparation should be used, but these can take up to 6 weeks before they are fully dispersed across the coat.

- *Foot care*
  o The feet of all goats should trimmed on entry to the quarantine facilities and carefully inspected.
  o *Dichelobacter nodosus*, the bacterium responsible for footrot, can be carried by apparently sound goats, particularly in dry weather.
  o Any goats where footrot is suspected should be footbathed at least twice during the quarantine period, using a 10% zinc sulphate solution footbath (Chapter 7).
- *Vaccination*
  o Purchased animals should be vaccinated according to their new herd's protocols.

Replacements or additions to an existing herd should have a similar, or preferably higher, disease status than the animals already in the herd.

Existing herds

Possible exposure to disease can be reduced by maintaining a *closed herd*, using artificial insemination and/or embryo transfer to introduce new genetics. Embryos and semen should be sourced from donors that are certified free of infectious disease, particularly CAE and scrapie.

Most herds will need to introduce new animals, particularly males, at some time. A quarantine and testing programme should be developed for all incoming animals, as discussed above.

Showing animals is a high-risk activity. Any animals taken to shows should be isolated when they return to the farm and throughout the show season. At the end of the show season, they should undergo quarantine and testing before reintroduction to the herd.

Other animals already on the holding or coming on to the holding
- Sheep potentially pose a serious health risk to goats because of disease shared between the two species (external and internal parasites, infectious abortions, scrapie, footrot, etc.) and should be kept well separated from goats.
- Cattle diseases such as Johne's disease and some internal parasites represent a risk to goats.
- Feral cats pose a problem because of diseases such as toxoplasmosis. Aim to prevent cats breeding and

maintain a stable, limited population of neutered animals for rodent control.

Dogs can transmit eggs of the tapeworm *Taenia multiceps*, which are ingested by the goat, producing 'gid' (Chapter 12). Dogs should be prevented from consuming raw goat or sheep brain and offal and the products of abortion.

Cats and dogs should be wormed regularly.

- Avoid stacking poultry waste near the goat unit.
- Horses represent a low risk and mixed grazing may be beneficial.

Milk and colostrum brought on to the farm

- Diseases like CAE can be introduced with milk or colostrum. As a general rule, goat milk or colostrum from goats out-with the herd should never be fed.
- Cow's colostrum can be used as an alternative to goat colostrum as part of a disease eradication programme, but can itself present a risk of introducing infection and should be introduced with care.

Feed and bedding

- Purchased feed and bedding, such as hay and straw, can be responsible for introducing diseases like salmonellosis and toxoplasmosis.
- Buying from arable farms, without livestock, is likely to be safer than obtaining supplies from livestock farms.

Water

- Piped mains water is safer than water from natural sources, such as streams, which may have been grazed by other animals upstream.

Other biosecurity measures

- *Approved disinfectants* should be available and suitable facilities for cleaning and disinfecting boots/clothing, vehicles and machinery.
- *Staff* who live or work on other farms, such as relief milkers, should wear dedicated clothing kept on the farm.
- *Limit visitors to the farm*.
  o Farm access should be restricted to only those people deemed essential.
  o Visitors should wear boots or disposable overshoes, disinfect them prior to entering the farm and

preferably not have been on another farm for at least 24 hours. Boots (or disposable overshoes) and single-use disposable overalls should be supplied by the farm to ensure compliance.

- *Limit vehicle traffic.*
  o Only vehicles essential for farm business should be allowed on the farm.
  o Provide a concrete area on the boundary of the farm to disinfect tyres and clean vehicles and suitable delivery and pick-up points away from livestock.
- *Equipment* brought on to the farm, such as scanning and shearing equipment, poses a threat to biosecurity. Veterinary instruments should be sterilised between farms. In particular, instruments that may be contaminated with blood should be thoroughly cleaned and disinfected.
- *Control the access of wildlife, rodents, birds and domestic animals* to the farm. In particular, restrict their access to feed and bedding stores. Where appropriate, insect populations may also need controlling.
  o Buildings should be kept in good repair so that animals and birds cannot gain access.
  o All waste food should be stored in a manner that will not attract vermin.

Identification of disease already on the farm

An assessment needs to be made of the health status of the herd with respect to *chronic infectious diseases*.

Consider:

- Current herd status with respect to:
  o Johne's disease
  o Caprine arthritis encephalitis virus (CAEV)
  o Caseous lymphadenitis (CLA)
  o Mycoplasma (out-with the UK)
- Have these been confirmed by:
  o Serology?
  o Post-mortem examination?
- What is the level of infection?
  o Serological testing and segregation or culling may be cost-effective in herds with a low incidence of disease, whereas hygiene and isolation of infected animals, together with vaccination, where applicable, will be the main strategies in heavily infected herds.

Standard procedures for managing disease risks that have been identified can then be set out.

Control of chronic infectious diseases

- What are the goals for the herd?
- Are these achievable within the economic framework of the farm?

  Pasteurised rearing programmes and, in particular, serological and/or post-mortem surveillance have financial implications for the farm and need to be off-set by potential benefits such as increased production, value of young stock sales and a longer productive life of the herd.
- Are records adequate to allow prevention and management of chronic diseases?

  o Individual animal identification (tattoos, ear tags, neck tags, etc.) is needed before permanent accurate records can be maintained to monitor infectious disease status.

  o Management decisions regarding disease control grouping, treatment, production and culling should be based on accurate lifelong records on each animal.
- What is the risk from other species, particularly sheep (small ruminant lentiviruses, scrapie, caseous lymphadenitis, Johne's disease) and cattle (Johne's disease)?

  Control programmes need to include all species potentially infected. Caprine and ovine lentivirus control programmes should be considered together as part of a herd approach to CAEV control.
- Is the herd closed or are replacements bought in?

Bought-in animals both create additional risk and are at risk themselves if they come into an infected environment.

Control strategies

Control strategies are discussed under the sections for individual diseases. Different diseases will need different strategies:

- Serological testing and segregation or culling for CAEV.
- Serological testing and segregation or culling for herds with a low incidence of CLA; improved management and hygiene, vaccination and isolation of affected animals in herds heavily infected with CLA.
- Identification and culling of infected animals, improved management and hygiene and vaccination of kids (if not reared separately from the rest of the herd) for Johne's disease.
- Milking hygiene measures, routine milk cultures and segregation for mycoplasma control.

Kid rearing

Because most of the important chronic infectious diseases of goats are acquired shortly after birth, a sensible common kid-rearing strategy to minimise infection of the newly born kids will help control CAEV, Johne's disease, CLA and mycoplasmosis. A protocol for rearing kids on farms with chronic infective diseases is shown in Table 23.1.

Table 23.1 Rearing kids on farms with chronic infectious diseases.

- Batch-mate and induce parturition using prostaglandins to ensure attended birth.
- Remove kids from dams at birth before suckling or licking by the dam.
- Use teat tape on dams close to parturition as a backstop to prevent suckling if birth is not attended immediately.
- Isolate kids and house separately from adult goats.
- Feed cows' colostrum or goats' colostrum from a CAE and Johne's seronegative animal. Do not pool colostrum from multiple animals. Colostrum can be collected and frozen in small feeding size portions for later use.
- Commercial colostrum products can be used, but may not promote adequate levels of circulating IgG antibodies.
- Rear on pasteurised cows' milk, or calf, or kid milk replacer.
- **If goats' milk is fed, it must be pasteurised and come from a recently tested CAE and Johne's seronegative doe**.
- Blood-sample kids shortly after birth for CAEV to detect any possible passive transfer of antibody if the snatching was not done efficiently, then at 6 months and at 3-monthly intervals thereafter to detect possible virus carriers.
- Rear kids isolated from other goats, separated by a least 1.8 m with separate feeding/water utensils and no access to yards or grazing used by older animals.

Pasteurisation of colostrum and milk can never be guaranteed to kill 100% of infective organisms, so wherever possible milk from animals that have been tested negative for the diseases being controlled should be used. Herd biosecurity may be compromised by using milk from other goat or cow herds because their disease status may be uncertain. Feeding milk replacer is safer than feeding pasteurised goat milk.

If the availability of buildings and land permits, rearing kids in isolation can allow the establishment of a separate minimal-disease herd alongside the parent 'infected' herd, which can be culled as the 'clean' herd becomes productive, allowing producers to stay in production and maintain desirable genetics during the transition period.

Ongoing disease surveillance

Although an integrated approach to kid rearing will reduce the overall disease prevalence on the farm, controlling disease in the herd requires additional strategies depending on the disease(s) present and the money available to spend on control measures. Animals that show obvious clinical signs of disease are easily identified, but the identification of carrier animals and animals with subclinical disease is much more difficult, often problematic and expensive.

However, successful control of chronic diseases relies on continued disease surveillance:

- Post-mortem examination of selective herd culls.
- Post-mortem examination of animals that die naturally. Post-mortem examination allows the monitoring of diseases present in the herd, such as CAE, CLA, Johne's disease and gastrointestinal parasites, even if they are not the actual cause of death.
- Serological testing for disease – CAE, CLA. Serological tests require careful interpretation, particularly in vaccinated herds.
- Routine milk cultures – Mycoplasma.

Additional strategic monitoring of parasite burdens, anthelmintic resistance, trace element status, etc., may help identify concurrent disease problems, which exist out-with specific disease control programmes and help maintain a healthy productive herd.

Routine disease surveillance should also include the analysis of all other veterinary records and investigations, including laboratory results and clinical records.

> ### Pasteurisation of milk to control CAE and Johne's disease
>
> A higher temperature is required for treating milk that is possibly contaminated with *Mycobacterium avium* subsp. *paratuberculosis* (MAP) organisms than is required for CAE virus. A heat treatment protocol of 56–59°C for 1 hour is adequate for CAE, but will not kill sufficient numbers of MAP.
>
> For MAP, milk can be pasteurised by heating for 30 minutes at 63°C in a conventional 'batch' pasteuriser or 72°C for 15 seconds (flash pasteurisation) in a pressurised pasteuriser. A higher pasteurisation temperature of 74°C is required to control *Coxiella burnetti*. Although pasteurisation at these temperatures will kill almost 100% of infectious organisms, pasteurised milk from known carriers should never be fed.
>
> An accurate thermometer is important and the final temperature of the milk should be closely monitored. The milk should be stirred or kept in motion to ensure even heat distribution. It is recommended to use a water bath or double boiler to regulate the temperature more closely. Pasteurised milk can be marked with food colouring to minimise the risk of accidentally feeding unpasteurised milk to kids, particularly if several people are involved in the care of kids.
>
> #### Pasteurisation of colostrum
> Colostrum must be collected, stored and chilled under clean conditions.
>
> The thick viscous nature of colostrum makes it very difficult to pasteurise satisfactorily. Only conventional 'batch' pasteurisers should be used.
>
> If heated to temperatures >59°C, proteins, including IgG antibodies, will coagulate, reducing the value of colostrum, so that, unless 'high-quality' colostrum is used, the level of antibodies in the pasteurized product will be too low.
>
> If temperatures lower than 59°C are used, the number of MAP organisms will not be sufficiently reduced to ensure that feeding infected milk is safe. Under commercial conditions, it is probable that the value of the colostrum will be greater than the risk of MAP transmission – in those circumstances, it is essential to use colostrum from goats of known MAP infection status and to use young low-risk animals.

Vaccination

In addition to the routine vaccination for clostridial disease, vaccination can also be used to help control infectious diseases endemic to the farm, including Johne's disease, CLA, respiratory diseases, such as as pasteurellosis, and causes of abortion, such as toxoplasmosis and clamydophilosis.

Use of drugs

Drug use may be appropriate for short-term control of a particular problem, such as respiratory disease, but wherever possible other methods should be considered for long-term control on the grounds of welfare and cost and because of the danger of infectious agents developing resistance to treatment.

Official health schemes and disease-free acceditation

Many pedigree and some commercial herds have obtained disease-free accreditation through goat health schemes provided by government or other responsible bodies. These schemes involve testing and monitoring for specific diseases, together with movement controls on the animals entering the herd. In the United Kingdom, certification is available for scrapie (Scrapie Monitored Scheme) and CAE (Premium Sheep and Goat Health Scheme) under the auspices of Scotland's Rural College (SRUC) and CAE in the British Goat Society Monitored Herd Scheme. Australia has a National Johne's Disease Control Program (NJDCP) and the Goat Industry Council of Australia has a National Kid Rearing Plan for CAE and Johne's disease. The Norwegian Goat Health Service runs the Healthier Goats Programme with the aim of eradicating CAE, CLA and Johne's disease. Other countries have Johne's disease control programmes that target cattle, but not necessarily goats.

Further reading

1 Anzuino, K., Bell, N.J., Bazeley, K.J. and Nicol, C.J. (2010) Assessment of welfare on 24 commercial UK dairy goat farms based on direct observations. *Vet. Rec.* **167** (20), 774–780.

2 Battini, M. *et al.* (2014) Invited review: animal-based indicators for on-farm welfare assessment for dairy goats. *J. Dairy Sci.*, **97** (11), 6625–6648.

3 Hart, N. (2006) Ideas for a Dairy Goat Herd Health Plan. *Goat Vet. Soc. J.*, **22**, 45–50.

4 Hosie, B. and Clark, S. (2007) Sheep flock health security. *In Pract.*, **29**, 246–254.

5 Mahler, X. and Noordhuizen, J. (2008) Applying the HACCP principles to selected hazards during goat kids rearing on milking goat farms in western France. *Revue de Medecine Veterinaire*, **159** (1), 38–48.

6 Malher, X. and Noordhuizen, J.P.T.M. (2008) Application of the HACCP principles to milking goat farms in France. In: *Applying HACCP-Based Quality Risk Management on Dairy Farms* (eds Noordhuizen, J.P.T.M., Cannas da Sylva, J., Boersema, S.J. and Vieira, A.), pp. 199–217. Wageningen Academic Publishers, Wageningen, The Netherlands.

7 Muri, K., Stubsjøen, S.M. and Valle, P.S. (2013) Development and testing of an on-farm welfare assessment protocol for dairy goats. *Animal Welfare*, **22**, 385–400.

8 Muri, K., Leine, N. and Valle, P.S. (2015) Welfare effects of a disease eradication programme for dairy goats. *Animal*, **20**, 1–9.

9 Nagel-Alne, G.E. *et al.* (2014) The Norwegian Healthier Goats Programme – a financial cost–benefit analysis. *Prev. Vet. Med.*, **114** (2), 96–105.

10 Nagel Alne, G.E., Valle, P.S., Krontveit, R. and Sølverød, L.S. (2015) Caprine arthritis encephalitis and caseous lymphadenitis in goats: use of bulk tank milk ELISAs for herd-level surveillance. *Vet. Rec.* **176** (7), 173.

11 Noordhuizen, J.P.T.M. *et al.* (2008) *Applying HACCP-based quality risk management on dairy farms.* Wageningen Academic Publishers, Wageningen, The Netherlands.

12 Animal Health Australia, Farm Biosecurity. Available at: http://www.farmbiosecurity.com.au/industry/goat/.

13 Animal Health Australia, Johne's disease. Available at: http://www.animalhealthaustralia.com.au/wp-content/uploads/2011/04/GoatMAP-manual.pdf.

14 Canadian Food Inspection Agency: Biosecurity Planning Guide for Canadian Goat Producers. Available at: http://www.inspection.gc.ca/animals/terrestrial-animals/biosecurity/standards-and-principles/producer-guide-goats/eng/1375213342187/1375213659306?chap=1#s4c1.

15 Johne's Information Center, University of Wisconsin. Available at: www.johnes.org/goats.

CHAPTER 24

Anaesthesia

Worldwide only a limited number of drugs are licensed for sedation, analgesia or anaesthesia in any food-producing animal and fewer still licensed for use in goats. This generally means that extra label drug use (ELDU) is required in most surgical situations and it is the responsibility of the veterinary surgeon to ensure that the necessary requirements for extra label drug use are met. In the United Kingdom, the Cascade should be followed as closely as possible and, in the United States, the procedures laid out in the Animal Medicinal Drug Use Clarification Act (AMDUCA) should be adopted.

There is no provision in Europe for the use of many safe and effective anaesthetic agents. The veterinary surgeon has a dilemma, as best anaesthetic practice does not always match legal requirements when selecting which drugs to use. The practical effect of the provisions of the Cascade are that the active ingredient(s) of any medicine (including anaesthetics) used in goats must be listed in Table 1 of EU 37/2010. The only products in Table 1 likely to be of use, either alone or in combination, are: xylazine, detomidine, romifidine, isofluorane, ketamine, thiopental sodium, lignocaine/lidocaine, mepivicaine, procaine and butorphanol. At the time of publication, only ketamine (Anaestamine, Animalcare) was licensed for goats in the United Kingdom.

Atipamezole, commonly used to reverse the sedative effects of alpha2 agonist sedative agents, is not listed on EU37/2010 and therefore its use is not legally allowed.

In Europe, when lidocaine is administered under the cascade provision to cows, a minimum period of 15 days must be applied between administration of the lidocaine and taking milk for human consumption.

Hopefully, increased recognition by licensing authorities around the world of the problems facing small ruminant practitioners may soon lead to legislation that will allow them to practice good veterinary medicine within the law.

Initial clinical examination

A routine clinical examination should be carried out in all animals to determine the degree of anaesthetic risk.
- General condition – fat cover, anaemia, etc., age.
- Auscultation of heart and lungs:
  o Normal respiratory rate 15 to 20/minute.
  o Normal pulse rate 70 to 95/minute.
- Accurate assessment of weight (weigh if necessary) – it is very easy to overdose if the estimation is inaccurate.

Normal physiological parameters are listed in Table 24.1.

General anaesthesia

Careful pre-anaesthetic evaluation and preparation can prevent most anaesthetic-related complications.

Basic considerations
- How is the patient going to be handled before, during and after surgery?
- What problems may be encountered during anaesthesia and what should be done if problems do occur?
- Are the nursing staff fully conversant with the procedure to be undertaken?
- Select a breathing system suitable for the size of animal. A *T-piece system* is suitable for neonatal kids and a standard *small animal circle system* for goats weighing > 15–20 kg.
- Has the animal's weight been accurately measured (use dog scales)?
- Anaesthesia of neonates can result in hypothermia and hypoglycaemia, so be prepared to provide an external source of heat and fluid therapy if necessary.
- Adequate *analgesia* should be provided *before* induction of anaesthesia.

Diseases of the Goat, Fourth Edition. John Matthews.
© 2016 John Wiley & Sons, Ltd. Published 2016 by John Wiley & Sons, Ltd.

Table 24.1 Physiological parameters.

	Preanaesthesia	Anaesthetised
Body temperature	38.6–40.6 °C (102–104 °F) (average 39.3 °C)	
Heart rate	70–95/minute	80–150/minute
Respiratory rate	15–30/minute (adult) 20–40/minute (kid)	20–40/minute
Tidal volume	325 ml	325 ml
Mean arterial pressure		75–100 mmHg
Rumination	1–1.5/minute	

With the exception of neonatal kids, which are essentially monogastric, general anaesthesia of goats carries the same hazards as that of any other ruminant, namely:

- *Regurgitation.*
- *Salivation.*
- *Ruminal tympany.*
- *Cardiovascular and respiratory embarrassment* during lateral and dorsal recumbency.

These can be minimised by sensible routine precautions before and during surgery.

Pre-operatively

- *Starve the patient.*Except for young kids, goats should be routinely starved for about 18 hours pre-operatively if elective surgery is being undertaken. Longer periods of starvation may result in the rumen contents becoming more fluid, with a greater likelihood of regurgitation occurring, and may also predispose to the development of metabolic acidosis.

Kids under 4 weeks of age should have food and milk withheld for about 2 hours.

Kids 4 weeks to 6 months of age should be starved for 6 to 8 hours.

> Starvation means no food offered and no clean bedding, for example straw, either in the pen or in the vehicle used to transport the goat to the surgery.

Access to water should not be restricted for more than 12 hours prior to induction.

- Insert an indwelling *jugular catheter* (16 g for adult goats, 18 g for younger animals). It provides easy access for administration of sedatives, analgesics, induction agents and fluids (Plate 24.1). Alternatively, the *cephalic vein* can be catheterised (18g). The vein runs obliquely in comparison with a canine cephalic vein.

- *Sedate* the patient to give a tractable animal (Plate 24.2) who needs much less induction agent or can be masked down more easily.
- *Use fluid therapy routinely* for maintenance and replacement needs. Maintenance will be provided by a balanced electrolyte solution such as Lactated Ringers at a flow rate of *4–10 ml/kg/h.*

During prolonged surgery in kids under 12 weeks, check blood glucose during anaesthesia and infuse 5% dextrose 3–5 ml/kg/h where necessary.

- *Use analgesics pre- and post-operatively.*
- *Intubate with a cuffed endotracheal tube.*

> Endotracheal intubation with a cuffed tube is essential whenever general anaesthesia is induced in an adult goat, except for very short procedures such as dehorning.

During anaesthesia

- *Position the goat correctly on the operating table.*
  - The thorax and head should be raised if possible by tilting the table to lower the hindquarters, while the head is tilted downwards to allow free drainage of saliva (Plate 24.3).
    - Head down, allowing saliva to drain from the mouth.
    - Neck placed over a sandbag.
  - Hindquarters lowered – decreases pressure on the diaphragm and reduces the risk of regurgitation.
  - Place in sternal or left lateral recumbency whenever possible. Right lateral recumbency results in intra-abdominal pressure, pressure on the diaphragm and the collection of gas in the rumen by restricting eructation.

- *Keep all anaesthetic procedures as short as possible.*
- *Recumbency causes respiratory depression and hypoxaemia.*

The inspired gases should contain at least 30% oxygen (supply oxygen by mask if the goat is not incubated).

Intubation

Intubation is difficult in goats because the mouth does not open wide, the intermandibular space is narrow and the laryngeal opening difficult to visualise over the base of the tongue.

The oral cavity and the trachea must be held in a straight line by an assistant – a loop of bandage around the upper jaw helps to keep the mouth open – whilst the person placing the tube pulls the tongue forward, using a swab to hold the slippery tongue if necessary.

Intubation of goats can be performed with or without a long-bladed laryngoscope, but a laryngoscope is useful not only to visualise the larynx, but also to depress the tongue for easier access (Plate 24.4).

An endotracheal tube as large as possible should be used – endotracheal tubes about sizes 8 to 9 are generally suitable for adult goats. Comparatively, goats have a much smaller laryngeal opening than a dog and need relatively small tubes. An adequate depth of anaesthesia is essential for intubation. If a laryngoscope is not available, a technique of threading the tube through the larynx is relatively easy with experience. The goat is placed in lateral or dorsal recumbency and the tube inserted until the top touches the larynx; the larynx is then manipulated from the outside over the tube. A distinct click is usually felt as the tube passes into the laryngeal cartilages. The use of a *wire stiffener* in the tube makes intubation much easier – the rod from a wire cat carrier is eminently suitable (Plate 24.5).

Alternatively, a *guide tube* such as a canine urethral catheter can be inserted into the trachea and the endotracheal tube slipped over it.

Goats, especially kids, are prone to *laryngospasm*, generally following regurgitation at the time of intubation. Spraying the cords with lignocaine will reduce the hazard. In an emergency, a tracheotomy may be necessary.

Anaesthetic circuits

A *circle circuit* connected to a small animal anaesthetic machine is suitable for goats <200 kg. The breathing bag should have a volume of >20 ml/kg, meaning that a 2 or 3 litre bag is suitable for dairy goats.

Non-rebreathing systems such as a *modified Ayre's T-piece* is suitable for animals <10 kg.

Animals >200 kg will require a *large animal circle circuit* as used in horses.

Hazards of general anaesthesia
Regurgitation

General anaesthesia (or deep sedation) can lead to passive regurgitation and aspiration of rumen contents. The risk of regurgitation can be minimised by:

- Pre-operative starvation.
- Correct positioning of the goat on the operating table. The thorax and neck should be raised if possible by tilting the table to lower the hindquarters, while the head is tilted downwards to allow free drainage of saliva.
- If problems arise during intubation, a cuffed tube in the oesophagus will help to protect the airway from regurgitation.
- If regurgitation occurs, the pharynx should be drained, the trachea sucked out and atropine administered if there is a danger of bronchospasm.

Salivation

Like all ruminants, goats salivate copiously during anaesthesia and it is important that the saliva is allowed to drain freely from the mouth and not pool in the pharynx. Except for very short procedures the goat should be intubated with a cuffed inflated endotracheal tube.

Hypovolaemia and acidosis can occur through loss of alkaline saliva during long periods of anaesthesia (more than 2 to 3 hours). Therefore, during long periods of anaesthesia, the saliva should he collected and replaced on a volume for volume basis with *lactated Ringer's solution (Hartmann's solution) and sodium bicarbonate, 1 mmol/kg/h* (4.2% bicarbonate contains 0.5 mmol/ml = 2 ml/kg/h).

Ruminal tympany

Ruminal tympany becomes progressively more important with the length of the operation as continuous gas production puts pressure on the diaphragm, interfering with respiration and leading to hypoxia. In elective surgery, pre-operative starvation will reduce the risk of tympany, or in non-elective surgery, rumen contents can be emptied by stomach tube, the contents kept at 37 °C and then returned to the rumen post-operatively.

Removal of rumen contents by stomach tube may be possible if tympany occurs or the distension may be relieved by trocarisation using a 14 or 16 gauge needle.

Cardiovascular and respiratory embarrassment

During lateral and, particularly, dorsal recumbency the large mass of the rumen puts pressure on the diaphragm and great vessels, leading to decreased tidal volume and inadequate ventilation, with increased areas of lung tissue not ventilated and consequently respiratory acidosis and hypoxaemia. All anaesthetic procedures, particularly those requiring dorsal recumbency, should be kept as short as possible. Hypoxaemia can be prevented by the provision of at least 30% inspired oxygen and respiratory acidosis prevented by the use of intermittent positive pressure ventilation.

Fall in rectal temperature

Rectal temperature usually decreases during anaesthesia. Goats have difficulty regaining normal body temperature when the temperature falls below 36 °C.

Depth of anaesthesia

No single reflex is reliable enough to be used on its own to assess the depth of anaesthesia. The assessment must be based on a combination of:

- Response to surgery. The anaesthetist should monitor the heart rate, pulse, respiratory rate, colour of mucous membranes, gingival perfusion time (normally 1 to 2 seconds) and muscle relaxation.
- Experience with the drug being used.
- Examination of a number of reflexes:
  o *Jaw tension*: this decreases with an increasing depth of anaesthesia, but some tone persists even in deep anaesthesia. As the anaesthetic level lightens, swallowing or chewing movements can be elicited.
  o *Eye rotation*: unlike cattle, eye rotation is not a useful method of assessing the depth of anaesthesia.
  o *Pupils*: during surgical anaesthesia, the eye is normally *central* and the pupil moderately *constricted*. During both light and deep anaesthesia, the pupil is *dilated*.
  o *Palpebral reflex*: this usually (but *not* always) disappears as surgical anaesthesia is obtained.
  o *Limb withdrawal reflexes*: these are reduced during light anaesthesia with barbiturates or halothane and are generally absent under deep anaesthesia. However, they may persist if ketamine is used. (Generally,

they are not as good an indicator of the depth of anaesthesia as in dogs and cats).
  o *Corneal reflex*: this persists through all levels of anaesthesia.

Monitoring during anaesthesia

Respiratory system:

- Respiratory rate 20–40 breaths/min (rapid respiratory rate common).
- Hypoventilation is common.

Cardiovascular system:

- Mucous membranes should remain pink.
- Heart rate 60–100 (55 is bradycardia) – an oesophageal stethoscope is useful.
- The median and caudal auricular arteries or peripheral arteries on the lower fore or hind limbs can be catheterised for direct measurement of blood pressure. Mean arterial pressure should be above 65 mmHg.

Oxygen saturation:

- Haemoglobin oxygen saturation and pulse rate can be measured with a pulse oximeter. The probe can conveniently be placed on the tongue or between the digits.

Recovery

The vapouriser should be turned off, the rebreathing system flushed with oxygen and the patient kept connected to the system until signs of recovery, such as an active palpebral reflex, limb movement, chewing and swallowing are present. When strong swallowing reflexes are evident, the endotracheal tube should be removed *with the cuff inflated*, so any accumulated saliva or regurgitated material is removed. The animal should be placed and supported in sternal recumbency and supervised until it is completely recovered.

Sedatives

See Table 24.2.

Benzodiazepines
Diazepam, 0.25–0.5 mg/kg, 2–4 ml/40 kg slowly i.v.

- Gives tractable animal that requires less induction agent and can be masked down more easily if required.
- Provides 30 minutes of sedation, decreased anxiety and muscle relaxation but *no analgesia*.

Table 24.2 Premedicants and sedatives.

Drug	Dosage	Route of administration
Benzodiazipines		
Diazepam	0.25–0.5 mg/kg	i.v.
Midazolam	0.1–0.3 mg/kg	i.v.
Opioid analgesics		
Buprenorphine	0.01 mg/kg	i.m. or s.c.
Butorphanol	0.2–0.5 mg/kg	i.v., i.m. or s.c.
Pethidine hydrochloride	10 mg/kg	i.m. or s.c.
Alpha-2-agonists		
Detomidine	20–40 µg/kg	i.m.
Medetomidine	25–35 µg/kg	i.v. or i.m.
Xylazine	0.05 mg/kg (adult)	i.v.
	0.025 mg/kg (kids)	
	0.1 mg/kg	i.m.
Alpha-2 antagonists		
Atipamazole	125–175 µg/kg	half i.v. and half i.m.
Yohimbine	0.2 mg/kg	i.v.
Phenothiazines		
Acepromazine maleate	0.05–0.1 mg/kg	i.v.
Antimuscarinic drugs		
Atropine	0.6–1 mg/kg	s.c.

- It has minimal cardiovascular and pulmonary effects at therapeutic doses.
- Can be combined with ketamine as a pre-anaesthetic to improve muscle relaxation and to permit intubation for inhalation anaesthesia (see later).

> Diazepam and midazolam are the drugs of choice for sedation, prior to induction for general anaesthesia.

Midazolam, 0.2–0.4 mg/kg slowly i.v.

- Similar effects in goats to diazepam, with minimal cardiovascular depression.
- Provides 20–30 minutes of recumbency or sedation but no analgesia.
- Midazolam can also be given intramuscularly as it is non-irritant to tissues (unlike diazepam).

  Neither diazepam or midazolam are licensed for use in food-producing animals and no maximum residue limits (MRLs) are available.

Opioid analgesics

Opioids are potent analgesic agents although they are not licensed for use in food-producing animals and MRLs are not available.

Butorphanol, 0.2–0.5 mg/kg, 0.8–2 ml/40 kg i.v., i.m. or s.c.

- Analgesia only lasts 2–3 hours.
- Often combined with other drugs to provide additional analgesia.

Buprenorphine, 0.01 mg/kg, 1 ml/30 kg i.m. or s.c.

- Onset of sedation/analgesia is slow (i.e. 45 minutes minimum, but analgesia lasts 4 hours).
- Can be used as a pre-medicant and then given every 4 to 6 hours to provide post-operative analgesia.

Pethidine hydrochloride (Meperidine hydrochloride), 10 mg/kg, i.m. or s.c.

- Can be used as a pre-medication.
- Short-acting analgesia, so not suitable for long-term post-operative pain relief, as it needs repeating every 2 to 4 hours.
- Maximum plasma concentrations are achieved about 10 minutes after i.m. injection.

Alpha-2 agonists

The alpha-2 agonists xylazine, medetomidine and detomidine have *sedative, muscle relaxant* and *analgesic* properties in goats. Analgesia lasts for only 30 to 50% of the detectable duration of sedation.

Xylazine (2% solution), 0.05 mg/kg, 0.1 ml/40 kg slowly i.v. or 0.1 mg/kg, 0.2 ml/40 kg i.m.

- The standard *2% solution* can be diluted and administered via an insulin syringe to allow more accurate dosing.
- Be careful not to confuse 2% and 10% solutions!
- *Minute doses are required in young animals and it is very easy to overdose. In kids, 0.025 mg/kg i.m. is probably the maximum safe dose.*
- Angora goats are reported to require lower levels of the drug than dairy goats.
- Xylazine causes cardiovascular and respiratory depression and hyperglycaemia with resultant diuresis and a major increase in urine output. It also suppresses the release of antidiuretic hormone from the posterior pituitary. *It is contraindicated in animals with depressed*

cardiovascular function or urinary tract obstruction. It also causes rumen hypomobility, so goats should be fasted to reduce the risk of bloat.

- Xylazine is probably contraindicated in late pregnancy (last trimester), as it has been associated with abortion, because of an oxytocin-like effect on the gravid uterus.
- Often combined with ketamine as a pre-anaesthetic to permit intubation for inhalation anaesthesia (see later).
- Analgesia does not extend to the end of xylazine-induced sedation and painful procedures should be restricted to the initial 15 to 30 minutes after drug administration or else supplemental local or regional analgesia should be used.
- Severe pulmonary changes have been observed after the administration of xylazine, which seem to outlast the sedative effects of the drug. The cardiorespiratory system should be carefully monitored, both during sedation and recovery.

> The majority of anaesthetic deaths in goats are caused by xylazine overdose.

Medetomidine, 25-35 µg/kg, 1–1.5 ml/40 kg i.v. or i.m.

- Sedation is evident in 5 to 15 minutes.
  o Can be combined with *ketamine* (see later) and/or *butorphanol, 0.1–0.2 mg/kg.*

Detomidine, 20–40 µg/kg, 0.08–0.16 ml/40 kg i.v. or i.m.

- Quicker, better and deeper sedation is achieved when the drug is administered intravenously.
- At 20 µg/kg, mild sedation is produced, but the goat will remain standing with slight ataxia.
- 40 µg/kg will produce deeper sedation with sternal recumbency and some analgesia for about 70–110 minutes, with complete recovery in about 200 minutes.
- Pre-medication with detomidine can be followed by induction with thiopental, propofol or ketamine (see later). Maximum sedation should be allowed to develop before administration of the induction agent and this may take approximately 5 minutes.

- Used in combination with *opioid analgesics* to produce deeper and more reliable sedation, for example *butorphanol, 0.2mg/kg i.v. or i.m.*
- Safer than xylazine for pregnant goats at therapeutic doses as it does not have an Oxytocin effect on the uterus.

Reversion of the effects of alpha-2 agonists

> Overdosage of xylazine and other alpha-2 agonists can be reversed by Atipamezole.

Reversal also removes any analgesic benefits gained from alpha-2 administration. Reversal agents should be given slowly to avoid sudden awareness of pain and excitement.

- *Atipamezole* is an alpha-2 adrenoceptor blocking drug licensed to reverse medetomidine at 5 times the dose of medetomidine (i.e. the same volume of metomidine previously administered). It also effectively reverses the effects of detomidine and xylazine. Atipamezole is not listed on EU37/2010 and therefore its use is not legally allowed in the EU.

Atipamezole, 125–175 µg/kg, 1–1.5 ml/40 kg, half i.v. and half i.m.

Resedation may rarely occur if atipamezole is used a short time after administration of the sedative because the effect of atipamezole may subside before that of the sedative.

- *Yohimbine* and *Tolazoline* are also effective antagonists.

Yohimbine, 0.2 mg/kg very slowly i.v.

Tolazoline, 2 mg/kg very slowly i.v. (over 3 to 4 minutes), or i.m., or half i.v. and half i.m.

The intramuscular route is considered safer for tolazoline, unless administered very carefully intravenously.

Tolazine has mixed alpha-1 and alpha-2 adrenoreceptor antagonist activity. It can be used to antagonise xylazine-induced sedation and initiate arousal and also antagonises the less desirable side effects. Tolazine antagonises the sedative effects of epidural anaesthesia with xylazine while anaesthesia caudal to the injection site of the xylazine persists.

Phenothiazines
Acepromazine maleate, 0.05–0.1 mg/kg, 1–2 ml/40 kg slowly i.v.

- Provides mild sedation without analgesia.
- Smooths induction with barbiturates, but also greatly increases the risk of regurgitation and contraindicated in shocked animals because it produces a fall in blood pressure.
- Prolapse of the penis may occur in goats as in horses.

Antimuscarinic pre-anaesthetic medication
Atropine, 0.6–1 mg/kg, 1–1.5 ml/kg i.m.

- At this dose rate, atropine will reduce the flow of saliva but also render it more viscus, which may result in endotracheal tubes being blocked.
- Most authorities do not recommend that atropine be given routinely as a pre-medication, although recognising its use in situations where handling viscera may cause bradycardia (<55 beats/min) and possible cardiac arrest because of vagal inhibition.

Injectable anaesthetic agents

See Table 24.3.

Barbiturates
Thiopental sodium, 5%, 10–15 mg/kg, 8–12 ml/40 kg i.v.

- In general, the barbiturate drugs produce a marked respiratory depression, with delayed recovery if additional amounts are given to maintain anaesthesia. Regurgitation is particularly likely if thiopentaone is used. Their use as sole agents is thus limited, but they are very useful induction agents before intubation and maintenance with gaseous anaesthesia.
- The short-acting barbiturates give a rapid, smooth induction. Giving half the calculated amount (5 mg/kg) rapidly followed by the remainder over a 2 minute period may reduce the period of apnoea that occurs following rapid injection of the whole amount.
- Maintaining general anaesthesia with thiopentone for any longer than 15 minutes results in its progressive accumulation in body tissues, which may result in delayed recovery from anaesthesia.
- Pre-medication with diazepam will reduce the barbiturate dose.

Table 24.3 Anaesthetic drugs.

Drug	Dosage and route of administration	
Gaseous drugs		
Halothane	Induction 4%	
	Maintenance 2%	
Isofluorane	Induction 2–5%	
	Maintenance 0.25–5%	
Injectable drugs		
Thiopentone sodium 5%	10–15 mg/kg	i.v.
Alphaxalone 10 mg/ml	4.5 mg/kg	i.v.
Propofol	3–5 mg/kg	i.v.
Ketamine	3–5 mg/kg	i.v.
Ketamine + sedative combinations	See text	
Tiletamine-zolazepam	5.5 mg/kg	i.v.

Alphaxalone, 10 mg/ml, 4.5 mg/kg very slowly i.v. to effect, 4.5 ml/10 kg (Alphaxan, Vetoquinol)

- Smooth anaesthetic induction with good muscle relaxation.
- Rapid onset of action, rapid redistribution and uneventful recovery.
- Administer slowly over about 30 seconds.

Propofol, 3–5 mg/kg, 12–20 ml/40 kg slowly i.v.

- Propofol can be used to provide short duration anaesthesia with the advantage of rapid recovery or for induction followed by intubation.
- Induction apnoea can occur, especially if administered too rapidly and at high doses.
- Relaxation may be insufficient for intubation unless given pre-anaesthetic sedation, for example with diazepam or detomidine/butorphonal.
- Kids presented for disbudding require between 1 and 2 ml intravenously.

Ketamine, 10–15 mg/kg, 4–6 ml/40 kg slowly i.v.

- Ketamine does not depress cardiovascular function – as a result of central sympathetic stimulation, heart rate and arterial blood pressure increase.
- When ketamine is used on its own, there is inadequate muscle relaxation for abdominal procedures and excessive trembling.
- Ketamine has a short duration of action in ruminants.

- Better results are obtained by using ketamine in combination with diazepam or an alpha-2 adrenoceptor stimulant like xylazine, medetomidine or detomidine and/or butorphanol.

Ketamine + sedative combinations

- Sedatives can be used in combination with ketamine to provide better muscle relaxation and increased analgesia during surgery.
- Anaesthesia can be extended by additional injections of ketamine and sedative, although prolonged surgery (>1.5 hours) results in an unacceptably long recovery.
- The patient should be intubated, because the swallowing reflex is abolished or decreased and there is a risk of aspirating rumen contents.

> Ketamine is used in combination with alpha-2 agonists, diazepam and/ or butorphanol.

(1) Diazepam and ketamine

Diazepam, 0.25–0.5 mg/kg, 2~4 ml/40 kg slowly i.v., wait 2–3 minutes, then Ketamine, 4 mg/kg, 1.6 ml/40 kg i.v.

- The lower level of diazepam is used in larger animals.
- This combination provides adequate time for intubation and maintenance on gaseous anaesthesia.

(2) Xylazine and ketamine

Xylazine (2% solution), 0.1 mg/kg, 0.2 ml/40 kg i.m. followed by Ketamine, 10 mg/kg, 4 ml/40 kg i.m. or 5 mg/kg, 2 ml/40 kg i.v.

- The combination gives 15 to 20 minutes anaesthesia with good analgesia and intubation is not essential, although advisable for abdominal surgery in case of regurgitation or passive reflux.
- Lower doses of xylazine, *0.025 mg/kg*, should be used in kids.
- Anaethesia may be prolonged by an incremental intramuscular dose of ketamine at *2.5–5 mg/kg* or by use of gaseous anaesthetics such as halothane.
- May require inspired oxygen supplementation by mask or endotracheal tube during recumbency.

> KXB mixtures meet the legal requirements for use of anaesthetic drugs in the UK.

KXB mixture

1000 mg **K**etamine:100 mg **X**ylazine:10 mg **B**utorphanol

10 ml ketamine (100 mg/ml) + 1 ml xylazine (100 mg/ml) + 1 ml butorphanol (10 mg/ml), that is add 1 ml xyalazine 10% solution and 1 ml butorphanol to a 10 ml bottle of ketamine.

The solution is administered at *1 ml/50 kg i.v.*

- Gives 20 to 30 minutes anaesthesia; recovery takes about 20 minutes.
- The xylazine can be reversed with antisedan (see above).
- The amount of butorphonal can be increased to 20 mg (i.e. 2 ml) if required.

KXB kid mixtures

1000 mg **K**etamine:20 mg **X**ylazine:10 mg **B**utorphanol

10 ml ketamine (100 mg/ml) + 1 ml xylazine (20 mg/ml) + 1 ml butorphanol (10 mg/ml), that is add 1 ml xyalazine 2% solution (or 0.2 ml 10% solution) and 1 ml butorphanol to a 10 ml bottle of ketamine. The solution is administered at *0.1 ml/5 kg i.v.*

An alternative mixture is:

400 mg **K**etamine:8 mg **X**ylazine:8 mg **B**utorphanol

4 ml ketamine (100 mg/ml) + 0.4 ml xylazine (20 mg/ml) + 0.8 ml butorphanol (10 mg/ml). The solution is administered at *0.1ml/5kg i.v.*

Ketamine, xylazine and guaifenesin (KXG or Triple Drip)

200 mg **K**etamine + 2 mg **X**ylazine + 100 ml 5% **G**uaifenesin (5 g/100 ml) that is 2 ml ketamine + 0.1 ml xylazine 2% solution to 100 ml guaifenisin. The solution is administered at *1 ml/kg i.v.* for induction (50–75% of calculated dose first), then *2 ml/kg/h*, or to effect, for maintenance.

- Gives 30 minutes of surgical anaesthesia.
- Anaesthesia can be prolonged by incremental doses according to the patient's response but total surgical time should not exceed 60 minutes.

- The solution should be given through a jugular catheter as it is very irritating to tissues.

Note: guaifensin is available as a 15% solution licensed for induction of anaesthesia in horses in the United Kingdom.

Ketamine, xylazine and diazepam

Xylazine 0.2mg/kg i.m., wait 10 minutes then *ketamine 10 mg/kg + diazepam 0.3 mg/kg* in the same syringe i.v.

(3) Medetomidine and ketamine

Medetomidine, 25–35 mg/kg, 1–1.5 ml/40 kg, mixed in the same syringe with *ketamine, 1–1.5 mg/kg, 0.4–0.6 ml/40 kg i.m.*

- Adult animals require higher doses than young animals.
- Induction of anaesthesia takes 5 to 10 minutes and the combination provides 30 to 40 minutes of anaesthesia. *Butorphanol, 0.1–0.2 mg/kg*, can be added to the mixture.

The sedative effects of medetomidine can be reversed by *atipamezole, 125–175 ug/kg, 1–1.5 ml/40 kg, half i.v. and half i.m.*

Tiletamine-zolazepam

Tiletamine-zolazepam, 5.5 mg/kg i.v., is not available in the United Kingdom.

Note: The dosage is the sum of both drugs, that is tiletamine 50 mg/ml + zolazepam 50 mg/ml = 100 mg/ml total.

Telazol is a proprietary combination of tiletamine (dissociative) and zolazepam (benzodiazepine). Compared with ketamine, Telazol anaesthesia produces better muscle relaxation, more profound analgesia and longer lasting effects. It provides adequate anaesthesia for about 1 hour and anaesthesia can be extended by incremental doses at 0.5–1.0 mg/kg as needed.

Gaseous anaesthetic agents

> Human exposure to anaesthetic gases must be reduced by using active scavenging systems in a well ventilated environment. Particular care must be taken if mask induction is practised – masks must be close fitting.

Gaseous anaesthetic agents, such as *isofluorane*, in oxygen provide excellent safe anaesthesia, either via mask for induction and maintenance of kids for disbudding or for maintenance of older goats via endotracheal tube following induction by injection. Pre-medication with diazepam, or other sedative drug, reduces the amount of gaseous agent required and makes mask induction easier.

- An oxygen flow of 11 ml/kg/minute is adequate during maintenance (1 to 2 litres/min).
- During mask induction, the initial oxygen flow should be 4 to 6 litres/min to achieve denitrification.

Isoflurane

- Induction of anaesthesia 2 to 5%.
- Maintenance of anaesthesia 0.25 to 5%.

Faster recovery occurs after maintenance with isoflurane as compared with halothane.

Hepatotoxicity has not been reported in goats anaesthetised with isofluorane.

Isoflurane does not have specific MRLs for food-producing animals, but the European Medicines Agency (EMA) has concluded that residues in meat are most unlikely to occur because of its rapid elimination.

Halothane

- Induction of anaesthesia – gradually increase by 0.5% increments every 30 seconds until a 4% vapouriser setting is reached.
- Maintenance of anaesthesia – 2%.
- Halothane hepatotoxicity has been reported after prolonged (3 to 9 hours) anaesthesia (see Chapter 12).

Nitrous oxide

Nitrous oxide can be used during the induction of anaesthesia, but should then be discontinued, because it accumulates in the rumen and can potentiate ruminal tympany. When used for induction, nitrous oxide should be 50% of the total gas flow.

Local anaesthetic agents

Procaine 5% (Willcain, Dechra Veterinary Products) is the only local anaesthetic licensed for use in food-producing animals in the United Kingdom. The preparation available includes adrenaline. The dose rate for procaine and lidocaine is the same.

Lidocaine (lignocaine) 2% (20 mg/ml) produces local anaesthesia for about 0.75–2 hours. The addition of **adrenaline** prolongs the duration of anaesthesia.

Bupivacaine is approximately four times more potent than lidocaine, so that a 0.5% (5 mg/ml) bupivacaine solution is equivalent to a 2% lidocaine solution, and lasts for 4 to 8 hours.

Mepivacaine is used as a 2% (20 mg/ml) solution and lasts for 1.5 to 3 hours.

Maximum safe dose of local anaesthetics

- *Procaine, Lidocaine and Mepivacaine 5 mg/kg i.v. (10 mg/kg i.m.).*
- *Bupivacaine 2 mg/kg i.v.*

Paravertebral anaesthesia

Use

Flank laparotomy for caesarian section or other abdominal surgery. Desensitises the whole of the flank, so the incision can be extended as necessary. Allows better wound healing than local infiltration.

Technique

T13, L1, L2 and L3 are blocked. Figure 24.1a shows the area served by each of the nerves. The nerves run caudally at an angle.

- Clip and surgically scrub the skin over the area where the needles will be inserted.
- Inject 0.5 to 1.0 ml of local anaesthetic into the skin over the midpoint of each of the first, second and third lumbar processes. Subsequent injections are made through these desensitised areas after waiting for a few minutes.
- The sites for injection can be palpated. 'Walk' the needle over the anterior edge of the transverse process of the vertebra caudal to the nerve being blocked and inject approximately 2 cm from the midline, that is halfway between the midline and the tip of the transverse process. The transverse process is 4 to 5 cm deep.
- Use *5 ml of 5 % procaine or 2% lidocaine plus adrenaline*. Inject 2 ml into skin and muscle above the intertransverse ligament and 3 ml below the ligament.
- 6 cm 19 gauge or spinal needles are suitable.
- Onset of analgesia is about 5 minutes after injection and the flank should be anaesthetised after about 10 minutes.
- Duration of analgesia is approximately 1.5 hours.

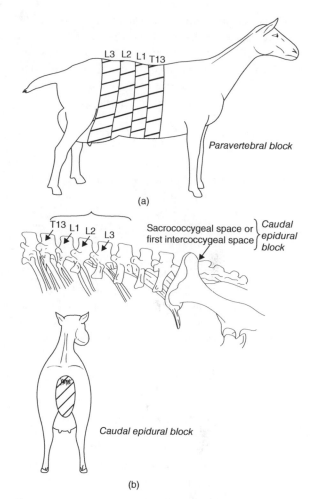

Figure 24.1 (a) Paravertebral block. (b) Caudal epidural block.

Caudal (sacrococcygeal) epidural anaesthesia

Use

Desensitises the perineal area, tail and vagina (see Figure 24.1b); is useful for perineal surgery, foe example replacement of rectal prolapses and perineal urethrostomies, and some obstetrical conditions, for example replacement of cervicovaginal or uterine prolapses, correction of dystocias.

Technique

The area over the tailhead is clipped and surgically prepared. The *first intercoccygeal space* or the *sacrococcygeal space* (preferred) is identified by digital palpation as the tail is moved gently up and down. In dairy goats, an 18 or 19 gauge × 2.5 cm needle is inserted vertically and cranially at an angle of 15 degrees. The correct position of the needle is determined by failure to strike bone and lack of resistance to injection of the anaesthetic solution. The local anaesthetic should be injected slowly.

Lidocaine, 2–4 ml 2% solution, depending on the size of the animal

The onset of analgesia occurs within 1 to 5 minutes and lasts for about 1 hour.

2 ml 2% lidocaine (0.5 mg/kg) + 0.25 ml xylazine (0.07 mg/kg)

Injection of a combination of xylazine and lignocaine provides adequate analgesia to permit replacement of rectal, vaginal or uterine prolapses after 5 to 10 minutes, although loss of tail tone and perineal sensation usually occurs within 2 minutes. Overdosage with lignocaine/xylocaine may cause pelvic limb parasis, which can persist for 36 hours or more.

Lumbosacral epidural anaesthesia

Use

Desensitises the abdominal wall caudal to the umbilicus, inguinal region, flank and perineal area, providing analgesia of the flank for caesarian section, for vasectomy and hindlimb surgery.

Technique

The lumbosacral space is located just caudal to the spinous process of the last lumbar vertebra; it can be palpated in thin goats as a depression 1 to 3 cm caudal to an imaginary line drawn between the cranial borders of the two iliac wings. The needle is inserted on the midline halfway between the spinous processes of L7 and the sacrum. The area is clipped and prepared surgically. Using a 23 g needle, inject 1 to 3 ml of 2% lidocaine subcutaneously. An 18 or 19 g × 5 cm (6.25 c)] needle* (or spinal needle) is inserted through the skin at a 90 degree angle and then slowly advanced until first the resistance of the interarcuate ligament over the epidural space and the ';pop' as this is penetrated is felt as the needle enters the epidural space. A slight vacuum should be noted on entering the epidural space. If blood or cerebrospinal fluid is encountered on aspiration, the needle is in the subarachnoid space and should be withdrawn. Local anaesthetic should be injected slowly over at least 30 seconds.

For *bilateral analgesia*, the animal should be prone or supine so that the spinal canal is horizontal; for *unilateral analgesia*, the animal should be in lateral recumbency with the side on which analgesia is required downwards. Do not allow the animal to 'dog sit' as this will prevent analgesia developing cranially.

5% procaine with adrenaline, 1 ml/5 kg very slowly

Note: data sheets indicate that 5% procaine is contraindicated for use in epidurals, but it is used by some anaesthetists with no reported ill-effects.

2% lidocaine with adrenaline, **1 ml/5 kg** very slowly
  0.5% bupivacaine, 1 ml/4 kg very slowly

- Analgesia and hindleg paralysis occurs after 5 to 15 minutes and lasts 1 to 2 hours with lidocaine.
- For caesarian section, lidocaine is preferred to bupivacaine as the extended hindlimb paralysis interferes with suckling by the kids.

Other drugs and combinations used to provide analgesia by lumbosacral epidural

Xylazine 0.05 mg/kg, 0.1 ml/40 kg (dilute with sterile saline to give 2.5 ml)

- Provides analgesia for surgery, either alone or as an adjunct to general anaesthesia.
- Hindlimb ataxia may be prolonged (up to 8 hours).

Morphine, 0.1 mg/kg as 10 mg/ml, 15 mg/ml, 20 mg/ml or 30 mg/ml, diluted in saline to give 0.15–0.20 ml/kg

- Provides analgesia in about 10 minutes, without loss of motor control to hind legs, and lasting for up to 6 hours.

---

*For kids and pygmy goats, a 22 g × 3.75 cm needle is suitable.

- Provides suitable post-operative analgesia for orthopaedic and abdominal surgery.
- Decreases requirement for general anaesthetic agents.

Morphine, 0.1 ml/kg + 2–4 ml 2% lidocaine

- Provides analgesia with loss of motor control to hind limbs for surgical procedures (castration, dystocia, caesarian section, limb amputation, cystotomy) within 10 minutes.

> Animals should be placed on deep bedding to avoid the risk of fracture if the animal falls suddenly and neuropathy if the animal remains recumbent for a long time.

Local infiltration

> Total dose of lidocaine by local infiltration should be <10 mg/kg.

Goats, particularly kids, are sensitive to the toxic effects of lidocaine, which include drowsiness and respiratory depression. *Convulsions occur at about 6 mg/kg i.v. or 10 mg/kg i.m.* Care must be taken not to exceed recommended doses, for example 30 ml of 2% solution in 45 to 70 kg goats and 40–50 ml in larger animals.

- Infiltration analgesia is useful for suturing wounds and as a line block for laparotomy where the anaesthetic is infiltrated along the line of the incision.
- *Inverted L block.* Local anaesthetic is injected as an inverted L into the skin and full thickness of the body wall, so as to block the nerves entering the operation site, creating an area of analgesia. The horizontal arm of the L is ventral to the transverse processes of the lumbar vertebrae and the vertical arm is posterior to the last rib (Figure 24.2a). This technique avoids oedema of tissues, with subsequent delayed wound healing in the area of the incision.

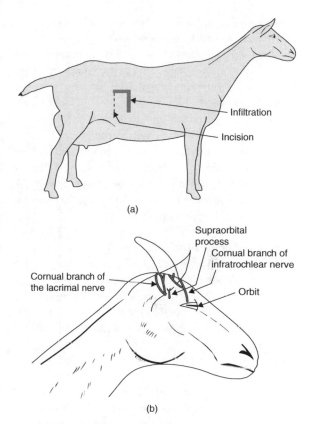

(a)

(b)

Figure 24.2 (a) Inverted L block and (b) local anaesthetic for dehorning.

Intravenous regional analgesia

Use: analgesia of the lower limb.

Sedation prior to injection is advisable as it limits movement of the limb, aiding injection of the anaesthetic.

First *5 ml of 2% lidocaine* (without adrenaline) is injected, via a 23 g needle, into any superficial vein such as the cephali or medial radial vein in the fore leg and the lateral saphenous vein or recurrent tarsal vein in the hind leg. The injection should be directed distally, with pressure on the injection site to avoid a haematoma. A tourniquet is applied above the carpus or hock to localise the effect of the lignocaine and prevent its leakage into the circulation. A roll of bandage below the tourniquet on the lateral surface of the hock allows better occlusion of the blood vessels.

The onset of analgesia is about 5 to 10 minutes after injection and persists for as long as the tourniquet is left in place. The tourniquet should not be removed for at least 20 minutes (to prevent the release of local anaesthetic into the systemic circulation) and should not be left in place for more than about 75 minutes.

Note: although many anaesthetists recommend the use of local anaesthetic without adrenaline, procaine or lignocaine with adrenaline can be used safely if the tourniquet is applied tightly and remains in place for the recommended 20 minutes.

Cornual nerve block

First *2-3 ml of 5% procaine or 2% lidocaine* are injected at each of the following sites (see Figure 24.2b):

- Cornual branch of the lacrimal nerve is blocked as in the calf using the supraorbital process as a landmark. Insert the needle as close as possible to the supraorbital process.
- Cornual branch of the infratrochlear nerve is blocked dorsomedial to the eye close to the orbit.
- In kids, use a maximum of 1 ml of 1.25 or 2.5% procaine or 0.5 or 1% lidocaine on each side. General anaesthesia is safer and easier for routine disbudding (see Chapter 25).

Wait 5 minutes for the anaesthetic to take effect.

Note: Under most conditions, general anaesthesia is to be preferred to local anaesthesia for dehorning. For the technique, see Chapter 25.

Further reading

Abrahamsen, E.J. (2008) Ruminant field anesthesia. *Vet. Clin. North Amer.: Food Anim. Pract.*, **24** (3), 429–441.

Aithal, H.P., Pratap, A.K. and Singh, G.R. (1997) Clinical effects of epidurally administered ketamine and xylazine in goats. *Small Rum. Res.*, **24** (1), 55–64.

Babalola, G.O. and Oke, B.O. (1983) Intravenous regional analgesia for surgery of the limbs in goats. *Vet. Q. J. Clin. Sci. Epidemiol.*, **5** (4), 186–189.

Barvalia, D.R., Patil, D.B., Kelawal, N.H., Parikh, P.V. and Parsania, R.R. (1998) Comparative study of lignocaine, ketamine and ketamine-lignocaine combination for epidural analgesia in goats. *Indian Vet. Med. J.*, **22** (4), 317–320.

Carroll, G.L., Hartsfield, S.M. and Hambleton, R. (1997) Anesthetic effects of tiletamine-zolazepam, alone or in combination with butorphanol, in goats. *J. Amer. Vet. Med. Assoc.*, **211** (5), 593–597.

Dzikiti, T.B. (2013) Intravenous anaesthesia in goats: a review. *Journal of the South African Veterinary Association, North America*, **84**, Feb. 2013. Available at: http://www.jsava.co.za/index.php/jsava/article/view/499.

Dzikiti, T.B. *et al.* (2015) Determination of the minimum infusion rate of alfaxalone during its co-administration with midazolam in goats. *Vet. Rec. Open*, **2** (1), e000065. DOI: 10.1136/vetreco-2014-000065.

Ewing, K.K. (1990) Anesthesia techniques in sheep and goats. *Vet. Clin. North Amer.: Food Anim. Pract.*, **6** (3), 759–778.

Galatos, A.D. (2011) Anesthesia and analgesia in sheep and goats. *Vet. Clin. North Amer.: Food Anim. Pract.*, **27**, 47–59.

Gray, P.R. and McDonell, W.M. (1986) Anaesthesia in goats and sheep. Part I. Local analgesia. *Comp. Cont. Ed. Pract. Vet.*, **8** (1), S33–39.

Gray, P.R. and McDonell, W.M. (1986) Anaesthesia in goats and sheep. Part II. General anaesthesia. *Comp. Cont. Ed. Pract. Vet.*, **8** (3), S127–135.

Hallowell, G., Potter, T. and Aldridge, B. (2012) Medical support for cattle and small ruminant surgical patients. *In Pract.*, **34**, 226–233.

Hodgkinson, O. and Dawson, L. (2007) Practical anaesthesia and analgesia in sheep, goats and calves. *In Pract.*, **29** (10), 596–603.

Kutter, A.P.N. *et al.* (2006) Cardiopulmonary effects of dexmedetomidine in goats and sheep anaethetised with sevroflurane. *Vet. Rec.*, **159**, 624–629.

Lin, H. and Walz, P (eds) (2014) *Farm Animal Anesthesia: Cattle, Small Ruminants, Camelids, and Pigs*. Wiley-Blackwell, Oxford.

Prassinos, N.N., Galatos, A.D. and Raptopoulos, D. (2005) A comparison of propofol, thiopental or ketamine as induction agents in goats. *Veterinary Anaesth. Analg.*, **32**, 289–296.

Scott, P. (2015) Anaesthesia and analgesia in small ruminants. *Goat Vet. Soc. J.*, **31**, 3–11.

Taylor, P. (1980) *Goat anaesthesia. Goat Vet. Soc. J.*, **1**, 4–11.

Taylor, P.M. (1991) Anaesthesia in sheep and goats. *In Pract.*, **13** (1), 31–36.

Thurmon, J.C. *et al.* (1999) Xylazine sedation antagonised with tolazoline. *Comp. Cont. Educ. Pract. Vet.*, **21**, S11–S19.

CHAPTER 25

Disbudding and dehorning

In the United Kingdom, the disbudding and dehorning of goats is considered in veterinary surgery under the provision of the Veterinary Surgeons Act 1966, as amended 1982. These procedures can therefore only be undertaken by a veterinary surgeon. The only exception is the trimming of the insensitive tip of an ingrowing horn, which, if left untreated, could cause pain or distress. The secondary legislation in the United Kingdom does not specifically require an anaesthetic to be administered when disbudding goats. However, disbudding should be carried out by veterinary surgeons in accordance with good practice and in such a way as to minimize pain and suffering caused to the animal, which should include use of an anaesthetic (see RCVS, 2012, *Veterinary Record*, which clarifies the legal position on disbudding goats).

Anatomy

- The horn bud in the kid is proportionately much larger than in the calf.
- Two nerves supply the horn:
  1 Cornual branch of the lacrimal nerve.
  2 Cornual branch of the infratrochlear nerve.
  See Figure 24.2b.

Disbudding of kids

Of all the domestic species, only kids are routinely anaesthetised so soon after parturition. Because they are alert and active and relatively large when compared to, say, an adult cat, it is easy for the veterinary surgeon to forget that they are dealing with a neonatal animal.

> Kids are the youngest animals most veterinary surgeons ever anaesthetise.

Disbudding is the commonest surgical procedure carried out in goats, but there are still too many horror stories of kids not recovering from the anaesthetic (these are usually related to overdosage with xylazine), suffering *disbudding meningioencephalitis* from overenthusiastic use of the disbudding iron, with subsequent death later, or poor technique resulting in the regrowth of unsightly scurs (Plate 25.1). Fitting in goats is more common than is reported in the literature and, in many cases, this is probably due to brain damage incurred at disbudding.

The essential ingredients for successful and safe disbudding are:

- Short time away from the mother.
- Short time in the surgery.
- Short-acting anaesthetic.
- Rapid recovery.
- Very hot disbudding iron.
- Short time of application of the iron (<20–25 seconds total).
- Large enough diameter head on the iron (minimum 2 cm).
- Horn buds small enough to remove with one application of the iron.
- Keep kids warm, dry and draught free before, during and after disbudding.
- Weigh the kid if injectable drugs are being used for induction.

Diseases of the Goat, Fourth Edition. John Matthews.
© 2016 John Wiley & Sons, Ltd. Published 2016 by John Wiley & Sons, Ltd.

Age

Kids should preferably be disbudded between 2 and 7 days of age, when the horn buds are small enough to remove with one application of the iron (Plate 25.2). This applies particularly to males where horn growth is rapid.

Do not attempt to use the disbudding iron to remove overlarge buds in older kids as it is stressful for both the kid and veterinary surgeon and the buds will *always* regrow. It is better to wait until the horns are big enough to be removed with a wire.

Selection of anaesthetic agent for disbudding kids.

Best anaesthetic practice is not always in accordance with legislation governing the use of anaesthetic agents in farm animals (see Chapter 24).

By mask

At the surgery, induction and maintenance with *isoflurane* in oxygen by mask is simple, quick and safe and recovery is very rapid, but there are Health and Safety implications for staff; use a close-fitting mask in a well ventilated environment; monitor gas levels. As oxygen supports combustion, the mask must be removed before disbudding if a gas disbudder is used.

By intravenous injection into the cephalic or jugular vein

Propofol, 3–5 mg/kg, 3-5 ml/10 kg slowly i.v.

- Propofol can be used to provide short duration anaesthesia with the advantage of rapid recovery or for induction followed by intubation.
- Kids presented for disbudding require between 1 and 2 ml intravenously.

Alphaxalone, 10 mg/ml, 4.5 mg/kg slowly i.v., 4.5 ml/10 kg

- Smooth anaesthetic induction with good muscle relaxation.
- Administer very slowly to effect over about 30 seconds.
- Kids presented for disbudding require between 1 and 2 ml intravenously.

Note: propofol and alphaxalone are not licensed for use in food-producing animals.

Local infiltration

> Local nerve blocks can be used for anaesthesia, but great care must be taken to avoid overdosing and **other methods of anaesthesia** are preferable – use propofol or mask down with isofluorane.

Like all neonates, kids are very sensitive to *procaine* and *lidocaine* – analgesic doses are very close to toxic doses – and overdosage will result in lethargy, unwillingness to feed and even death. The toxic dose is about 10 mg/kg, that is 2 ml of 2% lidocaine or 5% procaine for a 4 kg kid.

Two nerves supply each horn bud (see Figure 24.2b):
- The cornual branch of the lacrimal nerve is blocked, as in the calf, between the lateral canthus of the eye and the posterior aspect of the bud, using the supraorbital process as a landmark.
- The cornual branch of the infratrochlear nerve is blocked dorsomedial to the eye close to the orbit.

Add 3 ml of sterile water to:
- 1 ml of 2% lidocaine + adrenaline to give 4 ml of 0.5% lidocaine and then use a maximum of 1 ml of diluted (0.5%) *lidocaine* on each site or
- 1 ml of 5% procaine + adrenaline to give 4 ml of 1.25% procaine and then use a maximum of 1 ml of diluted (1.25%) *procaine* on each site.

Alpha-2 agonists

Xylazine is the commonest alpha-2 agonist used as an anaesthetic for disbudding kids. Unless reversed with atipamezole, it produces *prolonged recumbency* and because very small amounts are required, it is very easy to overdose the kid, sometimes with fatal consequences.

The ruminant dose is much less than that routinely used in the dog and cat and it is preferable to dilute the standard 2% solution. Xylazine can be combined with ketamine and butorphanol to produce a mixture that can be used on the farm when groups of kids need disbudding. The small amount of the mixture required means use of an insulin syringe for accurate measurement is essential and kids should be weighed as necessary.

The majority of anaesthetic deaths in kids are caused by xylazine overdose.

Xylazine (2% solution), 0.05 mg/kg, 0.01 ml/10 kg slowly i.v. or 0.1 mg/kg, 0.02 ml/10 kg i.m.

- The standard *2% solution* can be diluted and administered via an insulin syringe to allow more accurate dosing.
- Be careful not to confuse 2% and 10% solutions!
- *Minute doses are required in young animals and it is very easy to overdose. In kids, 0.025 mg/kg i.m. is probably the maximum safe dose.*

Overdosage of xylazine and other alpha-2 agonists can be reversed by Atipamezole, 125–175 µg/kg, 0.1–0.15 ml/10 kg, half i.v. and half i.m.

KXB kid mixture

1000 mg   **K**etamine:20 mg   **X**ylazine:10 mg **B**utorphanol
   10 ml ketamine (100 mg/ml) + 1 ml xylazine (20 mg/ml) + 1 ml butorphanol (10 mg/ml)

that is add 1 ml xyalazine 2% solution and 1 ml butorphanol to a 10 ml bottle of ketamine. The solution is administered at *0.1 ml/5 kg i.v.*

Analgesia

Non-steroidal analgesics are not generally recommended for neonates, although meloxicam at 0.5 mg/kg has been shown to reduce pain for the first 24 hours after disbudding when compared to untreated kids
   Butorphonal 0.2 mg/kg i.v. is suitable for kids and provides analgesia for >2 hours.

Equipment

Calf disbudding irons are quite adequate for disbudding small kids, provided they reach a *satisfactory temperature* and have a *large enough diameter head* (minimum 2 cm, preferably 2.5 cm or 2.8 cm for male kids).

In this respect gas irons are probably better than electric irons. Dehorning irons, heated in a gas blowtorch to 600 °C, are also suitable. A technique for disbudding kids using a tubular cutting edge has been described by Boyd (1987).

Procedure

- Clip the hair from around the horn bud.
- With larger buds clip off the tip of the buds with scissors or bone forceps if necessary.
- Apply the iron to the bud with an even action to ensure the whole bud tissue is Destroyed. It is important to use a *hot* iron for the *minimum* time necessary to remove the bud. It is the heat of the iron that destroys the bud, rather than pressure. Excessive pressure or prolonged application of the iron may result in cortical necrosis, cerebral oedema and a brain-damaged kid or even fracture of the skull.
- The whole bud is best removed, rather than just burnt around, as this reduces the risk of infection.
- Where the disbudding iron has a recessed head or the iron is not very hot, scraping the burnt-out area with a scalpel blade and then briefly reapplying the iron ensures the tissue is destroyed.
- If the cauterised area is not large enough, a further ring of tissue can be removed with a scalpel blade or, even better, with an electric cautery knife. Several superficial vessels, especially the superficial temporal artery on the lateral side of the horn, may require recauterising.
- Spray the cauterised areas with tetracycline spray.
- Give broad spectrum antibiotics and tetanus antitoxin.
- Keep the kids warm, dry and draught free during their recovery and observe them regularly.

Note: large buds are best removed with embryotomy wire as described in dehorning. Where kids are presented at about 3 or 4 weeks, it is extremely difficult to remove successfully all horn tissue with a calf disbudding iron. In these cases it may be best to wait for a few more weeks until the horn can be removed with wire.

Take time to reexamine older kids to determine the success of your disbudding technique.

Descenting of kids

The sebaceous *scent glands* are located caudomedially behind the horn buds, so that burning a semicircular area caudomedially behind the buds will also remove the scent glands from the area, reducing to some extent buck odour (see Figure 25.1). However, the presence of musk cells in other parts of the tin-body and the habit of spraying urine means that even 'descented' males will still smell during the breeding season.

Dehorning of adult goats

Before an adult goat is dehorned, the whole procedure should be discussed with the owner and possible psychological and medical problems carefully explained.

Surgery is best carried out on a dry, non-pregnant goat during the autumn, winter or early spring.

> Removal of large horns from mature animals is probably contraindicated and should be undertaken with trepidation (Plate 25.3).

Psychological effect of dehorning

Horned goats, particularly when running with hornless animals, are often dominant within the herd. Dehorning can thus have profound psychological implications for the goat, involving loss of status, reduced milk yields or impaired fertility.

Possible complications from surgery include:

- Haemorrhage
- Sinusitis (Chapter 17)
- Myiasis
- Tetanus

Removal of the horns exposes variable size openings into the frontal sinuses, which extend into the hollow base of the horn. Even relatively small horns have a large base (Plates 25.4 and 25.5). After surgery, breathing can be seen to occur through the frontal sinuses and haemorrhage may occur down the nostrils.

It is important that the openings are kept as clean as possible after surgery by treating regularly with antibiotic powders or sprays, feeding hay from the floor rather

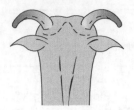

Figure 25.1 Incision line for scent gland removal.

than a rack and housing the goat in clean surroundings. The head is likely to remain tender for a month or more.

Anaesthesia

See Chapter 24.

With general anaesthesia, intubation should be considered, but it is not usually necessary if the operation is performed quickly on a starved animal.

Surgical technique

If the horns are relatively small, as for instance in a large kid or yearling animal, there is no need to suture the skin over the exposed area of the frontal sinuses, provided the area can be kept clean post-surgically, as the hole will heal naturally within a few days and the skin will grow back over the area fairly quickly. In mature animals, particularly males, the exposed area of the frontal sinuses should be closed by suturing the skin across the wound.

- *Smaller horns.* The area around both horns is clipped and routinely prepared for surgery and the skin incised in a ring about 1 cm from the base of the horn. The horns are removed in turn with embryotomy wire, working from the back of the horn forward and leaving the wire as low as possible to avoid leaving scurs. Any haemorrhage should be controlled by cautery.

    Bandaging of the head is sometimes recommended or the holes can be covered in Stockholm tar.

- *Larger horns.* The area around both horns is clipped and prepared for surgery and the skin incised about 1 cm from the base of the horns. The skin incision starts on the cranial aspect of the horn, encircles the horn and is then directed caudally towards the ear. It is important to leave plenty of skin to make closure easier, using the loose skin around the ears. The edges of the skin are undermined using sharp dissection with scissors and horns removed as above. After horn removal, the skin is undermined for an additional 2 to 3 cm to permit closure.

The surgical site is flushed with sterile saline and the skin closed with interrupted horizontal mattress sutures, using a non-absorbable material. The wound is dressed and the head bandaged until suture removal after 10 to 14 days, with the bandage changed after 4 days.

Antibiotics should be given for 5 to 7 days, together with tetanus antitoxin. A non-steroidal anti-inflammatory drug, carprofen or flunixin, should be given daily for 2 or 3 days.

Note: in the absence of infection overzealous cleaning of the area after dehorning will *delay* healing.

Descenting of adult goats

Descenting of polled, horned or disbudded adult males can be carried out under general anaesthesia.

A triangular skin flap is made, with the base of the triangle approaching the caudal aspect of the head and the apex 3 to 4 cm in front of a line between the horns or polls (Figure 25.1). The skin flap is separated from the underlying tissue and folded caudally to its base. The large scent glands, which generally lie within the borders of the triangle are exposed, grasped with forceps and removed with scissors or a scalpel blade, taking care to remove all glandular tissue. The skin flap is replaced with simple interrupted sutures. Antibiotic cover and tetanus antitoxin should be given.

Further reading

Alvarez, L. *et al.* (2009) Physiological and behavioural alterations in disbudded goat kids with and without local anaesthesia. *Appl. Anim. Behavioural Sci.*, **117**, 190–196.

Anon (1984) Disbudding. *Goat Vet. Soc. J.*, **5** (2), 32–33.

Anzuino, K. (2014) Disbudding goat kids and pain. *Goat Vet. Soc. J.*, **30**, 3–11.

Boyd, J. (1987) Disbudding of goat kids. *Goat Vet. Soc. J.*, **8** (2), 77–78.

Buttle, H.L. *et al.* (1986) Disbudding and dehorning of goats. *In Pract.*, 63–65.

Hague, B.A. and Hooper, R.N. (1997) Cosmetic dehorning in goats. *Veter. Surg.*, **26** (4), 332–334.

Ingvast-Larsson, C., Högberg, M., Mengistu, U. , Olsén, L. *et al.* (2011) Pharmacokinetics of meloxicam in adult goats and its analgesic effect in disbudded kids. *J. Vet. Pharmacol. Therap.*, **34** (1), 64–69.

Johnson, E.H. and Steward, T. (1984) Cosmetic descenting of adult goats. *Agri. Pract.*, **5** (9), 16.

Mobini, S. (1991) Cosmetic dehorning of adult goats. *Small Rum. Res.*, **5**, 187–191.

RCVS (2012) *Veterinary Record*, **171** (8), 186.

Taylor, P. (1983) Goat anaesthesia. *Goat Vet. Soc. J.*, **1**, 4–11.

Turner, A.S. and McIlwraith, C.W. (1982) Dehorning the mature goat. In: *Techniques in Large Animal Surgery*, pp. 317–319. Lea and Febiger, Philadelphia, PA.

CHAPTER 26

Surgical techniques

Considerations before surgery

Compared to other domestic species, there is a paucity of references to surgical techniques in goats. There are no textbooks dealing specifically with surgery in small ruminants, although most general large animal surgical texts contain references to the goat.

Unfortunately, many veterinary surgeons still approach surgery in the goat with trepidation. In part, this is fear of the unknown and partly because goats have the reputation of being poor patients. Stress on both surgeon and patient can be reduced by:

■ *Using familar techniques*. This may mean a different preferred surgical approach between a veterinary surgeon used to dealing with companion animals and one in farm practice.
■ *Using familiar drugs*. For instance, isofluorane and xylazine are useful anaesthetic agents in goats.
■ *Basic preparation beforehand*:
  o How is the patient going to be handled before, during and after surgery?
  o What problems may be encountered during anaesthesia and what should be done if problems do occur?
  o Are the nursing staff fully conversant with the procedure to be undertaken?
■ Routine use of fluid therapy for maintenance and replacement needs:
  o Maintenance will be provided a balanced electrolyte solution at a flow rate of *4–10 ml/kg/h*.
  o During prolonged surgery in kids under 12 weeks, check blood glucose during anaesthesia and infuse 5% dextrose 3–5 ml/kg/hour where necessary.
■ *Routine use of analgesics pre- and post-operatively.*
■ *Knowledge of the anatomy of the area concerned.*

Table 26.1 Clinical signs of post-operative pain.

■ Increased heart rate
■ Rapid and shallow breathing
■ Changes in facial expression
■ Decreased appetite
■ Cessation of cudding
■ Teeth grinding
■ Grunting
■ Changes in gait or posture
■ Violent reaction to handling or rigid posture designed to immobilise the painful region

Pre- and post-operative pain management

Pre-surgical parameters, including respiratory rate, heart rate, amount of vocalisation and activity, and general appearance and attitude should be recorded to be used as a basis for post-surgical evaluation (Table 26.1). Pre-operatively analgesia should be provided whenever possible by an *opioid analgesic* (Table 26.2) and/or a *non-steroidal anti-inflammatory (NSAID) drug* (Table 26.3) or a *local block* using a local anaesthetic agent such as procaine, together with an NSAID. The alpha-2 agonists xylazine, medetomidine and detomidine all have analgesic properties, but the duration of action of many opioid analgesics is generally longer and a combinations of alpha-2 agonists and opiod analgesics will provide better analgesia. Five main NSAIDs are licensed for use in cattle in the United Kingdom and can therefore be used in goats under the cascade system. They can be given parenterally, usually by intravenous or subcutaneous injection (Table 26.2), or orally.

Diseases of the Goat, Fourth Edition. John Matthews.
© 2016 John Wiley & Sons, Ltd. Published 2016 by John Wiley & Sons, Ltd.

Table 26.2 Opioid analgesics.

Drug	Dose	Route
Buprenorphine	0.01 mg/kg	i.m. or s.c.
Butorphanol	0.2–0.5 mg/kg	i.v., i.m. or s.c
Morphine	Up to 10 mg total	i.m.
Pentazocine	2 mg/kg every 4 hours	i.m. or slow i.v.
Pethidine hydrochloride (Meperidine hydrochloride)	10 mg/kg	i.m. or s.c.

Table 26.3 Injectable NSAIDs licensed for food-producing animals in the United Kingdom.

Drug	Dose	Route
Carprofen	1.4 mg/kg repeat once after 48–72 hours	s.c. or i.v.
Flunixin meglumine	2 mg/kg sid for 3–5 days	i.v.
Ketoprofen	3 mg/kg sid for 3–5 days	i.m. or i.v.
Meloxicam	2 mg/kg initially, followed by 0.5 mg/kg every 36 hours	s.c. or i.v.
Tolfenamic acid	2–4 mg/kg repeated once after 48 hours	s.c. or i.v.

Post-operatively some animals will show obvious signs of pain such as grunting, grinding of the teeth, guarding of painful areas and vocalisation on movement or palpation, but evaluation of the animal should include close monitoring for more overt and subtle signs of pain, such as an increased heart rate, rapid shallow breathing and changes in facial expression. The goat might also appear dull and lethargic with little interest in its surroundings and a depressed appetite, with cessation of cudding. Post-surgical analgesia should be continued for at least 3 days after major surgery, usually with *NSAIDs* (Table 26.1), but *opiates* can be used if appropriate.

Neuroleptanalgesics like fentanyl have also been used. Intravenous administration of fetanyl results in a relatively short half-life (1 to 2 hours) that limits its use for pain management in the goat, but can be used as an intravenous loading dose, *fentanyl*, **2.5** *µg/kg i.v.,* before application of a transdermal patch. *Fentanyl transdermal patches (50 µg/h)* are applied to shaved skin on the neck, where they cannot be chewed by the patient, and taped and stapled in place. The goat should be kept separate from other animals. Transdermal administration of fentanyl results in variable plasma concentrations detectable between 1 and 8 hours, with peak concentration ranging from about 8 to 18 hours.

Caudal analgesia can also be provided by administering drugs by saccrococygeal and lumbosacral epidural injection (Chapter 24).

> In almost all situations, pain relief should be administered routinely for at least 3 days after major surgery.

Castration

Goats are commonly castrated if they are to be:
- Kept for meat for longer than 4 months.
- Retained as wethers for fibre production.
- Kept as pets.
- Used as pack animals or harness goats.

Castration renders the animal infertile and prevents the development of male odour and unpleasant secondary sexual behaviour, such as spraying urine.

Uncastrated kids show better growth rate, efficiency of feed utilisation and carcase yield than castrated kids, but, in older kids, the meat is likely to be darker and more strongly flavoured. Early castration may lead to a greater risk of urolithiasis, because the urethra remains relatively small. It may be better to delay castration in animals that are to be kept for work or as pets, but an uncastrated male should never be sold as a pet, without full discussion with the new owner and arrangements for castration having been made.

In the United Kingdom, there is a difference in the law regarding the castration of lambs and kids; kids over 2 months of age must be castrated by a veterinary surgeon using anaesthesia (Table 26.4), whereas lambs up to 3 months of age can be castrated surgically by a lay person without anaesthesia.

Rubber rings

Very young kids can be castrated with elastrator rings placed round the neck of the scrotum using a special applicator. The ring constricts the blood flow to and from the testes and scrotum, which wither and drop off in about 2 to 6 weeks. It is essential to confirm that both testicles are fully trapped within the scrotal sac

Table 26.4 Castration of kids.

Age of animal	Technique	Person who may perform castration	Anaesthetic required?
1st week of life	Rubber ring	Any	No
	Burdizzo	Any	No
<2 months	Surgical	Any	No
>2 months	Surgical	Veterinary surgeon	Yes

beneath the ring or an induced inguinal cryptorchid may be produced. Conversely, placing the ring too high can trap the urethra – ensure that the teats are proximal to the ring.

There is a risk of infection around the ring and also of tetanus. Kids castrated by rings show behavioural evidence of acute pain for at least 3 hours. There is evidence in lambs that a combined technique of rubber ring and bloodless castrator, or Burdizzo emasculator (see below), causes less acute pain. The Burdizzo emasculator is applied for 10 seconds, just distal to the rubber ring, across the full width of the scrotum.

Emasculator (Burdizzo)

Each spermatic cord is crushed in turn using the emasculator, depriving the testicle of its blood supply and causing the testicle to atrophy and become non-functional after several weeks, whilst leaving the scrotum intact. By staggering the placing of the emasculator on the two cords, the skin in the middle of the scrotum is left undamaged, retaining sufficient blood supply to retain scrotal viability.

Each cord is generally crushed twice, with the second crush below the first, although a single application for 6 to 10 seconds of a correctly functioning emasculator should be effective. The scrotum should be carefully palpated before application of the emasculator to check both testicles are descended and that there is no scrotal hernia.

This technique is less painful than using a rubber ring, at least in the first few hours after castration.

Surgical (open) castration

Kids

The scrotum is cleaned and scrubbed with chlorhexidine or povidone-iodine, the bottom of the scrotum pulled downwards and the distal third removed with a scalpel blade. In very young kids, each testicle is grasped individually, the testicle and spermatic cord with intact tunica freed from the fascia by traction and blunt dissection and the cremaster muscle and tunica then ruptured by continuing controlled traction. Traction to the spermatic vessels produces rupture in the inguinal area as the testicle is removed. Ligation of the spermatic vessels is unnecessary in newborn kids, but is recommended in kids over a few days of age. Kids mature rapidly and are sexually mature by 3 months of age. Older kids, even pygmies, have relatively large testicles.

Adults

An emasculator with catgut ligation can be used in adult animals. The ventral third of the scrotum is removed with a scalpel, as in kids, or an incision just shorter than the length of the testicle is made in the ventral scrotum. Each testicle is then individually exposed and the fascia bluntly separated from the spermatic cord. The vascular and non-vascular portions of the spermatic cord are identified. The non-vascular portion is crushed for about 10 seconds just proximal to the epididymis and then the vascular portion is crushed to remove the testicle, leaving the emasculator in place for at least 1 minute. A catgut suture is placed around the cord, 1 cm proximal to the emasculator blade. Before releasing the emasculator, an artery forceps is placed on the edge of the cord and a check made for haemorrhage before the cord is released.

Open castration should not be carried out in warm weather when fly strike may be a problem.

Prophylaxis against tetanus should always be given. After castration, the goat should be placed in a clean, dust-free environment and exercise encouraged.

Anaesthesia is desirable in all animals, although only legally required in kids over 2 months. Kids can be conveniently castrated at the same time as they are anaesthetised for disbudding. In other animals, general anaesthesia (see Chapter 24) or local infiltration with lignocaine and adrenalin can be used. Because goats are sensitive to the toxic effects of lignocaine, care should be taken not to exceed recommended doses – toxic effects occur at 10 mg/kg intramuscularly, that is 5 ml of 2% lignocaine in a 10 kg kid.

Umbilical hernias

Surgical resection

In cases in which the hernial ring is larger than 5 cm, surgical intervention should be carried out.

> *Anaesthesia.* sedation + local anaesthetic infiltration or general anesthesia

The area around the hernia is clipped and surgically prepared. The hernial sac is opened and the area carefully checked digitally to ensure that no viscera are adhered to the inner lining of the ring and that no enlarged or infected umbilical remnants are present. Excess skin is removed, the hernial sac everted into the abdominal cavity, the ring edges freshened and the defect in the abdominal wall closed by opposing the abdominal wall with horizontal mattress sutures using absorbable suture material. Subcutaneous tissue can be closed with a simple interrupted pattern using absorbable sutures and the skin with non-absorbable sutures. Prosthetic mesh may be required to close large defects in the body wall.

Animals should be given tetanus prophylaxis and antibiotics and then closely monitored for signs of sepsis and surgical failure. Exercise should be limited for 7 to 14 days after surgery.

If an abscess is present, the hernial sac can be resected at the junction with the hernial ring and the entire intact abscess and hernial sac resected and discarded, being careful not to break the abscess and contaminate the wound.

Surgical treatment of obstructive urolithiasis

See also Chapter 15.

> It is not possible to catheterise male goats as far as the bladder so surgical intervention is always necessary in cases of obstructive urolithiasis.

Treatment of urolithiasis presents major problems for the veterinary surgeon. Complete catheterisation to the bladder is anatomically impossible as catheters will not pass the ischial arch as they enter a diverticulum of the urethra, the urethral recess, so surgical intervention is usually inevitable and it is necessary to make rapid decisions so that the discomfort of the animal can be relieved once a diagnosis has been reached. Many of the techniques used have a problematical outcome and there is a high recurrence rate in many animals following surgery. *It is essential that the owner is fully involved in the discussion concerning the possible options for treatment and is aware of the costs and long-term prognosis before surgery is undertaken.* Stud males present particular problems, as surgery must not impair fertility, and in harness goats, the backward direction of urination following a urethrostomy can present major difficulties for the owner. Many owners may opt for euthanasia. Figure 26.1 attempts to provide a rational framework for surgery and Table 26.5 compares surgical techniques. How far each goat is taken down the surgical pathway will depend on the value of the goat, its future use and owner preference. *Early treatment is associated with a higher survival rate.*

Animals with obstructive urolithiasis are usually uraemic, with BUN levels often < 40 mmol/litre, and with elevated serum creatinine levels. *Dehydration and electrolyte abnormalities must be corrected before surgery.* Electrolyte abnormalities include *hyponatraemia, hypochloraemia* and *hyperglycaemia* and most animals show an elevated white cell count due to a *neutrophilia*.

Intravenous fluid therapy, using *0.9% saline solution,* should be given pre-operatively and for as long as necessary post-operatively to correct electrolyte imbalances. Potassium concentrations are variable, so potassium salts should only be given if hypokalaemia is established – males with chronic obstructions, metabolic acidosis and/or uroperitoneum are likely to be *hyperkalaemic.*

Hypophosphataemia is a common abnormality in caprine urolithiasis and if severe may cause general muscle weakness or cardiac abnormalities. *Hypocalcaemia* may occur secondary to bladder ruture.

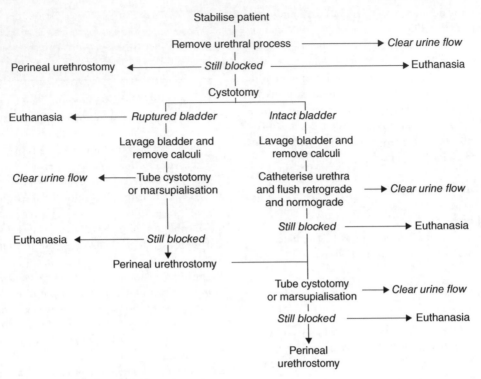

Figure 26.1 Treatment of obstructive urolithiasis.

Table 26.5 Comparison of surgical techniques in treatment of obstructive urolithiasis.

Surgical procedure	Anaesthesia	Pros	Cons
Urethral process amputation	+/–Sedation + LA	Simple Immediate resolution if sludge or calculi in process only	Most reobstruct in <36 hours as calculi enter urethra from bladder
Perineal urethrostomy	Sedation + LA Epidural	Short hospitalisation	Salvage procedure Stricture formation always occurs in <1 year
Tube cystotomy	GA	80+% success rate <20% recurrent obstruction Suitable for stud males	Expensive Long hospitalisation Catheter problems Adhesion formation
Bladder marsupialisation	GA	Salvage procedure	Expensive Urine scald Urinary tract infections Stricture Bladder mucosa prolapse
Cystotomy with lavage and urethral flushing		Shorter duration of hospitalization than tube cystotomy	Prolonged surgical time Risk of urethral rupture

After successful removal of the obstruction, BUN levels fall rapidly to below 20 mmol/litre within 24 hours and below 10 mmol/litre within 48 hours.

Pre-operative *cystocentesis* reduces pressure on the diaphragm during lateral or dorsal recumbancy, prevents spontaneous bladder rupture from fluid administration, slows the progression of azotaemia and elecrolyte imbalances and helps relax urethral spasm. A Bonanno catheter can be placed in the bladder, preferably under ultrasound guidance. Emptying the bladder allows surgery to be planned for a convenient time. The catheter consists of a straight trocar, which serves as a core and guide for a plastic tube with a curved end that is kept straight while it is inside the trocar. At the end of the plastic tube, a small flat plate is present that can be taped or sutured to the skin. When the trocar is removed the curved end keeps the catheter in the bladder. If surgery is not an option for the owner, the catheter can be left in place until patency is achieved, but the flow may become restricted, or the catheter kink, if it is left in for more than 36 to 48 hours. The Bonanno catheter is generally removed during the surgical preparation for a tube cystostomy or other surgical procedure. The hole in the bladder made by the catheter can be closed during surgery, but does not seem to cause a problem if the catheter is removed from goats that do not go to surgery.

Antibiotic cover should be given to prevent ascending infection – use penicillin, cephalosporins, ampicillin, amoxycillin, potentiated sulphonamides or fluoroquinolones. Temporary pain relief is achieved by use of caudal epidural anaesthesia (see Chapter 24).

Surgical removal of the urethral process

The urethral process should be examined in all cases of suspected urolithiasis as this is the commonest site of blockage. Gritty or sandy material can occasionally be milked out without resorting to surgery, particularly in kids and if the animal is sedated. If this is unsuccessful, amputation of the process may alleviate the blockage. Administration of a spasmolytic and analgesic agent (metamizole, hyoscine butylscopolamine, 0.5–5 ml i.v.) will relieve pain and aid passage of calculi. Alternatively, flunixin meglumine, 2 mg/kg, 2 ml/45 kg i.v. will provide analgesia and reduce inflammation.

Sedation will aid the exteriorisation of the penis and may provide sufficient muscle relaxation to allow a stone to be passed. Diazepam (0.25–0.5 mg/kg slowly i.v.) is the sedative of choice, although it does not provide analgesia. The diuretic effect of xylazine may worsen bladder distension if the urethral obstruction is complete.

If it is not possible to exteriorise the penis, it is possible to gain access to the penis by making a longitudinal incision through the prepuce, after anaesthetising the skin with a small amount of local anaesthetic. The urethral process can be exposed or, alternatively, if a blockage has been detected by palpation or ultrasound in the shaft of the penis, the obstructed area can be elevated and an incision made over the stones, allowing them to be removed. Small incisions can be closed with surgical glue. Larger incisions may need closure of the mucosa with fine monofilament absorbable sutures.

Even if urethral patency is restored, recurrent urethral blockage may subsequently occur as additional calculi enter the urethra from the bladder.

Where further stones are present or the blockage is not at the urethral process, surgery will be necessary to locate and remove the obstruction.

> The urethral process should be examined and removed in all cases of urethral blockage.

Tube cystotomy

Tube cystotomy is the treatment of choice for relief of obstructive urolithiais in valuable animals, if the male is to be used for breeding and in animals where a ruptured bladder is suspected. It is expensive, involving a long period of hospitalisation or careful nursing at home and must be combined with dietary changes to prevent a recurrence of the problem. The insertion of an indwelling Foley catheter into the urinary bladder temporarily relieves the obstruction, providing immediate relief to the animal, by diverting urine flow from the blocked urethra. This gives time for the obstruction of the urethra to be resolved by eliminating urethral spasm associated with urethral pressure, allowing time for the urethritis to subside and the urinary calculi to dissolve. Dissolution of struvite calculi can be helped by altering the urinary pH by dietary change and by dosing with ammonium chloride. Calcium carbonate stones will not dissolve in the acidified urine but the formation of new stones will be prevented. Ideally, all the calculi will be removed during surgery by careful flushing of the bladder and urethra but some calculi may be firmly embedded in the urethral mucosa, preventing removal.

Anaesthesia: general anaesthesia

The goat is placed in dorsal recumbency and the abdomen clipped and routinely prepared for surgery. A 10–15 cm paramedian incision is made midway between the scrotum and the distal prepuce, 3 cm to the left or right of the midline. The penis and prepuce are reflected and the abdomen opened through the linea alba. The bladder is exteriorised and packed off from the abdomen with moist swabs.

If the bladder is intact, two stay sutures are placed on the ventral aspect of the bladder and a cystotomy performed, with a full thickness incision at the apex of the bladder. Urine is aspirated, any calculi removed and the bladder lavaged with sterile isotonic saline. Careful removal of all possible calculi will reduce the risk of further obstruction later.

Calculi are flushed from the urethra with sterile saline, (a) *retrograde* by means of a urinary catheter (8–10 fg) passed through the neck of the bladder into the urethra and (b) *normograde* by means of a urinary catheter inserted into the distal opening of the urethra (easier if the urethral process has been amputated). Care should be taken not to exert excessive pressure on the urethra during flushing as *overenthusiastic flushing can lead to rupture of the urethra.*

If the bladder is ruptured, the bladder wall is repaired with a 2 metric synthetic absorbable suture, using a continuous inversion suture (Lembert or Cushing) or simple continuous suture, followed by a continuous Lembert suture.

The bladder is thoroughly lavaged with isotonic saline and any residual calculi removed. Any calculi in the peritoneal cavity are harmless. As many calculi as possible are removed from the urethra by retrograde and normograde flushing. This is especially important with calcium carbonate stones, which do not dissolve in acidified urine. An 8–20 fg silicone treated latex Foley catheter is placed through a small incision lateral to the paramedian incision and tunneled subcutaneously a short distance before entering the abdominal cavity. The end of the catheter is passed through a stab incision into the bladder, where it is secured by two purse-string sutures. The balloon of the catheter is inflated *with 10 ml saline* (air escapes) and traction applied to the distal portion of the catheter to draw the bladder closer to the body wall, although in most cases it does not come into direct contact with the wall. The abdominal incision is closed and the catheter sutured to the skin, using Chinese finger cuff ligatures or tape tabs.

A 1% acetic acid solution can be used to flush the bladder, via the Foley catheter. This can be produced by diluting a standard commercial vinegar product, containing 4 to 8% acetic acid, 1 part in 5 (20% solution of vinegar). Keeping the catheter plugged for 30–60 minutes will give time to dissolve crystals or stone still in the bladder and some pass into the urethra to help dissolve any crystals there.

Stones that dissolve when placed in a tube of 1% acetic acid are most likely to be struvite. If the stones dissolve, there is better prognosis for the resolution of a urethral obstruction.

Broad-spectrum antibiotics should be given before surgery until 3 to 5 days after the catheter is removed and urethral inflammation reduced by giving flunixin meglumine, 1.1 mg/kg, 1 ml/45 kg i.v. every 12 hours until the urethral obstruction is resolved.

The catheter needs to be left in situ for a minimum of 7 to 10 days to allow time for a fibrinous or omental seal to form around the cystotomy site. After this time, the catheter can be removed without urine leakage occurring.

The catheter is left open for 3 to 4 days after surgery and then intermittently closed to determine if the urethra is patent. If the animal shows signs of discomfort such as straining or crying, the catheter is again opened and the process repeated the following day. When urine starts to drip from the urethra, the catheter is incrementally closed for longer periods, until a steady stream of urine is produced. Once urination has been normal for 24 hours, the catheter can be removed.

The time to dribbling of urine varies between 1 day and 4 weeks and the time to a steady stream of urine between 4 days and 5 weeks. Goats seem to tolerate the catheters very well and do not normally need restraint or an Elizebethan collar to prevent the removal of the catheter. The greatest risk for unwanted removal is generally other goats. Dissolution of struvite calculi can be encouraged by:

■ Dosing the animal with *ammonium chloride orally* daily or twice daily to acidify the urine. The dose should be titrated for the individual goat, with urinary pH being determined using a pH meter or urine strips; *10 g* is a reasonable starting point for a daily dose, but substantially higher levels may be necessary in large animals to ensure that the urine pH remains <6.0 for 24 hours. The salt can be dissolved in 40 ml of water for drenching and sweetened with sugar if necessary. Most goats readily take the necessary dose in orange juice.

- *Ammonium chloride* can be fed at *40 mg/kg* daily in feed, but is not very palatable and will need disguising in molassed food.
- Infusing the bladder daily with *200 ml of Walpole's Buffer Solution* through the Foley catheter.
- Urine pH should be monitored daily wherever possible (goats will often urinate when a stranger enters the pen). *The urine pH should be stabilised at 5.5 to 6.0.*
- Human drugs such as *hemiacidrin* (Renacidin, Guardian Labs) have also been used to acidify the urine and dissolve struvite calculi. It does not work well if the stones have a significant calcium oxalate component; 30 ml of undiluted solution are instilled into the bladder and left for 30 to 60 minutes. The catheter is then allowed to drain. This is repeated 4 to 6 times daily until dissolution of stones is achieved. The solution is irritating if it leaks out of the bladder or urethra, so it should not be used in patients with urinary tract infection or urethral/bladder rupture and use is delayed for five days following surgery to allow the seal to form around the cystotomy site. During this time, uroliths obtained during surgery can be placed in a solution of the drug to see if they dissolve *in vitro*.

An intact urethral process, absence of abdominal fluid and a serum potassium level <5.2 mEq/litre have all been associated with an improved survival rate. Tube cystotomy may not be successful in a small number of animals. In these animals, a urethrostomy should be carried out or euthanasia considered.

Percutaneous tube cystotomy

Percutaneous tube cystotomy provides a cheaper option for the owner. However, because it does not permit the removal of calculi by lavage of the bladder and catheterisation of the urethra, it is more suited to the treatment of phosphate (struvite) induced blockages, which will dissolve in acidic urine, rather than those produced by calcium carbonate calculi, which do not dissolve.

Anaesthesia: caudal epidural or general anaesthesia

The goat is placed in right lateral recumbency with the hind limb tied caudodorsally. The bladder is identified by ultrasound in the left prepubic region, making sure that there is no viscera between the abdominal wall and the bladder. A 12 fg sleeved trochar is thrust into the bladder under ultrasound guidance and a 10 fg Foley catheter inserted into the bladder through the sleeve. The balloon of the bladder is inflated with 10 ml saline, the sleeve removed from the abdomen, the balloon pulled towards the left abdominal wall and the catheter sutured in place. The catheter is left in situ for a variable length of time (see tube cystotomy above).

Bladder marsupialisation

Bladder marsupialisation involves the creation of a permanent stoma between the bladder mucosa and the skin of the ventral abdomen, bypassing the urethra so urine flows directly from the bladder to the exterior. It can be used as the primary corrective procedure for urethral blockage, as well as a salvage option for animals where previous attempts at surgery have been unsuccessful. In some large, deep-bodied animals, it may be difficult to bring the bladder into contact with the abdominal wall, so the procedure may be contraindicated in these animals.

Anaesthesia: lumbosacral epidural or general anesthesia

The animal is placed in dorsal recumbency and a 10–15 cm laparotomy incision is made 3 cm lateral to and parallel with the prepuce. Urine is aspirated from the bladder and two stay sutures are placed beside the apex of the bladder. A 3–4 cm, longitudinal cystotomy incision is made on the ventral aspect of the bladder apex. Any remaining urine is drained and calculi removed by lavage and suction.

The apex of the bladder is then positioned against the peritoneal surface of the opposite abdominal wall, as far cranially as possible without producing excessive tension on the bladder. A 4 cm paramedian, longitudinal incision is made in the abdominal wall, aligned optimally with the bladder, the bladder apex repositioned through the second incision and the stay sutures repositioned. Four simple interrupted sutures of 2 metric synthetic absorbable suture material are placed through the external rectus sheath of the incision and into the seromuscular layer of the bladder at the 12, 3, 6, and 9 o'clock positions, so that the opening into the bladder is level with the skin. The seromuscular layer of the bladder around the cystotomy incision is sutured to the external rectus sheath, using 2 metric synthetic absorbable material in an interrupted horizontal mattress pattern. The edges of the cystotomy incision are then sutured circumferentially to the skin, using 3 metric synthetic absorbable material in a simple continuous pattern to appose the bladder mucosa to the skin. The abdomen is lavaged with isotonic saline and the laparotomy incision is closed routinely. Post-operative antibiotic therapy is continued for approximately one week.

Long-term post-operative complications include the inevitable *urinary incontinence* and *urine scalding* of the ventral abdomen, possible fibrosis and chronic stenosis of the marsupialisation site, *cystitis* and *bladder mucosal prolapse*.

Clipping the hair on the abdomen, periodic cleaning of the site and the judicious use of protective ointments such as petroleum jelly will reduce the effects of urine scald.

Cystotomy

Cystotomy, together with thorough lavaging of the bladder and bidirectional flushing of the urethra with saline to remove calculi, is often successful in relieving the obstruction, but prolonged surgical time (2–3 hours) is required for the urethral flushing and there is a risk of urethral rupture at the site of obstruction.

Anaesthesia: general anaesthesia

The goat is placed in dorsal recumbency and the abdomen clipped and routinely prepared for surgery. A 10–15 cm paramedian incision is made midway between the scrotum and the distal prepuce, 3 cm to the left or right of the midline.The penis and prepuce are reflected and the abdomen opened through the linea alba. The bladder is exteriorised and packed off from the abdomen with moist swabs.

If the bladder is ruptured, a tube cystotomy should be considered (see below).If the bladder is intact, two stay sutures are placed on the ventral aspect of the bladder and a cystotomy performed, with a full thickness incision at the apex of the bladder. Urine is aspirated, any calculi removed and the bladder lavaged with sterile isotonic saline. Careful removal of all possible calculi will reduce the risk of further obstruction later. Calculi are flushed from the urethra with sterile saline, (a) retrograde by means of a urinary catheter (8–10 fg) passed through the neck of the bladder into the urethra and (b) normograde by means of a urinary catheter inserted into the distal opening of the urethra (easier if the urethral process has been amputated). Care should be taken not to exert excessive pressure on the urethra during flushing as *overenthusiastic flushing can lead to rupture of the urethra*.

If the urethral obstruction is cleared by flushing, the bladder is closed with 2 metric synthetic absorbable suture, using a continuous inversion suture (Lembert or Cushing), or simple continuous suture followed by a continuous Lembert suture. The linea alba is closed with 3metric synthetic absorbable suture in a simple interrupted pattern, the subcutaneous tissue closed in a simple continuous pattern and the skin sutured with non-absorbable material.

If the urethral blockage cannot be cleared, the surgical options are 1) a perineal urethrostomy or 2) a tube cystotomy.

Urethrotomy

Urethrotomy should be considered an emergency procedure to relieve the pressure on the goat and the surgeon, giving time to consider the options for the long-term surgical solution of the problem. Amputation of the urethral process should be carried out at the same time as the urethrotomy to prevent the possibility of a smaller calculus causing obstruction later.

If the blockage is in the distal portion of the urethra, a low urethrotomy, with or without urethral closure, may relieve the obstruction, at least temporarily. Although plain or contrast radiography or ultrasound studies may help to locate calculi and determine the numbers of calculi present, in many cases it is difficult to establish the precise location of the calculi and several calculi may be present at different sites, so that the urethra may subsequently become obstructed again as additional calculi travel down the urethra. Postsurgical fibrosis and chronic stenosis commonly occur and result in even smaller calculi causing reobstruction.

Anaesthesia: caudal epidural or general anaesthesia

The surgical site is clipped and routinely prepared for surgery. A skin incision is made directly over the penis at the site of the obstruction and the penis located by blunt dissection of the underlying subcutaneous adipose tissue and elastic tissue surrounding the penis. A small incision is made in the ventral surface of the penis, directly over the calculus (calculi) and the calculus (calculi) removed.

A catheter is passed proximal and distally up the urethra as far as possible to ensure urethral patency.

The urethral wall may be sutured with an absorbable material, using simple interrupted or continuous sutures, but urine often seeps through the incision and it is preferable to leave both urethra and skin to heal by secondary intention.

Broad-spectrum antibiotics should be given before and for several days after surgery.

Perineal urethrostomy

Perineal urethrostomy is a salvage procedure, unsuitable for breeding males. Even with good surgical techniques, the long-term prognosis is poor, with less than 20% of animals surviving more than a year without stricture or recurrent obstruction.

Anaesthesia: caudal epidural or general anaesthesia

The skin from the anus to scrotal neck is routinely prepared for surgery and a midline skin incision is made from the dorsal aspect of the ischium distally for about 10 cm. A relatively high site encourages urine to be expelled caudally, reducing urine scald of the hind legs, which is often a major long-term problem post-operatively.

The penis is exposed by blunt dissection of the subcutaneous tissues and then incised longitudinally in the midline, separating the bulbourethral and ischiocavernosus muscles, so that the urethra, surrounded by the corpus cavernosum urethrae, is exposed. Adequate mobilisation of the urethra is important to ensure that the urethral mucosa and skin are well apposed and the sutures are not under tension. Apart from urine scald, the commonest complication of perineal urethrostomy is stricture formation.

A 1–2 cm incision is made in the urethra, releasing a flow of urine if the urethra is patent distal to the incision and the urethral mucosa and a small amount of underlying fibrous tissue sutured to the skin with 2 or 3 metric polyglycolic acid is attached to a swaged-on needle. The initial sutures are placed dorsally and ventrally, and then the lateral sutures. An indwelling urinary catheter (8–10

fg) is placed in the bladder, sutured to the skin using a tape tab and left in situ for 3 days.

Broad-spectrum antibiotics should be given before surgery and continued for 3 days after catheter removal.

Vasectomy

Anaesthesia: sedation and local anaesthesia or lumbosacral epidural anaesthesia

Effective analgesia makes surgery much easier. Lumbosacral epidural anaesthesia provides superior anaesthesia compared with infiltration of the spermatic cord with local anaesthetic – the buck is relaxed and exteriorising of the spermatic cord is relatively easy as the cremaster muscle is flaccid

The scrotum is prepared for surgery. A longitudinal incision is made in the neck of the scrotum over the spermatic cords. Separate incisions can be made for each testicle or a bilateral vasectomy can be performed through a single midscrotal incision. The spermatic cord is exteriorised by blunt dissection and the vas deferens is identified as a firm white cord and carefully dissected free from the adjacent blood vessels, avoiding damaging the blood vessels with resultant haemorrhage. Each end of the vas deferens is ligated to prevent recanalisation and at least 5 cm of the vas deferens removed. There is no need to suture the vaginal tunics. The skin is closed with absorbable or non-absorbable sutures. Portions of the removed vas deferens can be submitted for histopathology if confirmation of removal is required or stored in formol saline in case confirmation is required later. Allow 30 days post-vasectomy before assuming that the male is infertile.

Caesarian section

Indications

Dystocia (see Chapter 4), pregnancy toxaemia (see Chapter 4), as an aid to disease control (e.g. CAE)

A caesarian section in the goat can be successfully carried out using a variety of surgical approaches – flank, ventral abdominal midline, ventral abdominal paramedian – and with the goat in lateral or dorsal recumbency or standing. It is important that the surgeon adopts an approach with which he/she is comfortable and this may depend on whether the surgeon's experience is based

Table 26.6 The pros and cons of left flank and ventral midline laparatomy.

Left flank laparotomy

Pros:	local anaesthesia; less risk of wound breakdown; goat conscious so readily mothers kids; kids not depressed by anaesthetic
Cons:	difficult to exteriorise and isolate uterus to prevent contamination of the abdominal cavity when kids are dead and putrified

Ventral midline laparotomy

Pros:	easier access to gravis uterus; easier to prevent abdominal contamination
Cons:	general anaesthesia; greater risk of wound breakdown in active animal or from interference by suckling kids

---

largely on small or large animals. The most common surgical approaches are either a left flank or a ventral midline laparotomy. The right flank offers no advantage over the left flank, since it is easier for a single surgeon to hold the rumen in than to keep the intestines in place (Table 26.6).

In general, goats are less amenable than sheep to being restrained and restraint in lateral recumbency is much easier than in dorsal recumbency. A flank approach can be undertaken with minimal restraint under local anaesthesia, whereas a midline laparotomy will usually require general anaesthesia.

Left flank laparotomy

Anaesthesia: local infiltration or inverted L block or paravertebral regional anaesthesia (Table 26.7)

The goat is placed in right lateral recumbency and the surgical site in the mid-left paralumbar fossa routinely prepared for surgery. Most surgeons use a muscle incisional approach, although a grid or muscle-splitting approach can be used if preferred. The skin, internal and external abdominal oblique muscles, transversus abdominis muscle and peritoneum are incised and the uterus exposed. The abdominal muscles are fairly thin and easily incised. Muscle layers should be carefully identified to avoid penetrating the abdominal contents. The peritoneum should be incised by puncturing it and enlarging the incision with scissors. The exposed horn of the uterus is packed off with swabs. The usual site for incision into the uterus is over the greater curvature of one horn, which will usually allow all the fetuses to be removed from one site and avoids major blood vessels, so reducing haemorrhage. In the case of a live, uncontaminated fetus, the uterus can be opened within the abdomen if necessary, but if the fluids are contaminated, the portion of uterus to be opened must be exteriorised. The incision into the uterine muscle should be large enough to permit delivery of the kids without causing tearing of the uterus. It may be possible to deliver a kid from the other horn through the same

Table 26.7 Choice of anaesthesia for caesarian section.

	Advantages	Disadvantages
Local anaesthesia		
Line infiltration	Doe conscious so readily mothers kids	Poor muscle relaxation
or	Kids not depressed by anaesthetic	Wound healing may be compromised with infiltration
Inverted L block	Easy technique	Risk of haematomas at infiltration site
		Poor anaesthesia of peritoneal membrane
Paravertebral	Good relaxation	Needs experience of technique
	Doe readily mothers kids	More difficult in fat animals
	Kids not depressed	
Epidural anaesthesia	Good relaxation	Doe may be off hind legs for 24 hours
	Good anaesthesia of caudal flank	Mothering kids difficulty
		Needs 1 hour to become effective
General anaesthesia	Good relaxation	Hazards of general anaesthesia
	Good anaesthesia and analgesia	Kids may be depressed
		Preferably done at practice

incision, but often a second incision is necessary in the other horn.

If the umbilical cord does not break during delivery, it is clamped with two pairs of forceps and broken between them. Ligation is not usually necessary but should be considered if haemorrhage is excessive. The placental membranes are removed from the uterus if they come away easily. Closely attached membranes are left in situ. Intrauterine antibiotics are of limited value and should not be used routinely.

The uterine incision is closed using an inverting suture, such as Lembert or Cushing, with 3 metric catgut or synthetic absorbable material swaged on an atraumatic needle. Any tears in the uterine horn should be carefully sutured. Entry of uterine fluid into the abdominal cavity does not present a problem, unless there is intrauterine infection associated with an emphysematous kid. In cases of grossly infected fluids, removal should be attempted by swabs, lavage and aspiration. In all cases, the uterus should be swabbed to remove excessive blood and fetal fluids before returning it to the abdominal cavity, as this will help prevent adhesions during healing.

The transversus abdominis muscle and peritoneum are closed using a 3.5 or 4 metric absorbable suture material in a simple continuous or interrupted pattern, followed in turn by the internal and external abdominal oblique muscles and the subcutaneous truncus muscle and fascia. The skin is closed with a non-absorbable suture, using a simple interrupted or horizontal mattress suture pattern.

Ventral midline laparotomy

Anaesthesia: general anaesthesia (Table 26.7)

The goat is placed in dorsal recumbency and the surgical site, from the umbilicus to just in front of the udder, is routinely prepared for surgery. The incision is made through the skin, subcutaneous tissues and linea alba. The greater omentum is pushed cranially and the gravid uterine horn exteriorised. The surgical procedure is then as for the flank incision. The peritoneum and linea alba are closed with a continuous mattress eversion suture of 5 metric absorbable synthetic material. Bury this layer with a continuous simple layer of absorbable suture material and then suture the skin and subcutis with interrupted mattress sutures of 4 or 5 metric

monofilament nylon. Leave the ends long so the sutures are easier to find for suture removal.

Following caesarian section

If surgical sterility is doubtful or in cases of uterine infection, *broad spectrum antibiotics* should be given parenterally for 3 to 5 days and *tetanus antitoxin* should be given routinely if the goat is not vaccinated.

Perioperative pain relief is very important and will greatly speed recovery:

- *Carprofen, 1.4 mg/kg, 1 ml/35 kg i.v.*
- *Flunixin meglumine, 2 mg/kg, 2 ml/45 kg i.v.*

If necessary, milk letdown can be encouraged by administering oxytocin:

- *Oxytocin, 2–10 i.u.; 0.2–1.ml i.m. or s.c.*
  0.5–2.5 i.u. (diluted 1 in 10 with water for injection) slowly i.v.
- *Pituitary extract (posterior lobe), 20–50 i.u.; 2–5 ml i.m. or s.c.*

There are no figures available for post-operative fertility following caesarian section but levels appear to be close to those following normal parturition.

Care of kids following caesarian section

> Have assistance available to deal with the kids.

Live kids should be dried thoroughly with towels and placed in a warm environment with their mother as soon as she is sufficiently recovered to respond to them. A live kid will usually produce a positive response even from a very weak dam and may be the deciding factor in a goat that is deciding whether to live or die! As soon as the kid is delivered, ensure that the respiratory tract is clear of mucus. Towelling will help stimulate respirations or respiration can be encouraged by using a respiratory stimulant:

- *Doxapram hydrochloride, 5–10 mg, sublingually or by s.c. or i.v. injection*

Where necessary the umbilical cord should be shortened and then treated with strong tincture of iodine or antibiotic spray.

Blood concentrations of drugs such as medetomidine and ketamine cross the placenta readily, producing blood concentrations in the kid similar to those in the dam. Reversal drugs, such as antisedan, should be administered to any kids that seem slow or depressed after being delivered. Care of the newborn kid is discussed in Chapters 4 and 5.

Exploratory laparotomy to examine the uterus and ovaries

Anaesthesia: general anaesthesia

The goat is placed in dorsal recumbency and a midline incision is made through the skin, subcutaneous tissues and linea alba. The incision starts as close to the pelvis brim as possible (and may need to extend on to the udder septum) and extends cranially for about 5 or 6 cm. Tilting the table cranially makes finding the uterus easier (but increases pressure on the diaphragm from the abdominal contents and may compromise respiration).

The uterine horns and ovaries of a non-pregnant animal can be completely exteriorised through the incision by inserting a finger into the abdominal cavity, hooking it round the uterus and applying gentle traction. The uterus should be handled gently to avoid unnecessary trauma that might lead to adhesions forming. Talc on gloves has also been implicated in causing adhesions.

Mastectomy

> As with all surgery, prior knowledge of the anatomy of the area is recommended – watch for those large blood vessels!

Mastectomy is a straightforward procedure, but is major surgery so far as the animal is concerned and intravenous fluid therapy is indicated during surgery.

Indications

Chronic mastitis or gangrenous mastitis, pendulous udder.

Anaesthesia: general anaesthesia

The goat is placed in dorsal recumbency if a bilateral mastectomy is being carried out or lateral recumbency, with the hind leg pulled caudally, for a unilateral mastectomy. The site is routinely clipped and prepared for surgery. The weight of the udder can be supported by attaching Allis tissue forceps to the teats and suspending the udder above the table from a hook or drip stand (Plate 26.1).

An elliptical incision is made around the base of the udder, *leaving as much skin as possible* to facilitate closure. The gland is separated from the skin and underlying tissue by blunt dissection. After incising the skin, the incision is extended through the lateral suspensory ligament of the udder, exposing the external pudendal artery and vein, which lie just underneath.

Identification of the blood vessels in the area is essential. Several major blood vessels will require ligating during the dissection. These include the external pudendal artery (which should be *double ligated*), the external pudendal vein, the subcutaneous abdominal vein and the perineal vein. Ligating the external pudendal artery before any of the venous system allows the blood contained in the udder to drain back into the circulation.

After ligating all the blood vessels, the medial suspensory ligament is incised close to the body wall. In the case of unilateral mastectomy, the gland is separated medially from the medial suspensory ligament of the remaining half. The mammary lymph glands, which lie caudal and dorsal to each gland, should be removed at the same time as the gland.

As much dead space as possible is reduced by means of several rows of absorbable simple continuous subcutaneous sutures and drains should be used if necessary. The skin is closed with simple interrupted sutures using 3 metric non-absorbable material.

Periparturient complications, such as prolonged labour and poor cervical dilation, have been reported in does that are mated after mastectomy, probably because of the absence of hormones such as oestradiol-17ß, which are normally produced by the mammary gland during the final few days of gestation. This, together with the lack of milk for the kids, means that goats should not be mated after a mastectomy.

Teat injuries

Partial-thickness lacerations have a better prognosis than full thickness lacerations into the teat cistern and fresher lacerations have a better prognosis than older ones – ideally repair should be undertaken within 6 hours after the injury. Lacerations nearer the udder heal better than those near the teat tip, particularly if the teat sphincter is involved. Vertical lacerations heal better than horizontal lacerations. Skin flaps with the base towards the teat tip are likely to be poorly vascularised and should be trimmed before suturing where necessary.

Goats with teat injuries are at increased risk of mastitis.

Damage to the teat end is best treated conservatively. Provided the goat can be milked carefully, most teat injuries will heal in about 14 days. A teat cannula can be used at each milking (apply local anaesthetic cream if necessary) and the teat dipped after each milking. The casing of an intramammary tube can be used as a cannula – remove the contents and the plunger – and can be used repetitively if carefully sterilised after each milking. Intramammary and systemic antibiotics should be administered as necessary. Lacerations more than three days old are best left to heal by secondary intention, with the resulting fistula being closed in three layers later.

Lacerations to the teat that do not penetrate the mucosa will usually heal by secondary intention after cleaning and application of topical treatment, but teat lacerations that penetrate the mucosa of the teat require suturing to maintain normal teat function for milking and to prevent the development of teat fistulae or mastitis. The mucosa will need to be sutured separately.

Anaesthesia: sedation + local anaesthetic ring block or general anaesthesia

As aseptic a technique as possible should be used to reduce the risk of mastitis. Thoroughly cleanse the teat and surrounding udder, debride the wound and carefully freshen the wound edges. The tissue lining the teat should be carefully sutured to obtain a milk-tight seal in a continuous pattern using fine absorbable suture material with a swaged-on atraumatic needle. A further continuous suture layer is placed in the submucosal tissue and the skin then sutured with vertical mattress sutures using a fine, synthetic, non-absorbable suture material. Sutures should not be left in place for longer than 9 days to reduce the chance of fibrosis developing.

If milking is likely to traumatise the wound, milk can be drained with a cannula for a few days. The tip of the teat should be swabbed with alcohol before inserting the cannula.

Rumenotomy

Indications
To remove impacted ingesta in treating rumen impaction; to remove ruminal contents in rumen acidosis; to remove a foreign body.

Pre-operatively
Antibiotic administration because of expected contamination of the incision site with rumen microflora even with careful surgery. Penicillin is the antibiotic of choice, because rumen microflora are predominantly anaerobic bacteria – sodium benzylpenicillin (10 mg/kg) can be given intravenously initially, followed by procaine penicillin, 10 mg/kg i.m. daily for 3–5 days. Perioperative pain relief should be provided using a non-steroidal anti-inflammatory drug.

Anaesthesia: general anaesthesia or sedation and local infiltration of the incision site
Rumenotomy is performed through a 15 cm left paralumbar incision, 5 cm caudal and parallel to the last rib (it is essential to leave sufficient tissue caudal to the last rib for suturing). The site is clipped and surgically prepared and the incision extended through the skin and underlying muscle layers – the muscle layers are fairly thin and care must be taken not to penetrate the rumen or intestines.

The rumen is then pulled through the incision and sutured to the skin with a simple continuous suture around the whole of the incision, so that contamination of the abdominal musculature and peritoneum is avoided so far as is possible during the rumenotomy.

The rumen is incised with a scalpel, making a large enough incision so the interior of the rumen can be explored without traumatising the rumen wall. When the rumen contents have been investigated/emptied, the rumen incision is closed with a row of continuous inverting sutures (Cushing, Lembert, etc.) using 3.5 or 4 metric absorbable suture material. The whole area is then irrigated with warm, sterile isotonic saline and the surgeon rescrubs and gloves before completing the surgery. The suture securing the rumen to the skin is removed, the area irrigated again with saline and the abdominal and subcutaneous layers closed with 3.5 or 4 metric absorbable sutures using simple continuous patterns. The skin is closed with a non-absorbable suture, using a simple interrupted or horizontal mattress suture pattern.

Treating dog bite wounds

The severity of bite wounds may be difficult to assess initially by looking at the puncture wounds because:

- The teeth may have penetrated abdominal organs leading to leakage and peritonitis.
- Compression trauma produces compromised tissues and, due to loss of blood supply, release of cytoxins, etc., tissue damage often worsens for several days after the initial attack.
- Osteomyelitis due to periosteal damage is generally not radiographically visible for 1–2 weeks.
  Do:
- Surgically open puncture wounds where the skin is undermined, so that the true extent of the damage can be determined.
- Provide good pain management (NSAIDs, opiates, butorphanol) as well as antibiotic cover.
- Debride necrotic tissue as necessary (and for as long as necessary) before allowing large wounds to heal by secondary intention.

Fracture management

First aid advice to the owner

- Restrict movement:
  o A temporary pen can be constructed with hurdles or straw bales.
- Cover any wounds with a clean dressing.
- Splint the fracture leg if there is a delay in attending the animal or for transport (see Table 26.8). Nerve and vascular injury can be minimised by appropriate fracture immobilisation prior to transporting the animal. Fractures below mid-radius or mid-tibia are easier to splint satisfactorily without a fulcrum effect developing and causing more damage because of leverage of the proximal end of the splint. Adequate splinting stabilises the fracture, reduces pain, reduces soft tissue trauma and damage to neurovascular structures and may prevent a simple fracture from becoming further displaced or compounded. Splints can be constructed from any suitable material, including lengths of timber, broom handles or PVC

guttering. The leg should initially be padded with any suitable available material such as cotton wool, towelling or bandages and the splint secured to the leg with duct or gaffer tape. The injury should be centred within the splints with as much support proximal and distal to the injury as possible.

- The goat should only be transported if it can be done without excessive discomfort and the fracture is adequately stabilised. Space in the vehicle should be restricted with bales or tyres to reduce unnecessary movement and the goat positioned with two sound legs towards the front of the vehicle as acceleration is more controlled than braking. If animals *must* be transported without adequate stabilisation, they must be carefully loaded on to the trailer and encouraged to lie down before moving.

Fractures in kids

Fractures in kids are usually relatively simple to treat with casts or splints (Table 26.8) and heal relatively quickly (often under 4 weeks in neonates). Fractures distal to the carpus or tarsus normally only require splinting with suitable materials, depending on the size of the kid. Commercially available small animal splints are suitable for smaller kids; a PVC pipe cut in half can be used for larger kids. Splints must be sufficiently long to prevent movement of the joints above and below the fracture. Fractures above the carpus and tarsus may require a cast. The splints should be well padded and attached to the leg with conforming bandage and self-adhesive bandage tape. The proximal and distal ends of the tape can be covered in duck-tape

Table 26.8 Fracture splinting.

Frontleg	
Fracture between foot and distal radius/ulna	1 lateral splint , 1 splint palmar aspect, ground to elbow
Fracture between distal radius and elbow	1 lateral splint from ground to shoulder joint
Hindleg	
Fracture between foot and proximal metatarsus	1 lateral splint, 1 on plantar aspect, ground to shoulder
Fracture between hock and stifle joints	1 lateral splint from ground to hip joint
Fractures proximal to either elbow or stifle	
Do not use splints	

Table 26.9 Suitable orthopaedic procedures for caprine fractures.

Metacarpal/metatarsal	
Distal	Cast - foot to point just distal to carpus/tarsus
Proximal or comminuted	Cast - full limb (+ - transfixation pins)
Carpus/tarsus	
Uncomtaminated	Cast - full limb
Contamination of joint	Cast - full limb (+ window for local treatment)
Radial	
Distal	Cast - full limb
Proximal	External fixator, transfixation (hanging-pin) cast, modified Thomas splint (to above elbow), internal fixation (plate & screws)
Tibial	
Distal	Cast - full limb
Proximal	Cast - full limb (+ transfixation pins)
	External fixator
Humerus/femur	Internal fixation (plates, screws, intramedullary pins)

to discourage chewing. Splints should be changed as necessary every 2 to 3 weeks to allow for the rapid growth of the kid.

Fractures in older goats

Older, heavier goats are likely to require more substantial casts, with or without transfixation pins, or some form of internal fixation (Table 26.9). Most small animal orthopaedic procedures, including amputation, can be transferred directly to caprine fractures, with the primary limiting factor in most cases being cost. Amputation should be considered with open or severely comminuted fractures. Goats generally adapt well to having only three legs.

The type of treatment chosen will depend on a number of factors:
- *Client related:* cost, likelihood of successful repair, economic and genetic value of the animal.
- *Animal related*: size, weight and temperament. The prognosis is generally better in young animals – more mobile, less weight, better bone healing.
- *Fracture related*: location and type of fracture, closed or open fracture, presence of soft tissue or neurovascular damage, contamination of wound. The prognosis is generally better with fractures of the distal limb, with closed rather than open and simple rather than comminuted fractures.

Is fracture reduction possible closed or is internal reduction necessary?

Can the fracture be immobilised successfully using external co-aptation or is internal fixation, with or without external support, required?

In addition, the experience of the veterinary surgeon with different types of repair will affect the choice of technique. Suitable orthopaedic procedures are listed in Table 26.9.

Open fractures carry a worse prognosis than closed fractures. Thorough cleaning of the fracture site, debridement and pressurised lavage of the wound using large volumes of an isotonic solution, together with the use of appropriate broad-spectrum antimicrobial drugs will reduce the bacterial load of the tissue and minimise the risk of sepsis. Antimicrobial therapy should be reassessed following bacterial culture of tissue sample taken at the time of surgery – common pathogens are coliforms, *Staphylococcal* species, *Streptococcal* species and *Trueperella pyogenes*. Microbial cultures should be performed on all open fractures if economic considerations allow.

Radiography

Wherever possible radiography should be taken to assess the location and type of fracture, alignment of distal and proximal segments in relation to each other and possible joint involvement: two views (dorsopalmar/plantar and lateromedial) are necessary for long bone fractures.

Follow-up radiographs are necessary to demonstrate callus formation, union and possible complications like osteomyelitis.

Complications of fracture repair

The most common complications of fractures are sepsis, nerve damage and vascular injury. Furthermore, delayed or non-union, osteomyelitis, abnormal bone growth, compromise of the blood supply distal to the fracture site and disuse atrophy with extended immobilisation can all follow fracture repair. The type of repair can lead to additional complications. With external skeletal fixators these include instability at the fracture site, pin loosening, pin tract infections and osteolysis. With casting and splinting, cast or splint sores can develop at specific sites of bony protruberances if they have been insufficiently protected or the cast has been too tight – between the claws, around the accessory digits, medial and lateral tibial malleolus, calcaneous and over the proximal aspect of the cast. Angular lamb deformity can occur if the reduction is not initially completely stable.

Sedation and analgesia

Until the bone is stabilised, fractures are extremely painful and adequate analgesia is required before transport or splinting and before and after fracture repair, using NSAIDs. Additional analgesia is provided by the use of butorphanol as part of the sedative/anaesthetic mix (see Chapter 24).

Deep sedation or anaesthesia is required for adequate manipulation of the limb to achieve good bone alignment.

Cast application

External coaptation, using a cast, is suitable for the majority of closed distal fractures up to the level of the carpus or proximal metatarsus, where the joints either side of the fracture can be included.

The leg is covered in a light layer of protective bandage, using stockinette or cotton cast paddings, with additional padding only in the interdigital space, over the accessory digits to prevent skin ulceration or sloughing of the digits and the top of the cast and for full-limb casts over bony protruberances. Excessively thick padding over the whole limb will become compressed, allowing the limb to move within the cast. Use excess padding in young animals that are more likely to get cast sores because of limb growth within the cast.

The thickness of the cast depends on the size and weight of the animal. Fibreglass resin cast material is lighter, faster setting and more resistant to breaking than plaster-of-paris. Additionally, it does not weaken when wet. Embryotomy wire, threaded through a sleeve of drip tubing, placed between the padding and the cast on the medial and lateral aspect of the leg allows the cast to be removed easily without using an oscillating saw.

In growing animals the cast should end just below the coronary band, so the foot is not included in the cast, and the cast should be changed after about 3 weeks because cast sores can be induced by the compression caused by growth. In adults, the cast can be left in place for 4 to 6 weeks if no complications occur. The cast should be checked daily; complications may be indicated by increased pain in the limb, leading to increased lameness following a period of weight bearing, pyrexia, increased heat in the limb, malodour or wet spots, which indicate exudate leaking through the fibreglass.

In adult goats, stability of the fracture site should be established with a fibrocartilaginous callus after three weeks, with mineralisation visible on radiographs at about 6 weeks when the cast is changed. Splitting the cast into two halves at this time allows further use as a splint or half-cast. Fractures should heal in 8 to 10 weeks, although complete clinical union may take longer and it is important to provide prolonged support of decreasing strength after cast/fixation removal, using a Robert-Jones bandage or splint or by removing ESF pins gradually.

Thomas splint and cast combination

A modified Thomas splint can be used for repair of fractures of the radius and ulna, which cannot be stabilised by external coaptation alone. With the animal standing, the required length of the splint is determined by measuring the normal limb. The fracture is reduced and a full limb cast applied. The modified Thomas splint is then placed on the limb. To allow maximum weight transference, the ring of the splint must be placed firmly into the axilla or groin – the ring needs to be of sufficient diameter so movement of the elbow or hip is not impaired and needs to be well padded to avoid abrasions. The splint is then attached to the cast with additional cast material or tape.

Transfixation pin cast (hanging pin cast)

Transfixation pin casts (hanging pin casts) are an intermediary between external coaptation and external skeletal fixation. Two or three transfixating pins are placed in the proximal bone above the fracture site, extending from one side of the bone to the other, helping to stabilise the fracture by transferring the loading forces from the ground to the pins. The foot must be included in the cast with this technique so that all the weight is transferred on to the cast.

The pin insertion and exit sites are protected with non-adherent bandage and gauze dressing and the pins are included in the cast with the initial layers of casting material pushed over the end of the pins to lie close to the leg. Six to eight layers are applied to provide a cast thickness of 6–7 mm. The pins are cut to an appropriate length and the ends protected with suitable beading or polymethylmethacrylate (PMMA).

The technique is useful for comminuted fractures or where the distal fragment is very small or close to a joint, as an alternative to external skeletal fixation.

External skeletal fixation (ESF)

External skeletal fixation is useful for managing comminuted and open fractures as it allows direct access to the site, but requires general anaesthesia to ensure proper placement of the pins. Two or three transcortical pins are placed proximally and distally to the fracture and connected by sidebars, which should be as close as possible to the skin for maximum strength.

Internal fixation

With suitable fractures, techniques using ASIF screws and plates, intramedullary pins and cerclage wires are readily adapted from small animal surgery if the expense and surgical facilities permit.

Closed fractures of the phalanges can be treated by applying a 2.5–3 cm height block to the sole of the healthy digit, with stall confinement for 6 to 8 weeks.

Amputation of a digit

Indications

Septic pedal arthritis; traumatic damage.

Anaesthesia: intravenous regional anaesthesia; general anaesthesia

The distal limb is thoroughly cleaned and given a surgical scrub, although full surgical preparation is unnecessary. The skin incision is made, starting in the interdigital space, and extending along the abaxial and axial surfaces of the coronary band. A length of embryotomy wire is place in the incision in the interdigital space and the digit removed at an angle of 15° to the horizontal plane with the abaxial side higher. Once the digit has been removed, any excess tissue, particularly if necrotic or infected, should be removed. In the absence of infection, as much of the skin flap as possible can be sutured down, but this is often not possible and infected wounds should be left to drain ventrally.

The wound can be sprayed topically with an oxytetracycline spray and then covered with a suitable non-absorbent dressing and a pressure bandage applied tightly. Post-operative analgesia should be given, using NSAIDs. The dressing should be changed after 3 or 4 days and the wound redressed regularly until healing has occurred.

Eye enucleation

Indications

Intraocular neoplasia, severe keratitis with a perforating ulcer, severe trauma.

Anaesthesia: general anaesthesia

Sedation and local anaesthesia with lignocaine using a four-site retrobulbar block by injecting through the eyelids (dorsally, ventrally and at the medial and lateral canthi). Topical 0.5% proparacaine can be used to desensitise the cornea and conjunctivae before injecting the lignocaine.

The eyelids are sutured together using a monofilament non-absorbable suture material, leaving the ends long and the lids clipped and surgically prepared. A transpalpebral incision is made around the orbit, 3 to 4 mm from the eyelid margins. Blunt dissection is then used circumferentially around the orbit with curved scissors to undermine the ocular muscles, adipose tissue and fascia, so that the eyeball is free apart from its attachment at the optic stalk. The optic nerve and vessels are clamped with a curved artery forcep, ligated tightly and then transected, so that the contents of the orbit along with the eyelids can be removed.

The orbit should be lavaged with sterile saline containing antibiotic. Considerable dead space remains after the removal of the eye from the orbit and, despite adequate ligation of the optic vessels, a haematoma may form. The subcutaneous tissues are closed with an absorbable continuous suture and the skin closed using simple interrupted sutures using non-absorbable suture material. Systemic antibiotics and anti-inflammatory drugs should be given for a minimum of 5 days after surgery.

Further reading

Amputation of a digit

Scott, P. (1995) Amputation of the ovine digit. *In Pract.*, **17**, 80–82.

Analgesia

Carroll, G.L., Hooper, R.N., Boothe, D.M., Hartsfield, S.M. and Randoll, L.A. (1999) Pharmacokinetics of fentanyl after intravenous and transdermal administration in goats. *Amer. J. Vet. Res.*, **60** (8), 986–991.

Coetze, J.F. (2013) A review of analgesic compounds used in food animals in the United States. *Vet. Clin. North Amer.: Food Anim. Pract.*, **29** (1), 11–28.

Hendrickson, D.A., Kruse-Elliott, K.T. and Broadstone, R.V. (1996), A comparison of epidural saline, morphine, and bupivacaine for pain relief after abdominal surgery in goats. *Vet. Surg.*, **25** (1), 83–87.

Plummer, P.J. and Schleining, J.A. (2013) Assessment and management of pain in small ruminants and camelids. *Vet. Clin. North Amer.: Food Anim. Pract.*, **29** (1), 185–208.

Caesarian section

Mueller, K. (2011) Caesarian section in the doe. *Goat Vet. Soc. J.*, **27**, 34–38.

Fracture management

Anderson, D.E. and St Jean, G. (1996) External skeletal fixation in ruminants. *Vet. Clin. North Amer.: Food Anim. Pract.*, **12** (1), 117–152.

Joy, B. and Venugopal, S.K. (2014) Complications in fracture healing using external skeletal fixation in goats. *Int. J. Rec. Sci. Res.*, **5** (7), 1298–1299.

Mueller, K. (2015) Goat orthopaedics – bone sequestrum and fractures. *Goat Vet. Soc. J.*, **31**, 54–59.

Mulon, P.-Y. (2013) Management of long bone fractures in cattle. *In Pract.*, **35**, 265–271.

Vogel, S.R. and Anderson, D.E. (2014) External skeletal fixation of fractures in cattle. *Vet. Clin. North Amer.: Food Anim. Pract.*, **30**, 127–142.

General surgery

Hallowell, G., Potter, T. and Aldridge, B. (2012) Medical support for cattle and small ruminant surgical patients. *In Pract.*, **34**, 226–233.

Mueller, K. (2010) Common surgical procedures in goats. *Goat Vet. Soc. J.*, **26**, 9–14.

Mueller, K. (2015) Soft tissue surgery, urethrotomy, tube cystotomy, dehorning and caesarian section. *Goat Vet. Soc. J.*, **31**, 67–71.

Mastectomy

Cable, C.S. *et al.* (2004) Radical mastectomy in 20 ruminants. *Vet. Surg.*, **33** (3), 263–266.

Kerr, H.J. and Wallace, C.E. (1978) Mastectomy in a goat. *Vet. Med., Small Anim. Clin.*, **73** (9), 1177–1181.

Obstructive urolithiasis

Ewoldt, J.M. *et al.* (2006) Short- and long-term outcome and factors predicting survival after surgical tube cystotomy for treatment of obstructive urolithiasis in small ruminants. *Vet. Surg.*, **35**, 417–422.

Ewoldt, J.M., Jones, M.L. and Miesner, M.D. (2008) Surgery of obstructive urolithiasis in ruminants. *Vet. Clin. North Amer.: Food Anim. Pract.*, **24** (3), 455–465.

Fortier, L.A. *et al.* (2004) Caprine obstructive urolithiasis: requirement for 2nd surgical intervention and mortality after percutaneous tube cystotomy, surgical tube cystotomy or urinary bladder marsupialization. *Vet. Surg.*, **33** (6), 661.

George, J.W. *et al.* (2007) Serum biochemical abnormalities in goats with uroliths: 107 cases (1992–2003). *J. Amer. Vet. Med. Assoc.*, **230** (1), 101–106.

Halland, S.K., House, J.K. and George, L.W. (2002) Urethroscopy and laser lithotripsy for the diagnosis and treatment of obstructive urolithiasis in goats and potbellied pigs. *J. Amer. Vet. Med. Assoc.*, **220**, 1831–1834.

Haven, M.L. *et al.* (1993) Surgical management of urolithiasis in small ruminants. *Cornell Vet.*, **83**, 47–55.

Hunter, B.G., Huber, M.J. and Riddick, T.L. (2012) Laparoscopic-assisted urinary bladder marsupialization in a goat that developed recurrent urethral obstruction following perineal urethrostomy. *J. Amer. Vet. Med. Assoc.*, **241** (6), 778–781.

Janke, J.J. *et al.* (2009) Use of Walpole's solution for treatment of goats with urolithiasis: 25 cases (2001–2006). *J. Amer. Vet. Med. Assoc.*, **234** (2), 249–252.

May, K.A. *et al.* (1998) Urinary bladder marsupialization for treatment of obstructive urolithiasis in male goats. *Vet. Surg.*, **27** (6), 583–588.

Rakestraw, P.C. *et al.* (1995) Tube cystotomy for treatment of obstructive urolithiasis in small ruminants. *Vet. Surg.*, **24**, 498–505.

Stone, W.C. *et al.* (1997) Prepubic urethrostomy for relief of urethral obstruction in a sheep and a goat. *J. Amer. Vet. Med. Assoc.*, **210** (7), 939–941.

Tobias, K.M. and Amstel, S.R. (2013) Modified proximal perineal urethrostomy technique for treatment of urethral stricture in goats. *Vet. Surg.*, **42** (4), 455–462.

Van Metre, D.C. *et al.* (1996) Obstructive urolithiasis in ruminants: medical treatment and urethral surgery. *Comp. Contin. Educ. Pract. Vet.*, **18**, 317–327.

Orthopaedics

Mueller, K. (2010) Goat orthopaedics – bone sequestrum and fractures. *Goat Vet. Soc. J.*, **31**, 54–59.

Reproductive system

Noakes, D.E. (1985) Surgical answers to reproductive problems in the female goat. *Goat Vet. Soc. J.*, **6** (2), 61–63.

Teat surgery

Couture, Y. and Mulan, P.-Y. (2005) Procedures and surgery of the teat. *Vet. Clin. North Amer.: Food Anim. Pract.*, **21** (10), 173–204.

Umbilical surgery

Baird, A.N. (2008) Umbilical surgery in calves. *Vet. Clin. North Amer.: Food Anim. Pract.*, **24** (3), 467–477.

Appendix: Drugs for goats

Because goats are a minority species in most Western countries, there are few drugs specifically licensed for use in goats, so that is generally necessary to use drugs licensed for use in other species of farm animals.

Although the exact regulations vary from country to country, regulatory authorities expect that a genuine veterinarian–client relationship exists and that animals are under the clinical control of the veterinary surgeon before drugs are prescribed 'off-label'. In the United Kingdom, a veterinary surgeon, or someone acting under his direction, may only administer a product to a food-producing animal if it contains substances found in a product authorised for use in other food-producing animals and other countries have similar restrictions on the use of drugs. Furthermore, so far as most regulatory authorities are concerned, *all* goats are food-producing animals and they do not recognise a separate category of 'pet goat', which will never enter the food-chain.

Under UK Regulations, where no authorised veterinary medicine exists in the United Kingdom for a condition in an animal, in order to avoid unacceptable suffering, a veterinarian responsible for the animal may exercise their clinical judgement whereby they select in the following order:

(1) A veterinary medicine authorised in the United Kingdom for use in another animal species or for another condition in the same species or (2) if, and only if, there is no such product that is suitable, either (i) a medicinal product authorised in the United Kingdom for human use or (ii) a veterinary medicinal product not authorised in the United Kingdom but authorised in another EU member state for use with any animal species that is a food-producing species.

In addition to the above legislation, if the animal is a food-producing animal, the treatment in any particular case is restricted to a single holding. Veterinarians should keep adequate case records, including details of medicines used for the treatment of animals and the circumstances, including justifications, of their use. The Regulations require that records must be kept when prescribing, administering and supplying medicines for food-producing animals under the cascade. The veterinarian must specify an appropriate withdrawal period. *Pharmacologically active substances which are not contained in products currently authorised for food-producing species, must not be administered to food-producing animals under the cascade.* It is the reader's responsibility to ensure that he/she is legally entitled to use any drug mentioned in this book.

All drugs, which are not specifically licensed for goats, carry a mandatory *7 day withholding time for milk and 28 day withholding time for meat*, but in some instances these times will not be long enough, for example with dry-cow intra-mammary tubes and avermectins. If in doubt, drug manufacturers should be consulted about suitable withholding times.

Australia/New Zealand

McDougall, S. and Millar, A (2011) If it's not on the label, what do I do? Off-label drug use. Australian College of Veterinary Scientists, Chapter of Veterinary Pharmacology Science Week 2011 Session Proceedings, pp. 3–11.

Canada

Policy on Extra-Label Drug Use (ELDU) in Food Producing Animals. http://www.hc-sc.gc.ca/dhp-mps/vet/label-etiquet/poleldu-umdde-eng.php.

Diseases of the Goat, Fourth Edition. John Matthews.
© 2016 John Wiley & Sons, Ltd. Published 2016 by John Wiley & Sons, Ltd.

United Kingdom

Guidance on the Use of Cascade – Veterinary Medicines Guidance Note 13. https://www.vmd.defra.gov.uk/pdf/vmgn/VMGNote13.pdf.

United States

Animal Medicinal Drug Use Clarification Act (AMDUCA). https://www.avma.org/KB/Resources/Reference/Pages/AMDUCA.aspx.

Fajt, V.R. (2011) Drug laws and regulations for sheep and goats. *Vet. Clin. North Amer.: Food Anim. Pract.*, **27**, 1–21.

The Food Animal Residue Avoidance Databank (FARAD) has current label information including withdrawal times for all drugs approved for use in food-producing animals in the United States (www.farad.org).

The USA Food and Drug Administration's interactive website is available at: http://www.accessdata.fda.gov/scripts/animaldrugsatfda/index.cfm?gb=1.

Drug doses

Manufacturers should also be consulted about suitable drug doses for goats. Drug metabolism shows species variation, with the result that dose rates and excretion times for goats cannot be simply extrapolated from sheep and cattle data.

The elimination half-life of some drugs, including many anthelmintics that are eliminated mainly by hepatic metabolism is, in goats, about half that for sheep. Meloxicam has an elimination half-life of 24 hours in cattle, 10.85 hours in sheep, but only 6.73 hours in goats. The dosage interval of 48 hours, recommended for calves when an intravenous or subcutaneous dose of 0.5 mg/kg is used, is thus likely to be too long for effective treatment of goats.

Furthermore, there are species differences between breeds of goats. Pygmy goats are reported to metabolise sulphonamides, chloramphenicol and probably other drugs that are metabolised by hepatic microsomal enzymes faster than other breeds.

In the EU only approved pharmacologically active substances should be administered to a food-producing animal. These are listed in the allowed substances table in the annex 'Pharmacologically active substances and their classification regarding maximum residue limits (MRL) of Commission Regulation (EU) No. 37/2010'. A copy of the Regulation is available on the Veterinary Medicines Directorate's website: www.vmd.defra.gov.uk/public/vmr_legislation.aspx. Another table lists substances that are actively prohibited.

Administration of drugs

(1) Intramuscular injections

Lameness, sometimes permanent, is a common sequel to intramuscular injections.

Because the goat has relatively small muscle masses in the hind leg, particularly the gluteal region, temporary lameness is common after injections of irritant substances such as tetracyclines and fluoroquinolones. More permanent lameness may result from damage to the sciatic nerve, if the gluteal muscle mass is used, or to the peroneal nerve, if the injection is in the caudal thigh region.

An alternative site for intramuscular injections is the cleido-occipitalis muscle in the mid-neck region, but induced pain in this region may result in the goat being unwilling to feed. A preferable site in the neck is the triangular area bordered by the vertebral column ventrally, the nuchal ligament dorsally and the shoulder caudally. The triceps muscle mass and the longissimus muscles of the back in the lumbar region can also be used.

The volume of drug administered at one site should never be more than 5 ml, using a needle of 18 g or less and 25 to 38 mm in length in adult goats. Smaller amounts and shorter needles should be used in kids.

It is always safer to use the subcutaneous route rather than give intramuscular injections and this route should be adopted wherever possible.

Note: drug persistence in the body is much more variable after subcutaneous than intramuscular administration, so care should be taken when considering milk and meat withhold times.

(2) Subcutaneous injections

Subcutaneous injections are normally given on the chest wall just behind the elbow or in the loose skin of the neck just in front of the shoulders.

(3) Intravenous injections

Intravenous injections are generally given via the external jugular vein:
- Animal is held standing with head restrained by hand on the nose.
- Clip hair over jugular furrow at approximately mid-point of neck.
- Clean site with surgical spirit or iodophor.
- Apply external pressure with fingers or tourniquet on the jugular groove in the lower part of the jugular furrow to dilate the external jugular vein.
- An 18 g × 38 mm (1.5 inches) is suitable for adult goats, 20 g × 25 mm (1 inch) for smaller animals; pucture the vein, blood should flow through the needle.
- Infuse drug slowly.

(4) Oral medication

Oral medication can be given relatively easily by means of syringes, drenching guns or boluses, if the goat is properly restrained. Back the animal into a corner with one side against a wall, then either straddle the animal or stand against the shoulder in a larger animal. The head should be held normally in a horizontal position, and not tilted, to reduce the chance of inducing aspiration pneumonia. Holding the lower jaw with one hand, the syringe or drenching gun is slipped into the corner of the mouth at the commissure of the lips, so that the tip is just over the base of the tongue.

Goats are generally tolerant of the passage of a stomach tube but tend to bite through it unless a suitable gag is available. Any of the varieties of sheep gag are suitable or use a block of wood with a hole drilled through it.

Closure of the reticular groove

The absorption of many drugs from the rumen is problematical. Closure of the reticular groove, allowing orally administered drugs to pass straight to the abomasum, can be achieved by:
- Oral administration of 5 ml of a solution of copper sulphate (a tablespoonful in a litre of water).
- Injection of 0.25 IU/kg lysine-vasopressin i.v.
- In cattle, oral administration of 60 ml of sodium bicarbonate 10% causes reticular groove closure.

Anaesthetics, sedatives and pre-medications

(1) Benzodiazepines

Diazepam	0.25–0.5 mg/kg slowly i.v.
Midazolam	0.2–0.4 mg/kg slowly i.v.

(2) Alpha-2 agonists

Detomidine	20–40 µg/kg i.v. or i.m.
Medetomidine	25–35 µg/kg i.v. or i.m.
Xylazine (2% solution)	0.05 mg/kg slowly i.v or 0.1 mg/kg i.m.

Overdosage of xylazine and other alpha-2 adrenoceptor stimulants can be reversed by:

Atipamezole	125–175 µg/kg half i.v. and half i.m.
Tolazoline	2 mg/kg slow i.v.
Yohimbine	0.2 mg/kg slow i.v.

(3) Phenothiazines
Acepromazine maleate	0.05–0.1 mg/kg slowly i.v.

(4) Antimuscarinic pre-anaesthetic medication
Atropine	0.6–1 mg/kg i.m.

(5) Injectable anaesthetics

Barbiturates
Thiopental sodium 5%	10–15 mg/kg, 8–12 ml/40 kg i.v.

Other drugs
Alphaxalone	10 mg/ml, 4.5 mg/kg very slowly i.v. to effect, 4.5 ml/10 kg
Ketamine	10–15 mg/kg, 4–6 ml/40 kg slowly i.v
Propofol	3–5 mg/kg, 12–20 ml/40 kg slowly i.v.
Tiletamine -zolazepam	5.5 mg/kg i.v. (not available in the UK)

(6) Ketamine + sedative combinations

Diazepam and ketamine
Diazepam	0.25–0.5 mg/kg, 2~4 ml/40 kg slowly i.v., wait 2–3 minutes, then
Ketamine	4 mg/kg, 1.6 ml/40 kg i.v.

Xylazine and ketamine
Xylazine (2% solution)	0.1 mg/kg, 0.2 ml/40 kg i.m. followed by
Ketamine	10 mg/kg, 4 ml/40 kg i.m. or 5 mg/kg, 2 ml/40 kg i.v.

Ketamine, xylazine and diazepam
Xylazine	0.2 mg/kg i.m., wait 10 minutes then
Ketamine + Diazepam	10 mg/kg + 0.3 mg/kg in the same syringe i.v.

Medetomidine and ketamine
Medetomidine	25–35 mg/kg, 1–1.5 ml/40 kg , mixed in same syringe with
Ketamine	1–1.5 mg/kg, 0.4–0.6 ml/40 kg i.m.
Butorphanol	0.1–0.2 mg/kg can be added to the mixture

Analgesics and anti-inflammatory drugs

(1) Opioid analgesics

Butorphanol	0.2–0.5 mg/kg i.v., i.m. or s.c.
Buprenorphine	0.01 mg/kg i.m. or s.c.
Pethidine hydrochloride (Meperidine hydrochloride)	10 mg/kg i.m. or s.c.

(2) Non-steroidal anti-inflammatory drugs

Injectable drugs

Carprofen	1.4 mg/kg s.c. or i.v., repeat once after 48–72 hours
Flunixin meglumine	2.2 mg/kg i.v. daily for 3–5 days
Ketoprofen	3 mg/kg i.m. or i.v. daily for 3–5 days
Meloxicam	2 mg/kg loading dose then
	0.5 mg/kg s.c. or i.v. every 36 hours
Phenylbutazone[a]	4 mg/kg i.v. daily
Tolfenamic acid	2–4 mg/kg s.c. or i.v., repeat once after 48 hours

Oral drugs

Aspirin[b]	50–100 mg/kg every 12 hours
Carprofen	1–2 mg/kg once daily
Meloxicam	2 mg/kg initial dose
	1 mg/kg daily until pain controlled
	0.5–1 mg/kg every other day long term
Phenylbutazone[a]	10 mg/kg for 2 days, then once daily for 3 days, then every other day or as needed

[a]Under present legislation, phenylbutazone is banned from use in food-producing animals in the EU and its extra-label use is strongly discouraged in the United States.
[b]Aspirin is not licensed for food-producing animals in the United Kingdom and its use is discouraged in the United States. Aspirin is poorly absorbed from the rumen so relatively high doses are needed.

(3) Corticosteroids

Dexamethasone	0.1 mg/kg i.v.
Methylprednisolone	10–30 mg/kg i.v. every 4 to 6 hours for 24 to 48 hours

(4) Other anti-inflammatory drugs

The following have all been used empirically in non-lactating pet goats with dose rates extrapolated from those for other species as there are no published results of clinical trials in goats. They are not licensed for food-producing animals in the United Kingdom.

Pentosan polysulphate sodium	3 mg/kg s.c. weekly for 4 weeks, then a single injection every 4 to 6 months	Do not use concurrently with steroids or non-steroidal anti-inflammatory drugs, including aspirin and phenylbutazone
Polysulphated glycosaminoglycan	125 mg, 1.25 ml i.m. weekly for 4 weeks, then a single injection every 4–6 months	Large animals may need an increased amount
Sodium hyaluronate	20 mg, 2 ml i.v.	

Anthelmintics

Dose rates for sheep cannot be directly extrapolated to goats. Higher dose rates are often required in goats than sheep. The half-life of some drugs that are eliminated mainly by metabolism in the liver is, in goats, about half that for sheep. Therefore, in general, a dose 1.5 to 2.0 times the ovine anthelmintic dose is recommended for goats.

However, idiosyncratic reactions to levamisole have been noted in individual fibre-producing goats. In general, the *oral* route is recommended for all groups of anthelmintics.

(1) Benzamidazoles	>2 times sheep dose rate	
Albendazole, Febental, Fenbendazole, Oxfendazole	7.5–10 mg/kg orally	20 mg/kg has been recommended as a quarantine drench
Mebendazole	22.5 mg/kg orally	
Netobimin	11.25 mg/kg orally	

(2) Levamisole	1.5 times sheep dose rate	
Levamisole	12 mg/kg orally	Do not exceed this rate as levamisole is toxic in goats at dose rates approaching 20 mg/kg; do not use injectable preparations; do not use during the last 3 weeks of pregnancy or in

(3) Avermectins/Milbemycin	2 times sheep dose rate
Ivermectin, Doramectin and Moxidectin	400 micrograms/kg orally or s.c.

(4) Monepantel	2 times sheep dose
Monepantel	5 mg/kg

Drugs for flukes (trematodes)

(1) Chronic fascioliasis

		Effective against adult fluke	Effective against immature fluke
Albendazole	10 mg/kg orally 15–20 mg/kg orally	76–92% 90%	No
Clorsulon	2mg/kg s.c. (combined with ivermectin 200 mg/ml)	Yes	No
Closantel	10 mg/kg orally	Yes	From 3 to 4 weeks
Nitroxynil	10 mg/kg s.c.	Yes	No
Oxyclozanide	15 mg/kg orally (combined with levamisole)	Yes	No
Triclabendazole	10 mg/kg orally	Yes	Yes

(2) Acute and subacute fascioliasis

		Effective against immature fluke
Triclabendazole	10 mg/kg orally	From 2 days old to adults
Closantel	10 mg/kg orally	23–73% of 3–4 week >90% of 6–8 week
Nitroxynil	10 mg/kg s.c	Moderately effective from 8 to 9 weeks old

Drugs for tapeworms (cestodes)

Albendazole	10 mg/kg orally	
Febantel	7.5 mg/kg orally	
Fenbedazole	15 mg/kg orally	
Oxfendazole	10 mg/kg orally	
Praziquantel	3.75 mg/kg orally 5 mg/kg s.c.	Injectable form not licensed in UK

Antibiotics

Only Baytril 100 mg/ml solution for injection (Bayer) is currently licensed specifically for goats in the United Kingdom. In general, it is safe to extrapolate from recommendations for sheep or cattle, but it cannot always be assumed that the pharmokinetics of a particularly drug will be the same in the goat as in other species, for example oxytetracycline is more rapidly excreted in the goat than in cattle.

Milk withdrawal times in goats after using dry cow therapy can be substantially different from that recommended for cows. The antibiotic screening tests in common use by dairies are extremely sensitive and antibiotic residues have been detected in goats' milk many months after treatment with some products, resulting in major loss of income from discarded milk

Do not use tilmicosin (Micotil, Elanco) in goats, as injection has been fatal.

Anticonvulsants

Diazepam	0.25–0.5 mg/kg i.v. to effect
Phenobarbitone	0.04 ml/kg i.v.

Coccidiosis

(1) Treatment

Sulphadimethoxine	75 mg/kg orally for 4–5 days
Sulphamethoxypyridazine	20 mg/kg s.c. once only
Sulphadimidine	200 mg/kg initial dose then 100 mg/kg s.c. or i.v. (preferred) daily for up to 5 days total
Sulphadiazine + Trimethoprim	30 mg/kg daily s.c. or slow i.v.
Sulphadoxine + Trimethoprim	15 mg/kg daily s.c. or slow i.v.
Diclazuril	1 mg/kg orally
Toltrazuril	20 mg/kg orally
Decoquinate	100 g/tonne feed or 1 mg/kg for 28 days
Amprolium	50 mg/kg orally daily for 3–5 days Only licensed for use in poultry in the UK.

(2) Prophylaxis

Decoquinate	100 g/tonne feed or 1 mg/kg for 28 days to kids	
Decoquinate	50 g/tonne feed or 0.5 mg/kg for 28 days to does	
Monensin	10–30 g/ton of feed	Banned in the UK Non-lactating goats only in the USA

Drugs acting on the digestive tract

Spasmolytic

Metamizole, hyoscine butylbromide	2.5 ml/50 kg i.v.

External parasites

(1) Amidines

Amitraz	0.025% solution, by spray or wash

(2) Pyrethrins and synthetic pyrethroids

Cypermethrin	1.25% solution, 0.25 ml/kg (maximum 20 ml) by pour-on	There are also many preparations containing permethrin marketed for use in dogs and cats as shampoos and powders that can be used on pet and pygmy goats, if regulations permit
Deltamethrin	1%, 'spot-on'	
Permethrin	4%, 'pour-on'	
Pyrethrins		Dog and cat sprays and powders containing pyrethrins and piperonyl butoxide can be used on pet and pygmy goats, where regulations permit

(3) Avermectins/milbemycin

Abamectin, Doramectin Ivermectin, Moxidectin,	200 micrograms/kg 10 mg/50 kg, 1 ml/50 kg s.c.	400 µg/kg are now recommended for anthelmintic use
Eprinomectin	500 micrograms/kg, 1 ml/10 kg pour-on	Although pour-on preparations are not generally recommended for the control of endoparasites, eprinomectin pour-on has been shown to be effective for the targeted treatment of ectoparasites

(4) Fipronil

Suitable for pygmy goats or individual pet goats as expensive!   Not licensed for use in food-producing animals in the UK

(5) Dips

Fibre goats can be dipped, using products approved for sheep, such as synthetic pyrethroid (cypermethrin) or organophosphorus preparations (diazinon).

Fertility

(1) Prostaglandins

Dinaprost	5–10 mg, i.m. or s.c.
Clorprostenol	62.5–125 µg, i.m. or s.c.

(2) Oxytocin

Oxytocin	2–10 units , i.m. or s.c.
Pituitary extract (posterior lobe)	20–50 units, i.m. or s.c.

(3) Chorionic gonadotrophin

	500 i.u., i.m.	At time of service
	1000 i.u., i.m.	For cystic ovaries

(4) Gonadotrophin releasing hormone (GnRH)

Gonadorellin	0.25 mg i.m.
Buserelin	0.010 mg i.m., s.c. or i.v

(5) Serum gonadotrophin

PMSG	400–700 i.u.	Varies with size of goat, milk yield and season

Fungal treatments

(1) Topical fungicides

Eniliconazole	0.2% solution by wash or spray, every 3 days for 3 or 4 applications	
Natamycin	0.01% solution locally, repeat after 4 or 5 days and again after 14 days if required	
Griseofulvin	*7.5 mg/kg orally for 7 days*	Under present EU legislation, griseofulvin cannot be used in food-producing animals

Further reading

Anatomy

Garrett, P.D. (1988) *Guide to Ruminant Anatomy Based on the Dissection of the Goat*. Iowa State University Press, Iowa.

Owen, N.L. (1977) *The Illustrated Standard of the Dairy Goat*. Dairy Goat Publishing Corporation, Lake Mills, Wisconsin.

Fluid therapy

Jones, M. and Navarre, C. (2014) Fluid therapy in small ruminants and camelids. *Vet. Clin. N. Amer.: Food Anim. Pract.*, **30** (2), 441–453.

Haematology and biochemistry

Davies, D.M. and Sims, B.J. (1985) Welsh and Marches Goat Society survey to determine normal blood biochemistry and haematology in domestic goats. *Goat Vet. Soc. J.*, **6** (1), 38–42.

Jones, M. L. and Allison, R.W. (2007) Evaluation of the ruminant complete blood cell count. *Vet. Clin. North Amer.: Food Anim. Pract.*, **23** (3), 377–402.

Mews, A. and Mowlem, A. (1981) Normal haematological and biochemical values in the goat. *Goat Vet. Soc. J.*, **2** (1), 30–31.

Russell, K.E. and Roussel, A.J. (2007) Evaluation of the ruminant serum chemistry profile. *Vet. Clin. North Amer.: Food Anim. Pract.*, **23** (3), 403–426.

Cornell University College of Veterinary Medicine online textbook on Veterinary Clinical Pathology, eClinPath: http://www.eclinpath.com/.

Management

Gall, C. (ed.) (1981) *Goat Production*. Academic Press, London.

Guss, S.B. (1977) *Management and Diseases of Dairy Goats*. Dairy Goat Publishing Corporation, Lake Mills, Wisconsin.

Mackenzie, D. (revised and edited by R. Goodwin) (1993) *Goat Husbandry*, 5th edn. Faber and Faber, London.

Mowlem, A. (1992) *Goat Farming*, 2nd edition. Farming Press Books, Ipswich.

Peacock, C. (1996) *Improving Goat Production in the Tropics*. Oxfam/Farm-Africa, Oxford.

Medicine and surgery

Baxendell, S.A. (1988) *The Diagnosis of the Diseases of Goats*. Vade Mecum Series No. 19. University of Sydney Post-Graduate Foundation in Veterinary Science, Sydney, Australia.

Dunn, P. (1994) *The Goatkeeper's Veterinary Book*, 3rd edition. Farming Press Books, Ipswich.

Ermilio, E.M. and Smith, M.C. (2011) Treatment of emergency conditions in sheep and goats. *Vet. Clin. North Amer.: Food Anim. Pract.*, **27** (1), 33–45.

Goats No. 73 (1984) *Proceedings of University of Sydney Post-Graduate Foundation in Veterinary Science*, Sydney, Australia.

Goat Health and Production No. 134 (1990) *Proceedings of University of Sydney Post-Graduate Foundation in Veterinary Science*, Sydney, Australia.

Howe, P.A. (1984) *Diseases of Goats*. Vade Mecum Series No. 5. University of Sydney Post-Graduate Foundation in Veterinary Science, Sydney, Australia.

Linklater, K.A. and Smith, M.C. (1993) *Colour Atlas of the Diseases and Disorders of the Sheep and Goat*. Mosby-Wolfe, London.

Lloyd, S. (1982) Goat medicine and surgery. *Br. Vet. J.*, **138**, 70–85.

Pugh, D.G. and Baird, A.N. (eds) (2012) *Sheep and Goat Medicine*, 2nd edition. Elsevier-Saunders, Maryland Heights, MO.

Smith, M.C. (ed.) (November 1983) Sheep and goat medicine. *Vet. Clin. North Amer.: Large Anim. Pract.*, **5** (3) (whole book).

Smith, M.C. (ed.) (November 1990) Advances in sheep and goat medicine. *Vet. Clin. North. Amer.: Large Anim. Pract.*, **6** (3) (whole book).

Smith, M.C. and Sherman, D.M. (2009) *Goat Medicine*, 2nd edition. Wiley-Blackwell, Blackwell Publishing, Ames, Iowa.

Nutrition

AFRC Technical Committee on Responses to Nutrients Report No. 10 (1998) *The Nutrition of Goats*. CAB International, Wallingford, UK.

British Goat Society (1997) *Feeding Goats, a Modern Guide to Healthy Nutrition*. British Goat Society, Bovey Tracey.

Committee on the Nutrition Requirements of Small Ruminants, National Research Council (2007) *Nutrition Requirements of Small Ruminants, Sheep, Goats, Cervids and New World Camelids*. The National Academies Press, Washington, DC.

Orskov, B. (1987) *The Feeding of Ruminants, Principles and Practice*. Chalcombe Publications, Canterbury.

Pain

Coetze, J.F. (2013) A review of analgesic compounds used in food animals in the United States. *Vet. Clin. North Amer.: Food Anim. Pract.*, **29** (1), 11–28.

Plummer, P.J. and Schleining, J.A. (2013) Assessment and management of pain in small ruminants and camelids. *Vet. Clin. North Amer.: Food Anim. Pract.*, **29** (1), 185–208.

Reproduction

Artificial Breeding in Sheep and Goats No. 96 (1987) *Proceedings of University of Sydney Post-Graduate Foundation in Veterinary Science*, Sydney, Australia.

Embryo Transfer/Goats and Sheep No. 127 (1989) *Proceedings of University of Sydney Post-Graduate Foundation Veterinary Science*, Sydney, Australia.

Evans, G. and Maxwell, W.M.C. (1987) *Salomon's Artificial Insemination of Sheep and Goats*. Butterworths, London.

Index

Mycoplasma mycoides, 109, 191, 263
Mycoplasma ovipneumoniae, 263, 297
Mycoplasma ovis, 280
Mycoplasma putrefaciens, 109, 191
Mycoplasma spp., 30, 109, 188, 191–192, 263, 297
Mycoplasma argini, 191, 263, 297
Mycotic dermatitis, 91–92, 155
Mycotoxin binders, 330
Mycotoxins, 128, 230, 323, 329–331
  and abortion, 33
  clinical signs, 329–330
Myelofibrosis, 66, 282
Myiasis, 148–149
Myopathy, lupinosis-associated, 322

N

Nasal discharge, 261, *Plates 17.1, 17.2, 17.3*
  differential diagnosis, 259
Navel ill, 65, 162
Nematodiasis, cerebrospinal, 179
Nematodirus spp., 213, 215
Nematophagus fungi, 223
Neospora caninum, 28–29
Neosporosis, 29
  and abortion, 29
Neotyphodium coenophialum, 330
Nerve injuries
  peroneal, 97
  radial, 96
  sciatic, 97
Nervous diseases, 158–184
  clinical examination, 158
  clinical signs, 159–160
  initial assessment, 158
  kids, 2–7 months,166
  kids 7 months to adult, 166–182
  kids up to 1 month, 162–166
  laboratory investigation, 160
  neonatal kids, 162–163
  and plant poisoning, 308, 324–327
  postmortem examination, 161
  treatment, 161–162
Nitrite/nitrate poisoning, 309, 318–319
Nitrous oxide, 354
Nonsteroidal antiinflammatory drugs (NSAIDs), 82, 162, 206, 337, 388
  and diarrhoea, 206
  and lameness, 82, 337
  and nervous disease, 162
  and osteoarthritis, 82, 337
Normal goat, 1
  cerebrospinal fluid, 179
  female, 1
  physiological values, 347
  red blood cell parameters, 276
  reproductive data, 1
  rumination, 347
  temperature, 347
Nutrition
  early lactation, 43–44
  geriatric, 335
  kid, 75–76
  late gestation, 42–43

over and under feeding in pregnancy, 41
Nymphomania, 7

O

Ochratoxin A, 329
Oesophageal obstruction, 253
Oesophagoscopy, 260
  indications for, 260
Oesphagostomum venulosum, 213, 215
Oestrone sulphate assay for pregnancy diagnosis, 8
Oestrus
  determination of, 3
  duration, 1
  and plant poisoning, 309, 328
  during pregnancy, 8
  signs of, 3
  silent, 6–7
Oestrus cycles
  long, and infertility, 6–7
  regular, and infertility, 7–8
  short, and infertility, 7
Oestrus ovis, 179
Onchocerca, 150
Onions, and anaemia, 281, 320
Ophthalmic diagnostic test values, 301
Opioid analgesics, 350, 365
Opisthotonus, 159
Oral medication, 386
Orchitis, 37, *Plate 3.1*
Orf, 37, 92, 137, *Plates 10.8, 10.9, 10.10*
Organophosphate poisoning, 181, 288
Orthobunyaviruses
  and abortion, 31
  and angular limb deformity, 106
Osteoarthritis, 98, 336
  and CAE, 99, 336
Osteodystrophia fibrosa, 111–112, 136, *Plates 8.1, 8.2*
Osteomyelitis, vertebral, 162–163, 179
Osteopetrosis, 97–98
Otitis media/interna, 180
Out of season breeding, 12–16
Ovarian follicular cysts, 7
Ovarian malfunction, 6
Ovarian tumours
  and infertility, 7
Ovaries, cystic, 7
Overextension stifle and hock, 105
Ovulation, 1
  delayed, 7
Oxalate poisoning, 315–316
  and urolithiasis, 240–241, 316

P

Pain, clinical signs post-operatively, 364
Pain management
  butorphanol, 186, 350, 353
  caudal analgesia, 355–356
  morphine, 356–357
  neuroleptanalgesics, 365
  NSAIDs, 82, 162, 206, 337, 365, 388
  opioid analgesics, 187, 350, 365
  pre-and post-operatively, 364–365, 375
Parainfluenza virus, 267